LASIK

REFRACTORY SURGERY

Series Editors

Dimitri T. Azar, M.D.

*Massachusetts Eye and Ear Infirmary
Schepens Eye Research Institute
and Harvard Medical School
Boston, Massachusetts*

Douglas D. Koch, M.D.

*Cullen Eye Institute
Baylor College of Medicine
Houston, Texas*

1. *LASIK: Fundamentals, Surgical Techniques, and Complications*, edited by Dimitri T. Azar and Douglas D. Koch

ADDITIONAL VOLUMES IN PREPARATION

Hyperopia and Presbyopia, edited by Kazuo Tsubota, Brian S. Boxer Wachler, Dimitri T. Azar, and Douglas D. Koch

LASIK

Fundamentals, Surgical Techniques, and Complications

edited by

Dimitri T. Azar

Massachusetts Eye and Ear Infirmary
Schepens Eye Research Institute
and Harvard Medical School
Boston, Massachusetts, U.S.A.

Douglas D. Koch

Cullen Eye Institute
Baylor College of Medicine
Houston, Texas, U.S.A.

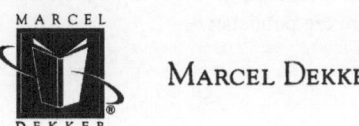

MARCEL DEKKER, INC.   NEW YORK • BASEL

Transferred to Digital Printing 2005

Library of Congress Cataloging-in-Publication Data
A catalog record for this book is available from the Library of Congress.

ISBN: 0-8247-0797-4

Headquarters
Marcel Dekker, Inc.
270 Madison Avenue, New York, NY 10016
tel: 212-696-9000; fax: 212-685-4540

Eastern Hemisphere Distribution
Marcel Dekker AG
Hutgasse 4, Postfach 812, CH-4001 Basel, Switzerland
tel: 41-61-260-6300; fax: 41-61-260-6333

World Wide Web
http://www.dekker.com

The publisher offers discounts on this book when ordered in bulk quantities. For more information,
write to Special Sales/Professional Marketing at the headquarters address above.

To Nathalie, Alexander, Nicholas, and Lara—for all the joyful moments that we share.

DTA

To my wife, Marcia, who makes it all so much more meaningful—and fun.

DDK

Preface

Dov'é mio figlio? . . . più non lo vedo:

In te più Alfredo–trovar non so

For decades, the majority of ophthalmologists have been embarrassed by and highly suspicious of refractive surgery, at times with good justification. They have been repelled by its tactics in patient recruitment, uneasy about its seemingly cavalier use without long-term data, eager to defend its unsuspecting victims, and deeply concerned that its short-term benefits are outweighed by its burdensome long-term consequences. And so the words of Germont, uttered pursuant to the most dramatic moment in Verdi's La Traviata, echo the extreme and oftentimes passionate contempt expressed by so many colleagues and close friends towards academically oriented ophthalmologists who marched among the van-guards of laser refractive surgeons. Their repudiation was not unlike Germont's scorn of his son Alfredo for offending Violetta and for making himself worthy of disdain:

Where is my son? . . . no more do I see him.

I am unable to see Alfredo in you.

The ophthalmological peer-reviewed publications and textbooks prior to the late 1980s reflected this disinterest in or hostility toward refractive surgery. Unfortunately, in the pre-LASIK era, there were relatively few high-quality peer-reviewed reports on refrac-tive surgery. Criticisms of the scientific rigor with which clinical studies were conducted were often justified, which, in turn, discouraged academically bound graduates of ophthal-mology training programs from dedicating their careers to this subspecialty. Comprehen-sive textbooks of ophthalmology in the pre-LASIK era also kept refractive surgery at arm's length, relegating it to a minor chapter on the topic. Refractive surgery was viewed as an outlier of great potential but little practical merit in mainstream ophthalmology. But this has all changed with the advent of LASIK!

This book is the first in a series dedicated to Refractive Surgery by Marcel Dekker, Inc. It will most certainly be judged by many as just another LASIK book. While there is abundant coverage of the topic in other books, this volume has several unique features. Its coverage of LASIK is relatively comprehensive, in that it is not limited to LASIK history, surgical techniques, complications, and their management. New aspects of lasers, optics, refraction, diagnostics, and instrumentation are combined with the science and general principles of LASIK, and indications for its use. Although not meant to be encyclopedic, key references abound. They are intended to serve as a guide to the literature on the topic. Thus, this book is not so much a chronicle of LASIK, as an attempt to serve as a source of information relevant to clinical practice.

We are indebted to the students, residents, and colleagues who have made valuable contributions to this book. Several have included original work and analysis in their chapters. It is evident that the authors have attended diligently to their assignments. We are grateful for their effort in integrating the sometimes limited information in peer-reviewed literature with the knowledge derived from their clinical experiences and interactions with colleagues. We hope that this has resulted in a text that is both clinically relevant and as evidence-based as possible.

We thank Dr. Geoffrey Greenwood and Elizabeth Curione of Marcel Dekker, Inc., for their commitment to this project and Drs. Tsubota, Boxer Wachler, Hoang-Xuan, Ang, and Gatinel for their assistance in future books in this series. Special thanks go to Leona Greenhill, for her editorial assistance, and to Rhonda Harris, who managed this project with care and precision. Her attention to detail and her dedication have enabled us to work coherently in the face of adversity.

We take the opportunity to acknowledge the pioneering surgeons and researchers in the field of refractive surgery. Their work and vision have provided the basis not only for current refractive developments that we can offer to our patients, but also for future advances to be made by the next generation of thoughtful contributors to this important field.

Dimitri T. Azar
Douglas D. Koch

Contents

Preface   *v*
Contributors   *xi*

1. **Refractive Errors and Their Treatment**   1
   Liane Clamen Glazer and Dimitri T. Azar

2. **History of LASIK**   21
   Ioannis Pallikaris and Thekla Papadaki

3. **Lasers in LASIK: Basic Aspects**   39
   Rodrigo Torres, Robert T. Ang, and Dimitri T. Azar

4. **Microkeratomes**   57
   Sandeep Kakaria, Thanh Hoang-Xuan, and Dimitri T. Azar

5. **Adjunctive Instrumentation in LASIK**   71
   Robert T. Ang and Dimitri T. Azar

6. **LASIK Indications, Contraindications, and Preoperative Evaluation**   91
   Richard E. Braunstein, Marc Winnick, and Kenneth A. Greenberg

7. **Preoperative Optical Considerations in LASIK: Refractive Errors,
   Monovision, and Contrast Sensitivity**   101
   Balamurali K. Ambati, Leon Strauss, and Dimitri T. Azar

8. **Corneal Topography and LASIK Applications**   111
   *Li Wang, Douglas D. Koch, Dimitri T. Azar, Robert T. Ang,
   and Rengin Yildirim*

9. **Wavefront Technology and LASIK Applications** 139
Naoyuki Maeda

10. **Preoperative Considerations: Diagnosis, Classification, and Avoidance of Keratoconus Complications** 153
Paul Chung-Shien Lu and Dimitri T. Azar

11. **Corneal Stability and Biomechanics After LASIK** 163
Esen Karamursel Akpek, Rana Altan-Yaycioglu, and Walter J. Stark

12. **LASIK Techniques** 175
Dimitri T. Azar, Kathryn Colby, and Douglas D. Koch

13. **Microkeratomes and Laser Settings** 189
William J. Lahners and David R. Hardten

14. **Centration of LASIK Procedures** 199
Marsha C. Cheung, Chun Chen Chen, and Dimitri T. Azar

15. **Surgical Caveats for Managing Difficult Intraoperative Situations** 229
Samir G. Farah and Dimitri T. Azar

16. **Bilateral Simultaneous LASIK: Advantages, Disadvantages, and Surgical Caveats** 243
David R. Hardten, Elizabeth A. Davis, Richard L. Lindstrom, and William J. Lahners

17. **Postoperative Management Protocols for Uncomplicated LASIK Procedures** 255
Melanie A. R. Graham and Dimitri T. Azar

18. **Visual Outcomes After Primary LASIK** 265
Samir G. Farah and Dimitri T. Azar

19. **Quality of Vision After LASIK** 277
Patrick C. Yeh and Dimitri T. Azar

20. **LASIK for Hyperopia, Hyperopic Astigmatism, and Presbyopia** 285
Neal A. Sher

21. **LASIK Retreatments** 297
Ayman F. El-Shiaty and Brian S. Boxer Wachler

22. **LASIK Following Radial Keratotomy and Photorefractive Keratectomy** 313
Natalie A. Afshari and Dimitri T. Azar

23. **LASIK After Penetrating Keratoplasty**   319
    Glenn C. Cockerham and Natalie A. Afshari

24. **Bioptics: Combined LASIK and Phakic Intraocular Lens Surgery**   329
    José L. Güell, Mercedes Vázquez, Fortino Velasco, and Felicidad Manero

25. **LASIK and Intrastromal Corneal Ring Segments (ICRS)**   335
    Jonathan D. Primack, Samir G. Farah, and Dimitri T. Azar

26. **Intraoperative Complications**   351
    Li Wang, Manjula Misra, and Douglas D. Koch

27. **Postoperative Complications of LASIK**   365
    Samir G. Farah, Jae Bum Lee, and Dimitri T. Azar

28. **Optical Aberrations After LASIK**   387
    Samir A. Melki, Cinthia E. Proano, and Dimitri T. Azar

29. **Posterior Segment Complications of LASIK**   397
    Ron Afshari Adelman and Natalie A. Afshari

30. **Management of Topographical Irregularities Following LASIK**   403
    Jeffrey Johnson, Roselyn Jeun, and Dimitri T. Azar

31. **LASIK and TopoLink for Irregular Astigmatism**   421
    Michael C. Knorz

32. **Management of Flap Complications in LASIK**   431
    Manolette R. Roque, Samir A. Melki, Dimitri T. Azar, and Emily Yeung

33. **Management of Interlamellar Epithelium**   463
    Nan Wang and Douglas D. Koch

34. **Management of Infections, Inflammation, and Lamellar
    Keratitis After LASIK**   477
    *Bilal F. Khan, Margaret Chang, Sandeep Jain, Kathryn Colby,
    and Dimitri T. Azar*

35. **The Future of LASIK**   491
    Nan Wang and Douglas D. Koch

Index   *495*

Contributors

Ron Afshari Adelman, M.D. Massachusetts Eye and Ear Infirmary, Boston, Massachusetts, and Yale University Eye Center, New Haven, Connecticut, U.S.A.

Natalie A. Afshari Cornea Service, Duke University Eye Center, Durham, North Carolina, U.S.A.

Esen Karamursel Akpek, M.D. Cornea and External Disease Service, The Wilmer Eye Institute, Johns Hopkins University School of Medicine, Baltimore, Maryland, U.S.A.

Rana Altan-Yaycioglu, M.D. Cornea and External Disease Service, The Wilmer Eye Institute, Johns Hopkins University School of Medicine, Baltimore, Maryland, U.S.A.

Balamurali K. Ambati, M.D. Massachusetts Eye and Ear Infirmary and Department of Opthalmology, Harvard Medical School, Boston, Massachusetts, U.S.A.

Robert T. Ang, M.D. Cornea and Refractive Surgery Service, Massachusetts Eye and Ear Infirmary and Harvard Medical School, Boston, Massachusetts, U.S.A., and Asian Eye Institute, Makati, The Philippines

Dimitri T. Azar, M.D. Cornea and Refractive Surgery Service, Massachusetts Eye and Ear Infirmary, Schepens Eye Research Institute, and Harvard Medical School, Boston, Massachusetts, U.S.A.

Brian S. Boxer Wachler, M.D. Refractive Surgery Service, Jules Stein Eye Institute at UCLA, Los Angeles, California, U.S.A.

Richard E. Braunstein, M.D. Department of Ophthalmology, Columbia University College of Physicians and Surgeons, and Harkness Eye Institute, New York, New York, U.S.A.

Margaret Chang   Columbia University College of Physicians and Surgeons, New York, New York, U.S.A.

Chun Chen Chen, M.D.   Cornea and Refractive Surgery Service, Massachusetts Eye and Ear Infirmary, Schepens Eye Research Institute, and Harvard Medical School, Boston, Massachusetts, U.S.A.

Marsha C. Cheung   Massachusetts Eye and Ear Infirmary and Harvard Medical School, Boston, Massachusetts, U.S.A.

Glenn C. Cockerham, M.D.   Department of Surgery, Allegheny Ophthalmology and Orbital Associates, Pittsburgh, Pennsylvania, U.S.A.

Kathryn Colby, M.D., Ph.D.   Cornea and Refractive Surgery Service, Department of Opthalmology, Massachusetts Eye and Ear Infirmary, Schepens Eye Research Institute, and Harvard Medical School, Boston, Massachusetts, U.S.A.

Elizabeth A. Davis, M.D., Ph.D.   Department of Ophthalmology, University of Minnesota, and Minnesota Eye Consultants, Minneapolis, Minnesota, U.S.A.

Ayman F. El-Shiaty, M.D.   Department of Ophthalmology, Faculty of Medicine, Cairo University, Cairo, Egypt, and Jules Stein Eye Institute at UCLA, Los Angeles, California, U.S.A.

Samir G. Farah, M.D.   Massachusetts Eye and Ear Infirmary, Boston, Massachusetts, U.S.A.

Liane Clamen Glazer, M.D.   Massachusetts Eye and Ear Infirmary and Department of Ophthalmology, Harvard Medical School, Boston, Massachusetts, U.S.A.

Melanie A. R. Graham, M.D.   Greater Baltimore Medical Center, Baltimore, Maryland, U.S.A.

Kenneth A. Greenberg, M.D.   Department of Ophthalmology, Columbia University College of Physicians and Surgeons, New York, New York, U.S.A.

José L. Güell, M.D., Ph.D.   Instituto de Microcirugía Ocular, Barcelona, Spain

David R. Hardten, M.D.   Department of Ophthalmology, University of Minnesota, and Department of Medicine, Minnesota Eye Consultants, Minneapolis, Minnesota, U.S.A.

Thanh Hoang-Xuan, M.D.   Fondation Ophtalmologique Adolphe de Rothschild, and Paris University, Paris, France

Sandeep Jain, M.D.   Cornea and Refractive Surgery Service, Massachusetts Eye and Ear Infirmary, Schepens Eye Research Institute, and Harvard Medical School, Boston, Massachusetts, U.S.A.

Roselyn Jeun, O.D.   Massachusetts Eye and Ear Infirmary, Boston, Massachusetts, U.S.A.

Jeffrey Johnson, O.D. Massachusetts Eye and Ear Infirmary, and Department of Ophthalmology, Harvard Medical School, Boston, Massachusetts, U.S.A.

Sandeep Kakaria, M.D. Department of Ophthalmology, Cornell University Medical Center, New York, New York, U.S.A.

Bilal F. Khan, M.D. Massachusetts Eye and Ear Infirmary and Department of Ophthalmology, Harvard Medical School, Boston, Massachusetts, U.S.A.

Michael C. Knorz, M.D. University of Heidelberg, Heidelberg, Germany, and Baylor College of Medicine, Houston, Texas, U.S.A.

Douglas D. Koch, M.D. Department of Ophthalmology, Cullen Eye Institute, Baylor College of Medicine, Houston, Texas, U.S.A.

William J. Lahners, M.D. University of South Florida, Tampa, and Center for Sight, Sarasota, Florida, U.S.A.

Jae Bum Lee Cornea and Refractive Surgery Service, Massachusetts Eye and Ear Infirmary, Schepens Eye Research Institute, and Harvard Medical School, Boston, Massachusetts, U.S.A.

Richard L. Lindstrom, M.D. Department of Ophthalmology, University of Minnesota, and Department of Medicine, Minnesota Eye Consultants, Minneapolis, Minnesota, U.S.A.

Paul Chung-Shien Lu, M.D. Department of Ophthalmology, Chang Gung Memorial Hospital, Taipei, Taiwan, and Harvard Medical School, Boston, Massachusetts, U.S.A.

Naoyuki Maeda, M.D. Departments of Ophthalmology and Medical Robotics and Image Sciences, Osaka University Medical School, Osaka, Japan

Felicidad Manero Instituto de Microcirugía Ocular, Barcelona, Spain

Samir A. Melki, M.D., Ph.D. Cornea and Refractive Surgery Service, Massachusetts Eye and Ear Infirmary, and Boston Cornea Center, Harvard Medical School, Boston, Massachusetts, U.S.A.

Manjula Misra, M.D. Cullen Eye Institute, Baylor College of Medicine, Houston, Texas, U.S.A.

Ioannis Pallikaris, M.D. Department of Ophthalmology, University of Crete Medical School, and Ophthalmology Clinic, University Hospital of Heraklion, Heraklion, Crete, Greece

Thekla Papadaki, M.D. Refractive Surgery Service, Vardinoyannion Eye Institute of Crete, University of Crete Medical School, Heraklion, Crete, Greece

Jonathan D. Primack, M.D. Massachusetts Eye and Ear Infirmary, Boston, Massachusetts, U.S.A.

Cinthia E. Proano, M.D.   Cornea and Refractive Surgery Service, Massachusetts Eye and Ear Infirmary and Harvard Medical School, Boston, Massachusetts, U.S.A.

Manolette R. Roque, M.D.   Massachusetts Eye and Ear Infirmary and Department of Ophthalmology, Harvard Medical School, Boston, Massachusetts, U.S.A.

Neal A. Sher, M.D., F.A.C.S.   Department of Ophthalmology, University of Minnesota Medical School, and Department of Surgery, Phillips Eye Institute, Minneapolis, Minnesota, U.S.A.

Walter J. Stark, M.D.   Cornea, Cataract and Refractive Services, The Wilmer Eye Institute, Johns Hopkins University School of Medicine, Baltimore, Maryland, U.S.A.

Leon Strauss, M.D., Ph.D.   The Wilmer Eye Institute, Johns Hopkins University School of Medicine, Baltimore, Maryland, U.S.A.

Rodrigo Torres   Massachusetts Eye and Ear Infirmary and Harvard Medical School, Boston, Massachusetts, U.S.A.

Mercedes Vázquez, M.D   Instituto de Microcirugía Ocular, Barcelona, Spain

Fortino Velasco   Instituto de Microcirugía Ocular, Barcelona, Spain

Li Wang, M.D.   Cullen Eye Institute, Baylor College of Medicine, Houston, Texas, U.S.A.

Nan Wang   Cullen Eye Institute, Baylor College of Medicine, Houston, Texas, U.S.A.

Marc Winnick, M.D.   Department of Ophthalmology, Columbia University College of Physicians and Surgeons, and Harkness Eye Institute, New York, New York, U.S.A.

Patrick C. Yeh   Cornea and Refractive Surgery Service, Massachusetts Eye and Ear Infirmary, Schepens Eye Research Institute, and Harvard Medical School, Boston, Massachusetts, U.S.A.

Emily Yeung, M.D.   Massachusetts Eye and Ear Infirmary, Schepens Eye Research Institute, and Harvard Medical School, Boston, Massachusetts, U.S.A.

Rengin Yildirim, M.D.   Refractive Surgery Department, Cerrahpasa Medical School, University of Istanbul, Istanbul, Turkey

Refractive Errors and Their Treatment

LIANE CLAMEN GLAZER

*Massachusetts Eye and Ear Infirmary and Harvard Medical School,
Boston, Massachusetts, U.S.A.*

DIMITRI T. AZAR

*Massachusetts Eye and Ear Infirmary, Schepens Eye Research Institute,
and Harvard Medical School, Boston, Massachusetts, U.S.A.*

A. LASIK: DEFINITION AND OVERVIEW

Laser in-situ keratomileusis (LASIK) involves creating a corneal flap so that midstromal tissue can be ablated directly and reshaped with an excimer laser beam (1,2). The procedure allows the ophthalmologist to surgically reshape the cornea in an attempt to obviate the need for corrective lenses (Fig. 1.1). LASIK is a modification of Colombian José Barraquer's ingenious innovations. In 1949, Barraquer first described his technique, and in 1964 he published clinical results of his attempts to achieve emmetropia by shaving and reshaping the cornea (3–5). With Barraquer's technique of keratomileusis (i.e., carving the cornea), a lamellar button (lenticule) of the patient's cornea was excised with a manual microkeratome. Barraquer then reshaped the lenticule so that the central corneal curvature was flattened and the refractive power of the cornea decreased. He then replaced the lenticule in position, either with or without sutures. Barraquer's specific attempts to correct myopia were called cryolathe keratomileusis, because they involved freezing and reshaping the removed lenticule with a cryolathe.

Troutman and Swinger introduced cryolathe keratomileusis to the United States in 1977 (6). While keratomileusis produced good results when performed by experienced surgeons, the procedure was technically very difficult and the results were therefore variable (7–11). Innovations to this procedure, however, eventually led to the creation of the more highly refined procedure of LASIK.

The introduction of the "excited dimer" (excimer) 193 nm UV laser allowed for the

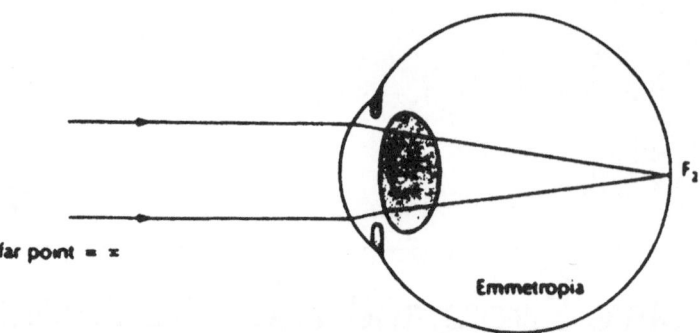

Figure 1.1 Schematic diagram of emmetropia. In emmetropia, the far point is optical infinity, and the secondary focal point (F_2) is at the retina. Parallel rays of light focus on the retina. (From Ref. 115.)

development of LASIK. The argon–fluoride excimer laser is capable of precise ablation of corneal tissue with minimal disruption of adjacent tissue. The excimer laser's effect on the cornea was first studied in animal models in 1983 (12). In 1989, Peyman first used a laser to remove corneal stroma from a lamellar bed in animals (13). Shortly thereafter, similar attempts were made in human eyes (14,15). This early work supported the theory that in situ keratomileusis was better than surface ablation because it induced less activation and proliferation of stromal keratocytes, thereby avoiding both haze and regression. In addition, the excimer laser allowed for more accurate tissue removal, thereby eliminating one of the main deterrents to lamellar surgery (see Chap. 2).

The LASIK procedure, in its current refined state, involves increasing the eye's intraocular pressure to at least 65 mmHg with a suction device, and then using a microkeratome to create a corneal flap that is at least 6 mm in diameter and 150 microns thick. This flap, which allows the Bowman's-layer epithelial complex to remain intact, is then carefully lifted to expose the layers of the cornea that will be reshaped by the excimer laser. The size of the optical zone and the depth and profile of the laser ablation will determine the correction achieved (Fig. 1.1).

B. THE EPIDEMIOLOGY OF LASIK

Refractive surgery is a young and rapidly growing field. In 1998, 400,000 Americans underwent refractive surgical procedures. This represents an increase over 1997 of approximately 100% (16). Despite the many refractive surgeries that have been performed, the target population for laser vision correction at the turn of the century is still an estimated 44 million people. Currently, approximately 3,000 ophthalmologists have been trained to perform refractive surgery. This number is increasing at a rate of 500 to 1,000 surgeons per year. Industry observers predict that the number of trained surgeons will approach 6,000 to 8,000, or approximately 50% of the U.S.-based ophthalmologists (16).

LASIK produces good refractive results for low, moderate, and high myopia (see Chap. 18). Recent reports for low myopia show postoperative uncorrected visual acuities of 20/40 or better in 100% of patients, and 20/20 or better in 81% of patients (17).

Potential complications of LASIK include halos, interface inflammation, haze, and regression. However, significant complications causing a loss of two or more lines of best corrected visual acuity (BCVA) are rare (1,18,19). In addition, with improved instrumentation and increasing surgeon experience, LASIK complication rates continue to fall.

C. REFRACTIVE ERRORS THAT ARE TREATABLE WITH LASIK

Three components of the eye work together to determine the refractive power of the eye: the shape of the cornea, the power of the lens, and the length of the eye. The overall refracting power of the eye is approximately 60 diopters: the cornea contributes about 45 diopters of power, while the lens provides approximately 15 diopters of refractive power to the eye. When the cornea, lens, and length of the eye combine and produce no refractive error, emmetropia is achieved. In the instance of emmetropia, a ray of light parallel to the optical axis and limited by the pupil focuses at a point on the retina. In other words, the secondary focal point is located on the retina. In addition, the "far point" (i.e., the furthest point at which the eye can see clearly) is optical infinity (Fig. 1.2). Because the cornea accounts for approximately two-thirds of the refractive power of the eye, it is logical that most refractive surgeries attempt to change the shape of the cornea. Other methods of refractive surgery include implanting intraocular lenses.

Traditionally, four major types of naturally occurring ametropias, or refractive errors, have been described: myopia, hyperopia, astigmatism, and presbyopia. Wavefront analysis of human eyes after correction of these optical abnormalities often show additional irregularities that have been classified using Zernike polynomials into complex subgroups that may be simplified into lower- and higher-order aberrations.

In myopia, the secondary focal point is anterior to the retina. In other words, the refractive power of the eye is greater than that required for emmetropia; parallel rays of light entering the eye are in focus at a location in the vitreous, rather than on the retina. Refractive myopia is due to steep corneal curvature or high lens power. Axial myopia is due to an eye that is too long (i.e., longer than 22.6 mm). For every millimeter of axial elongation of the globe, there are 3 diopters of myopia. When myopia is corrected with spectacles, contact lenses, or refractive surgery, the parallel rays of light entering the eye come into focus on the retina, which is consistent with a far point at infinity. The prevalence of physiologic myopia in the general population is approximately 25% (20). LASIK corrects for myopia by removing tissue in the center of the cornea, thereby flattening the cornea and decreasing the refractive power of the eye.

A hyperopic eye's secondary focal point is posterior to the retina. In other words, parallel rays of light entering the eye come into focus at a location posterior to the retina. Refractive hyperopia is due to a flat cornea (less corneal refracting power), or a lens with lower power. Axial hyperopia is due to a short axial length. While hyperopia affects approximately 40% of the adult population, it is clearly less visually significant than myopia (21). This is because accommodation may produce enough additional plus power to bring the parallel rays of light to focus on the retina. Thus young hyperopes may compensate and see well until their accommodative power weakens and they begin to experience manifest hyperopia in their mid to late 30s. LASIK corrects for hyperopia by removing a ring of tissue around the center of the cornea, thereby making the cornea steeper.

Astigmatism refers to a refractive error in which the curvature of the cornea, or less commonly the curvature of the lens, varies in different meridians. In other words, patients with astigmatism have two focal lines formed by the convergence of rays of light. The first focal line, created by the more powerful corneal meridian, is closer to the cornea. The second focal line, formed by the less powerful meridian, is further away. Dioptrically midway

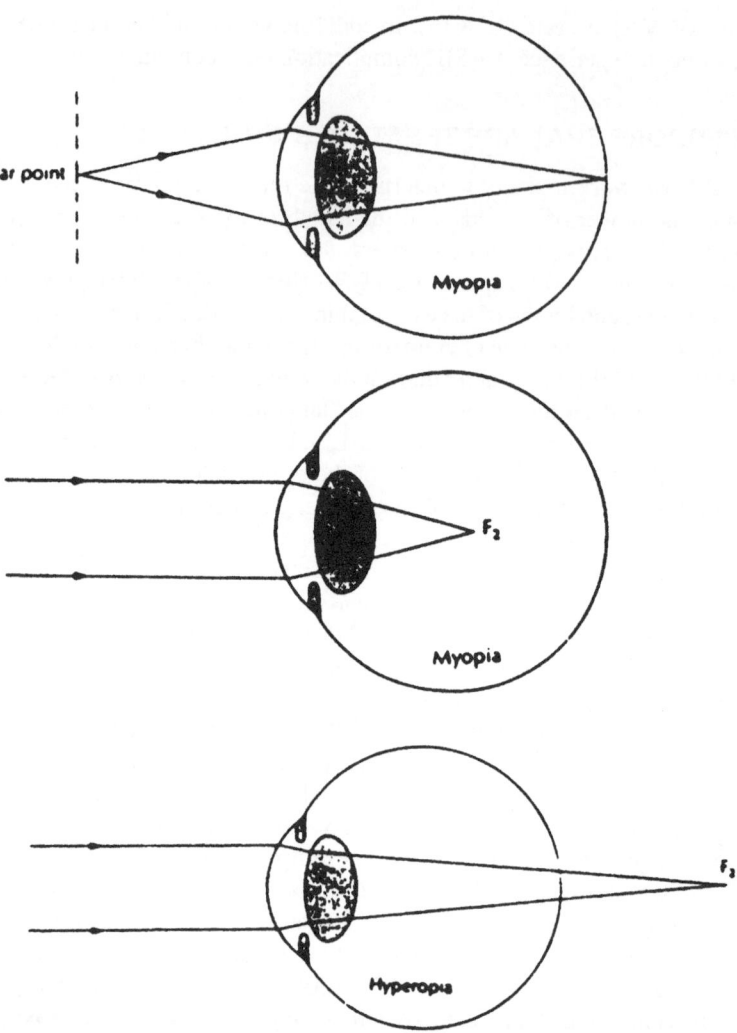

Figure 1.2 Schematic diagrams of myopia and hyperopia. In myopia, the far point is in front of the eye (top), and the secondary focal point (F_2) is anterior to the retina, in the vitreous (middle). In hyperopia (bottom), the rays of light are in focus at a point behind the retina. (From Ref. 115.)

between the two focal lines is the circle of least confusion. A proper refractive correction will place the circle of least confusion on the retina.

While astigmatism is clinically detectable in up to 95% of eyes, astigmatism of less than 0.50 diopters rarely requires optical correction (22). However, 10% of the general population has naturally occurring astigmatism greater than 1 D. Since an astigmatic refractive error of 1.00 to 2.00 D can decrease uncorrected vision to the 20/30 to 20/50 level, this degree of astigmatism causes an unacceptably poor quality of uncorrected visual acuity (23,24).

Regular astigmatism refers to corneal curvatures that are different but symmetrical, with principal meridians 90 degrees away from each other. For regular astigmatism, one can achieve a refractive correction with cylindrical or spherocylindrical lenses. LASIK can correct regular astigmatism by removing more tissue from the steeper side of the cornea.

Irregular astigmatism refers to a condition in which the principal meridians change from point to point across the pupil, or in which the amount of astigmatism changes from one point to another. Examples of irregular astigmatism include keratoconus or traumatic corneal scars. LASIK is contraindicated in eyes with irregular astigmatism. Often, rigid contact lenses are the best way to improve the visual acuity for eyes with irregular astigmatism. The use of Zernike polynomials to analyze the wavefront in patients with irregular astigmatism has allowed, at least in theory, the incorporation of this information into the laser treatment algorithm in LASIK and paved the way for custom corneal treatments.

Presbyopia refers to the age-related loss of accommodative response. Presbyopia typically sets in at approximately 40 years of age. The condition results from either a loss of lens elasticity or an anatomic change in the position of the lens equator to the ciliary body position. Presbyopia is an important issue to discuss during the informed consent of patients seeking refractive surgery. Some physicians give their patient the option of monovision, in which one eye is corrected for near vision and the other for distance vision.

D. ETIOLOGY, EPIDEMIOLOGY, AND LASIK ALTERNATIVES

1. Corneal Subtractive Procedures

a. Lamellar Procedures

Lamellar refractive keratoplasty refers to the placement of a lenticule on or within the cornea to change its refractive power, typically by altering its anterior curvature. As described above and in Chap. 2, Jose Barraquer's introduction of lamellar refractive surgery and of cryolathe keratomileusis were followed by Ruiz' introduction of the concept of in situ keratomileusis (25). He introduced a microkeratome propelled by gears that could create the corneal flap and allow one to perform intrastromal tissue subtraction. When advances in instrumentation allowed the lamellar keratoplasty to be performed more accurately, the procedure became known as automated lamellar keratoplasty (ALK) (Figure 1.3). The initial results of ALK for myopia showed improvement over previous lamellar techniques. Results described postoperative uncorrected visual acuities of 20/40 or better in 86% of patients, with a 6% loss of two or more lines of best spectacle corrected visual acuity (26,27). However, ALK outcomes were not significantly better than the results achieved with contemporary radial keratotomy (RK) techniques (28,29). The accuracy of ALK is limited by the imprecise nature of mechanical cutting.

Hyperopic ALK uses a very deep lamellar pass, cutting more than 70% of the stromal depth (versus the 40% of stromal depth that is used for myopic ALK or for LASIK). The intraocular pressure causes the thinned cornea to bow forward, and thus the central cornea steepens (Figure 1.4). As one may imagine, this procedure was often unpredictable and occasionally led to progressive ectasia. Long-term results published in 1998 reported instability of the postoperative refraction with a progressive myopic shift. Even worse, 26% of eyes developed "iatrogenic keratoconus," and 16.4% required penetrating keratoplasty (30,31). Hyperopic ALK is now considered unsafe due to the risk of progressive corneal ectasia.

b. Surface Laser Ablation (PRK and LASEK)

Another form of refractive surgery that utilizes corneal subtractive procedures is photorefractive keratectomy (PRK). PRK is more accurate than ALK because it makes use of the

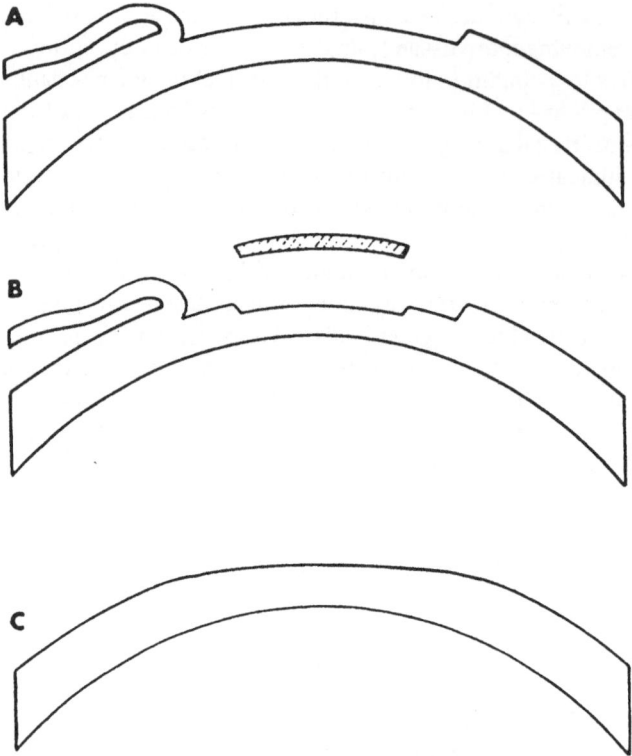

Figure 1.3 Myopic automated lamellar keratoplasty. (A) A microkeratome is used to create a hinged flap in the cornea. (B) A second microkeratome is used to remove a parallel-faced disc of tissue from the corneal bed. (C) The initial flap is replaced, leaving a flattened central cornea. (From Ref. 116.)

193 nm argon fluoride (ArF) excimer laser. Like LASIK, PRK utilizes the excimer laser to flatten the cornea by ablating the central cornea. Unlike LASIK, no corneal flap is made; rather, the central corneal epithelium is simply removed with a spatula or with the laser itself (Fig. 1.5). While there are three distinct techniques for performing excimer laser PRK for myopia, the most widely used technique applies wide-area surface ablation with a large-diameter beam. Most of the published results of PRK are based on PRK performed in this manner. It is primarily in Europe that PRK is performed with the two other techniques: scanning slit and flying spot lasers. A modification of PRK, first performed at the Massachusetts Eye and Ear Infirmary by Azar and Abad in 1996, was the use of 20% alcohol to create an epithelial flap which was repositioned to cover the stromal ablation bed. Since then, several investigators have started to use this laser epithelial keratomileusis (LASEK) technique, but it is not clear whether LASEK offers any advantages over PRK.

PRK has been shown to be safe and efficacious for the treatment of low to moderate myopia. Several national studies of PRK demonstrated that 90 to 100% of patients had 20/40 or better uncorrected visual acuity, and 78 to 98% had postoperative refractions within 1.0 D of the target outcome (32–34). Refractive results of PRK in patients with more than 6 D of myopia tend to be highly variable and undergo more regression. Another disadvantage of PRK is a prolonged recovery time: while the corneal epithelium is healing,

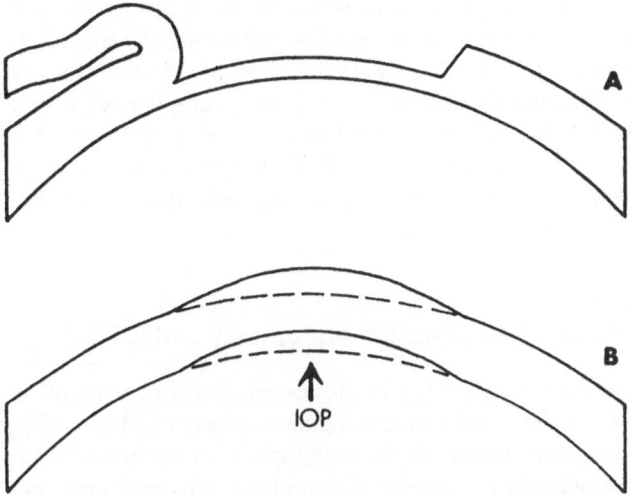

Figure 1.4 Hyperopic automated lamellar keratoplasty. (A) A hinged flap, approximately 70% of corneal thickness, is created with a microkeratome. (B) Intraocular pressure displaces the very thin posterior layer and overlying flap anteriorly, causing central corneal steepening. The original shape of the cornea is shown with dotted lines. (From Ref. 116.)

patients may experience discomfort and blurry vision. In addition, potential complications include postoperative haze, halos, induced astigmatism, diplopia, and keratitis (32,35–37).

Although PRK was the first widely accepted laser vision correction procedure, it has been largely supplanted by LASIK as the refractive procedure of choice not just for high myopia but even for low and moderate myopia. This is partly because LASIK provides faster visual rehabilitation and decreased time for wound healing (38–43).

While LASIK is often the refractive procedure of choice for myopes, PRK may be preferable to LASIK for patients who are hesitant to undergo incisional surgery, or for patients who have contraindications to LASIK. Such contraindications would include corneal

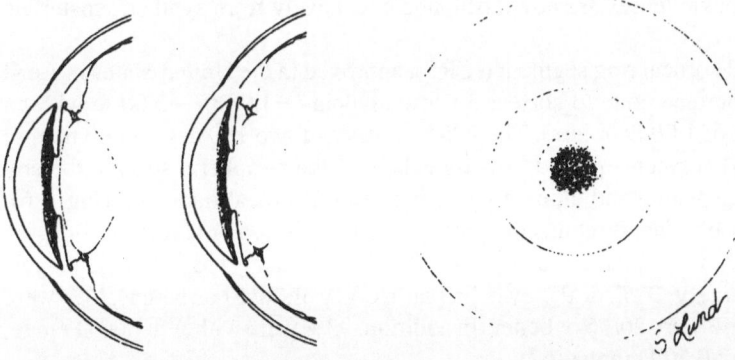

Figure 1.5 Schematic illustration of photorefractive keratectomy. The excimer laser is used to remove anterior stroma (left), causing corneal flattening (middle). The region of tissue subtraction is designated by the shaded area. (From Ref. 115.)

thinning, in which less than 200 to 250 microns of tissue would be left in the corneal bed, and epithelial anterior basement membrane dystrophy, because this carries the risk of epithelial ingrowth. PRK is also competitive with LASIK in the arena of treatment for low hyperopia. A recent review of 65 eyes with +1.00 to +4.00 D of hyperopia documented that 92% of the eyes were within ±1.00 D of the intended manifest SE at 18 months follow-up (44). Other reports support the use of hyperopic PRK (H-PRK) for treating low degrees of hyperopia (45–48). H-PRK for the treatment of higher degrees of hyperopia is less predictable and may result in greater regression (45).

2.   Biologic and Synthetic Tissue Addition: Epikeratoplasty and ICRS

One can alter the shape, and thus the refractive index, of the cornea by adding material either to the surface of the cornea or into the corneal stroma. Epikeratoplasty involves adding a lenticule with power (i.e., carved donor tissue) to the deepithelialized surface of Bowman's layer. Also called epikeratophakia or lamellar keratoplasty, this technique has proven problematical. First, the refractive results have been disappointing: only 33% of eyes achieved 20/40 or better uncorrected visual acuity, 15% lost two or more lines of best corrected visual acuity (BCVA), and regression was more than 2 D in 17.6% of patients at 5 months' follow-up (49–51). Secondly, 2.5–3.5% of patients who underwent this procedure had delayed reepithelialization, which in some cases led to infections and graft melting (49,52–55). Almost 8% of grafts had to be removed due to failure of epithelialization, haze, glare, irregular astigmatism, epithelial ingrowth, epithelial interface cysts, melt, infection, stromal infiltrates, and wound dehiscence (49,53–54,56–57). After the lenticules were removed, many patients were left with central corneal scarring and loss of BCVA (58,59). Because of the disappointing outcomes and unfortunate complications, epikeratoplasty has been abandoned as a technique for the correction of myopia. However, epikeratoplasty is still occasionally used to diminish the myopia and irregular astigmatism of keratoconus or other corneal thinning disorders (60). This procedure is also sometimes used for the treatment of pediatric and adult aphakia.

Keratophakia is a procedure in which a lens is placed within the corneal stroma to alter the cornea's refractive power. While lenses used to be fashioned from donor human corneas (homoplastic), these lenses had variable outcomes and a high incidence of complications (61). Keratophakic lenses are now fashioned exclusively from synthetic materials (alloplastic).

The intrastromal corneal ring segment (ICRS), approved in the United States in April 1999, is a keratophakic technique to correct for low myopia (−1.00 to −3.00 D with an astigmatic component of 1.00 D or less). The ICRS consists of two 160 degree polymethyl methacrylate (PMMA) segments placed in two pockets of the peripheral stroma, thereby inducing peripheral steepening and indirectly causing central corneal flattening (Fig. 1.6). The procedure is unique in that it retains the potential to be adjusted or reversed.

Two-year results of the phase II and phase III FDA trial analyzed 358 patient eyes. At 24 months after surgery, 97% of the eyes had an UCVA of 20/40 or better, 76% were 20/20 or better, and 55% were 20/16 or better. In addition, 93% were within ±1.00 D range, and 73% were within ±0.50 D range (62).

Potential disadvantages with the procedure include accidental perforation into the anterior chamber, surface perforation of the epithelium anteriorly, and induced astigmatism, which can result from postoperative movement of the intracorneal ring segments (63).

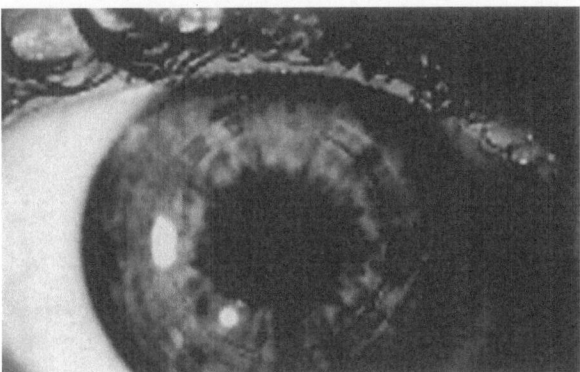

Figure 1.6 Intrastromal corneal ring segments. (From Ref. 63.)

3. Corneal Surface Remodeling: Incisional Surgery, Thermal Surgery, and Orthokeratology

a. Incisional Surgery: Radial Keratotomy

Radial keratotomy (RK) is a procedure that treats myopia by making deep and radial corneal stromal incisions to weaken the peripheral and paracentral cornea and thereby flatten the central cornea (Figs. 1.7 and 1.8). Experimenting on rabbits' corneas, Dutch ophthalmologist Lendert Jan Lans first demonstrated that nonperforating corneal incisions parallel to the limbus cause peripheral bulging and central flattening (Fig. 1.7) (64,65). Japanese ophthalmologist Tsutomu Sato first performed anterior and posterior keratotomies to treat myopia after observing that patients with keratoconus who had experienced breaks in Descemet's membrane and hydrops subsequently developed corneal flattening (66–67). Sadly, the role of the corneal endothelium was not understood when Sato was performing his keratotomies. Later follow-up showed that of 170 eyes that underwent a keratotomy by Sato's group, 121 (71%) developed bullous keratopathy, and only 49 eyes (21%) retained clear corneas. The average time between the procedure and the onset of edema was 20 years (68). The posterior keratotomy was abandoned for anterior keratotomies once the physiological importance of the corneal endothelium had been established.

In 1960, Svyatoslav Fyodorov of the Soviet Union visited Japan, where Akiyama taught him Sato's technique of radial keratotomy (Sato himself had recently died). Fyodorov improved upon Sato's techniques by devising improved instrumentation and by developing mathematical formulas to improve the reproducibility of RK (69–70). Fyodorov also showed that paracentral incisions were more effective than peripheral, scleral incisions. In addition, he demonstrated that the diameter of the central clear zone is inversely proportional to the magnitude of refractive correction.

In the United States, the first RK was performed by Bores at the Kresge Eye Institute in November 1978. It was at about this time that the 20 year follow-up data of Sato's posterior keratotomy patients was revealing the 75% incidence of bullous keratopathy. Because the newer anterior procedure had scarce follow-up data, the National Eye Institute chose to fund two large nationwide studies to examine RK: the Prospective Evaluation of Radial Keratotomy (PERK) and the Analysis of Radial Keratotomy.

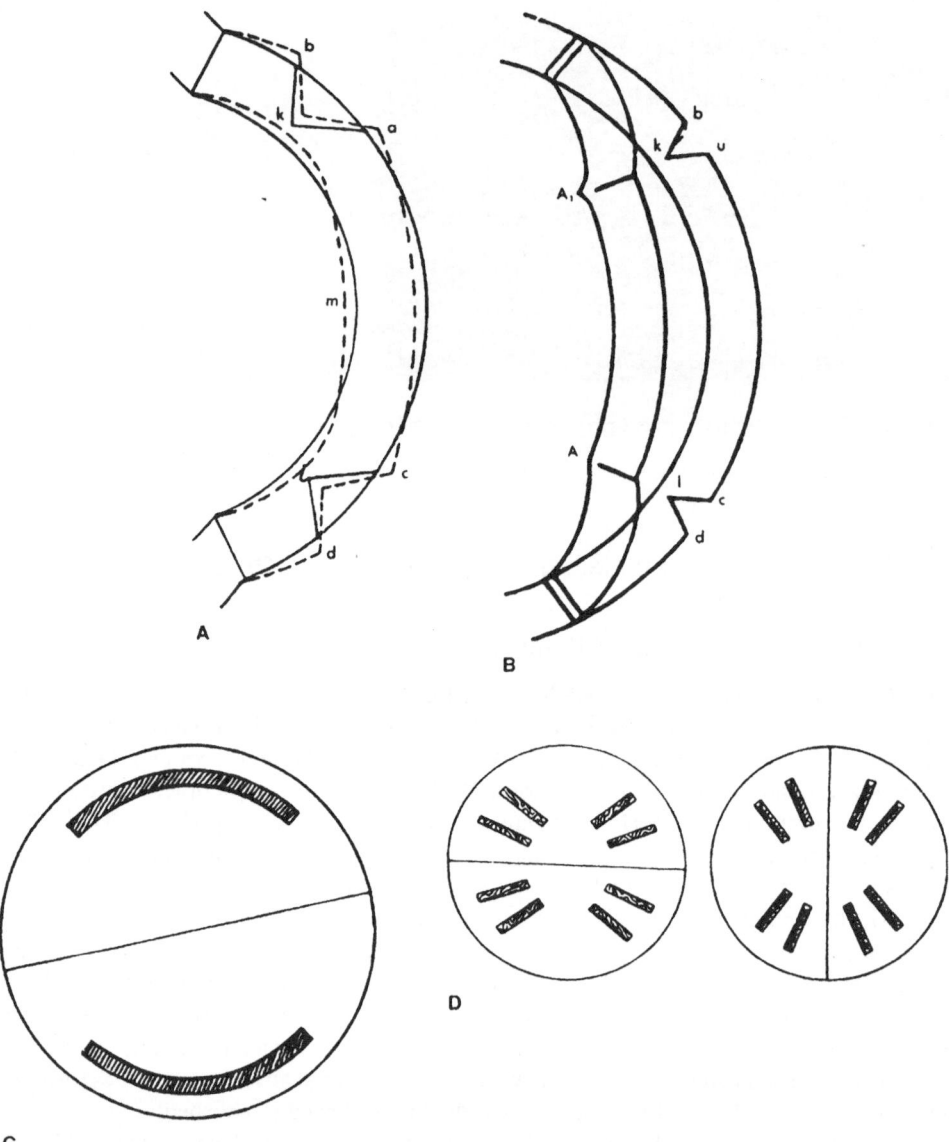

Figure 1.7   The development of radial and astigmatic keratotomy. Illustrations of Lans's studies showing peripheral corneal bulging (A) and subsequent scarring (B) after astigmatic keratotomy (C) and radial keratotomy (D). (From Ref. 117.)

The PERK study showed that 10 years after surgery, 53% of the patients had 20/20 or better uncorrected vision, 85% had 20/40 or better, and 63% of patients younger than 40 years old were spectacle-independent. Low myopes did better than moderate myopes: 94% of patients with low myopia (−2.00 to −3.12 D) had an uncorrected visual acuity (UCVA) of 20/40 or better, while 79% of moderate myopes (−3.25 to −4.37) had 20/40 or better UCVA. The 10-year PERK results also revealed a long-term instability of refractive errors:

43% of eyes demonstrated a hyperopic shift of one diopter or more (71). Of note, the PERK study employed eight-incision surgery (Fig. 1.8). In lower myopes, the four oblique incisions may be sufficient to achieve the desired result.

The concept of standardized RK was introduced by Casebeer in the early 1990s. Using his "cookbook" method, even novice surgeons have been able to perform RK, but the safety and stability of this approach was controversial, for it was not studied with the same rigor that was used in the PERK study (72–75).

Approximately 250,000 RK operations were performed each year in the United States in the early 1990s (71–76). There were advantages of RK over more modern forms of refractive surgery; RK utilized relatively inexpensive equipment, the procedure did not involve incisions in the optical zone, and RK had more long-term follow-up data than several other contemporary refractive procedures. In the early days of excimer laser surgery, RK was generally reserved for patients who had low and moderate myopia (up to 5 D) who

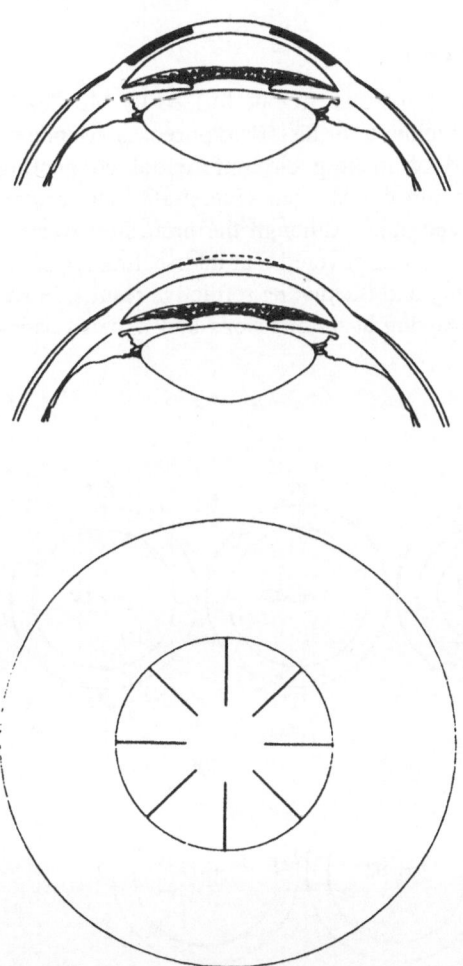

Figure 1.8 Eight-incision radial keratotomy. A diagram highlights the optical zone (top) and the central flattening (middle) after performing an RK with eight incisions (bottom). (From Ref. 117.)

were willing to accept initial undercorrections because they had the best long-term results with RK.

b. Incisional Surgery: Astigmatic Keratotomy

Astigmatic keratotomy (AK) is a procedure that attempts to correct astigmatic refractive errors in patients with greater than 1.5 D of astigmatism. AK involves performing arcuate or transverse (also called tangential, or T) incisions that parallel the limbus, flattening the meridian in which they are placed and steepening the unincised meridian 90 degrees away.

The first AK was performed by Schiotz, a Norwegian ophthalmologist, in 1885. He performed a 3.5 mm penetrating incision at the limbus in the steep meridian of a post cataract patient. The patient's astigmatism was reduced from 19.5 to 7 D (77). Since then, many incision configurations and techniques have been described, with variable outcomes (78–80). In general, deeper and longer incisions produce greater effect, but cuts greater than 75 degrees are not recommended. In addition, the effects of the cuts increase with age. Both new instruments and nomograms for AK such as Lindstrom's have improved results (Fig. 1.9).

c. Incisional Surgery: Hexagonal Keratotomy

The first incisional surgery for the treatment of hyperopia was performed by Mendez in 1985 (81–82). Discussion of this procedure is included for historical purposes. Mendez's "hexagonal keratotomy" procedure consisted of making circumferential connecting hexagonal peripheral cuts around a 4.5 to 6.0 mm optical zone (Fig. 1.10). The central cornea then bulged forward, correcting the hyperopia. Although the procedure was reported to be successful in early studies, it was soon discovered that intersecting incisions caused corneal instability with poor predictability and fluctuating refractive results. In addition, many patients experienced excessive scarring at the incisions and induced astigmatism (83).

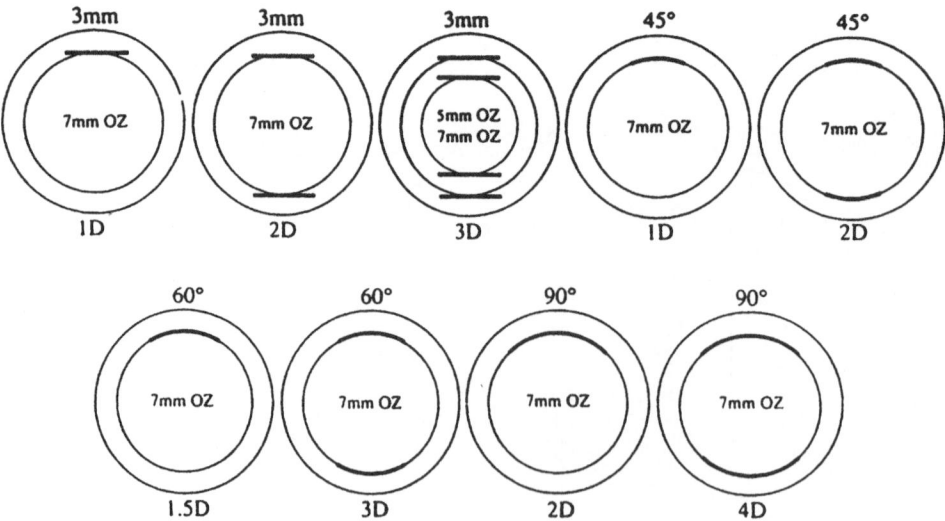

Figure 1.9 Lindstrom's nomogram for astigmatic keratotomy. (From Ref. 118.)

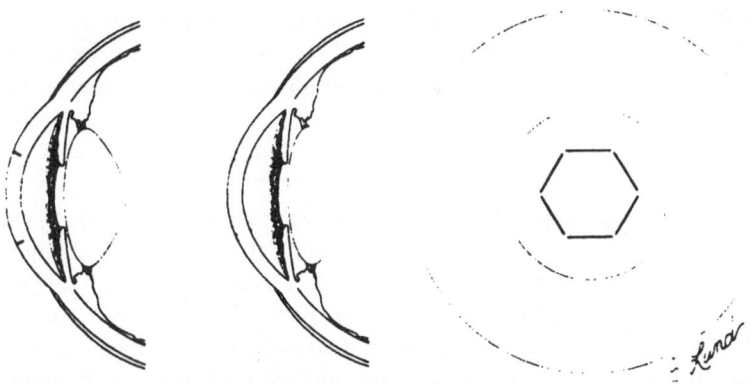

Figure 1.10 Hexagonal keratotomy. (From Ref. 115.)

In 1989, Jensen and Mendez attempted to improve upon the technique with shorter, nonintersecting hexagonal incisions (84). Despite these modifications, corneal scarring, optical aberrations, irregular astigmatism, perforation after minimal trauma, keratitis, and endophthalmitis were complications that plagued this procedure (85–87). It was soon determined that hexagonal keratotomy was "an unpredictable, unsafe surgical procedure with a high complication rate . . ." (87). As such, the procedure has largely been abandoned.

d. Thermal Surgery

Thermal keratoplasty (TK) was first performed by Lans in 1898 to treat astigmatism (64). Lans applied thermal energy via a cautery to alter the structure of the corneal stromal collagen and change the anterior corneal curvature. Heat was later applied by means of radio frequency waves with instruments like the Los Alamos thermal keratoplasty probe (88). Because it was difficult to control the amount of energy applied, TK using simple cauteries and probes resulted in unpredictable results and regression (89,90).

Interest in TK was rekindled with the introduction of lasers that could heat the cornea in a more controlled manner. In 1990, Seiler first reported the use of the holmium:yttrium aluminum garnet (Ho:YAG) laser for hyperopia, a technique called laser thermokeratoplasty (LTK) (91). Ho:YAG LTK delivers infrared radiation that is focused on the midstroma, thereby avoiding damage to the epithelium. Two types of Ho:YAG LTK delivery systems were developed: contact and noncontact.

Contact LTK was performed by applanating the cornea with a probe that applied energy pulses to achieve local, peripheral flattening and subsequent central steepening. In the early 1990s, the procedure underwent Food and Drug Administration (FDA) trials. Regression and undercorrection plagued the procedure, and contact LTK was withdrawn from US FDA trials (92).

Noncontact LTK is performed by projecting simultaneously up to eight spots onto the cornea through a slit lamp-mounted fiberoptic delivery system. FDA phase IIa clinical trials with two years of follow-up showed a mean change in refraction of -0.53 to -1.48 D, with UCVA at two years improved by one or more lines of Snellen visual acuity in 19 (73%) of 26 treated eyes (93). The problem with noncontact LTK is regression. Studies have shown 31.5 to 40% regression (94,95). Another problem apparent with LTK is the induction of irregular astigmatism (95,96). Despite these imperfections, noncontact

Ho:YAG LTK recently received approval by the FDA. Some investigators are attempting to improve upon the current pulsed Ho:YAG LTK with a new continuous wave diode laser that can achieve similar effects on the cornea, without the peaks and troughs of the pulsed laser (97).

e. Orthokeratology

Orthokeratology is the programmed application of contact lenses to reduce or eliminate refractive anomalies, primarily myopia. An orthokeratology lens is flatter, looser, and larger than a conventional lens. Theoretically, the lens mechanically alters the central corneal contour over time. In 1963, Grant and May introduced this practice to the United States. They fitted a rigid PMMA lens that was 0.37 diopters flatter than the patients' flattest corneal median. As the cornea flattened, new lenses were applied, each time 0.37 D flatter than the flattest meridian. The patients wore their lenses for 12 to 15 hours a day and were followed at regular intervals. During the first phase of treatment, the adaptive phase, an average of six pairs of lenses was prescribed over a period of 18 to 24 months. When unaided vision reached 20/20 or refraction stabilized to plano $\pm$ 0.50 diopters, the retainer phase began and patients would then wear a retainer lens to maintain the permanence of the procedure (98,99).

While many anecdotal reports describe the myopia-reducing benefits of orthokeratology, there are no scientific studies to support claims that this practice is a viable alternative to refractive surgery. For example, one randomized, controlled clinical trial did demonstrate an improvement in uncorrected visual acuity from 20/100 to 20/50 in 36.6% of the orthokeratology group compared with 20.8% of the cosmetic lens wearers who improved the same amount. However this trial had no long-term follow up; results were from data at the very end of the 14 month (on average) treatment period (100).

4. Altered Index of Refraction: Phakic IOLs

Most types of refractive surgeries alter the cornea; however, the refractive power of the eye can also be adjusted by implanting an intraocular lens (IOL), with or without extraction of the crystalline lens. Barraquer implanted the first phakic intraocular lens in the 1950s (101). Unfortunately, many of these anterior chamber lenses were poorly finished and had sharp edges. After Barraquer implanted almost 500 lenses, significant complications such as corneal edema occurred, and over 300 of the lenses had to be removed (102). Because of experiences like this, interest in phakic IOLS waned until the labs were better able to guarantee the quality of IOLs.

Modern IOLs are of much better quality than those used in the 1950s. A recent study used a scanning electron microscope to analyze the surface quality of new generation phakic IOLs; the study showed that these lenses did not have any defects that would contraindicate their use as phakic IOLs (103). This study examined the three major types of lenses used as phakic IOLs today: anterior chamber lenses, iris-fixated anterior chamber lenses, and posterior chamber lenses (Fig. 1.11). Even in IOLs with smooth surfaces, however, there is still a risk of progressive corneal endothelial cell loss with the use of phakic IOLs (104–108). Other complications include cataract formation, endopthalmitis, and retinal detachments (109–112).

While phakic IOL implantation does have risks, this procedure enjoys many advantages for the correction of refractive errors: the procedure is both highly predictable and reversible, it can correct higher refractive errors than LASIK and other types of refractive surgeries, and it can be performed by most ophthalmologists. In addition, phakic IOLs, while currently used to treat myopia, may soon be approved to correct hyperopia. A recent Phase I trial of silicone plate posterior chamber lenses, implanted in hyperopes, reported 100% of patients with 20/40 or better UCVA, and 70% with 20/20 or better UCVA (113).

The field of refractive surgery has changed significantly since Sato introduced radial keratotomy and Barraquer performed his first cryolathe keratomileusis. Advances in instrumentation, and in research and understanding of the eye and wound healing, and constant surgical innovation, will surely keep the field changing and improving as the years progress.

In the twenty-first century, LASIK has crossed the genre from medical procedure to star-endorsed "miracle treatment." The public is familiar with the litany of celebrities who have had success with the procedure. When a sports celebrity or an eye surgeon is willing to bet with such high stakes, perhaps the general public feels more comfortable taking a risk as well. More than one million Americans have had LASIK procedures, and predictions estimate that 1.2 million Americans will undergo LASIK in the year 2001 (2).

Some decry LASIK as a shift from disease-driven to demand-driven procedures. There are, however, individuals (such as athletes, firefighters, and military personnel) for whom spectacles or contact lenses are hindering or even dangerous. In addition, people with a high degree of myopia may find glasses to be inadequate due to image minification, or they may be intolerant of contact lenses. The visual disability of high myopes can reduce their quality of life so much that some studies suggest that refractive surgery for high myopes should be provided under health plans like Great Britain's National Health Service.

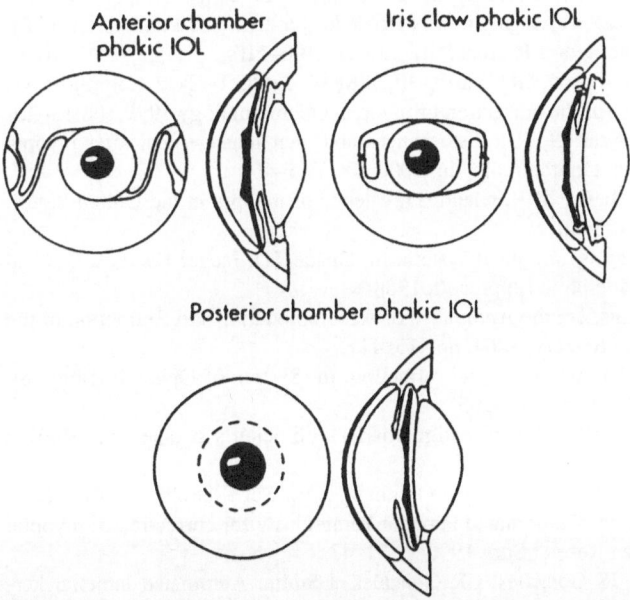

Figure 1.11 Phakic IOLs. Drawings illustrating the three major types of phakic intraocular lenses in use today. (From Ref. 119.)

REFERENCES

1. SG Farah, DT Azar, C Gurdal, J Wong. Laser in situ keratomileusis: literature review of a developing technique. J Cataract Refract Surg 1998;24:989–1006.
2. K Chang. Laser Eye Surgery's Turf War. The New York Times. August 1, 2000; F1, F5.
3. JI Barraquer. Queratoplastia refractiva. Estudios Inform Oftal Inst Barraquer 1949;10:2–21.
4. JI Barraquer. Queratomileusis para la correcion de la myopia. Arch Soc Am Oftalmol Optom 1964;5:27–48.
5. JI Barraquer. Keratomileusis for myopia and aphakia. Ophthalmology 1981;88:701–708.
6. RC Troutman, C Swinger. Refractive keratoplasty: keratophakia and keratomileusis. Trans Am Ophthalmol Soc 1978;76:329–339.
7. JI Barraquer. Keratomileusis. Int Surg 1967;48:103–117.
8. JI Barraquer. Results of hypermetropic keratomileusis, 1980–1981. Int Ophthalmol Clin 1983;23:25–44.
9. C Barraquer, AM Gutierrez, A Espinosa. Myopic keratomileusis: short-term results. Refract Corneal Surg 1989;5:307–313.
10. L Nordan. Myopic keratomileusis: 74 consecutive non-amblyopic cases with one year follow-up. J Refract Surg 1986;2:1224–1228.
11. CA Swinger, BA Barker. Prospective evaluation of myopic keratomileusis. Ophthalmology 1984;91:785–92.
12. SL Trokel, R Srinivasan, B Braren. Excimer laser surgery of the cornea. Am J Ophthalmol 1983;96:710–715.
13. GA Peyman, C Beyer, J Kuszak, B Khoobehi, M Shahsavari, R Badaro. Long-term effect of erbium-YAG laser (2.9 microns) on the primate cornea. Int Ophthalmol 1991;15:249–258.
14. IG Pallikaris, ME Papatzanaki, EZ Stathi, O Frenschock, A Georgiadis. Laser in situ keratomileusis. Lasers Surg Med 1990;10:463–468.
15. L Buratto, M Ferrari, C Genisi. Myopic keratomileusis with the excimer laser: one-year follow up. Refract Corneal Surg 1993;9:12–19.
16. BS Maller. Market trends in refractive surgery. Int Ophthalmol Clin 2000;40(3):11–19.
17. M Montes, A Chayet, L Gomez, R Magallanes, N Robledo. Laser in situ keratomileusis for myopia of −1.50 to −6.00 diopters. J Refract Surg 1999;15:106–110.
18. RD Stulting, JD Carr, KP Thompson, GO Waring III, WM Wiley, JG Walker. Complications of laser in situ keratomileusis for the correction of myopia. Ophthalmology 1999;106:13–20.
19. SA Melki, CE Proano, DT Azar. Optical disturbances and their management after myopia laser in situ keratomileusis. Int Ophthalmol Clin. 2000;40(1):45–46.
20. RD Sperduto, D Seigel, J Roberts, M Rowland. Prevalence of myopia in the United States. Arch Ophthalmol 1983;101:405–407.
21. A Sorsby. Biology of the eyes as an optical system. In: Duane TD, Jaeger EA, eds. Clinical Ophthalmology, rev ed. Philadelphia: Lippincott, 1988.
22. RC Donders, WD Moore, trans. On the Anomalies of Accommodation and Refraction of the Eye. London: New Sydenham Society, 1864, pp 415–417.
23. ESS Duke, D Abrams. Ophthalmic optics and refraction. In: System of Ophthalmology. St. Louis, MO: Mosby, 1970, Vol. 5, pp 274–295.
24. RL Lindstrom. The surgical correction of astigmatism: a clinician's perspective. Refract Corneal Surg 1990;6:441–454.
25. L Ruiz, J Rowsey. In situ keratomileusis. Invest Ophthalmol Vis Sci 1988;29 (suppl):392.
26. WA Lyle, GJ Jin. Initial results of automated lamellar keratoplasty for correction of myopia: one-year follow-up. J Cataract Refract Surg 1996;22:31–43.
27. FW Price Jr., WE Whitson, JS Gonzales, CR Gonzales, J Smith. Automated lamellar keratomileusis in situ for myopia. J Refract Surg 1996;12:29–35.
28. R Lindstrom. Minimally invasive radial keratotomy: mini-RK. J Cataract Refract Surg 1995;21:27–34.

29. TP Werblin, GM Stafford. The Casebeer system for predictable keratorefractive surgery. One-year evaluation of 205 consecutive eyes. Ophthalmology 1993;100:1095–1102.

30. WA Lyle, GJ Jin. Hyperopic automated lamellar keratoplasty: complications and visual results. Arch Ophthalmol 1998;116:425–428.

31. GO Waring III. A cautionary tale of innovation in refractive surgery. Arch Ophthalmol 1999; 117:1069–1073.

32. PS Hersh, RD Stulting, RF Steinert, GO Waring III, KP Thompson, M O'Connell, K Doney, OD Schein. Results of phase III excimer laser photorefractive keratectomy for myopia. The Summit PRK Study Group. Ophthalmology 1997;104:1535–1553.

33. SC Schallhorn, CL Blanton, SE Kaupp, J Sutphin, M Gordon, H Goforth Jr, FK Butler Jr. Preliminary results of photorefractive keratectomy in active-duty United States Navy personnel. Ophthalmology 1996;103:5–22.

34. SI Shah, PS Hersh. Photorefractive keratectomy for myopia with a 6-mm beam diameter. J Refract Surg 1996;12:341–346.

35. T Seiler, A Holschbach, M Derse, B Jean, U Genth. Complications of myopic photorefractive keratectomy with the excimer laser. Ophthalmology 1994;101:153–160.

36. T Seiler, PJ McDonnell. Excimer laser photorefractive keratectomy. Surv Ophthalmol 1995;40:89–118.

37. RF Steinert, S Bafna. Surgical correction of moderate myopia: which method should you choose? PRK and LASIK are the treatments of choice. Surv Ophthalmol 1998;43:157–179.

38. MA El Danasoury, GO Waring, A El Maghraby, K Mehrez. Excimer laser in situ keratomileusis to correct compound myopic astigmatism. J Refract Surg 1997;13:511–520.

39. Z Wang, J Chen, B Yang. Comparison of laser in situ keratomileusis and photorefractive keratectomy to correct myopia from −1.25 to −6.00 diopters. J Refract Surg 1997;13:528–534.

40. DG Kent, KD Solomon, Q Peng, SB Whiteside, SJ Brown, DJ Apple. Effect of surface photorefractive keratectomy and laser in situ keratomileusis on the corneal endothelium. J Cataract Refract Surg 1997;23:386–397.

41. T Latvala, C. Barraquer-Coll, K Tervo, T Tervo. Corneal wound healing and nerve morphology after excimer laser in situ keratomileusis in human eyes. J Refract Surg 1996;12:677–683.

42. Q Peng, KD Solomon, DG Kent, OF Ahmad, DJ Apple. Comparison of keratocyte activation in laser in situ keratomileusis and photorefractive keratectomy. Invest Ophthalmol Vis Sci 1996;37(3):S63.

43. K Tervo, JJ Perez-Santonja, JL Alio-Sanz, T Latvala, T Tervo. Nerve morphology after LASIK in rabbit corneas. Invest Ophthalmol Vis Sci 1996;37(3):S64.

44. WB Jackson, E Casson, WG Hodge, G Mintsioulis, PJ Agapitos. Laser vision correction for low hyperopia. An 18-month assessment of safety and efficacy. Ophthalmology 1998;105: 1727–1738; discussion 1737–1738.

45. D Dausch, R Klein, E Schroeder. Excimer laser photorefractive keratectomy for hyperopia. Refract Corneal Surg 1993;9:20–28.

46. D Dausch, Z Smecka, R Klein, E Schroder, S Kirchner. Excimer laser photorefractive keratectomy for hyperopia. J Cataract Refract Surg 1997;23:169–176.

47. DP O'Brart, CS Stephenson, K Oliver, J Marshall. Excimer laser photorefractive keratectomy for the correction of hyperopia using an erodible mask and axicon system. Ophthalmology 1997;104:1959–1970.

48. SM Daya, FR Tappouni, NE Habib. Photorefractive keratectomy for hyperopia: six-month results in 45 eyes. Ophthalmology 1997;104:1952–1958.

49. MB McDonald, HE Kaufman, JV Aquavella, DS Durrie, DA Hiles, JD Hunkeler, RH Keates, KS Morgan, DR Sanders. The nationwide study of epikeratophakia for myopia. Am J Ophthalmol 1987;103(3 Pt 2):375–383.

50. WR Schlichtemeier, KD Arbegast. Long-term loss of effect of myopic epikeratophakia. J Refract Surg 1987;3:46–49.

51. JT Woodhams. Regression of myopic epikeratophakia effects [letter]. J Cataract Refract Surg 1987;13:343–344.

52. TP Werblin, HE Kaufman. Epikeratophakia: the surgical correction of aphakia. II. Preliminary results in a non-human primate model. Curr Eye Res 1981;1:131–137.

53. PS Binder, EY Zavala. Why do some epikeratoplasties fail? Arch Ophthalmol 1987;105:63–69.

54. MB McDonald, HE Kaufman, JV Aquavella, DS Durrie, DA Hiles, JD Hunkeler, RH Keates, KS Morgan, DR Sanders. The nationwide study of epikeratophakia for aphakia in adults. Am J Ophthalmol 1987;103(3 Pt 2):358–365.

55. KS Morgan, MB McDonald, DA Hiles, JV Aquavella, DS Durrie, JD Hunkeler, HE Kaufman, RH Keates, DR Sanders. The nationwide study of epikeratophakia for aphakia in children. Am J Ophthalmol 1987;103(3 Pt 2):366–374.

56. DS Durrie, DL Habrich, TR Dietze. Secondary intraocular lens implantation vs. epikeratophakia for the treatment of aphakia. Am J Ophthalmol 1987;103(3 Pt 2):384–391.

57. M Busin, A Cusumano, M Spitznas. Epithelial interface cysts after epikeratophakia. Ophthalmology 1993;100:1225–1229.

58. PS Musco, JV Aquavalla. Reversibility of epikeratoplasty. J Refract Surg 1988;4:15–17.

59. FW Price Jr, PS Binder. Scarring of a recipient cornea following epikeratoplasty. Arch Ophthalmol 1987:105:1556–1560.

60. DJ Schanzlin, EM Sarno, JB Robin. Crescentic lamellar keratoplasty for pellucid marginal degeneration. Am J Ophthalmol 1983:96:253.

61. RC Troutman, C Swinger, M Goldstein. Keratophakia update. Ophthalmology 1981;88:36–38.

62. EJ Linebarger, D Song, J Ruckhofer, DJ Schanzlin. Intacs: the intrastromal corneal ring. Int Ophthalmol Clin 2000;40(3):199–208.

63. B Cochener, G Savary-LeFloch, J Colin. Effect of intrastromal corneal ring segment shift on clinical outcome: one year results for low myopia. J Cataract Refract Surg 2000;26:978–986.

64. LJ Lans. Experimentelle Untersuchungen über Entstehung von Astigmatismus durch nichtperfoririende Corneawunden. Arch fur Ophthalmologie 1898;45:117–152.

65. BH Schimmelpfennig, GO Waring. Development of refractive keratotomy in the nineteenth century. In: Waring GO, ed. Refractive Keratotomy for Myopia and Astigmatism. St, Louis: Mosby-Year Book, 1992, p 174.

66. T Sato. Treatment of conical cornea (incision of Descemet's membrane). Acta Soc Ophthalmol Jpn 1939;43:544–555.

67. T Sato, K Akiyama, H Shibata. A new surgical approach to myopia. Am J Ophthalmol 1953;36:823–829.

68. K Akiyama, H Shibata, A Kanai, S Akiyama, T Yamaguchi, A Nakajima, GO Waring. Development of radial keratotomy in Japan, 1939–1960. In Waring GO, ed. Refractive Keratotomy for Myopia and Astigmatism. St Louis: Mosby—Year Book, 1992, p 212.

69. SN Fyodorov, Durnev VV. Operation of dosaged dissection of corneal circular ligament in cases of myopia of mid degree. Ann Ophthlmol 1979;11:1185–1190.

70. SN Fyodorov, AA Agranovsky. Long-term results of anterior radial keratotomy. J Ocular Therapy Surg 1982;1:217–223.

71. GO Waring III, MJ Lynn, PJ McDonnell. Results of the prospective evaluation of radial keratotomy (PERK) study 10 years after surgery. Arch Ophthalmol 1994;112:1298–1308.

72. JC Casebeer. New techniques for radial keratotomy. Eur J Implant Refract Surg 1994;6:237–238.

73. TP Werblin, GM Stafford. The Casebeer system for predictable keratorefractive surgery. One-year evaluation of 205 consecutive eyes. Ophthalmology 1993;100:1095–1102.

74. TP Werblin, GM Stafford. Hyperopic shift after refractive keratotomy using the Casebeer system. J Cataract Refract Surg 1996;22:1030–1036.

75. TP Werblin, GM Stafford. Three year results of refractive keratotomy using the Casebeer system. J Cataract Refract Surg 1996;22:1023–1029.

76. GO Waring, MJ Lynn, A Nizam, MH Kutner, JW Cowden, W Culbertson, PR Laibson, MB McDonald, JD Nelson, SA Obstbaum. Results of the evaluation of radial keratotomy (PERK) study five years after surgery. Ophthalmology 1991;98:1164–1176.

77. LJ Schiotz. Hinfall von hochgradigem Hornhautsastigmatismus nach Staarextraction, Besserung auf operativem Wege. Arch Augenheilkd 1885;15:178–181.

78. LT Nordan. Quantifiable astigmatism correction: concepts and suggestions. J Cataract Refract Surg 1986;12:507–518.

79. EG Faktorovich, RK Maloney, FW Price Jr. Effect of astigmatic keratotomy on spherical equivalent: results of the Astigmatism Reduction Clinical Trial. Am J Ophthalmol 1999;127: 260–269.

80. RL Lindstrom. The surgical correction of astigmatism: a clinician's perspective. Refract Corneal Surg 1990;6:441–454.

81. A Mendez. Correcão da hipermetropia pela ceratotomia hexagonal. In: Guimarares R, ed. Cirugia Refractive. Rio de Janeiro, Brazil: Piramide Livro Medic Editora Ltda, 1987, pp. 267–279.

82. A Mendez. Advances in hyperopic correction with hexagonal keratotomy. Presented at the American Society of Cataract and Refractive Surgery Meeting, April 1986, Los Angeles, CA.

83. A Neumann, G McCarty. Hexagonal keratotomy for correction of low hyperopia: preliminary results of a prospective study. J Cataract Refract Surg 1988;14:265–269.

84. JC Casebeer, SG Phillips. Hexagonal keratotomy. An historical review and assessment of 46 cases. Ophthalmol Clin North Am 1992;5:727–744.

85. R Jensen. Hexagonal keratotomy: clinical experience with 483 eyes. Int Ophthalmol Clin 1991;31:69–73.

86. P McDonnell, J Lean, D Schanzlin. Globe rupture from blunt trauma after hexagonal keratotomy. Am J Ophthalmol 1987;103:241–242.

87. WL Basuk, M Zisman, GO Waring III, LA Wilson, PS Binder, KP Thompson, HE Grossniklaus, RD Stulting. Complications of hexagonal keratotomy. Am J Ophthalmol 1994; 117:37–49.

88. JJ Rowsey, JD Doss. Preliminary report of Los Alamos keratoplasty technique. Ophthalmology 1981;88:755.

89. H Stringer, J Parr. Shrinkage temperature of eye collagen. Nature 1964;204:1307.

90. AC Neumann, D Sanders, M Raanan, M DeLuca. Hyperopic thermokeratoplasty: clinical evaluation. J Cataract Refract Surg 1991;17:830–838.

91. T Seiler, M Matallana, T Bende. Laser thermokeratoplasty by means of a pulsed holmium:YAG laser for hyperopic correction. Refract Corneal Surg 1990;6:335–339.

92. DS Durrie, DJ Schumer, TB Cavanaugh. Holmium:YAG laser thermokeratoplasty for hyperopia. J Refract Corneal Surg 1994;10:S277–280.

93. DD Koch, T Kohnen, PJ McDonnell, R Menefee, M Berry. Hyperopia correction by noncontact holmium: YAG laser thermal keratoplasty: U.S. phase IIA clinical study with 2-year follow-up. Ophthalmology 1997;104:1938–1947.

94. JL Alio, MM Ismail, JL Sanchez Pego. Correction of hyperopia with non-contact Ho:YAG laser thermal keratoplasty. J Refract Surg 1997;13:17–22.

95. MK Tutton, PKM Cherry. Holmium: YAG laser thermokeratoplasty to correct hyperopia: two years follow-up. Ophthalmic Surg Lasers 1996;27(5 suppl):S521–S524.

96. DS Durrie, DJ Schumer, TB Cavanaugh. Holmium:YAG laser thermokeratoplasty for hyperopia. J Refract Corneal Surg 1994;10(2 suppl):S277–S280.

97. T Bende, B Jean, T Oltrup. Laser thermal keratoplasty using a continuous wave diode laser. J Refract Surg 1999;15:154–158.

98. SC Grant, CH May. Orthokeratology—control of refractive errors through contact lenses. J Am Opt Assoc 1971;42:1277–1283.

99. CH May, SC Grant, J Norlan. Orthokeratology, a Synopsis of Techniques. San Diego: International Society of Orthokeratology, 1972.

100. KA Polse. Corneal changes accompanying orthokeratology. Arch Ophthalmol. 1984;101: 1873–1878.

101. J Barraquer. Anterior chamber plastic lenses. Results of and conclusions from five years of experience. Trans Ophthalmol Soc UK 1959;79:393–424.

102. RC Drews. The Barraquer experience with intraocular lenses. 20 years later. Ophthalmology 1982;89:386–393.

103. T Kohnen, M Baumeister, G Magdowski. Scanning electron microscopic characteristics of phakic intraocular lenses. Ophthalmology 2000;107:934–939.

104. M Landesz, JGR Worst, G van Rij. Long-term results of correction of high myopia with an iris claw phakic intraocular lens. J Refract Surg 2000;16:310–316.

105. F Mimouni, J Colin, V Koffi, P Bonnet. Damage to the corneal endothelium from anterior chamber intraocular lenses in phakic myopic eyes. Refract Corneal Surg 1991;7:277–281.

106. JJ Saragoussi, J Cotinat, G Renard, M Savoldelli, A Abenhaim, Y Pauliquen. Damage to the corneal endothelium by minus power anterior chamber intraocular lenses. Refract Corneal Surg 1991;7:282–285.

107. JJ Perez-Santonja, MT Iradier, L Sanz-Iglesias, JM Serrano, MA Zato. Endothelial changes in phakic eyes with anterior chamber intraocular lenses to correct high myopia. J Cataract Refract Surg 1996;22:1017–1022.

108. JL Menezo, AL Cisneros, V Rodriguez-Salvador. Endothelial study of iris-claw phakic lens: four-year follow-up. J Cataract Refract Surg 1998;24:1039–1049.

109. F Trindade, F Pereira. Cataract formation after posterior chamber phakic intraocular lens implantation. J Cataract Refract Surg 1998;24:1661–1663.

110. PH Brauweiler, T Wehler, M Busin. High incidence of cataract formation after implantation of a silicone posterior chamber lens in phakic, highly myopic eyes. Ophthalmology 1999;106:1651–1655.

111. JM Ruiz-Moreno, JL Alio, JJ Perez-Santonja, F de la Hoz. Retinal detachment in phakic eyes with anterior chamber intraocular lenses to correct severe myopia. Am J Ophthalmol 1999; 127:270–275.

112. JJ Perez-Santonja, JM Ruiz-Moreno, F de la Hoz, C Giner-Gorriti, JL Alio. Endophthalmitis after phakic intraocular lens implantation to correct high myopia. J Cataract Refract Surg 1999;25:1295–1298.

113. K Rose, R Harper, C Tromans, C Waterman, D Goldberg, C Haggerty, A Tullo. Br J Ophthalmol 2000;84:1031–1034.

114. DR Sanders, RG Martin, DC Brown, J Shepherd, MR Deitz, M DeLuca. Posterior chamber phakic intraocular lens for hyperopia. J Refract Surg 1999;15:309–315.

115. MD Mead, DT Azar. Terminology, Classification, and Definitions of Refractive Surgery. Connecticut: Appleton and Lange, 1997, pp. 3–18.

116. CA Swinger, A Chou. History and principles of automated lamellar keratoplasty and laser in situ keratomileusis. In: RS Brightbill, ed. Corneal Surgery: Theory, Technique and Tissue. 3rd ed. New York: Mosby, 1999, pp. 762–770.

117. EW Kornmehl. Radial keratotomy: operative techniques. In: DT Azar, ed. Refractive Surgery. Connecticut: Appleton and Lange, 1997, pp. 255–272.

118. YR Chu, DR Hardten, RL Lindstrom. Concepts in astigmatic keratotomy. In: Brightbill RS, ed. Corneal Surgery: Theory, Technique and Tissue. 3rd ed. New York: Mosby, 1999, pp. 650–655.

119. H Leibowitz, G Waring. Corneal Disorders. Philadelphia: Saunders, 1998.

2

History of LASIK

IOANNIS PALLIKARIS

University of Crete Medical School and University Hospital of Heraklion
Heraklion, Crete, Greece

THEKLA PAPADAKI

Vardinoyannion Eye Institute of Crete, University of Crete Medical School
Heraklion, Crete, Greece

A. INTRODUCTION

Modern lamellar refractive surgery has its roots in the pioneer work of Professor José Ignacio Barraquer of Colombia. In 1949, Barraquer suggested that by adding or removing corneal tissue, it was possible to manipulate surgically the curvature of the air/tear film interface, where the two thirds of the refractive power of the eye is located (1). From the very beginning, he realized the importance of preserving each layer of the cornea, and so corneal lamellar techniques started to develop.

During the past 50 years, lamellar corneal refractive surgery has undergone a long evolutionary process. Various different methods have been suggested to remove and/or shape corneal tissue, in order to enhance the accuracy and predictability of lamellar procedures. Laser in situ keratomileusis (LASIK) is the most recent step in this process and combines well-established lamellar surgical techniques with the precision of excimer laser photoablation. Although it enjoys, at present, great popularity among refractive surgeons, LASIK is still a developing procedure in terms of technique and perioperative patient management.

In this chapter we are going to follow the steps that led from Barraquer's first experiments to LASIK. Reviewing the history of refractive surgery is essential, because it provides the fundamental principles which form the basis for better understanding and refining the currently used techniques.

B. FROM KERATOMILEUSIS TO ALK

In order to describe lamellar techniques, Barraquer used the term keratomileusis, which is derived from the Greek roots *keras* (hornlike = cornea) and *smileusis* (carving).

Myopic keratomuleusis (MKM) was introduced in 1949 (1). The initial procedure involved creating a lamellar corneal disc approximately 300 μm in depth (lamellar keratectomy) and removing tissue from the residual stromal bed or the disc (refractive keratectomy). When the disc was replaced, the anterior corneal curvature was flattened, thus reducing the refractive power of the eye and correcting myopia (Fig. 2.1). Both keratectomies were initially performed freehand with a Paufique knife. Removing stroma from the bed freehand proved to be so difficult technically and so inaccurate that Barraquer temporarily abandoned the in situ technique.

Instead, he focused on refining the lamellar keratectomy and perfecting the carving of the lamellar disc. He discovered that the relation between IOP and resection diameter directly affected the depth of keratectomy (2). Based on this knowledge, Barraquer designed the first manual microkeratome, applanator lenses, and suction rings of various heights. He also discovered that a slow passage speed and constant contact between the microkeratome and the suction ring during the cut were essential for a smooth, even keratectomy (3). He was now able to achieve lamellar discs of predetermined thickness and diameter (2). Barraquer's early work provided the principles of lamellar keratectomy and set the basis for the development of the modern automated microkeratomes.

In order to achieve more precise shaping of the resected corneal disc, Barraquer thought of freezing the tissue and carving it using a modified contact lens cryolathe in a procedure named freeze-myopic keratomileusis (F-MKM) (2). After the disc was excised with the microkeratome, its thickness was determined using an American Optical radiuscope. Using a certain formula, Barraquer could calculate the required curvature to correct the ametropia, given the original corneal radius of curvature and the dioptric correction (4). The lathe was preground for the required radius of curvature. The disc was stained with Kiton green 0.5%, to allow visualization during the procedure, and placed epithelial side-down on the lathe lap. The lap and disc were frozen to −30°C by liquid nitrogen. The stro-

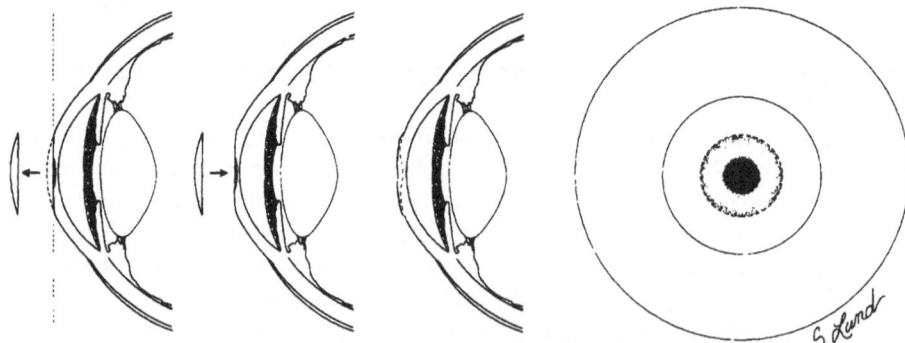

Figure 2.1 Myopic keratomileusis (MKM). A lamellar corneal disc approximately 300 μm in depth is created (lamellar keratectomy) and tissue is removed from the residual stromal bed (refractive keratectomy). Once the disc is replaced, the anterior corneal surface is flattened, thus reducing the refractive power of the eye and correcting myopia. (Reprinted with permission from D. T. Azar. Refractive Surgery. Appleton & Lange, 1997.)

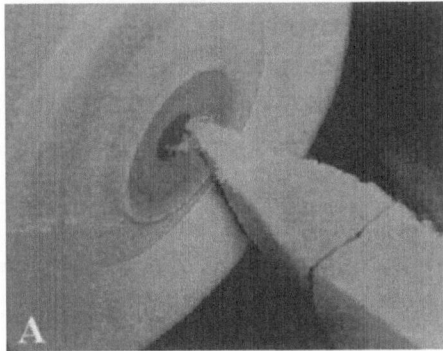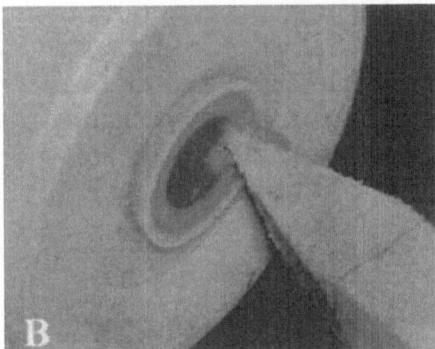

Figure 2.2 Free keratomileusis. The dyed corneal disc is placed on the lathe, epithelial side down, and frozen by liquid nitrogen (A). A frozen tool is then used to lathe the disc (B). (Courtesy of Dr. José Ignacio Barraquer.)

mal surface was then lathed with more tissue removed from the center than the periphery in the myopic cases so as to flatten the central corneal curvature (Fig. 2.2). For hyperopic correction the disc was treated in the opposite way to achieve steepening of the central corneal curvature (Fig. 2.3). After thawing, the carved disc was placed back on to the cornea and held in place with sutures. This was the first time a part of a human organ was removed from the body to alter its function and then returned.

Barraquer also thought he could achieve steepening of the central corneal curvature more effectively by implanting a preprocessed stomal tissue lenticle (allograft) within the recipient's stroma (5). To create the lenticle, a lamellar corneal disc was resected from fresh or preserved donor's cornea, using a microkeratome. The epithelium, Bowman's layer and the anterior stroma were removed. The remaining stromal tissue was preserved by a variety of means (refrigeration, freezing, and freeze drying) and processed on the lathe in a way

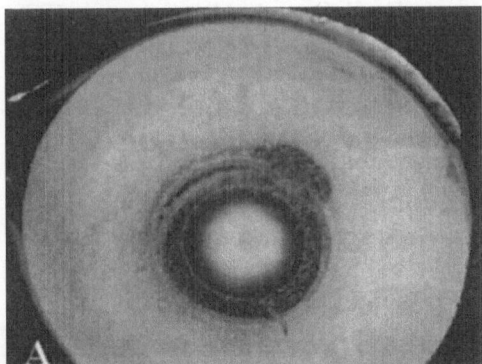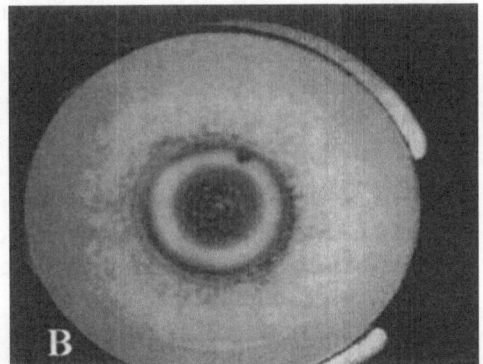

Figure 2.3 Freeze keratomileusis for myopia and hyperopia. As more tissue is removed centrally than peripherally (A), the plano corneal disc is converted to a concave (negative) lens, capable of correcting myopia. For hyperopic correction, more tissue is removed from the periphery of the disc to achieve steepening of the central curvature (B). (Courtesy of Dr. José Ignacio Barraquer.)

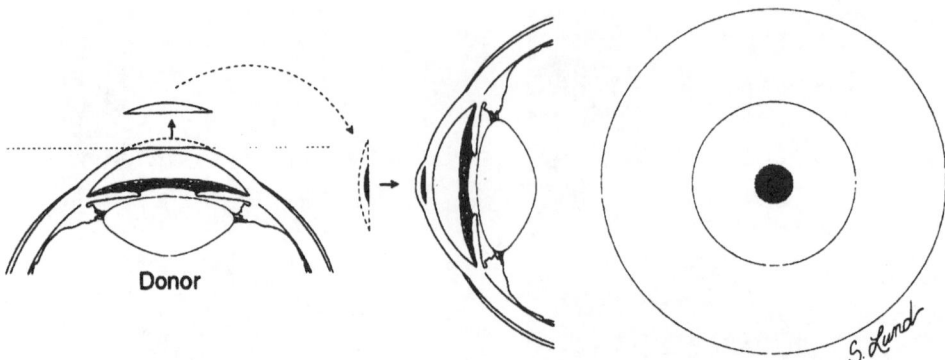

Figure 2.4 Keratophakia (KF) is the procedure in which a corneal lenticle is removed from a donor's cornea. After a lamellar resection is performed on the recipient's cornea, the lenticule is inserted underneath the resected corneal cap. As the cap is sutured back, a new steepend anterior corneal curvature is formed. (Reprinted with permission from D. T. Azar. Refractive Surgery. Appleton & Lange, 1997.)

similar to that in F-KM, to create a converge lenticle capable of correcting aphakia and high hyperopia. Keratophakia (KF) was the term employed to describe the procedure in which a lamellar keratectomy was performed on the recipient's cornea, the lenticle was placed intrastromally, and the lamellar disc was sutured in place (Fig. 2.4). The lenticle diameter and thickness varied, depending on the initial refractive error and the target correction. KF was first reported in 1958 as having the potential to correct aphakia (5). With this report Barraquer introduced his work to the ophthalmic community.

The first report on F-MKM followed in 1967 (2). First results revealed visual improvement in 80% of the patients and indicated that refinement of the procedure should proceed. Over the next decade significant advantages in the cutting and shaping of the tissue improved the predictability of the procedure but could not help overcome its major drawbacks. These were the use of very complicated technology and the steep learning curve required for the procedure, together with the prolonged visual recovery time and the high rate of complications such as scarring and irregular astigmatism (6).

Troutman and Swinger brought the concepts of KF and KM to the United States in 1978 (7). KF attracted the attention of the ophthalmic community as a possible solution for the treatment of aphakia after cataract extraction (8–10). However, with the advent of IOL technology, interest in KF subsided. Though early results on MKM were encouraging (11,12), the technical difficulty, the steep learning curve, and the potential of sight-threatening complications, which were attributed mainly to tissue damage during freezing and lathing (12–15), discouraged many ophthalmic surgeons, and the technique failed to be popularized.

In an attempt to simplify lamellar refractive surgery and make it safer, Kaufman, Werblin, and Klyce of the Louisiana State University Eye Center introduced epikeratophakia (epikeratoplasty or epi) in 1979 (16–18). The procedure involved deepithelialization of the recipient cornea and preparation of a peripheral annular partial-thickness keratotomy. A lyophilized preshaped corneal tissue lenticle (consisting of Bowman's layer and the anterior stroma) was reconstituted and sutured into the keratotomy site, creating a new shape for the anterior corneal surface (Fig. 2.5). The major advantage of this procedure was that it avoided the problems of using a microkeratome to cut across the optical zone and lathing the corneal tissue intraoperatively (19). Epi was intended for use in the treatment of aphakia, high myopia, or hyperopia (20,21). Plano epilenticles were also employed to flatten the cornea in keratoconus and provide a more regular surface for contact lens wear (22). Unfortunately, the initial reports proved that the procedure was neither predictable nor safe (23–24). The most common complications of epi included irregular astigmatism, persistent epithelial defects, and delayed visual recovery (25–27). These were mainly attributed to the heavy processing of the graft tissue (28). Several modifications of the initial procedure were employed (29–30), among them the application of nonfreezing techniques to shape the graft lenticle (31). Altman reported on using a spot excimer laser beam to shape the corneal tissue, mounted on a movable platform (32). Buratto and Ferrari used the Barraquer–Krumeich–Swinger technique (described below) to shape epilenticles without freezing. Predictability was still low, but visual recovery was significantly faster than with regular freezing techniques (33). Despite the efforts, epi never gained approval from the FDA and was withdrawn from the market (34). However, the ease of epi compared to MKM prompted the development of nonfreeze keratomileusis techniques.

The Barraquer–Krumeich–Swinger (BKS) refractive system was introduced in 1985 (35). This included an improved microkeratome (the BKS 1000), a set of dies, and a suction stand. The microkeratome was used to excise a lamellar corneal disc. The disc was then placed epithelial side down on one of the suction dies, and the second refractive cut was performed on the stromal aspect of the disc, using the microkeratome. The curvatures of the dies varied, depending on the amount of the attempted correction of myopia or hyperopia (Figs. 2.6 and 2.7). When a convex die was used, the keratome removed a central part of the stroma, thus flattening the anterior surface of the cornea. For hyperopia correction, the lenticle was placed on a concave die, and the microkeratome removed a peripheral portion of the stroma, steepening the central cornea. The sculptured lamellar disc was finally sutured back to the bed. Despite its technical difficulty, nonfreeze keratomileusis proved to have a major advantage: the rapid and comfortable visual recovery of the patients. This was

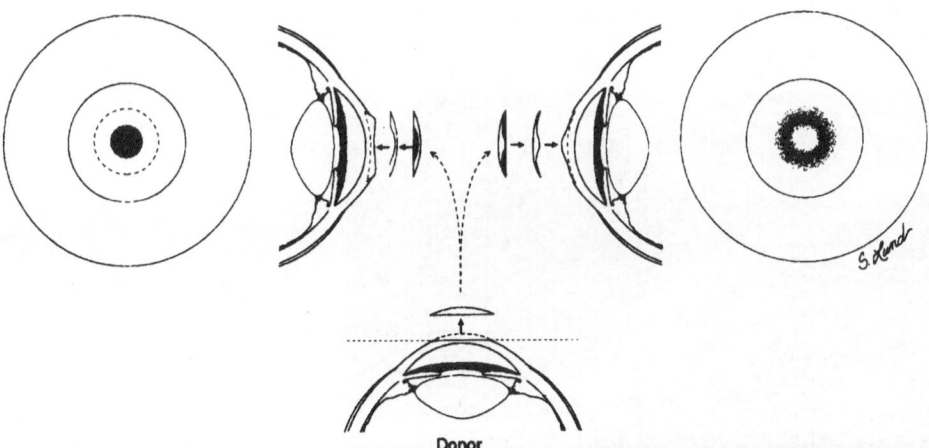

Figure 2.5 Epikeratophakia or epikeratoplasty. A preprocessed donor lenticle is fixed onto the corneal surface. A peripheral circumferential keratectomy allows fixation of the lenticle into the host cornea. For correction of hyperopia (right), a positive lens is used to steepen the anterior corneal curvature. A negative lens (left), on the contrary, would flatten the anterior corneal curvature, resulting in correction of myopia. (Reprinted with permission from D. T. Azar. Refractive Surgery. Appleton & Lange, 1997.)

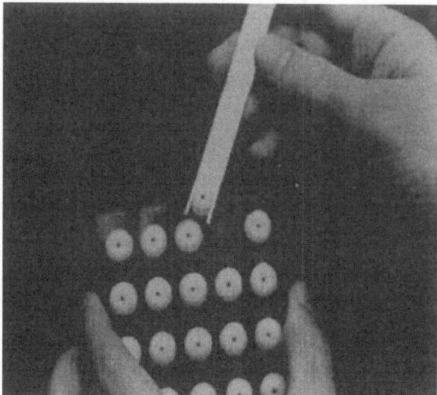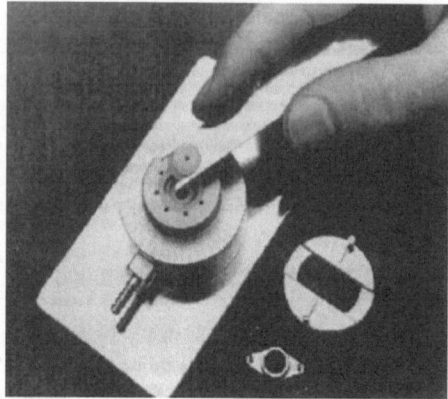

Figure 2.6 The Barraquer–Krumeich–Swinger (BKS) nonfreeze keratomileusis technique. Apart from the microkeratome, the BKS system includes a set of suction dies (left) and a suction stand. After the corneal cap is resected it is placed, epithelial side down, on the proper suction die, selected according to the amount of attempted correction of myopia or hyperopia. The die bearing the corneal cap is then fixed onto the suction stand for the refractive, second, cut to be made at the stromal side of the cap (right).

attributed to the preservation of fibroblasts and corneal epithelium. However, significant amounts of irregular astigmatism could not be avoided, as the refractive cut could not be centered with precision, and there was always the risk of trauma to the disc during manipulation. More important, the thickness of the lamellar disc determined completely the accuracy of the technique, which was ineffective for more than 16 diopters of myopia (36). It was now evident that carving of the corneal disc should be eliminated, in order to reduce the complication rate and achieve more predictable corrections of high myopia. Thus research turned once again towards keratomileusis in situ.

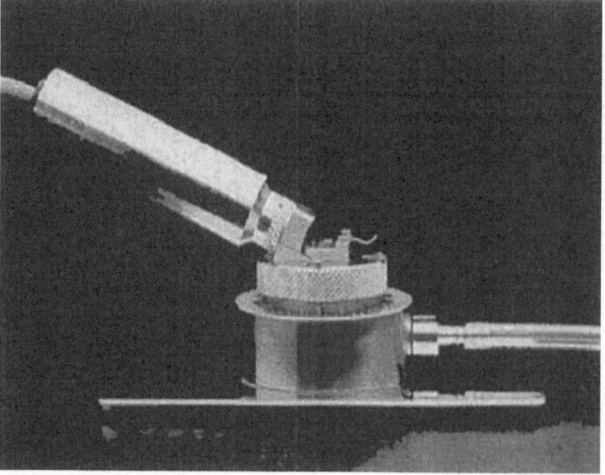

Figure 2.7 The Barraquer–Krumeich–Swinger (BKS) system for nonfreeze keratomileusis. The BKS microkeratome and the suction stand.

As mentioned previously, Barraquer introduced KM in situ in the late 1940s (1) but had to abandon the technique very soon due to the many technical difficulties inherent in the use of a manual microkeratome. Ruiz and Rowsey revised the idea of KM in situ in the late 1980s, taking advantage of the BKS system cutting properties (37). The initial keratectomy was performed as in the BKS technique. Subsequently, by using suction rings of different heights, Ruiz would perform the refractive cut on the stromal bed instead of the stromal aspect of the disc. The thickness of the cut was proportional to the degree of myopia to be corrected and was calculated using a nomogram that Ruiz proposed. The advantage of the procedure, compared to classic KM, was that carving the stromal bed allowed for larger optical zones and widened the range of potential correction (38,39). In 1987, Leo Bores performed the first KM in situ in the US (40) and initiated the investigation of the technique. KM in situ with the use of a manual microkeratome, however, was reported as being not technically safe, precise, or predictable and was adopted by a very small number of surgeons (38,39). The desire to improve the reproductability and accuracy of the in situ technique prompted research in developing new improved microkeratomes (41).

In the late 1980s, Luis Ruiz gave impulse to lamellar refractive surgery, by developing an automated geared microkeratome (Fig. 2.8). A suction device stabilized the keratome head on the eye, and the speed of the keratome passage could be controlled using a foot pedal, so that more even, consistent cuts were obtained. The microkeratome would also automatically reverse at the end of the procedure, without disturbing the lamellar cut. This automatic corneal shaper (ACS) led to the introduction of automated lamellar keratoplasty (ALK) in the field of lamellar refractive corneal surgery. The procedure involved resection of the initial lamellar disc using ASC. For myopic corrections a second, plano refractive cut was subsequently performed on the bed. The depth of the second cut was adjusted by altering the height of the suction ring. In the end the anterior lamellar disc was replaced on the stromal bed, with or without sutures (Fig. 2.9). In hyperopic ALK no refractive cut was performed, as the initial cut generated ectasia of the residual stroma adequate to correct up to 6 diopters of hyperopia. This ectasia was maintained after the anterior lamellar disc was replaced. For higher hyperopic corrections, homoplastic ALK was

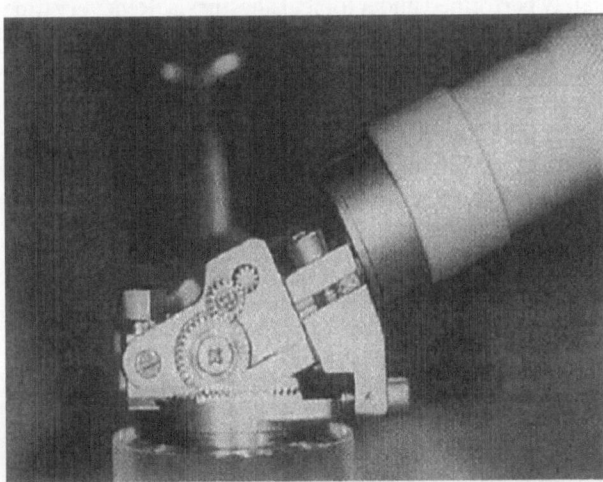

Figure 2.8 The Ruiz automated microkeratome is geared, so that the same motor that moves the blade also drives the microkeratome across the eye.

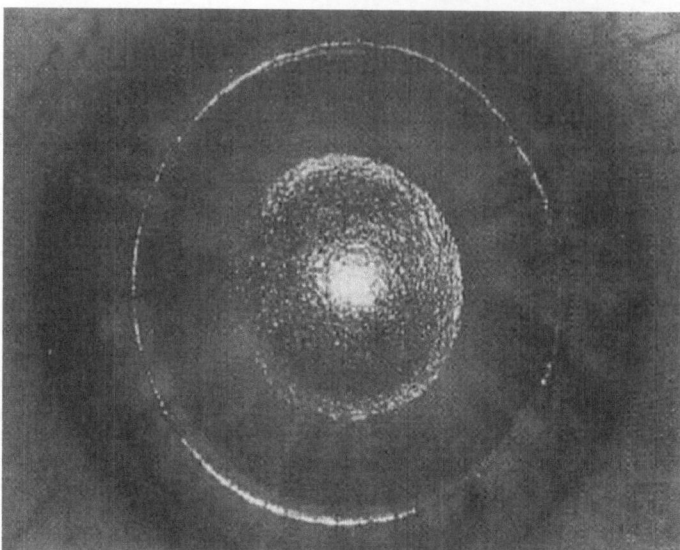

Figure 2.9   The Automated Lamellar Keratoplasty (ALK) is based on the same concept as keratomileusis in situ. The use of the automated microkeratome has increased dramatically the safety and effectiveness of the procedure. This photo shows the actual corneal bed after the two lamellar resections. The even sharp concentric borders of the lamellar cuts, as well as the smooth surface of the remaining stroma, are evident. (Reprinted with permission from J. Machat. Excimer Laser Refractive Surgery. Slack, 1996.)

invented (42). The procedure involved excision of a small, very thin anterior lamellar disc, which was discarded and replaced by a 300–400 μm thick donor lenticle (processed also using ACS).

ALK has been a breakthrough in lamellar surgery. The total operative time was reduced, and the procedure could be safely performed under topical anesthesia. Recovery time improved. ALK became very popular, as many surgeons who found it difficult to use the manual microkeratomes adopted ACS. The first clinical trials on ALK revealed its advantages: ease of use, rapid visual recovery, stability of refraction, and efficacy in th correction of high myopia (43). There were major disadvantages, however; a relatively high rate for irregular astigmatism (2%) and poor predictability of the procedure (within 2 D) (44). The latter was attributed to the imprecision of the depth obtained with the second lamellar resection. It became obvious that ALK could never overcome its inherent drawback: the refractive cut was not truly "refractive"—it was resection of a plano disc from the stromal bed. Investigators now started exploring ways to improve the accuracy of the second refractive cut. That time coincides with the beginning of the excimer laser era in ophthalmology.

C.   THE DEVELOPMENT OF THE EXCIMER LASER

Excimer is a term used to describe lasers with output in the ultraviolet (UV) range of the electromagnetic spectrum. In 1973, Charles Brau, James Ewing, and Donald Setser started working on using rare gas–halide mixtures to produce laser action. Two years later, in 1975, Stuart Searles produced the first excimer laser action by bombarding a medium of xenon bromide with an electron beam gun. In 1976, argon fluoride (ArF) was found to lase at 193.3 nm when excited in an electron beam (45).

The first laboratory excimer lasers required a great amount of energy to excite the rare gas–halide complex. Therefore their usefulness for biological experiments was limited. Later on, it was shown to be possible to achieve laser action in a more compact device, using a transverse electrical discharge as the energy source. Tachisto made the first commercial system in 1979 (45). Within only a year, excimer lasers improved in reliability and output energy and became suitable for general laboratory use. As a consequence, research on the possible applications of excimer lasers and their potential hazards started to evolve.

The United States Air Force (USAF) School of Aerospace Medicine started investigating the use of these new lasers on the eye. In 1981, Taboada reported that ArF laser light produces an immediate but temporary indentation of the corneal epithelium, which takes on the shape of the beam, without causing any opacification to the adjacent epithelium or stroma (46,47).

IBM researcher R. Srinivasan further studied the interaction of a 193 nm laser with organic materials. He suggested the term photoablative decompensation (later referred to as photoablation) to describe the mechanism of ablation with the 193 nm excimer lasers, and by creating grooves in human hair he demonstrated the high precision of the ablation technique. He suggested the possibility of optical control of the corneal surface by removing tissue and set the basis for further studies (48).

Stephen Trokel first experimented on the cornea with excimer photoablation and described its surgical potential. In 1983 Trokel reported, "UV light at 193 nm, ablated corneal tissue at a predictable rate, producing minimal thermal damage to the surrounding tissues" (49). These properties of excimer laser photoablation are the foundation of excimer laser refractive surgery. Separate patents on photorefractive keratectomy (PRK) were filed by Stephen Trokel and Francis L'Esperance. Studies on animal corneas as early as 1984 revealed that only 5 μm of corneal tissue had to be removed to lower the refractive power of a 4 mm corneal optical zone by 1 D (50). Early attempts to perform phototherapeutic keratectomy (PTK) showed that the ablated surface would heal without scarring (51,52). Thus the ophthalmologic community overcame the belief that the preservation of Bowman's membrane was essential to preserve corneal topography and clarity. Based on that evidence, the use of the excimer laser to alter directly the cornea curvature was made possible and PRK was introduced. In 1985, Theo Seiler of Germany was the first to perform excimer laser PTK in a sighted eye (53). Laser companies such as Meditec GmbH (Germany), VISX (Santa Clara, CA), and Summit Technologies (Waltham, MA) began to emerge. In 1987 Francis L'Esperance performed the first PRK in the U.S. on a blind eye (53). In 1988, FDA clinical trials on PRK began. Marguerite McDonald achieved the first successful refractive correction with PRK in a normally sighted myope, as part of an FDA trial (54). At the same time, C. Munnerlyn and his colleagues published a computer-based algorithm that relates ablation zone diameter and thickness to the required amount of dioptric change (50).

In 1995 FDA issued approval of the Summit and VISX lasers for PTK and the Summit laser for PRK. In 1996 FDA approved the VISX laser for PRK (53).

As the use of the 193 nm excimer laser in refractive surgery increased, it was revealed that, for the correction of more than 6 D of myopia, PRK resulted in significant central corneal haze, regression of the refractive effect, and poor predictability (55). To achieve more accurate corrections of high myopia, investigators began to use the excimer laser in combination with intrastromal techniques.

D. LASIK DEVELOPMENT

As a modality, LASIK was designed and developed at the University of Crete. In 1988, Ioannis Pallikaris and colleagues introduced the term laser in situ keratomileusis (LASIK) to describe excimer laser ablation performed under a hinged corneal flap (Fig. 2.10) (56). Pureskin first suggested the idea of raising a corneal flap and removing stromal tissue from the bed, back in 1967. He attempted to create the flap manually and cut out the in situ part with a trephine in a procedure that he termed stromectomy (57).

In LASIK the automated microkeratome is used to create a hinged corneal disc (i.e., flap), which consists of epithelium Bowmans layer and anterior stroma. The laser beam is then applied directly to the stroma, to remove a predetermined amount of tissue, depending on the target correction. Once ablation is completed, the flap is repositioned and held in place with the action of the endothelial pump (Fig. 2.11).

The idea for the LASIK procedure was based on the histological observation that during surface photoablation (PRK) the corneal neural network is also ablated and takes several months to reconstitute (58). The initial hypothesis was that destruction of both Bowman's layer and the superficial corneal nerves during PRK would have an adverse effect on the healing response. It was thus theorized that creation of a flap instead of a lamellar disc would assure better fitting of tissues after the ablation and would not affect the anatomic integrity of the cornea mainly by preserving Bowman's layer and the superficial corneal nervous net. Other important advantages would be reduction of surgical manipulations and total time required for the operation (56).

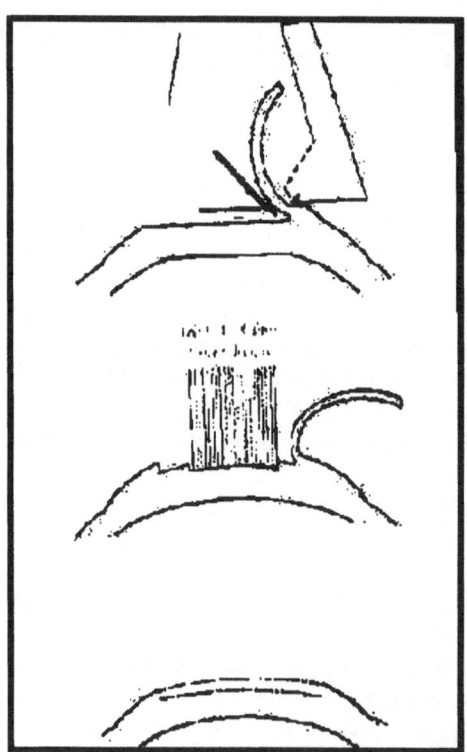

Figure 2.10   The first published diagram for LASIK. (Pallikaris 1989.)

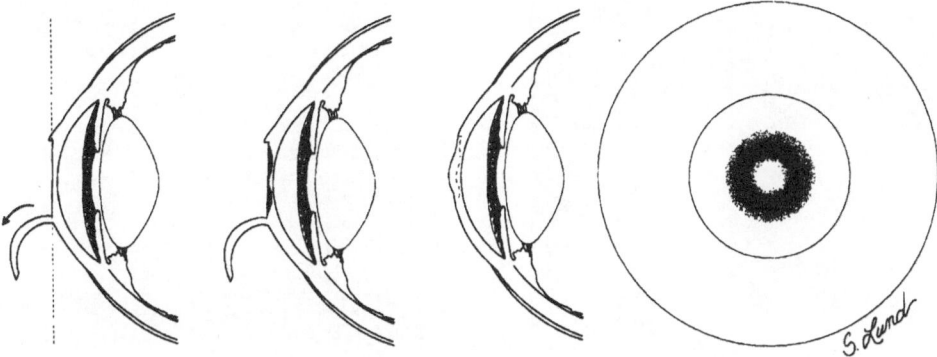

Figure 2.11 In laser in situ keratomileusis (LASIK) for hyperopia, the automated microkeratome is used to create a hinged corneal disc (i.e., flap), which consists of epithelium and anterior stroma. The laser beam is then applied directly to the stroma to remove a predetermined amount of tissue, depending on the target correction. Once ablation is completed, the flap is repositioned and held in place with the action of the endothelial pump. (Reprinted with permission from D. T. Azar. Refractive Surgery. Appleton & Lange, 1997.)

To support this hypothesis, animal studies to determine wound-healing reactions after LASIK began in 1987. A Lambda Physik excimer laser was used, along with a manual microkeratome that was designed to produce a 150 micron flap instead of a total cup (Fig. 2.12). The first published results regarding wound-healing reactions after LASIK on rabbit eyes revealed that the neural network is reestablished within a month after the procedure and no significant haze was present (58). These findings suggested that stromal ablation could avoid the regression of effect and stromal haze related to PRK, as the epithelium remains intact and the ablated area is hidden from the normal healing process of the eye that takes place at the epithelium/stromal interface. Gholam Peyman reported in 1989 an ani-

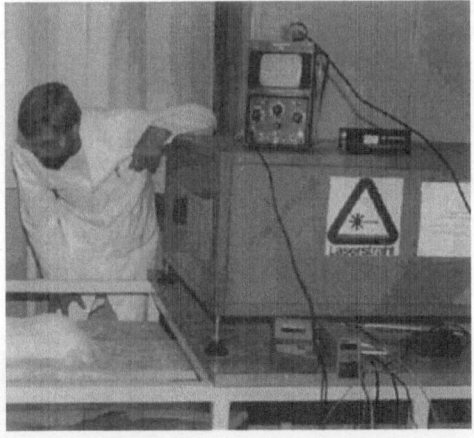

Figure 2.12 The first animal studies to determine wound healing after LASIK. University of Crete, 1987.

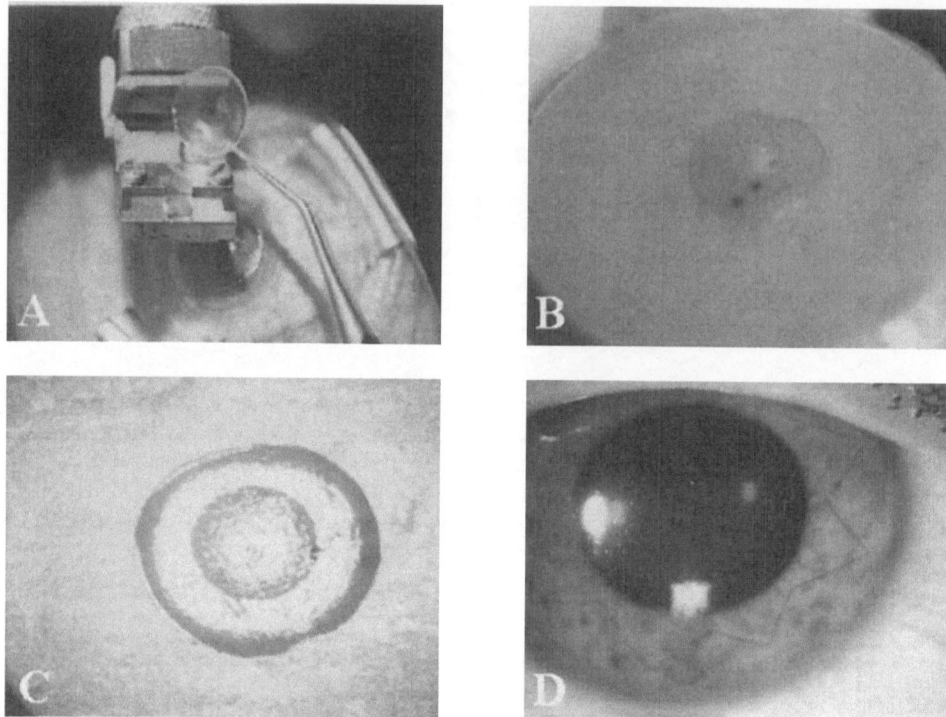

Figure 2.13   Excimer laser intrastromal keratomileusis. After the lamellar cap is harvested (A), it is positioned, epithelial side down, under the laser beam for photoablation (B). The ablated disc (C) is then sutured back in place (D). (Courtesy of Dr. Lucio Buratto.)

mal study in which an erbium-Yag laser was successfully used to remove the stroma from a lamellar bed as well as the corneal surface. Peyman's work, however, focused on the use of the erbium-Yag laser for experimental PRK (59).

In 1990 Lucio Buratto independently attempted to use the excimer laser to perform the second cut in KM. He introduced the technique of excimer laser intrastromal keratomileusis or photokeratomileusis (PKM), in which a 300 μm thick lamellar disc was excised, inverted, and ablated on its stromal aspect (Lucio Buratto, personal communication: First International Meeting on Keratomileusis, Venice, Italy, June 1990) (Fig. 2.13). First results on a large series of human eyes proved that this technique was effective for myopia up to 25 D, yet not safe (60). The complication rate was comparable to that of MKM, and so PKM was finally abandoned in favor of LASIK.

E.   LASIK MILESTONES

In June 1989, the first LASIK on a blind human eye was performed in the University of Crete, as part of an unofficial blind eye protocol. A specially modified BKS 1000 microkeratome was used for the operation.

Human studies begun in 1990 (61,63). The first blind eye study accessed the effect of flap creation on both the corneal healing response and the topographic pattern. It was revealed that, three months following the flap technique, corneal transparency was maintained and no significant irregular astigmatism was noted on corneal topography. The safety of sutureless LASIK was also suggested at that time (61). It was recognized that adequate adhesion between the flap and the stromal bed was possible even without sutures. The absence of irregular astigmatism, the elimination of sutures, and the invention of the automated geared microkeratome by Luis Ruiz (described previously) were the three most important developments that made LASIK widely accepted.

In 1992, Stephen Slade and Stephen Brint performed the first LASIK in the U.S.

In 1993, Slade used the automated microkeratome to create the flap. He termed the procedure excimer ALK (E-ALK) or flap and zap (64).

In 1994, Pallikaris and colleagues published their early experience in the use of LASIK on sighted eyes, as well as the first study comparing LASIK and PRK (65,66). LASIK proved superior to PRK in terms of stability and predictability for the correction of myopia greater than 10 diopters.

In 1997, Buratto suggested the down–up LASIK, which involves positioning the flap hinge superiorly instead of nasally. This modification of the procedure was thought to minimize the risk for flap dislodgment during the early postoperative term. A superior hinge would also allow for wider ablation profiles, which are crucial in cases of hyperopic and astigmatic corrections. The advantages of down–up LASIK over the classic technique are currently under investigation (67).

In 1999, the FDA approved the Summit Excimer Laser (Summit Technologies, Waltham, Mass.) for use in LASIK (68).

F. LASIK VS. PRK

As the use of the excimer laser in refractive surgery increased, it became obvious that wide area surface PRK was neither predictable nor accurate for the correction of more than 6 diopters of myopia (55). Thus, in the beginning, LASIK was suggested as a more precise alternative for the correction of high myopia. To date, several clinical studies published in peer-reviewed journals point out its advantages over PRK (69–90). These include:

1. Early recovery of visual function
2. Minimal postoperative pain
3. Lack of adverse healing phenomena such as haze formation
4. Increased range of efficacy over PRK in high myopia, hyperopia, and astigmatism
5. The ability to combine with previous refractive surgery, such as PRK, PTK, or RK.

However, the technique has also well-recognized disadvantages and limitations. These include:

1. Expense and complexity of instrumentation
2. Lack of a standardized nomogram for tissue ablation
3. Steep learning curve and potentially sight-threatening complications for the beginning surgeon

The refractive results of LASIK are far from optimum. A review of the current bibliography on LASIK by Farah and coauthors suggests that LASIK is, up to now, the best procedure to correct myopia greater than 6 D (91). It has acceptable visual outcomes and complication rates. It also appears effective for lower levels of hyperopia below 6 D. Its role in the treatment of low myopia and astigmatism remains to be investigated.

G. FUTURE TRENDS

For the foreseeable future, LASIK should remain the surgical treatment of choice for low and moderate refractive errors. The most serious alternative to LASIK may be the use of phakic intraocular lenses for high and moderate myopia.

For LASIK to be the first-choice procedure in the correction of high ametropias, its accuracy and postoperative quality of vision must improve to reach that of an IOL implantation (93). Continuous evolution in the field of microkeratome and excimer laser technology is the only way to achieve that goal.

Currently there is great interest in refining refractive surgery by identifying and reducing optical aberrations that degrade the optical image and limit visual acuity potential (94). Corneal topography guided ablations and wavefront technology are used to develop customized laser ablation patterns in an effort to improve optical performance after photoablation. The primary results of their application are encouraging (95, 96). Possibly, as the use of customized ablation increases, we will be able to improve the best-corrected visual acuity in many eyes.

It has been suggested recently that many variables play a role in the surgical effect obtained after LASIK (91). Currently used nomograms are far from perfect, as they consider only the depth and the diameter of the ablation zone. Improved nomograms that incorporate multiple variables are under development and will soon be available in clinical practice. We hope that their application will increase the accuracy of the procedure.

One area of advancement in LASIK may also be the development of nonexcimer lasers to cut corneal flaps, which could reduce or eliminate microkeratome-related complications.

Furthermore, intrastromal ablation with picolasers may eliminate the need for the microkeratome. Solid-state picosecond lasers are infrared lasers that can penetrate tissues without being absorbed. Thus such lasers can theoretically achieve intrastromal ablation without disturbing the overlying epithelium and Bowman's layer. Animal studies are by far encouraging, but extensive investigation is required before picosecond laser intrastromal ablation becomes an acceptable keratorefractive procedure (97).

Continuing evolution in the current techniques is the only way to approach the ultimate goal, which should be to offer our patients better vision in terms of quality and quantity.

REFERENCES

1. JI Barraquer. Oueratoplastia refractiva. Estudios Inform 1949;10:2–21.
2. JI Barraquer. Keratomileusis. Int Surg 1967;48:103–107.
3. JI Barraquer. Results of myopic keratomileusis. J Refract Surg 1987;3:98–101.
4. H Littman. Optic of Barraquer's keratomileusis. Arch Oftal Optom 1966;6:1.
5. JI Barraquer. Method for cutting lamellar grafts in frozen corneas: new orientations for refractive surgery. Arch Soc Am Ophthalmol 1958;1:237.
6. JI Barraquer. Keratomileusis for myopia and aphakia. Ophthalmology 1981;88:701–708.
7. RC Troutman, CA Swinger. Refractive keratoplasty: keratophakia and keratomileusis. Trans Am Ophthalmol Soc 1978;76:329–339.
8. D Taylor, A Stern, K Romanchuck. Keratophakia: clinical evaluation. Ophthalmology 1981; 88:1141–1150.
9. MH Friedlander, TP Werblin, HE Kaufman. Clinical results of keratophakia and keratomileusis. Ophthalmology 1981;88:716–720.
10. JV Jester, MM Rodrigues, RA Villasenor, DJ Schanzlin. Keratophakia and keratomileusis: histopathologic, ultrastructural and experimental studies. Ophthalmology 1984;91:793–805.

11. CA Swinger, BA Barker. Prospective evaluation of myopic keratomileusis. Ophthalmology 1984;91:785–792.
12. LT Nordan, MK Fallor. Myopic keratomileusis: 74 consecutive nonamblyopic cases with one-year follow-up. J Refract Surg 1986;2:124–128.
13. LJ Maquire, SD Klyce, H Sawelson, MB McDonald, HE Kaufman. Visual distortion after myopic keratomileusis: computer analysis of keratoscope photographs. Ophthalmic Surg 1987;18:352–356.
14. LT Nordan. Keratomileusis. Int Ophthalmol Clin 1991;31:7–12.
15. C Barraquer, A Guitierrez, A Espinoza. Myopic keratomileusis: short term results. Refract Corneal Surg 1989;5:307–313.
16. HE Kaufman. The correction of aphakia. XXXVI Edward Jackson Memorial Lecture. Am J Ophthalmol 1980;89:1–10.
17. TP Werblin, SD Klyce. Epikeratophakia: the correction of aphakia. I. Lathing of corneal tissue. Curr Eye Res 1981–1982;1:591–597.
18. JI Barraquer. Modification of refraction by means of intracorneal inclusions. Int Ophthalmol Clin 1966;6:53–78.
19. TP Werblin. Epikeratophakia: techniques, complications and clinical results. Int Ophthalmol Clin 1983;23:45–58.
20. TP Werblin, HE Kaufman, MH Friedlander, KL Sehon, MB McDonald, NS Granet. A prospective study of the use of hyperopic epikeratophakia grafts for the correction of aphakia in adults. Ophthalmology 1981;88:1137–1140.
21. TP Werblin, JE Blaydes, HE Kaufman. Epikeratophkia: the correction of astigmatism—preliminary experimental results. CLAO J 1983;9:61–63.
22. HE Kaufmann, TP Werblin. Epikeratophakia: a form of lamellar keratoplasty for the treatment of keratoconus. Am J Ophthalmol 1982;93:342–347.
23. MB McDonald, HE Kaufman, JV Aquavella, DS Durrie, DA Hiles, JD Hunkeler, RH Keates, KS Morgan, DR Sanders. The nationwide study of epikeratophakia for aphakia in adults. Am J Ophthalmol 1987;103:350–365.
24. MB McDonald, HE Kaufman, JV Aquavella, DS Durrie, DA Hiles, JD Hunkeler, RH Keates, KS Morgan, DR Sanders. The nationwide study of epikeratophakia for myopia in adults. Am J Ophthalmol 1987;103:375–383.
25. JJ Reidy, MB McDonald, SD Klyce. The corneal topography of epikeratophakia. Refract Corneal Surg 1990;6:26–31.
26. DR Wilson, AH Keeney. Corrective measures for myopia. Surv Ophthalmol 1990;34:294–304.
27. JD Goosey, TC Prager, CB Goosey, ME Allison, TL Marvelli. Stability of refraction during two years after myopic epikeratoplasty. Refract Corneal Surg 1990;6:4–8.
28. MH Friedlander, LF Rich, TP Werblin, HE Kaufman, N Granet. Keratophakia using preserved lenticles. Ophthalmology 1980;87:687–692.
29. JD Goosey, TC Prager, TL Marvelli, ME Allison, SR Hook, KA Carlson. Epikeratophakia without annular keratectomy. Ann Ophthalmol 1987;19:388–391.
30. SG Slade, GH Strauss. Use of tissue adhesive (Tisseel) in epikeratophakia. Invest Ophthalmol Vis Sci 1990;31:30.
31. EY Zavala, J Krumeich, PS Binder. Laboratory evaluation of freeze vs. non freeze lamellar refractive keratoplasty. Arch Ophthalmol 1987;105:1125–1128.
32. J Altmann, G Grabner, W Husinsky, S Mitterer, I Baumgartner, F Skorpik, T Asenbauer. Corneal lathing using the excimer laser and a computer-controlled positioning system. Part I—lathing of epikeratoplasty lenticles. Refract Corneal Surg 1991;7:377–384.
33. L Buratto, M Ferrari. Retrospective comparison of freeze and non-freeze myopic Epikeratophakia. Refract Corneal Surg 1989;5:94–97.
34. American Academy of Ophthalmology. Ophthalmic procedure assessment: epikeratoplasty. Ophthalmology 1996;103(6):983–988.

35. CA Swinger, J Krumeich, D Cassiday. Planar lamellar refractive keratoplasty. J Refract Surg 1986;2:17–24.

36. J Colin, F Mimouni, A Robinet. The surgical treatment of high myopia: comparison of epiker-atoplasty, keratomileusis and minus power anterior chamber lenses. Refract Corneal Surg 1990;6:245–251.

37. L Ruiz, J Rowsey. In situ keratomileusis. Invest Ophthalmol Vis Sci 1988;29(suppl):392.

38. E Arenas-Archila, JC Sanchez-Thorin, JP Naranjo-Uribe, A Hernandez-Lozano. Myopic keratomileusis in situ: a preliminary report. J Cataract Refract Surg 1991;17:424–435.

39. M Bas, H Nano. In situ keratomileusis—results in 30 eyes at 15 months. Refract Corneal Surg 1991;7:223–231.

40. L Bores. Lamellar refractive surgery. In: L Bores, ed. Refractive Eye Surgery. Boston: Blackwell, 1993, pp 324–392.

41. RF Hofmann, SJ Bechara. An independent evaluation of second-generation suction microkeratomes. Refract Corneal Surg 1992;8:348–354.

42. JH Krummeich, CA Swinger. The planar non-freeze lamellar refractive keratoplasty techniques. In: BF Boyd, ed. Highlights of Ophthalmology, 30th anniversary ed. Refractive Surgery with the Masters. Coral Gables, FL, 1987, pp. 2–28.

43. SG Slade et al. Keratomileusis in situ: a prospective evaluation. Ophthalmology 1993; 100(suppl).

44. SG Slade, SA Updegraff. Complications of automated lamellar keratectomy (comment). Arch Ophthalmol 1995;113(9):1092–1093.

45. S Trokel. History and mechanism of action of excimer laser corneal surgery. In: JJ Salz, ed. Corneal Laser Surgery. St Louis: Mosby - Year Book, 1995, pp 1–7.

46. J Taboada, GW Mikesell, RD Reed. Response of corneal epithelium to KrF excimer laser pulses. Health Phys 1981;40:677–683.

47. J Taboada, CJ Archibald. An extreme sensitivity in the corneal epithelium to far UV ArF excimer laser pulses, Proceedings of the Scientific Program of the Aerospace Medical Association, San Antonio, 1981.

48. R Srinivasan. Kinetics of the ablative photodecomposition of organic polymers in the far ultraviolet (193 nm). J Vac Sci Technol Bull 1983;4:923–926.

49. S Trockel, R Shrinivasan, B Braren. Excimer laser surgery of the cornea. Am J Ophthalmol 1983;94:125.

50. CR Munnerlyn, SJ Koons, J Marshall. Photorefractive keratectomy: a technique for laser refractive surgery. J Cataract Refract Surg 1988;14:46–52.

51. RR Krueger, SL Trokel, HD Schubert. Interaction of ultraviolet light with the cornea. Invest Ophthalmol Vis Sci 1985;26:1455–1464.

52. SL Trokel. The cornea and ultraviolet laser light. Laser in der Ophthalmologie, Vol. 113. Stuttgart: Bucherei des Augenarztes. Ferdinand Enke, 1988.

53. J Talamo. Excimer laser landmarks. In: J Talamo, RR Krueger, eds. The Excimer Manual. Little, Brown. Boston, MA, 1997, p. xxv.

54. MB McDonald, HE Kaufman, JM Frantz, S Shofner, B Salmeron, SD Klyce. Excimer laser ablation in a human eye. Arch Ophthalmol 1989;107:641–642.

55. T Seiler, PJ Mc Donnell. Excimer laser photorefractive keratectomy. Surv Ophthalmol 1995;40(2):89–118.

56. I Pallikaris, M Papatzanaki, EZ Stathi, O Frenschock, A Georgiadis. Laser in situ keratomileusis. Lasers Surg Med 1990;10:463–468.

57. N Pureskin. Weakening ocular refraction by means of partial stromectomy of the cornea under experimental conditions. Vestn Oftalmol 1967;80:1–7.

58. I Pallikaris, M Papatzanaki, A Georgiadis, O Frenschock. A comparative study of neural regeneration following corneal wounds induced by argon fluoride excimer laser and mechanical methods. Lasers Light Ophthalmol 1990;3:89–95.

59. G Peyman, C Beyer, J Kuszak, B Khoobehi, M Shahsavari, R Badaro. Long-term effect of erbium-YAG laser (2.9 m) on the primate cornea. Int Ophthalmol 1991;15:249–258.

60. L Buratto, M Ferrari, P Rama. Excimer laser intrastromal keratomileusis. Am J Ophthalmol 1992;113:291–295.

61. IG Pallikaris, ME Papatzanaki, DS Siganos, MK Tsilimbaris. A corneal flap technique for laser in situ keratomileusis. Arch Ophthalmol 1991;109(12):1699–1702.

62. IG Pallikaris, ME Papatzanaki, DS Siganos, MK Tsilimbaris. Tecnica de colajo corneal para la queratomileusis in situ mediane laser. Estudios en humanos. Arch Ophthalmol (ed esp). 1992;3(3):127–130.

63. DS Siganos, IG Pallikaris. Laser in situ keratomileusis in partially sighted eyes. Invest Ophthalmol Vis Sci 1993;34(4):800.

64. T Salah, G Waring, A El-Maghraby. Excimer laser keratomileusis. In: JJ Salz, ed. Corneal Laser Surgery. St Louis: Mosby—Year Book, 1995, pp. 187–189.

65. IG Pallikaris, DS Siganos. Excimer laser in situ keratomileusis and photorefractive keratectomy for the correction of high myopia. J Refract Corneal Surg 1994;10(15):498–510.

66. IG Pallikaris, DS Siganos. Corneal flap technique for excimer laser in situ keratomileusis to correct moderate and high myopia: two-year follow-up. Best papers of sessions. ASCRS Symposium on Cataract, IOL and Refractive Surgery, 1994, pp. 9–17.

67. L Buratto, M Ferrari. Indications, techniques, results, limits and complications of laser in situ keratomileusis. Curr Opin Ophthalmol 1997;8(4):59–66.

68. http://www.FDA.com

69. AM Bas, R Onnis. Excimer laser in situ keratomileusis for myopia. J Refract Surg 1995; 11(suppl):S229–S233.

70. DC Fiander, F Tayfour. Excimer laser in situ keratomileusis in 124 myopic eyes. J Refract Surg 1995;11(suppl):S234–238.

71. MC Knorz, A Liermann, H Steiner. Laser in situ keratomileusis to correct myopia of −6 to −29 diopters. J Refract Surg 1996;12:575–584.

72. T Salah, GO Waring III, A El Maghraby, K Moadel, SB Grimm. Excimer laser in situ keratomileusis under a corneal flap for myopia of 2 to 20 diopters. Am J Ophthalmol 1996;121: 143–155.

73. JL Guell, A Muller. Laser in situ keratomileusis (LASIK) for myopia ranging from −7 to −18 diopters. J Refract Surg 1996;12:222–228.

74. JJ Perez-Santonja, P Bellot Claramonte, MM Ismail, J Alio. Laser in situ keratomileusis to correct high myopia. J Cataract Refract Surg 1997;23:372–385.

75. MA El Danasoury, GO Waring, A El Maghraby, K Mehrez. Excimer laser in situ keratomileusis to correct compound myopic astigmatism. J Refract Surg 1997;13:511–521.

76. A Marinho, MC Pinto, R Pinto, F Vaz, MC Neves. LASIK for high myopia: 1-year experience. Ophth Surg Lasers 1996;27:S517–S520.

77. JC Casebeer, GM Kezirian. Outcomes of spherocylinder treatments in the comprehensive refractive surgery LASIK study. Semin Ophthalmol 1998;3(2):71–78.

78. CJ Argento, MJ Cosentino. Laser in situ keratomileusis for hyperopia. J Cataract Refract Surg 1998;24(8):1050–1058.

79. JD Carr, RD Stulting, Y Sano, KP Thompson, W Wiley, GO Waring III. Prospective comparison of single-zone and multizone laser in situ keratomileusis for the correction of low myopia. Ophthalmology 1998;105(8):1504–1511.

80. MC Knorz, B Wiesinger, A Liermann, V Seiberth, H Liesenhoff. Laser in situ keratomileusis for moderate and high myopia and myopic astigmatism. Ophthalmology 199;105(5):932–940.

81. JM Davidorf, R Zaldivar, S Oscherow. Results and complications of laser in situ keratomileusis by experienced surgeons. J Refract Surg 1998;14(2):114–122.

82. O Ibrahim. Laser in situ keratomileusis for hyperopia and hyperopic astigmatism. J Refract Surg 1998;14(2 suppl):179–182.

83. F Lavery. Laser in situ keratomileusis for myopia. J Refract Surg 1998;14(2 suppl):177–178.

84. AS Chayet, R Magallanes, M Montes, S Chavez, N Robledo. Laser in situ keratomileusis for simple myopic, mixed and simple hyperopic astigmatism. J Refract Surg 1998;14(2 suppl): 175–176.

85. A Maldonado-Bas, R Onnis. Results of laser in situ keratomileusis in different degrees of my-opia. Ophthalmology 1998;105(4):606–611.
86. S Goker, H Er, C Kahvecioglu. Laser in situ keratomileusis to correct hyperopia from +4.25 to +8.00 diopters. J Refract Surg 1998;14(1):26–30.
87. R Zaldivar, JM Davidorf, S Oscherow. Laser in situ keratomileusis for myopia from −5.5 to −11.50 diopters with astigmatism. J Refract Surg 1998;14(1):19–25.
88. DJ Salchow, ME Zirm, C Stieldorf, A Parisi. Laser in situ keratomileusis for myopia and my-opic astigmatism. J Cataract Refract Surg 1998;24(2):175–182.
89. RL Lindstrom, DR Hardten, YR Chu. Laser in situ keratomileusis (LASIK) for the treatment of low, moderate, and high myopia. Trans Am Ophthalmol Soc 1997;95:285–296; discussion 296–306.
90. GO Waring III, JD Carr, RD Stulting, KP Thompson. Prospective, randomized comparison of simultaneous and sequential bilateral LASIK for the correction of myopia. Trans Am Ophthalmol Soc 1997;95:271–284.
91. SG Farah, DT Azar, C Gurdal, J Wong. Laser in situ keratomileusis: literature review of a de-veloping technique. J Cataract Refract Surg 1998;24(7):989–1006.
92. LJ Maguire. Topographical principles in keratorefractive surgery. Int Ophthalmol Clin 1991; 31:1–6.
93. JT Holladay, TC Prager, RS Ruiz, JW Lewis, H Rosenthal. Improving the predictability of in-traocular lens power calculations. Arch Ophthalmol 1986;104:539–541.
94. SM MacRae. Supernormal vision, hypervision, and customized corneal ablation. J Cataract Re-fract Surg 2000;26(2):154–157.
95. G Alessio, F Boscia, MG La Tegola, C Sborgia. Topography-driven photorefractive keratec-tomy: results of corneal interactive programmed topographic ablation software. Ophthalmology 2000;107(8):1578–1587.
96. M Mrochen, M Kaemmerer, T Seiler. Wavefront-guided laser in situ keratomileusis: early re-sults in three eyes. J Refract Surg 2000;16(2):116–121.
97. M Ito, AJ Quantock, S Malhan, DJ Schanzlin, RR Krueger. Picosecond laser in situ ker-atomileusis with a 1053-nm Nd:YLF laser. J Refract Surg 1996;12:721–728.

3

Lasers in LASIK
Basic Aspects

RODRIGO TORRES

Massachusetts Eye and Ear Infirmary and Harvard Medical School, Boston, Massachusetts, U.S.A.

ROBERT T. ANG

Massachusetts Eye and Ear Infirmary and Harvard Medical School, Boston, Massachusetts, U.S.A., and Asian Eye Institute, Makati, The Philippines

DIMITRI T. AZAR

Massachusetts Eye and Ear Infirmary, Schepens Eye Research Institute, and Harvard Medical School, Boston, Massachusetts, U.S.A.

A. BASIC LASER PHYSICS

1. Definitions

Irradiance, mJ/cm^2. Energy/surface area. A measurement of the amount of light energy striking a given surface area. Conceptually it is the energy density transferred onto a surface from a laser pulse. Irradiance is a useful term, frequently correlated with corneal ablation rate in refractive surgery.

Fluence, mJ/cm^3. Energy/volume. Often confused with irradiance. In refractive surgery, fluence is not usually used to describe a laser. When fluence is mentioned, irradiance is often what is truly implied.

Energy, joule (J). Kg·m^2/s^2. Also measured in electron volts (eV). A force through a distance, or work. Energy is what is required for breaking chemical bonds.

Power, watt (W). J/s. Kg·m^2/s^3. Energy/time. The rate at which energy is delivered.

Intensity, Watt/surface Area. W/cm^2. Power density along a surface.

Homogeneity, the distribution of energy within the cross section of a laser beam. If a beam is perfectly homogeneous, the distribution of energy within the beam is uniform.

Coherence, monochromatic light waves perfectly in phase and parallel.

femtosecond, 10^{-15} seconds; *picosecond,* 10^{-12} seconds; *nanosecond,* 10^{-9} seconds.

2. Brief History of Lasers

Laser technology is just over forty years old. The theory of visible frequency lasers was first proposed by Schawlow and Townes in 1958 when they expanded upon an existing theory of microwave masers (1). In 1960, Maiman demonstrated the first experimental laser, a ruby crystal laser powered by a flashlamp (2). Since then, laser technology has grown exponentially.

The word laser comes from the acronym LASER, standing for light amplification by stimulated emission of radiation. The theory of stimulated emission is central to the generation of the laser beam. With stimulated emission, when a photon interacts with an excited atom capable of emitting an identical photon, the atom is stimulated to emit the photon so that it goes in the same direction and perfectly in phase with the incident photon. In this fashion, order is introduced to the normally chaotic process of electromagnetic emission. If enough of these coherent photons are recruited from the excited atoms, a beam of monochromatic, unidirectional, and in-phase photons is produced.

3. Laser Properties Relevant to Photorefractive Surgery

a. Frequency

The frequency of light determines where it falls within the electromagnetic spectrum (Fig. 3.1). The frequency of laser light determines what molecules or atoms are able to

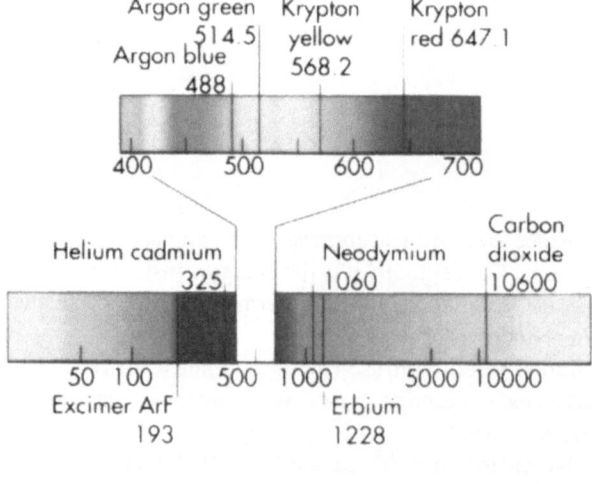

Figure 3.1   The electromagnetic spectrum. The 193 nm argon fluoride (ArF) excimer laser falls in the ultraviolet portion of the spectrum. (From Ref. 62.) [Color in original.]

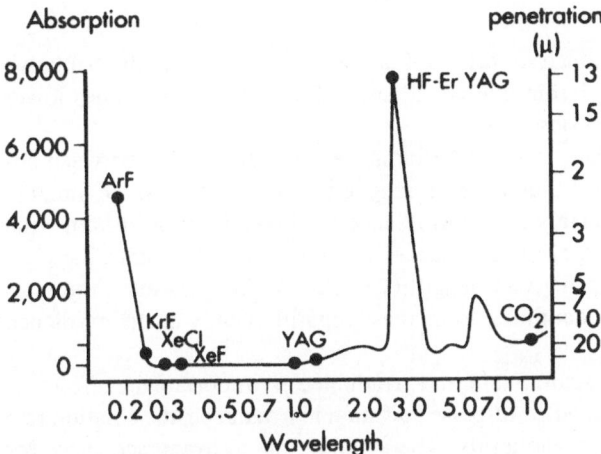

Figure 3.2 The argon fluoride excimer laser demonstrates high absorption and low penetration properties within the corneal surface. (From Ref. 63.)

absorb the radiant energy (Fig. 3.2). Other atoms are simply unaffected by the photons and let them pass by. By manipulating the frequency of light, we can choose whether we want the energy to affect water or biological tissue. Effectively, we can pick our molecular targets.

Lasers used in LASIK utilize ultraviolet wavelengths around 200 nm (0.2 μm), falling in the UV-C range of the spectrum. The dominant chromophore in cornea for the 193 nm and 213 nm wavelengths within this range is the peptide bond linking adjacent amino acids in collagen (3). Photons at these wavelengths carry in the range of 6.4 eV of energy each, an amount exceeding that in typical peptide bonds. The bonds are broken by the photon interaction. Ideally this process occurs with very little thermal generation, because the energy is used primarily in breaking bonds. The resulting fragments occupy a greater volume than the single polymer from which they originated and are imparted some kinetic energy from the irradiation. Both of these factors contribute to supersonic ejection of the material from the corneal surface (4,5). This process has been referred to as photochemical ablation, ablative photodecomposition (6), and photoablation (7–9). The choice of frequency determines whether photovaporization, photothermal shrinkage, or photochemical ablation occurs.

b. Homogeneity

A uniform distribution of energy in the beam cross section is termed beam homogeneity. Because no laser leaves the resonator with a uniform distribution, it is important to characterize the beam homogeneity. In the absence of homogeneity, ablation rates are expected to vary over the treatment zone, resulting in irregular tissue removal (10). Prior to beam manipulation, a gaussian distribution for the excimer laser is expected. With gaussian beam profiles, central overcorrection and peripheral undercorrection within the ablation zone have been reported (11–13). These distortions have been associated with the use of small ablation diameters and a nonuniform gaussian beam profile which is hotter centrally (12,14).

c.   Irradiance

Irradiance is central to studies of ablative threshold and ablative rate. The photoablative threshold at 193 nm wavelength is a minimum irradiance of 50 mJ/cm^2. At values lower than this, appreciable ablation is not observed.

Photoablative rate is also a function of the irradiance. The relationship between ablation rate and irradiance differs for different electromagnetic wavelengths. At 193 nm, the photoablative rate increases appreciably as the irradiance increases from 50 mJ/cm^2 (the photoablative threshold) to 150 mJ/cm^2; at irradiances greater than 150 mJ/cm^2, the photoablative rate tends to plateau for this wavelength (15). At 249 nm, however, the photoablative rate does not plateau but continues to increase logarithmically as the irradiance increases (Fig. 3.3).

The relationship between ablation rate and irradiance is important in refractive surgery. Because there is significant pulse-to-pulse variation in irradiance, the ablation rate must be fairly consistent despite this variability. The ablation rate to irradiance curve for the 193 nm wavelength is favorable because this curve plateaus at an irradiance of 150 mJ/cm^2.

Another important property related to ablation rate is ablation efficiency, which is the ablation rate divided by the irradiance. Maximizing ablation efficiency minimizes excess energy, which would otherwise contribute to shock waves, photochemical effects, and heating of sites local and distant to irradiation (16). The 160–180 mJ/cm^2 irradiance range is efficient for corneal ablation. At this range, ablation rates of 0.21–0.27 μm per pulse for the VISX laser and 0.26 μm per pulse for the Summit laser have been confirmed (17).

d.   Intensity

Irradiance is a measure of the amount of energy imparted onto a surface area, and intensity is a measure of the rate at which energy is imparted onto a surface area. Imparting energy at a rate greater than the rate at which it is absorbed by photoablation results in heating of

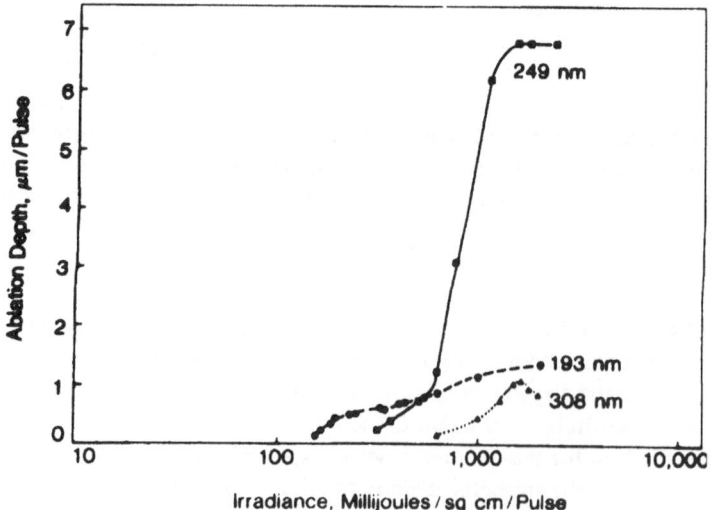

Figure 3.3   At irradiances greater than 150 mJ/cm^2, the curve plateaus for the 193 nm wavelength. The ablation rate remains fairly consistent despite a variability in irradiance. (From Ref. 15.)

collateral tissue. This heating can result in energy transduction into corneal surface shock waves, an undesirable outcome.

B. APPROACHES TO ABLATIVE DECOMPOSITION

Currently there are three approaches to refractive photoablative decomposition: scanning slit, wide area (broad beam), and flying spot (Fig. 3.4). A large diameter allows for the simpler wide area ablation approach, while smaller diameters rely on the scanning slit and flying spot approaches.

1. Wide Area (Broad Beam) Ablation

The wide area ablation method requires the use of a large-diameter beam and allows for simultaneous treatment of the entire operating field in a pulsatile fashion. By using diaphragms, a certain area of the operating field can be shielded from laser ablation, allowing for control of myopic and astigmatic correction patterns of ablation when using the wide area approach. This method has been in use longer than the other two and has generated the most clinical data.

Advantages of wide area ablation include a short operating time (often less than 30 seconds for low myopic photorefractive keratectomy), obviating the need for eye tracking. Also, because the entire treatment area is ablated simultaneously, there is no need for sophisticated scanning technology. Only a computer-controlled variable iris diaphragm is needed, which is simple to operate for the treatment of myopia and astigmatism.

Disadvantages of wide area ablation center on the need to produce a stable, homogeneous gaussian beam of large (about 6 mm) diameter in order to cover as much of the optic zone (treatable area) as possible. This requires the use of an excimer laser head because, to date, solid-state lasers cannot achieve ablative thresholds with homogeneous gaussian beams at such a large diameter (18). Excimer laser heads are large and bulky and use argon fluoride (ArF) gas, a toxic gas combination that introduces the risk of exposure. Furthermore, maintaining beam uniformity and homogeneity at such large beam diameters necessitates higher energy outputs, which translates to higher cost of operation. Greater acoustic shock waves are associated with the higher energy output. Higher energy output also puts increased strain on laser optics, increasing optical maintenance needs. Correction of hyperopia with the wide area approach has been technically challenging. Asymmetric astigmatisms cannot be corrected. Wide field ablation has also been known to carry some risk of steep central islands, in contrast to scanning slit and flying spot approaches.

Models available utilizing the wide field ablation approach include the VISX Star S2, Summit Apex Plus, Apex/OmniMed, and ExciMed; the Chiron-Technolas Keracor 116; and the Coherent-Schwind Keratom.

2. Scanning Slit Ablation

Scanning slit ablation uses a rectangular beam of light that is passed unidirectionally over the face of the cornea as laser pulses are passed through a slit-shaped diaphragm. In this fashion, a uniform layer of tissue can be removed from the cornea over the course of several pulses and slit positions. This is in contrast to the wide area ablation, which can treat the entire optical zone with each pulse.

Advantages of the scanning slit approach result from the fact that the beam energy does not have to be distributed over the entire treated area with each pulse. Specifically, the

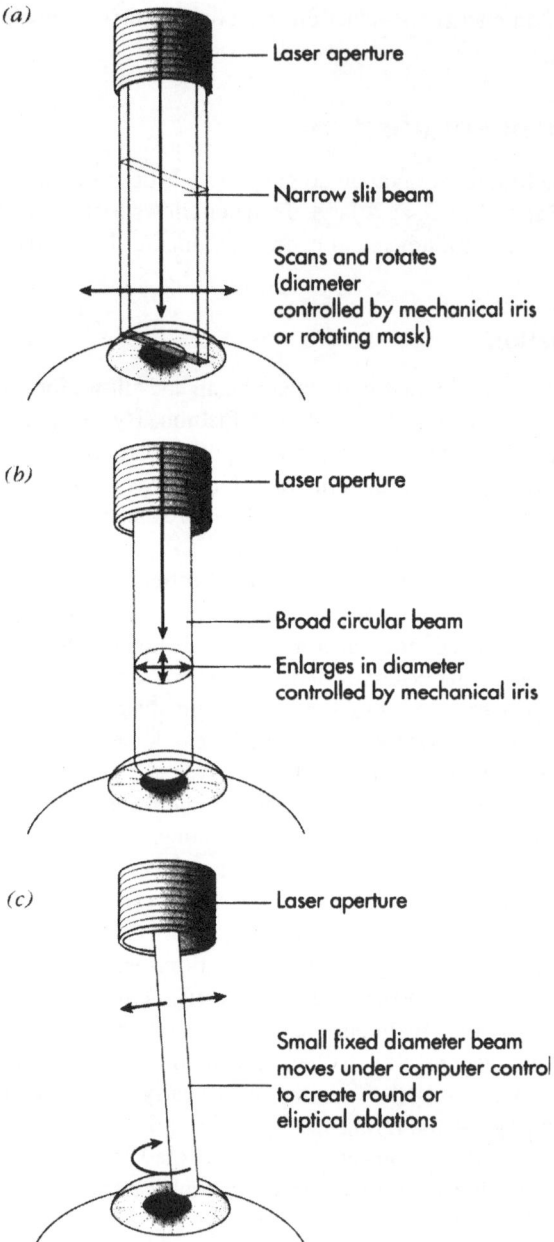

(a)

Laser aperture

Narrow slit beam

Scans and rotates
(diameter
controlled by mechanical iris
or rotating mask)

(b)

Laser aperture

Broad circular beam

Enlarges in diameter
controlled by mechanical iris

(c)

Laser aperture

Small fixed diameter beam
moves under computer control
to create round or
eliptical ablations

Figure 3.4 The three approaches to excimer laser photoablation. (a) Scanning slit. (b) Large or broad beam. (c) Flying spot. (From Ref. 64.)

smaller beam allows for ablation to occur at energy outputs less than those required for wide field ablation. Reduced acoustic shock waves and smoother ablative surfaces are possible compared with wide area ablation. Beam uniformity and homogeneity are much improved because of the smaller beam cross section. The incidence of steep central islands is much lower using the scanning slit approach. In contrast to wide area ablation, there are no optical zone (the size of the treated area) limitations for photorefractive keratectomy (PRK) or phototherapeutic keratectomy (PTK) with the scanning slit approach.

Disadvantages of the scanning slit technique include increased dependence upon complicated scanning systems and a longer operating time, compared with wide field ablation. Consequently, eye tracking and fixation become a concern with the scanning slit.

Some systems using this approach include the Nidek EC-5000 and the Meditec MEL 60.

3. Flying Spot Ablation

This approach utilizes a tightly focused beam to ablate very small areas of the cornea at a time. The small beam is redirected with x and y axis mirrors. Unlike the scanning slit approach, which requires scanning across the cornea in one direction, the flying spot is very versatile and can be maneuvered in multiple directions.

The small focal area of the flying spot permits ablation at lower energy outputs. This allows for smaller laser cavity size and reduced need for maintenance. Acoustic shock waves are reduced by lower energy outputs. Homogeneity requirements are less stringent, and fewer optics are needed for flying spot ablation. Spot placement is versatile, allowing for complicated sculpting of the cornea. This allows custom-designed patterns, permitting treatment of asymmetric astigmatism. Hyperopic correction is facilitated by this approach owing to the ease of creating peripheral annular ablation patterns. As with the scanning slit approach, there are no optical zone limitations for PRK or PTK. Another advantage of the flying spot approach is the flexibility in laser heads. Because a wide area beam is not necessary for ablation, it is possible to achieve ablation using solid-state laser heads. This offers the option of avoiding the risk of toxic gas exposure associated with excimer gas lasers.

Disadvantages associated with the flying spot approach include a longer operating time and consequently the need for a sophisticated eye-tracking device, in addition to the need for laser delivery (scanning) capability. Longer operating time also results in variations of corneal hydration, which has deleterious effects on surgical results.

Overall, flying spot technology is young but shows great promise for the future in that it allows for precise sculpting of the cornea. If current disadvantages can be minimized with technological advances, this may become the approach of choice.

Some of the flying spot lasers include the Bausch & Lomb Chiron Technolas 217, LaserSight Compak-200 Mini-Excimer Laser, Alcon Autonomous T-PRK and LadarVision 4000, and Novatec LightBlade (a solid-state laser).

C. TYPES OF LASER HEADS IN LASIK AND PRK

Laser heads can come in solid, liquid and gas phases. Liquid lasers have no immediate application to photorefractive refractive surgery. Gas lasers investigated for refractive surgery include the CO_2 and the excimer lasers, the latter being the most useful for refractive surgery.

1. Gas Lasers—Excimer Lasers

Excimer lasers, developed for their ability to produce ultraviolet laser frequencies, are a subclass of the gas laser heads. In 1975, excited xenon (Xe) atoms and halogen gas mixtures were found to emit ultraviolet radiation following the dissociation of an unstable xenon halide intermediary. By 1976, this type of interaction was noted with XeF, XeCl, XeBr, krypton fluoride (KrF), and (ArF) (19–22). The word excimer is a contraction of "excited dimer." Strictly speaking, a dimer is formed by two atoms of the same element. Because it was first thought that the intermediary structure for the excited state of these laser heads involved the formation of dimers (two atoms of the same element bound together), the term excimer was applied to these laser types. Now it is recognized that the activated intermediary is a rare gas halide, not a dimer. The name grew popular, however, and is universally accepted.

The ArF excimer laser has a wavelength of 193 nm, which imparts an energy of 6.4 eV per photon. This photon energy is adequate to break covalent bonds through the process of ablative decomposition. Krueger and colleagues compared the tissue effects of the ArF, KrF, XeF, and XeCl lasers and found that the 193 nm ArF wavelength provided for smoother results, more precise ablation, and decreased thermal damage to adjacent tissue (23). For these reasons the excimer ArF laser is the laser of choice for LASIK and PRK.

a. Safety of ArF Excimer Lasers

Mutagenicity of the 193 nm wavelength. Some frequencies of ultraviolet light carry mutagenic potential. Cyclobutyl pyrimidine dimers in DNA have been produced by irradiation with wavelengths under 280 nm, making the question of mutagenicity of excimer radiation a valid one (24). Results of a number of experimental studies have demonstrated that 193 nm radiation does not cause cytotoxic damage to DNA and mutagenicity (25–29).

In human skin, 193 nm ArF excimer radiation has led to no unscheduled DNA synthesis activity, in contrast to 248 nm KrF irradiation, which does induce such activity (30). Unscheduled DNA synthesis activity can be suggestive of activated excision repair mechanisms, commonly considered the most important mechanisms for removing damaged DNA. In comparison with the 248 and 254 nm wavelengths, the 193 nm wavelength results in little damage to DNA, and damage in 193 nm irradiated cornea is comparable to that in unirradiated cornea (26). It has been suggested that the potential for cataractogenicity is also very low, following the calculation of a very small lens exposure to excimer-induced ultraviolet fluorescence (31).

An explanation for the sparing of DNA damage by the 193 nm wavelength as opposed to other far-UV wavelengths lies in the high absorption of this wavelength by cytoplasm. A corneal epithelial cell has 1.5–3.0 μm of cytoplasm between the cell wall and the nucleus (27). After traveling through 1 μm of cytoplasm, 90% of the 193 nm radiation is absorbed, effectively shielding the nucleus from damage. Speculation of secondary UV exposure is not of great concern because this level of exposure is 10,000 times lower than the annual exposure to solar UV radiation (32).

Collateral damage by 193 nm wavelength ablative decomposition. Because the 193 nm wavelength is such an accurate tool for photoablation, collateral damage is mediated through indirect effects of the laser–tissue interaction. Shock waves, particulate ejection, and surface heating are the primary concerns in efforts to minimize collateral damage.

Shock waves result from high-pressure, high-temperature, expanding gas clouds above the surface of the cornea. They are estimated to travel at about 1 km/s, with variations in velocity dependent on the energy of ablation and the wavelength of the radiation. Pressures of up to 100 atmospheres can be generated, making corneal damage possible from shock waves. Thermal denaturation of surface collagen can result in pseudomembrane formation, currently considered a local protective effect (33). Structural changes beneath the corneal surface following ablation include stromal vacuoles and an increased number of keratocytes in later stages of wound healing (34).

Particulate ejection occurs as ablative decomposition renders polymers into multiple heated polymeric fragments that occupy a larger volume (Fig. 3.5). This forces particles into the air in a supersonic expanding plume (35) (Fig. 3.6). Particles in the plume include H_2O radicals, simple carbons, hydrocarbons, and some alkanes (36,37). The plume ejection results in a recoil surface wave that travels at several meters per second, although as yet this wave has not been demonstrated to induce corneal injury (38).

Corneal surface heating occurs secondary to ablative decomposition. Theoretically, ablative decomposition channels energy into breaking peptide bonds and not into heat, but the average corneal temperature has been observed to increase by 20°C during ablation (39). In theory, this increase in temperature could induce keratocyte injury.

Accuracy of the 193 nm excimer beam ablation. The 193 nm wavelength has subcellular levels of accuracy for photoablative decomposition. Typical ablation rates are 0.21–0.27 μm per pulse, which translates to roughly one twenty-eighth of the diameter of

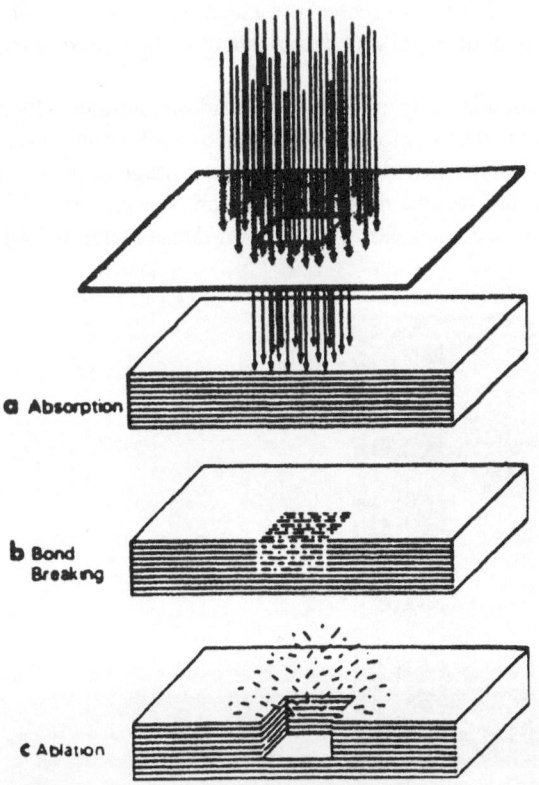

Figure 3.5 As laser energy is absorbed (a) peptide bonds are broken (b), resulting in increase in volume and subsequent ejection of particles (c). (From Ref. 7.)

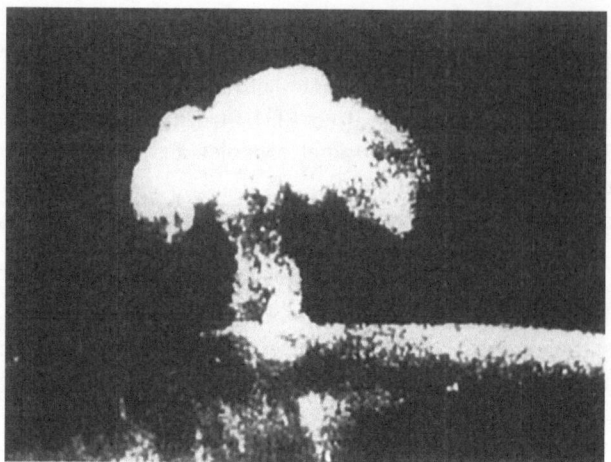

Figure 3.6 During excimer laser ablation of the cornea, the ejection of particles into the air is visible as an expanding plume. (From Ref. 35.)

a red blood cell (7 μm) of ablation per pulse. In a dramatic demonstration of the precision of the excimer laser, Srinivasan in 1983 used the ArF excimer to create grooves in a human hair strand (Fig. 3.7). Light microscopy of ablated areas show clean edges with no detectable traces of cellular injury other than in pale-staining cytoplasm of cells bordering the ablation.

One feature of this subcellular ablation is the formation of a pseudomembrane, which can be about 100 nm thick and is present at the ablation site. There is no cell membrane at this site, but the pseudomembrane is thought to provide a barrier to the passage of water as well as possibly provide a scaffolding for wound reepithelialization. On electron microscopy the pseudomembrane appears as a condensation of electron-dense material (40).

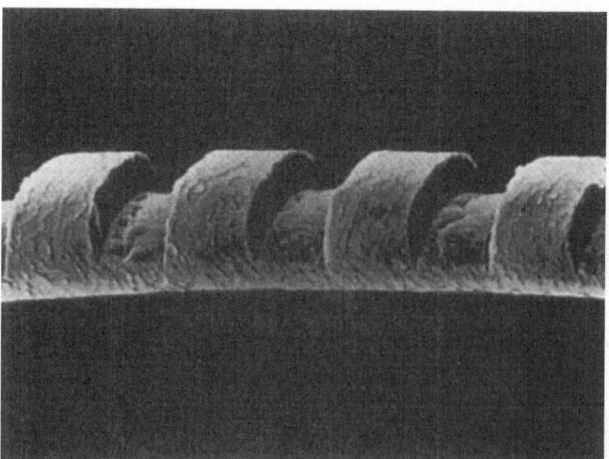

Figure 3.7 The clean, sharp edges of the grooves created by the excimer laser on a human hair demonstrate the accuracy and precision of the laser. (From Ref. 5.)

Not all corneas form pseudomembranes. It is not known what causes pseudomembrane formation, but the thermal effect and the uncoupling of organic double bonds during photoablation have been proposed as contributing to the phenomenon (41).

The 193 nm wavelength has the useful property of a relatively constant ablative rate at irradiances near the commonly used values of 160–180 mJ/cm^2. Because of this plateau, pulse-to-pulse variability in irradiance does not drastically affect the ablative rate, allowing for predictable ablative depths.

b. Other Advantages of the Excimer: Strong Beams with Large Diameters

An important advantage of the excimer ArF laser is the ability to produce a homogeneous, large-diameter beam (~6 mm), at ablative irradiances, capable of treating the entire optical zone simultaneously. This was especially important earlier in photorefractive surgery when eye tracking, eye fixation, and beam scanning made scanning slit and flying spot technologies more challenging to develop. As these technologies improve, reliance on large beam diameters may diminish, opening the door to nonexcimer laser types that initially were impractical for refractive purposes.

c. Disadvantages of Excimer Systems

Nonexcimer laser systems are desirable in the future owing to the several potential disadvantages of excimer laser systems. One disadvantage is the risk of toxic gas exposure. The gases are consumed by laser utilization and must be changed frequently, increasing the risk. The large size of the laser head and high energy requirements are also undesirable. Optics for beam homogenization can be complex and require frequent replacement. Finally, because the 193 nm wavelength is absorbed so avidly by cornea, the laser does not allow for intrastromal refractive surgery. This necessitates mechanical flap lifting for LASIK. Although there is currently no widely used alternatives to this approach for keratomileusis, in the future it would be desirable to minimize the invasiveness of the procedure with intrastromal keratomileusis.

2. Solid-State Lasers

Although the excimer gas lasers have made by far the most important contribution to photorefractive surgery, some solid-state lasers are showing promise for use in this capacity. Keeping in mind that the goal for refractive surgery is to change the shape of the cornea with precision and little collateral damage, it is important to remember that ablative decomposition is only one way to attain this goal. Any tissue-altering modality (photodisruption, photovaporization, collagen shrinking, photospallation) that alters tissue structure in a precise, localized, and predictable fashion has potential as a tool for refractive surgery.

a. Wavelength-Modulated Nd:YAG and Nd:YLF Lasers

The Nd:YAG and Nd:YLF lasers are infrared solid-state lasers. The active media are the neodymium-doped crystals of either yttrium-aluminum-garnet or yttrium-lithium-fluoride. The Nd:YAG and Nd:YLF lasers have fundamental wavelengths of 1064 nm and 1053 nm, respectively. When raised to the fifth harmonic, the wavelengths become 213 nm and 211 nm, respectively. These are very close to the 193 nm ArF excimer wavelength, suggesting that these lasers may be suitable for photoablative decomposition. Histological studies show that the damage zone created by the 213 nm Nd:YAG laser is less than 1 μm, which is similar to the results with the ArF laser (42). Furthermore, PRK with the 213 nm laser produces smooth surfaces and transitions, with a reepithelialization rate and histopathological findings similar to the results with the 193 nm excimer laser PRK in rabbit studies (43). This evidence supports the possibility that 213 nm photoablative decomposition is feasible and safe.

b.   Mutagenicity of the 213 nm Wavelength

The question of mutagenicity at the 213 nm wavelength has been addressed by in vitro studies (44). These studies measured free radical production in bovine corneas and in vitro bacterial survival following 193 and 213 nm irradiation at subablative irradiances. Evidence suggests that free radical production and species were identical for the two lasers, but the 213 nm wavelength clearly demonstrated increased bacterial cytotoxicity. If the differences in cytotoxicity apply to mammalian cells, corneal fibroblasts responsible for collagen repair would be much more affected by 213 nm irradiation (45). In vivo studies in rabbits do not provide clear evidence as to the safety of the 213 nm wavelength in PRK. In one study, the 213 nm radiation was found comparable to the 193 nm radiation (43), but in another study, the results were significantly worse at 213 nm (46). Increased postoperative complications observed in the latter study could be partially explained if the 213 nm wavelength were cytotoxic to mammalian keratocytes. More studies on the mutagenicity of the 213 nm wavelength will be an interesting area of future work.

In summary, the frequency-quintupled solid-state lasers do show promise as tools for refractive surgery. A solid-state laser on the market functioning at the 211 to 213 nm wavelength range is the Novatec Lightblade flying spot laser. Although these lasers are not as energy efficient as excimers, they show comparable ablative efficiency. As energy efficiencies of these systems improve, they may become available as wide-area ablation lasers, which would decrease operative time, improve intraoperative corneal hydration, and possibly produce superior surgical results. Also, as flying spot and eye tracking technology develop further, low-energy, small-beam solid-state lasers can also be expected to produce superior results. Although not as clinically developed, solid-state lasers have several advantages over the excimers. The frequency-quintupled Nd:YAG laser is less expensive and more compact than the ArF laser and does not require the use of toxic gases. Furthermore, solid-state lasers can provide increased reliability, robustness of design, safety, and lower operating costs than gas or dye lasers.

c.   Nd:Glass (Femtosecond) Lasers

The Nd:glass lasers have been investigated for their ability to generate femtosecond pulses. The technology for such generation has only recently become feasible. Because these pulses provide a much higher power output and a much shorter exposure time, they require only one-fourth to one-tenth the energy to produce corneal photodisruption compared with picosecond and nanosecond infrared laser pulses (47,48). By utilizing less radiant energy, the secondary shock wave and cavitation bubble size are reduced, allowing for closer packing of laser pulses and more contiguous photodisruption.

In a study using femtosecond pulses from a Nd:glass laser to produce an intrastromal spiral ablation in porcine and primate cadaver eyes, the pulses were focused 150–200 μm below the surface epithelium of the cornea and scanned in a spiral pattern to create a plane (49). The plane was extended to the surface to create a flap, and mechanical tissue plane separation was used to grade the contiguity of the intrastromal ablation. The results indicated that many of the shortcomings of picosecond technology (including incomplete tissue cutting, poor dissection, and surface quality) are significantly improved when the pulse duration is further reduced into the femtosecond region. The femtosecond pulses allow for very small cavitation bubbles, approximately 12 μm, which in turn allow for closer placement of pulses and smoother tissue dissection (47). Although results are encouraging, in vivo systems that closely reproduce the clinical situation must be investigated to establish clinical efficacy. An in vivo study in rabbits concluded that intrastromal photodisruption with femtosecond lasers produced consistent changes in corneal thickness without loss of corneal transparency (50). The study did not evaluate changes in corneal topography or specular microscopy, although no damage to the corneal endothelium was seen on histologic sections. This laser is now being used to create LASIK flaps in patients undergoing LASIK surgery with good results.

Advances in ultrafast laser design and the development of powerful laser diodes have finally made low-cost, reliable, diode-pumped, femtosecond laser systems possible (51). Femtosecond lasers are solid-state, enjoying all of the advantages of solid-state lasers over excimer lasers. Because infrared radiation is transmitted by corneal tissue (unlike excimer 193 nm radiation), infrared femtosecond lasers could allow for intrastromal refractive surgery that obviates the need for mechanical flap creation or epithelial disruption (50). It will be exciting to follow the advances in femtosecond laser technology and the applications it offers for corneal flap cutting, laser keratomileusis, corneal implant placement, and possible intrastromal keratectomy.

D. CALIBRATION AND ABLATION WITH THE EXCIMER LASER SYSTEMS

1. Causes of Beam Degradation

Excimer laser systems are high-maintenance systems that require frequent calibration to ensure high performance. Unlike other ophthalmic lasers, there is no modification of the laser energy based on any clinical indication of tissue response to ablation. This feature makes preoperative calibration an essential step in photorefractive surgery with the excimer (52).

a. Optics Degradation

Optics degradation is a natural consequence of laser energy interaction with the lens and mirror coatings. This leads to deterioration of beam quality and irradiance. Beam quality can be decreased by a reduction in beam homogeneity. A beam that loses its homogeneity is no longer an ideal surgical tool. Hot spots within the beam reduce ablation surface smoothness and can lead to poor refractive outcomes. Because broad beam systems have large beam diameters and high energy requirements to maintain beam homogeneity, their optical components can degrade fairly quickly. Furthermore, broad beam systems rely on complex optics (compared with scanning systems). On the other hand, scanning systems must use far more pulses to ablate a corneal surface than the broad beam lasers, which taxes the optics of the scanning systems. For these reasons, it is important to monitor the condition of optics with both broad beam and scanning systems.

b. Gas Impurities

Laser action releases contaminants into the laser head cavity. The fluorine gas reacts with contaminants within the laser cavity, further contaminating the cavity and reducing the availability of fluorine for stimulated emission. This reduces laser action. To maintain purity, the gas must be either constantly cleaned or frequently replaced. Cleansing of the gas involves precipitation of contaminants using a cryogenic device and liquid nitrogen. Alternatively, the chamber can be cleansed by flushing it with fresh gas to replace the contaminated gas. Improvements in laser construction have reduced the need for cryogenic gas purification and prolonged the lifetime of a single gas fill (6).

2. Calibration Techniques

It is important to check the laser ablation rate prior to surgery because if the output is too high, overcorrection is likely. If the output is compromised, undercorrection is a risk. This checking process is referred to as calibration. Calibration methods are generally based on measurement of energy (energy models) or measurement of ablation (ablation models). Energy models use direct measurement of the energy output of the laser with meters, which is accurate only within ±15% due to the extraordinarily high output of lasers (53). Furthermore, calibration of these meters requires sophisticated equipment that is difficult to use routinely in the field. For these reasons, the ablation models (ablation of Wratten filters, PMMA blanks, scanning profilometry) are used most frequently.

One approach to calibration involves ablation of a piece of plastic, forming a lens. The plastic used is PMMA, or polymethyl methacrylate, the plastic used for contact lenses. The power of the formed lens can be tested with a lensometer to assess laser irradiance, laser alignment, and laser beam profile. Distortions of the lens can indicate poor laser light distribution within the beam (6). Another approach to calibration involves counting the number of pulses necessary to perforate a plastic Wratten filter. This approach can be modified to ablate only 90% of the thickness of the plastic. The quality of light transmission through the plastic can be grossly assessed for uniformity.

The VISX laser is calibrated based on preoperative ablations performed on a PMMA block. Then the laser is reprogrammed to adjust the ablation rate to the desired value. The Summit laser can be checked by doing a 90% gelatin film ablation. The Chiron-Technolas laser is reprogrammed after counting the number of pulses needed to perforate a special foil. The Coherent-Schwind laser also uses a gelatin film for calibration, with reprogramming based on the number of pulses required for 10–90% perforation of the film. The LaserSight laser uses a patented device, ex-calibur, which employs commercially available corneal topography systems (54).

Broad beam excimer laser ablations are usually characterized by a relatively uniform distribution of surface power within the treated zone (55). Nonetheless, the hypothesis that corneal stromal ablation shape exactly matches the laser beam profile has been shown to be invalid (56). Rather, in uniform beams the ablation rate varies with the ablation diameter. This fact must be taken into account when attempting to calibrate by an energy model approach. Failure to correct for this variance can lead to central undercorrections and peripheral overcorrections, a phenomenon termed steep central islands. The underlying causes for spatially variable ablation rates across a uniform beam are unclear but may include differential hydration of the cornea, redeposition of ablated material as it lifts from the surface, photospallation effects, dependence upon proximity to an unablated area, and persistent ablation fog overlying the stromal surface.

Modifying the ablation algorithm to accommodate the spatial variance of corneal ablation has produced spherical enucleated eye PRK ablations. By analyzing the postoperative topography of PRK patients, the ablation algorithm was modified to produce a more spherical ablation in situ (56).

E. LASERS IN EYE TRACKING SYSTEMS FOR LASIK, LASEK, AND PRK

Eye tracking is of fundamental importance to the various ablation approaches because it allows for superior control of the surgical field. By tracking eye motion, the laser path can be redirected to ablate the desired portions of the cornea, regardless of involuntary saccades. This is especially important for the flying spot approach, where the beam is focused to ablate only a very small portion of the cornea at a time and where ablation of the entire cornea can take several minutes. Eye tracking is also especially important for complex asymmetrical ablation patterns, where each cornea can be custom-corrected based on regional irregularities as opposed to gross topographic irregularities. Furthermore, solid-state lasers, which show some promise of eventually replacing the bulkier, more dangerous excimer lasers, will most likely depend on flying spot approaches to ablation because of their limited beam diameter. In the future they will most likely rely heavily on adequate eye tracking technology to produce clinically maximized results. For these reasons, excellent eye tracking technology is a gateway to significant advances in photorefractive surgery.

Eye tracking can be active, passive, or a mixture of the two. Active eye tracking involves detection of a change in eye position. It also involves compensating for the change by redirecting the ablation laser beam to ablate the desired area, in its new location. Passive eye tracking is much simpler. Here a change in eye position is detected, and if the change is greater than a maximum acceptable limit, the laser ablation ceases until the eye is recentered. Then, ablation resumes where it had ceased. The speed at which changes in eye position can be detected and corrected is dependent upon the frequency at which the eye position is sampled and monitored. Frequency of sampling is determined by the type of technology used to monitor eye position.

Lasers can play an important role in the eye tracking systems used for LASIK, LASEK, and PRK. The laser head used for eye tracking is not any of the types we have considered previously for corneal ablation, quite simply because no ablation action is necessary. All the laser must do is detect changes in the eye position; no special laser-tissue interactions are necessary. By using a laser to monitor eye position, the frequency of sampling is very high, and eye tracking is much faster.

Traditionally, eye tracking has been performed by infrared video cameras. The frequency of sampling with this approach is limited by the camera frame capacity (images of the pupil's location are produced 60–120 times per second). Because lasers are capable of such high-frequency pulsing, the sampling frequency of a laser-based approach is much greater. One system, the Autonomous LADARVision excimer laser, uses this approach for eye tracking. The term LADAR stands for laser radar. This system uses a 905 nm diode laser to measure the position of the dilated pupillary edge at a sampling rate of 4,000 times per second (57). This signal is then conveyed to x and y axis tracking mirrors. Together the laser and mirrors can react with a response time of 600 radians per second. This means that redirection of the ablation beam to hit the desired target on the cornea can occur within 10 to 25 milliseconds of the change in eye position. This allows even the highest speed saccadic eye movements (up to 700°/s or approximately 150 mm/s) to be tracked with a peak position error of about 30 μm (58,59). Furthermore, this laser radar tracking system can detect and initiate a response over 50 times during a saccade and redirect the beam to its appropriate location before a new change occurs. This eye tracking feature is distinct from others in that it is mandatory for laser ablation function with the Autonomous LADARVision excimer laser. A disabled tracker will cause ablation to cease. In other tracking systems, the tracking function is optional. Similar tracking systems are available on most current laser systems, but the tracking is based on lower sampling frequencies, and with equally good outcomes.

A recent study used the LADARVision system to treat one eye of each of 102 patients with −1.5 to −6.25 D of spherical myopia (60). There was a 93% 1-year follow-up. The follow-up results reported uncorrected visual acuity of 20/40 or better in 99% of eyes, 20/20 or better in 70% of eyes, and BCVA of 20/25 in 100% of eyes. One eye lost two lines of BCVA (20/12.5 preoperative to 20/20 postoperative). No eyes lost more than two lines of BCVA, and corneal haze was trace or better for all patients. Results were within ±0.50 D of desired correction in 75% of eyes and within ±1.00 D in 93% of eyes. The results of this study were at least comparable, if not better, than those of a previous wide beam excimer laser clinical trial in which 63% of myopic eyes (baseline −1 to −6 D; $n = 342$) achieved visual acuity of ≥20/20 and 68% were within ±0.50 D of the desired refraction (57,61). The tracking systems on other laser platforms have also shown improved centration and improved visual outcomes (See ch. 14).

REFERENCES

1. AL Schawlow, CH Townes. Infrared and optical masers. Phys Rev 1958;112:1940–1949.
2. TH Maiman. Stimulated optical radiation in ruby. Nature 1960;187:493–494.
3. S Lerman. Radiant Energy and the Eye. New York: Macmillan, 1980, pp 43–59.
4. BJ Garrison, R Srinivasan. Microscopic model for the ablative photodecompensation of polymers by far ultraviolet radiation (193 nm). Appl Phys Lett 1984;44:849.
5. HH Jellinek, R Srinivasan. Theory of etching of polymers by far-ultraviolet, high-intensity pulsed laser and long-term irradiation. J Phys Chem 1984;88:3048.
6. S Trokel. History and mechanism of action of excimer laser corneal surgery. In: JJ Salz, ed. Corneal Laser Surgery. St. Louis: Mosby, 1995, pp 1–10.
7. R Srinivasan. Kinetics of the ablative photodecomposition of organic polymers in the far ultraviolet (193 nm). J Vac Sci Technol B 1983;1:923–926.
8. T Keyes, RH Clarke, JM Isner. Theory of photoablation and its implications for laser phototherapy. J Phys Chem 1985;89:4194–4196.
9. JM Krauss, CA Puliafito, RF Steinert. Laser interactions with the cornea. Surv Ophthalmol 1986;31:37–53.
10. PS Hersh, MD Wagoner. Excimer Laser Surgery for Corneal Disorders. New York: Thieme, 1998, p 5.
11. GM Kawesch, RK Maloney, M Derse, GO Waring, T Seiler. Contour of the ablation zone after photorefractive keratectomy. Invest Ophthalmol Vis Sci 1992;33(suppl):1105.
12. PS Hersh, BH Schwartz-Goldstein, The Summit Photorefractive Keratectomy Topography Study Group. Corneal topography of phase III excimer laser photorefractive keratectomy: characterization and clinical effects. Ophthalmology 1995;102:963–978.
13. T Seiler, A Holschbach, M Derse, B Jean, U Genth. Complications of myopic photorefractive keratectomy with the excimer laser. Ophthalmology 1994;101:153–160.
14. Summit Technology, ExciMed UV200LA Laser System User's Manual. Waltham, MA: Summit Technology, 1991, pp 5–25.
15. RR Krueger, SL Trokel. Quantitation of corneal ablation by ultraviolet laser light. Arch Ophthalmol 1985;103:1741–1742.
16. EA Davis, JC Abad, DT Azar. Excimer laser physics and biology. In: DM Albert, FA Jakobiec, eds. Principles and Practice of Ophthalmology. 2nd ed. Philadelphia: WB Saunders, 2000, pp 588–600.
17. HJ Huebscher, U Genth, T Seiler. Determination of excimer laser ablation rate of the human cornea using in vivo Scheimpflug videography. Invest Ophthalmol Vis Sci 1996;37:42–46.
18. GT Dair, WS Pelouch, PP van Saarloos, DJ Lloyd, SM Paz Linares, F Reinholz. Investigation of corneal ablation efficiency using ultraviolet 213-nm solid state laser pulses. Invest Ophthalmol Vis Sci 1999;40:2752–2756.

19. SK Searles, GA Hart. Stimulated emission at 281.8 nm from XEBR. Appl Phys Lett 27:243–245, 1975

20. JJ Ewing, CA Brau. Laser action on Sigma −2+1−2−] Sigma −2+1−2. Appl Phys Lett 1975;27:350–352.

21. CA Brau, JJ Ewing. 354-nm laser action on XEF. Appl Phys Lett 1975;27:435–437.

22. JM Hoffman, AK Hays, GC Tisone. High-power UV noble-gas–halide lasers. Appl Phys Lett 1976;28:538–539.

23. RR Krueger, SL Trokel, HD Schubert. Interaction of ultraviolet laser light with the cornea. Invest Ophthalmol Vis Sci 1985;26:1455–1464.

24. BM Sutherland, LC Harber, IE Kochevar. Pyrimidine dimer formation and repair in human skin. Cancer Res 1980;40:3181–3185.

25. S Jain, TW Hahn, RL McCally, DT Azar. Antioxidants reduce corneal light scattering after excimer keratectomy in rabbits. Laser Surg Med 1995;17(2):160–165.

26. RC Nuss, CA Puliafito, E Dehm. Unscheduled DNA synthesis following excimer laser ablation of the cornea in vivo. Invest Ophthalmol Vis Sci 1987;28:287–294.

27. J Trentacoste, K Thompson, RK Parrish II, A Hajek, MR Berman, P Ganjel. Mutagenic potential of a 193-nm excimer laser on fibroblasts in tissue culture. Ophthalmology 1987;94: 125–129.

28. CE Van Mellaert, L Missotten. On the safety of 193-nanometer excimer laser refractive corneal surgery. Refract Corneal Surg 1992;8:235–239.

29. IE Kochevar. Cytotoxicity and mutagenicity of excimer laser radiation. Lasers Surg Med 1989;9:440–445.

30. HA Green, R Margolis, J Boll, IE Kochevar, JA Parrish, AR Oseroff. Unscheduled DNA synthesis in human skin after in vitro ultraviolet-excimer laser ablation. J Invest Dermatol 1987;89:201–204.

31. MN Ediger. Excimer-laser-induced fluorescence of rabbit cornea: radiometric measurement through the cornea. Lasers Surg Med 1991;11:93–98.

32. HR Taylor, SK West, FS Rosenthal, B Muñoz, HS Newland, H Abbey, EA Emmett. Effect of ultraviolet radiation on cataract formation. N Engl J Med 1988;319:1429–1433.

33. J Marshall, S Trokel, S Rothery, H Schubert. An ultrastructural study of corneal incisions induced by an excimer laser at 193 nm. Ophthalmology 1985;92:749–758.

34. J Marshall, S Trokel, S Rothery, RR Krueger. Photoablative reprofiling of the cornea using an excimer laser: photorefractive keratectomy. Lasers Ophthalmol 1986;1:21.

35. CA Puliafito, D Stern, RR Krueger, ER Mandel. High-speed photography of excimer laser ablation of the cornea. Arch Ophthalmol 1987;105:1255–1259.

36. O Kermani, HJ Koort, E Roth, MV Dardenne. Mass spectroscopic analysis of excimer laser ablated material from human corneal tissue. J Cataract Refract Surg 1988;14:638–641.

37. G Kahle, H Städter, T Seiler, T Wollensak. Gas chromatographic and mass spectroscopic analysis of excimer and erbium: yttrium aluminum garnet laser-ablated human cornea. Invest Ophthalmol Vis Sci 1992;33:2180–2184.

38. Z Bor, B Hopp, B Rácz, G Szabó, I Ratkay, I Süveges, A Füst, J Mohay. Plume emission, shock wave and surface wave formation during excimer laser ablation of the cornea. Refract Corneal Surg 1993;9(suppl):S111–S115.

39. MW Berns, LH Liaw, A Oliva, JJ Andrews, RE Rasmussen, S Kimel. An acute light and electron microscopic study of ultraviolet 193-nm excimer laser corneal incisions. Ophthalmology 1988;95:1422–1433.

40. J Marshall, S Trokel, S Rothery, RR Krueger. A comparative study of corneal incisions induced by diamond and steel knives and two ultraviolet radiations from an excimer laser. Br J Ophthalmol 1986;70:482–501.

41. S Trokel. Evolution of excimer laser corneal surgery. J Cataract Refract Surg 1989;15:373–383.

42. Q Ren, RP Gailitis, KP Thompson, JT Lin. Ablation of the cornea and synthetic polymers using a UV (213 nm) solid-state laser. IEEE J Quant Electron 1990;26:2284–2288.

43. Q Ren, G Simon, J-M Legeais, J-M Parel, W Culbertson, J Shen, Y Takesua, M Savoldelli. Ultraviolet solid-state laser (213-nm) photorefractive keratectomy: in vivo study. Ophthalmology 1994;101:883–889.

44. MN Ediger, GH Pettit, LS Matchette. In vitro measurements of cytotoxic effects of 193 nm and 213 nm laser pulses at subablative fluences. Lasers Surg Med 1997;21:88–93.
45. DM Maurice. The cornea and sclera. In: H Davson, ed. The Eye. Vol. 1. New York: Academic Press, 1962, pp 289–368.
46. PG Soderberg, T Matsui, F Manns, J-H Shen, J-M Parel, J-M Legeais, M Savoldelli, I Drubaix, M Menashe, G Renard, Y Pouliquen. Three month follow up on changes in the rabbit cornea after photoablation with a pulsed scanning beam at 213 nm. In: JM Parel, Q Ren, KM Joos, eds. Ophthalmic Technologies V Proc. 1995;SPIE 2393:55–60.
47. T Juhasz, GA Kastis, C Suárez, Z Bor, WE Bron. Time-resolved observations of shock waves and cavitation bubbles generated by femtosecond laser pulses in corneal tissue and water. Lasers Surg Med 1996;19:23–31.
48. RM Kurtz, X Liu, VM Elner, JA Squier, D Du, GA Mourou. Photodisruption in the human cornea as a function of laser pulse width. J Refract Surg 1997;13:653–658.
49. RM Kurtz, C Horvath, H-H Liu, RR Krueger, T Juhasz. Lamellar refractive surgery with scanned intrastromal picosecond and femtosecond laser pulses in animal eyes. J Refract Surg 1998;14:541–548.
50. KR Sletten, KG Yen, S Sayegh, F Loesel, C Eckhoff, C Horvath, M Muenier, T Juhasz, RM Kurtz. An in vivo model of femtosecond laser intrastromal refractive surgery. Ophthalmic Surg Lasers 1999;30:742–749.
51. A Braun, H Liu, C Harvath, X Liu, T Juhasz, G Mourou. All solid-state, directly diode-pumped chirped-pulse amplification laser system. OSA Technical Digest 1997;11:323–324.
52. RR Krueger. Excimer laser: a step up in complexity and responsibility for the ophthalmic laser surgeon? J Refract Corneal Surg 1994;10:83–86.
53. JD Gottsch, EV Rencs, JL Cambier, D Hall, DT Azar, WJ Stark. Excimer laser calibration system. J Refract Surg 1996;12:401–411.
54. P Asbell, CF Beyer, MP Nevitt. LaserSight Compak-200 Mini-excimer laser. In: JH Talamo, RR Krueger, eds. The Excimer Manual: A Clinician's Guide to Excimer Laser Surgery. Boston: Little, Brown, 1997, pp 341–353.
55. SD Klyce, MK Smolek. Corneal topography of excimer laser photorefractive keratectomy. J Cataract Refract Surg 1993;19:122–130.
56. JK Shimmick, WB Telfair, CR Munnerlyn, JD Bartlett, SL Trokel. Corneal ablation profilometry and steep central islands. J Refract Surg 1997;13:235–245.
57. RR Krueger. In perspective: eye tracking and autonomous laser radar. J Refract Surg 1999; 15:145–149.
58. M McDonald, LC Van Horn. Autonomous T-PRK. In: JH Talamo, RR Krueger, eds. The Excimer Manual: A Clinician's Guide to Excimer Laser Surgery. Boston: Little, Brown, 1997, pp 355–368.
59. D Boghen, BT Troost, RB Daroff, LF Dell'Osso, JE Burkett. Velocity characteristics of normal human saccades. Invest Ophthalmol Vis Sci 1974;13:619–623.
60. IG Pallikaris, KI Koufala, DS Siganos, TG Papadaki, VJ Katsanevaki, V Tourtsan, MB McDonald. Photorefractive keratectomy with a small spot laser and tracker. J Refract Surg 1999;15:137–144.
61. VISX Excimer Laser System PRK Professional Use Information Manual, 1998.
62. DS Gartry. The development of excimer laser corneal surgery: beam tissue interactions. In: CNJ McGhee, HR Taylor, DS Gartry, SL Troke, eds. Excimer Lasers in Ophthalmology: Principles and Practice. Boston: Butterworth-Heinemann, 1997, p 33.
63. DS Gartry. The development of excimer laser corneal surgery: beam tissue interactions. In: CNJ McGhee, HR Taylor, DS Gartry, SL Trokel, eds. Excimer Lasers in Ophthalmology: Principles and Practice. Boston: Butterworth-Heinemann, 1997, p 33.
64. PP van Saarloos. Physical principles of excimer laser. In: CNJ McGhee, HR Taylor, DS Gartry, SL Trokel, eds. Excimer Lasers in Ophthalmology: Principles and Practice. Boston: Butterworth-Heinemann, 1997, p 18.

4

Microkeratomes

SANDEEP KAKARIA

Cornell University Medical Center, New York, New York, U.S.A

THANH HOANG-XUAN

*Fondation Ophtalmologique Adolphe de Rothschild, and Paris University,
Paris, France*

DIMITRI T. AZAR

*Massachusetts Eye and Ear Infirmary, Schepens Eye Research Institute,
and Harvard Medical School, Boston, Massachusetts, U.S.A.*

A. INTRODUCTION

Microkeratomes have evolved from suction rings and moving blades that were difficult to operate to more user-friendly devices currently utilized in LASIK refractive surgery. The early microkeratomes used by José Ignacio Barraquer were limited to the treatment of high myopia. Barraquer's technique, involving the creation of a central lenticule with a manual microkeratome, freezing this section, and carving the deep portion with a lathe, according to the amount of refractive error, had several technical limitations and was associated with numerous complications. Complications of this technique resulted from difficulties in mastering the microkeratome and cryolathe and included lenticular damage, persistent corneal haze, irregular astigmatism, under- and over-correction, and regression (1). Innovations to address this problem, including Swinger's technique, in which he did not freeze the back side of the lenticule (1–4), and Ruiz's in situ method for manually removing corneal stroma deep to the flap (5), were particularly important milestones that led to the development of current microkeratomes.

Burrato used argon-fluoride excimer laser ablation, previously reported for surface ablation by Trokel (6), in combination with the microkeratome on the deep portion of the lenticule (7). Pallikaris demonstrated that in situ ablation and refractive correction could be performed on the remaining stromal bed (8). With these advances and the increasing popularity of the excimer laser, the microkeratome still had its place, but it was no longer used for reshaping. Instead, its primary purpose was the creation of the corneal flap.

The microkeratomes of today have become safer and have been proven successful in performing corneal lamellar cuts; however, complications with their use continue to occur. These complications have been decreasing with surgical experience, advancements, and design elements incorporated into newer microkeratomes. The current microkeratomes are by no means close to being free of complications, nor do they approximately an ideal microkeratome, which would optimize the following parameters: safety, ease of use and sterilization, reliability, moderate increase in IOP and minimal structural deformation during surgery, smooth beds, regular edges, reproducible thickness, sufficient hinge width, suction ring stability, and reasonable cost of hardware and disposables. Although currently used microkeratomes incorporate several features of the ideal microkeratome, they nevertheless sacrifice some obviously useful features in order to achieve others.

Typical components of a modern microkeratome system include the following (9):

Motor
Microkeratome head
Applanator lenses to measure the diameter of the exposed cornea
Vacuum fixation ring used to secure the eye
Flap stop ring, which limits the travel of the microkeratome head through the fixation
    ring
Foot switch

B. MICROKERATOME TYPES

Although microkeratomes share several similarities, they can be divided into five basic categories:

1. Nondisposable horizontal
    A. Gear driven
    B. Automated sliding
    C. Manual
2. Nondisposable vertical
    A. Automated
    B. Manual
3. Disposable
    A. Cable driven
    B. Turbine driven
    C. Gear driven
4. Water jet
5. Laser microkeratomes (picosecond)

C. NONDISPOSABLE HORIZONTAL MICROKERATOMES

Automated horizontal microkeratomes include the Bausch and Lomb Surgical/Chiron Automated Corneal Shaper; Summit Krumeich-Barraquer (SKBM); Herbert Schwind; B.B.-I-T-I, Allergan, and Nidek (similar to Summit), Med-Logics, LaserSight Technologies Ultrashaper, and Innovative Optics Innovatome. Manual microkeratomes in this category

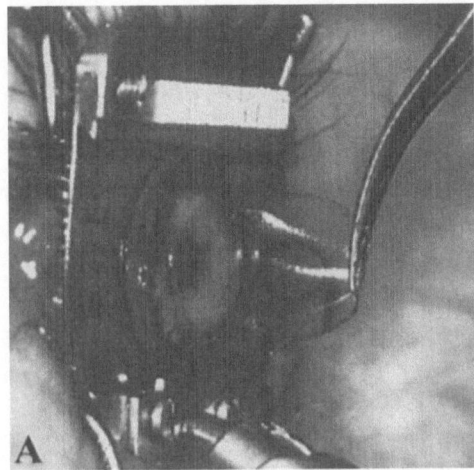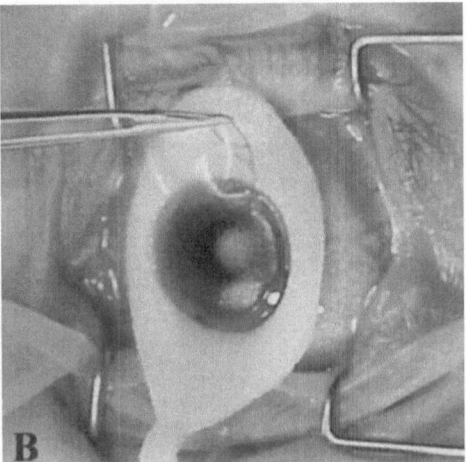

Figure 4.1 Hinge location. (A) Nasal hinge. The keratomileusis occurred in the temporal-to-nasal direction. (B) Superior hinge.

include the Moria LSK-1, the SCMD Turbokeratome by New United Development Corporation, and the Med-Logics Manual.

The automated sliding microkeratomes (SKBM, B.B.-I-T-I, Allergan, and Nidek) have virtually displaced all other horizontal microkeratomes in this category because they are surgeon-independent reliable units that require minimal assembly during surgery and have relatively high reproducibility of flap thickness.

1. Basics

Horizontal microkeratomes are derived from the original design by Barraquer. During the keratomileusis procedure, the turbines or electric motors of these instruments are located horizontally or to the side of the eye. Cuts are usually made with nasal hinges (Fig. 4.1A), although it is possible to position narrow versions of these microkeratomes to create superior hinges.

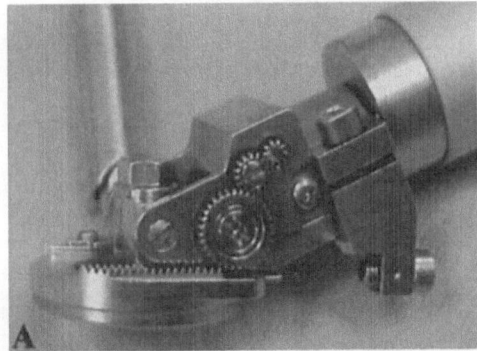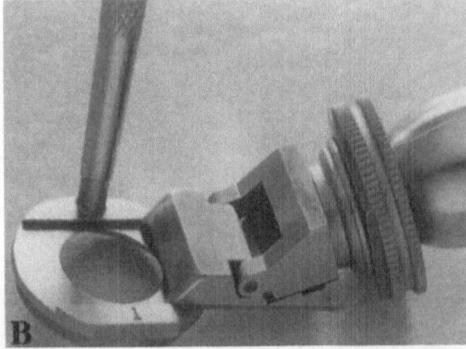

Figure 4.2 Gears vs. sliding mechanism in nondisposable horizontal microkeratomes. (A) The gears of the ACS head move through the geared tracks of the suction ring. (B) The SCMD slides through its track without the assistance of gears.

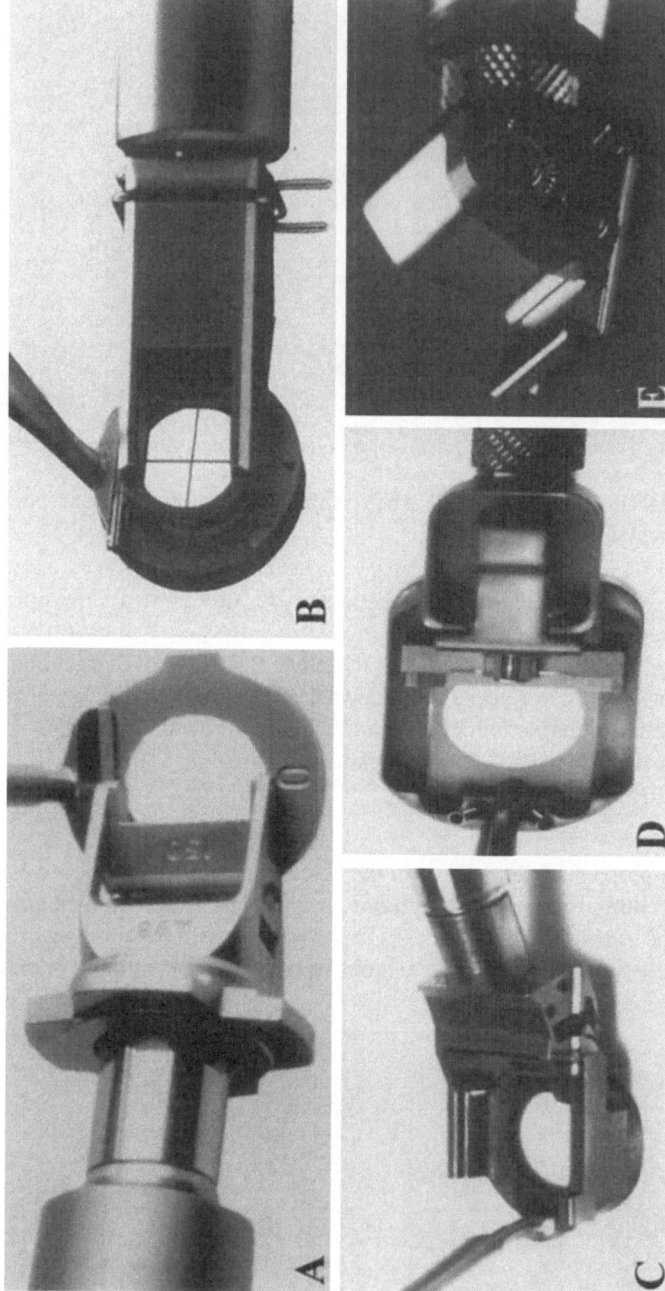

Figure 4.3 Other examples of nondisposable horizontal microkeratomes. Note that the microkeratome motor is not directly above the operating surface. (A) Moria Lamellar System for Keratoplasty-1. (B) Summit Krumeich-Barraquer. (C) Med-Logics Microkeratome. (D) Innovative Optics Innovatome. (E) LaserSight Technologies Ultrashaper.

2. Design

Automated horizontal microkeratomes may advance through the use of rotating gears between the microkeratome head and the suction ring (Fig. 4.2A) or through gearless sliding of the microkeratome head on the suction ring. Manual microkeratomes primarily consist of gearless sliding of the microkeratome head on the suction ring (Fig. 4.2B).

Gear-driven microkeratomes may have an increased likelihood of jamming due to operative debris and may also be more difficult to clean between procedures. Sliding designs may decrease these complications. The instances of microkeratome head slippage from the suction ring tracks in the manual microkeratomes have been practically eliminated in the newer automated sliding horizontal designs.

The ACS is a gear-driven nondisposable horizontal microkeratome, while the other instruments in this category utilize the sliding mechanism (Figs. 4.2B and 4.3). The Moria LSK-1 and the SCMD, both manual microkeratomes, run on a gas-turbine mechanism, while the others use an electric motor. Multiple flap sizes and depths are available. Technical features of individual nondisposable horizontal microkeratomes may be seen in Table 1.

3. Safety Issues

The original SCS microkeratome uses multiple components to ensure appropriate depths and flap size. Although this may allow flexibility, the incomplete, inappropriate tightening of this instrument may result in free caps (if stop is not screwed properly) or corneal perforation (if the depth plate is not tightened or mistakenly not inserted). Care must be taken

Table 1 Technical Features of Certain Nondisposable Horizontal Microkeratome

Manufacturer	Bausch and Lomb/Chiron	Summit	Med-Logics	LaserSight Technologies
Model Name	Automated Corneal Shaper	Krumeich-Barraquer	Med-Logics	Ultrashaper
Oscillation speed	7,500 rpm	≤20,000	8–13,000	7,500
Flap diameter	≥9.00 mm	8.0 to 10.0	8.00 to 10	7.2 and >
Depth	160 and 180 mm	130, 160, 180	160 and 180	160
Mechanism	Gear driven	Sliding	Sliding	Sliding
Automated/manual	Automated	Automated	Automated	Automated
Advance rate	3.7 mm/s	0.1–3.0 mm/s	3.5 mm/s	—
Motor	Electric	Electric	Electric	Electric

Manufacturer	Moria	BD	NIDEK	ALLERGAN
Model name	LSK-1	K-3000	MK-2000	Amadeus
Oscillation speed	15,000 rpm	12,000 rpm	9,000 rpm	9,000 to 20,000 rpm
Flap diameter	7.5 to >9.5 mm	8.5–10.0	9.0 or 10.0	8.5 or 9.55
Depth	130, 160, 180 μm	130, 168, 180	130, 160, 180	140, 160, 180
Mechanism	Sliding	Track & Reel	Dual Motors	Proprietary
Automated/manual	Manual	Automated	Automated	Automated
Advance rate	N/A	4.4 mm/s	2 mm/s	1.5–4.0 mm/s
Motor	Gas Turbine	Electric	Electric	Electric

in the use of all microkeratomes to ensure that a variable depth plate is tightened to the proper level or that fixed depth plates are always inserted prior to keratomileusis.

4. Oscillation and Advancement Rate

Automated microkeratomes allow advancement at a constant, appropriately slow speed throughout the keratomileusis procedure. Slow advance rates allow the blades to perform their shearing action with decreased chance of scraping, plowing, or producing areas of the flap that are thinner than others. When using manual microkeratomes, the surgeon must maintain a slow, steady advance rate throughout the cut to ensure consistent flap thickness.

Fast oscillation speeds allow for a cut that has reduced ridges or "chatter" in the stromal bed, while slow oscillation speeds have increased ridges. Gas turbines have allowed microkeratomes to oscillate at faster rates; however, they require large gas canisters to remain in the operating room.

Postoperative irregular astigmatism may be caused by variation in thickness throughout a flap or increased ridges created in the corneal stroma. Therefore, to minimize induced astigmatism, the surgeon should aim for a consistent flap thickness and minimal ridges or "chatter" especially when using a manual unit (10,11).

The manual horizontal microkeratomes that we have studied, Moria and SCMD, attempt to decrease the chance of induced astigmatism with a faster oscillation speed, while the automated microkeratomes decrease the complication by a programmed advance rate. It may be appropriate to hypothesize that the chance of induced astigmatism can be minimized by combining a fast oscillation with a consistent advance rate, which is the guiding principle of most of the newer automated sliding units.

D. NONDISPOSABLE VERTICAL MICROKERATOMES

These microkeratomes are available in automated and manual forms. The automated microkeratomes include the Carriazo-Barraquer and M-2 made by Moria and the Bausch and Lomb Surgical/Chiron Hansatome. Moria/Schwind also make manual versions of the Carriazo-Barraquer microkeratome.

1. Basics

In nondisposable vertical microkeratomes, the motor lies directly vertical or above the eye, rather than to the side of the eye. This instrument may be used to create a superior hinge (Fig. 1B). Vertical microkeratomes are equipped with a rotating head that travels to create the surgical arc (flap).

2. Designs

The primary difference between the two popular vertical microkeratomes is the presence of a geared track on the Hansatome compared to the smooth track of the Carriazo-Barraquer (Fig. 4.4). As with the ACS, the geared track may cause this instrument to be more susceptible to jamming from debris; however, it provides the microkeratome with more torque (torque=force* distance). Greater torque allows the microkeratome to perform its keratomileusis with minimal assistance from the surgeon. The Carrazo-Barraquer's lack

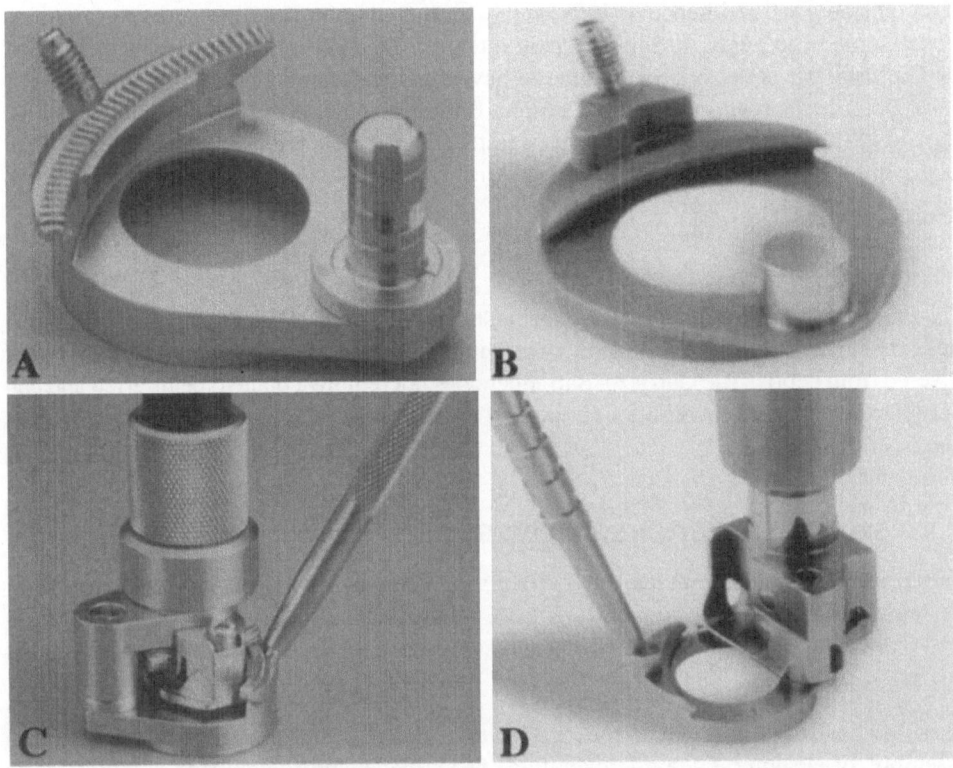

Figure 4.4 Examples of nondisposable vertical microkeratomes. Note that the microkeratome motor is directly above the operating surface. (A) The geared outer track of the Hansatome suction ring. (B) The smooth outer track of the Carriazo-Barraquer suction ring. (C) Fully assembled Hansatome with suction ring, plate, and head. (D) Fully assembled Carriazo-Barraquer with suction ring and head. Note the microkeratome head in B is smaller than A. The M-2 Moria Microkeratome has virtually replaced the Carriazo-Barraquer microkeratome because it avoids the problem of flap thickness variability.

Table 2 Technical Features of Nondisposable Vertical Microkeratomes

Manufacturer	Bausch & Lomb/Chiron	Moria and Schwind
Model name	Hansatome	Carriazo-Barraquer
Oscillation speed	14,000 rpm	15,000 rpm
Flap diameter	8.5 and 9.5 mm	7.0 mm and >
Depth	160 and 180 μm	130, 160, 180 μm
Mechanism	Outer gear	Only inner drive mechanism
Motor	Electric	Gas turbine or electric
Automated/manual	Automated	Both available
Advance rate	6.0 mm/s	3.7 mm/s
Hinge position	Superior	Anywhere

of an outside gear, and hence its inferior torque, may require the surgeon to push the microkeratome head gently to initiate keratomileusis. This causes the automatic version of the Carriazo-Barraquer microkeratome to have a manual component.

Both the Hansatome and the Carriazo-Barraquer operate at high oscillation speeds, close to 15,000 rpm. The Hansatome has a faster advancement rate, while the Carriazo-Barraquer has a greater selection of flap diameters. Technical features of nondisposable vertical microkeratomes appear in Table 2.

3. Safety Issues

The Hansatome has made a few advancements over the ACS. First of all, it will not operate if the plate is not inserted. Second, the number of gears is reduced and they are better covered from debris. The Carriazo-Barraquer does not require a plate to be inserted and can fit in narrower spaces. In addition, it may produce a hinge in any peripheral corneal location.

E. DISPOSABLE MICROKERATOMES

These microkeratomes include the Refractive Technologies Flapmaker, the LaserSight Technologies Unishaper, and the Moria LSK-1 Disposable.

1. Basics

These are horizontal microkeratomes that have the advantage of requiring no assembly, disassembly, or cleaning. Each microkeratome head, blade, and suction ring combination is sterile, used once, and then discarded.

2. Designs

In disposables, the blade is preassembled in the head, and the head is engaged in the track. The head and suction ring are made of clear plastic, and the instruments operate by utilizing a sliding (cable driven or turbine driven) or a gear driven mechanism (Fig. 4.5).

The Moria LSK-1 Disposable is a manual microkeratome and uses the same control unit as the other Moria microkeratomes. The Flapmaker and Unishaper are automated and use electric motors. Technical features of disposable microkeratomes appear in Table 3.

3. Safety Issues

Disposable systems have the advantage of requiring fewer components to be set up by the surgeon; they also have improved sterility, thus decreasing the chance of operational error or surgical infection. In addition, the clear plastic of the disposable systems ensures good visibility for the keratomileusis procedure.

F. WATER JET MICROKERATOMES

These instruments include the Medjet Hydrokeratome, the Medjet Hydrorefractive Keratectomy hydrokeratome, and the Visijet hydrokeratome.

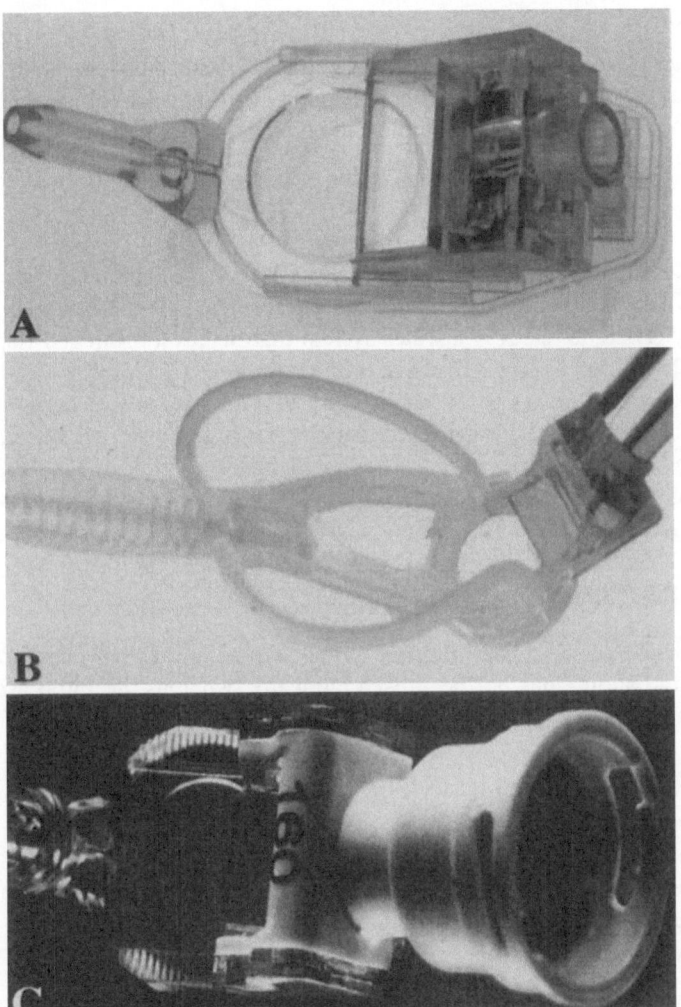

Figure 4.5 Examples of disposable microkeratomes. Note the pre-engaged plastic suction ring and head. See the smooth tracks of A and B and the geared track in C. (A) Refractive Technologies Flapmaker. (B) Moria LSK-1 disposable. (C) LaserSight Unishaper.

Table 3 Technical Features of Disposable Microkeratomes

Manufacturer	Refractive Technologies	Moria	LaserSight Technologies
Model name	Flapmaker	LSK-1 disposable	Unishaper
Oscillation speed	12,500 rpm	15,000 rpm	7,500 rpm
Flap diameter	8.5 and 10.5 mm	≤10 mm	8.5 mm and >
Depth	220, 200, 180, 160, and 130 μm	160 and 180 μm	160 μm
Design	Sliding	Sliding	Gear driven
Motor	Electric (cable)	Gas turbine	Electric
Automated/manual	Automated	Manual	Automated
Advance rate	6.8 mm/s	N/A	4.5 mm/s

1. Basics

The theory behind the water systems is that blades cause collateral tissue damage, while a beam of water can precisely cut between layers without leaving debris and provoking minimal wound response. In addition, the hydrokeratome can perform the cut without requiring an increase in intraocular pressure.

2. Designs

The Medjet Hydroblade Keratome uses a 30 μm beam, and advances at 6.7 mm/s. It has a fixed depth plate and can produce superior, temporal, or nasal hinges. The Medjet Hydrorefractive Keratectomy (HRK) System is a water system that makes a bi-hinged flap with a C-shaped needle. The system attempts to ablate without the need of a laser. Instead, the shape and pressure of the template can be changed, along with the scan rate, in order to remove different amounts of tissue. The Visijet Hydrokeratome is also a water jet system that uses a 36 μm beam and advances at 6.7 mm/s. It has a variable depth plate of 120–200 μm and a clear applanation lens for good visualization.

G. LASER MICROKERATOMES

These instruments include the Novatek Laser Microkeratome and the IntraLase Microkeratome. The Novatek microkeratome has not been used clinically, whereas the IntraLase Microkeratome (picosecond MK) has been in clinical use since early 2000 with outstanding results.

1. Basics

Laser systems create a precise flap with a laser or perform an intrastromal cavitation by carving a corneal lenticule with a laser beam. The vapor and fluid residues from intrastromal ablations dissipate a few hours after surgery.

2. Designs

The IntraLase Laser Microkeratome depends upon femtosecond pulses, so less energy is needed to photodisrupt corneal tissue, thus allowing more localized effects. It also allows a wide variety of corneal flap shapes. It also depends on an applanation plate to ensure consistent flap thickness. The Novatec Laser Systems Laser Microkeratome is expected to have eye tracking systems to monitor eye movements, giving a three-dimensional map for the laser's location within the cornea. The IntraLase Microkeratome has been continuously upgraded, so as to allow complete versatility and reproducibility, and may become the most commonly used system for corneal flaps in the future.

H. OTHER MICROKERATOMES

The Ophthalmic Technologies Inc./Loktal Medical Clear Corneal Molder allows for correction without photoablation. It can perform convex or concave cuts, thus correcting for myopia and hyperopia. It has minimal vibration, allowing use of steel or diamond blades. It also has gearless tracks, is a manual microkeratome, and has separate motors for oscillation and advancement. It is adjustable, 1–500 μm in depth, and the standard is fixed at 180 μm. Its blade speed is also adjustable to 24,000 rpm. It has a viewing window and automatically stops if suction is lost. In addition, it only cuts in forward motion.

Mastel Precision Surgical Instruments' Buzard Barraqueratome has a diamond blade and needs no assembly. It provides good visualization of the flap and is compact, so it can fit small eyes. It has a two-chambered vacuum, which acts on the cornea and sclera to allow for a lower IOP. The depth plate is fixed at 160 μm and the instrument makes nasally oriented flaps.

Hanna also makes a microkeratome. This instrument relies upon rotational motion and is known for the formation of a smooth bed.

I. DISCUSSION

Each of the above-mentioned microkeratomes attempts to decrease complications seen in LASIK surgery. Although no microkeratome is ideal, certain features are desirable in microkeratome systems and physicians should be encouraged to ask manufacturers about them:

Low level of flap complications
Consistent flap thickness
Good visibility
Fits into small eyes
Fixed depth plate
Loss of suction indicators

Table 4 Flap Combinations (Numbers indicate percent complication rates).

First author	Micro-keratome	# of eyes	Incomplete cut	Perorated lenticule	Short flap	Sliding flap	wrinkles (striae)	Free cap	Flap melt	Thin flap	Decentered flap	Cumulative
Brint	ACS	47		4.3								4.3
Bas	ACS	97	2.1									2.1
Fiander	ACS	124						9.7				9.7
Kremer	ACS	5					20					20.0
Guell	ACS	43						2.3				2.3
Helmy	ACS	40				0						0.0
Marinho	ACS	34			2.9	5.9		2.9				11.8
Salah	ACS	88						3.4				3.4
Condon	ACS	51					3.9					3.9
Perez-Santonja	ACS	143				0.7	3.5	0.7	8.0			12.9
Steinert	ACS	76	2.6					1.3				3.9
Waring	ACS	714	0.7	0.6		1.1	0.1	1.1		0.1		3.8
El-Maghraby	ACS	33				6.1	3.0					9.1
Stulting	ACS	1062	0.8	0.6		1.2	0.2	0.9		0.1		3.8
Gimbel	ACS	1000	1.2	0.3		1.2	0.6	0.1		0.3		3.7
Hersh	ACS	115	0.9					0.9		0.9		2.6
Dulany	ACS	124				2.4	4.8					7.3
Lindstrom	ACS	475				0.6		0.2				0.8
Knorz	ACS	42	2.4					7.1				9.5
Summary	ACS	4313	0.7	0.4	0.02	1.0	0.6	1.0	0.2	0.1		4.0
Velasco-Martinelli	Hansatome	400	1.0	0				0		1.3	2.3	4.5
Rosa	Hansatome	40					2.5				2.5	5.0
Summary	Hansatome	440	0.9	0			0.2	0		1.1	2.3	4.5

First and foremost, a suitable microkeratome should have a low level of flap complications. These complications depend on a multitude of factors, including experience and microkeratome safety features. As refractive surgeons know, there is a steep learning curve for LASIK, and regardless of microkeratome brand complications will decrease with time.

However, complications may be more apt to occur in certain microkeratomes (12–38). Farah's work quantitates flap complications, and by including data from further studies, one may see the number of flap complications that have occurred with different microkeratome designs (1), specifically the ACS and the Hansatome (Table 4). In these studies, serious flap-related complications occurred in 4% of the ACS cases and 1% of the Hansatome cases. The Hansatome studies contained less severe complications. There were no free caps in the 440 eyes analyzed, and 10 of the 20 complications were a decentered flap. Flap decentration appears to be an inherent possibility in the Hansatome cases. Oftentimes, suction ring application causes movement of the globe. The suction must be stopped and the area recentered. However, in some cases, scleral indentation occurs when the ring fixes on the globe on the first cut attempt and the indentation may prevent adjustment (12). In these cases, a different suction ring or repeated attempts at recentration will solve the problem.

Consistent flap thickness is also important in performing LASIK. Most surgeons aim to leave a minimum of 250 μm of residual cornea after ablation to prevent irreversible corneal edema. For patients whose residual corneal thickness is predicted to be close to 250 μm, according to refractive correction and preoperative pachymetry, a predictable flap thickness is essential. Many microkeratome companies have performed studies to indicate consistent flap thickness. Summit's two studies showed varied results on flap thickness. A 12 eye study with the Summit Krumeich–Barraquer microkeratome indicated a 190 ± 17 μm cut with the 160 μm head, while a 24 eye study indicated a 164 ± 13 μm cut with the same head. One study involving 93 eyes that underwent LASIK with the Moria LSK-1 microkeratome indicated that the 160 μm head averaged 159 ± 28 μm (13). Pineda's work on 25 eyes reveals a 117 ± 17 μm cut with the ACS, and his 21 eye study shows a 127 ± 29 μm cut with the Hansatome; both studies attempted a 160 μm cut (14). Pineda's work and our experience indicate that the ACS and Hansatome provide cuts that are more often thinner than expected.

In addition to consistent flap thickness, design features that offer good visibility are an asset to all surgeons, especially those who are still in the steep portion of the learning curve (15–38). Proper visibility allows the beginner to learn correctly the positions and technical details of microkeratome operation and aids the expert in avoiding debris in the surgical path. Also, designs that are slim have benefits, since they can fit into the widest variety of patients, such as those with narrow eyes or redundant eyelid skin.

Microkeratomes that rely on fixed depth plates, rather than heads that can achieve variable depths, are preferable. First, if a surgeon needs to cut at a different depth, he or she may still do so using a different head. Second, human error may occur when inserting the depth plate into variable depth systems, thus leading to corneal perforation with high intraocular pressure. Such a complication may cause damage to various structures in the eye, including the iris, the ciliary body, and the lens (37).

Finally, safety features such as alarms, automatic shut-sown buttons, or suction displays are very beneficial. If the microkeratome continues forward progress after suction is lost, an irregular cap can occur with a cut through the central cornea. Scarring in this location would be in the visual axis.

As for future methods to perform lamellar cuts, more accurate blades with consistent depths can be expected, along with laser systems that may cause less corneal disturbance. Time will tell where the future of microkeratomes lies, but one can be assured that microkeratome advances will continue (36–38).

REFERENCES

1. SG Farah, DT Azar, C Gurdal, J Wong. Laser in situ keratomileusis: literature review of a developing technique. J Cataract and Refract Surg 1998;24(7):989–1006.
2. O Gris, JL Guell, A Muller. Keratomileusis update. J Cataract Refract Surg 1996;22:620–623.
3. CA Swinger, J Krumeich, D Cassiday. Planar lamellar refractive keratoplasty. J Refract Surg 1996;2:17–24.
4. SF Brint, DM Ostrick, C Fisher, SG Slade, RK Maloney, R Epstein, RD Stulting, KP Thompson. Six-month results of the Multicenter Phase I Study of Excimer Laser Myopic Keratomileusis. J Cataract Refract Surg 1994;20:610–615.
5. L Buratto, M Ferrari. Indications, techniques, results, limits, and complications of laser in situ keratomileusis. Curr Opin Ophthalmol 1997;8(4):59–66.
6. SL Trokel, R Srinivasan, B Braren. Excimer laser surgery of the cornea. Am J Ophthalmol 1983;96:710–715.
7. L Buratto, M Ferrari, C Genisi. Myopic keratomileusis with the excimer laser: one year follow-up. Refract Corneal Surg 1993;9:12–19.
8. IG Pallikaris, ME Papatzanaki, DS Siganos, MK Tsilimbaris. A corneal flap technique for laser in situ keratomileusis; human studies. Arch Ophthalmol 1991;109:1699–1702.
9. M Duplessie. Surgical technique for laser-assisted in situ keratomileusis. International Ophthalmology Clinics 1996;36(4):45–51.
10. DT Azar. Refractive Surgery. In: SW Chang, L Ruiz, M Gomez, eds. Lamellar Refractive Surgery Instruments. New Jersey: Appleton and Lange, 1997, pp 239–251.
11. American Academy of Ophthalmology. Automated lamellar keratoplasty. Ophthalmology 1996;103(5):852–861.
12. EJ Velasco-Martinelli, FA Tarcha. Superior hinge laser in situ keratomileusis. J Refract Surg 1999;15(2S):S209–S211.
13. BJ Jacobs, TA Deutsch, JB Rubenstein. Reproducibility of corneal flap thickness in LASIK. Ophthalmic Surgery and Lasers 1999;30(5):350–353.
14. R Pineda. Comparative analysis of microkeratome flap thickness in LASIK. 21st Biennial Cornea Research Conference, Boston, 1999;21:45.
15. AM Bas, R Onnis. Excimer laser in situ keratomileusis for myopia. J Refract Surg 1995; 11S:S229–S233.
16. L Buratto, M Ferrari, P Rama. Excimer laser surgery of the cornea. Am J Ophthalmol 1992; 113:291–295.
17. PI Condon, M Mulhern, T Fulcher, A Foley-Nolan, M O'keefe. Laser intrastromal keratomileusis for high myopia and myopic astigmatism. Br J Ophthalmol 1997;81:199–206.
18. DD Dulaney, RW Barnet, SA Perkins, GM Kezirian. Laser in situ keratomileusis for myopia and astigmatism: 6 month results. J Cataract Refract Surg 1998;24(6):758–764.
19. A El-Maghraby, T Salah, GO Waring III, S Klyce, O Ibrahim. Randomized bilateral comparison of excimer laser in situ keratomileusis and photorefractive keratectomy for 2.50 to 8.00 diopters of myopia. Ophthalmology 1999;106(3):447–457.
20. DC Fiander, F Tayfour. Excimer laser in situ keratomileusis in 124 myopic eyes. J Refract Surg 1995;11S:S234–S238.
21. PS Hersh, SF Brint, RK Maloney, DS Durrie, M Gordon, MA Michelson, VM Thompson, RB Berkeley, OD Schein, RF Steinert. Photorefractive keratectomy versus laser in situ keratomileusis for moderate to high myopia. A randomized prospective study. Ophthalmology 1998;105(8):1512–1523.
22. HV Gimbel, EE Penno, JA van Westenbrugge, M Ferensowicz, MT Furlong. Incidence and

management of intraoperative and early postoperative complications in 1000 consecutive laser in situ keratomileusis cases. Ophthalmology 1998;105(10):1839–1848.

23. MC Knorz, A Liermann, V Seiberth, H Steiner, B Wiesinger. Laser in situ keratomileusis to correct myopia of −6.00 to −29.00 diopters. J Refract Surg 1996;12:575–584.

24. I Kremer, M Blumenthal. Myopic keratomileusis in situ combined with VISX 20/20 photorefractive keratectomy. J Cataract Refract Surg 1995;21:508–511.

25. RL Lindstrom, DR Hardten, YR Chu. Laser in situ keratomileusis (LASIK) for the treatment of low, moderate, and high myopia. Trans Am Ophthal Soc 1997;95:285–306.

26. A Marinho, MC Pinto, R Pinto, F Vaz, MC Neves. LASIK for high myopia: one year experience. Ophthalmic Surg Lasers 1996;27S:S517–S520.

27. JL Guell, A Muller. Laser in situ keratomileusis (LASIK) for myopia from −7 to −18 diopters. J Refract Surg 1996;12:222–228.

28. JJ Perez-Santonja, J Bellot, P Claramonte, MM Ismail, JL Alio. Laser in situ keratomileusis to correct high myopia. J Cataract Refract Surg 1997;23:372–385.

29. SA Helmy, A Salah, T Badawy, AN Sidky. Photorefractive keratectomy and laser in situ keratomileusis for myopia between 6:00 and 10:00 diopters. J Refract Surg 1996;12:417–421.

30. DS Rosa, JL Febbraro. Laser in situ keratomileusis for hyperopia. J Refract Surg 1999; 15(2S):S21–S215.

31. T Salah, GO Waring III, A El-Maghraby, K Moadel, SB Grimm. Excimer laser in situ keratomileusis under a corneal flap for myopia of 2 to 20 diopters. Am J Ophthalmol 1996;121: 143–155.

32. RF Steinert, PS Hersh. Spherical and aspherical photorefractive keratectomy and laser in-situ keratomileusis for moderate to high myopia: two prospective, randomized clinical trials. Summit technology PRK-LASIK study group. Trans Am Ophthalmol Soc 1998;197–227.

33. RD Stulting, JD Carr, KP Thompson, GO Waring III, WM Wiley, JG Walker. Complications of laser in situ keratomileusis for the correction of myopia. Ophthalmology 1999;106(1):13–20.

34. HV Gimbel, S Basti, GB Kaye, M Ferensowicz. Experience during the learning curve of laser in situ keratomileusis. J Cataract Refract Surg 1996;22:542–550.

35. Trends in technology: microkeratomes. Ocular Surg News 1998.

36. JI Barraquer. The history and evolution of keratomileusis. Int Ophthalmol Clin 1996;36(4):1–7.

37. SE Wilson. LASIK: management of common complications. Laser in situ keratomileusis. Cornea 1998;17(5):459–467.

38. GO Waring III, JD Carr, RD Stulting, KP Thompson, W Wiley. Prospective randomized comparison of simultaneous and sequential bilateral laser in situ keratomileusis for the correction of myopia. Ophthalmology 1999;106(4):732–738.

5

Adjunctive Instrumentation in LASIK

ROBERT T. ANG

*Massachusetts Eye and Ear Infirmary and Harvard Medical School,
Boston, Massachusetts, U.S.A., and Asian Eye Institute, Makati, The Philippines*

DIMITRI T. AZAR

*Massachusetts Eye and Ear Infirmary, Schepens Eye Research Institute,
and Harvard Medical School, Boston, Massachusetts, U.S.A.*

A. STANDARDIZED VISUAL ACUITY CHARTS

The measurement of visual acuity (VA) is an essential part of the ophthalmological examination, and it represents the most common useful test for assessing visual function. In clinical practice, the primary need is to document the occurrence or evolution of pathology; and in clinical trials or research projects, the need is to perform a reliable and reproducible baseline and evaluation of outcome. In refractive surgery, it is relevant to measure the best-corrected VA before and after surgery, to rule out any pathology other than refractive error, and to analyze differences and changes over time.

Charts with a regular progression of optotype size and spacing, with the same number of letters per row of approximately equal recognition difficulty (Landolt C or Sloan letters), are more useful for the standardization requirements. The Landolt ring has been consistently advocated as a standard test object since 1909 and was eventually adopted as the primary standard optotype by the National Academy of Sciences–National Research Council (NAS-NRC) Committee on Vision in 1980 (1). The Sloan and British Standard Institution optotype sets are substantially equivalent to the Landolt rings in terms of recognition difficulty (1). Optotype sizes must be reduced in a constant way in order to obtain an equal variation all over the scale extension. A logarithmic progression in steps of 0.1 logUnits corresponds to a geometric progression in which each row contains optotypes about 1.26 times smaller than the preceding one. Optotypes must also be quite far apart to avoid the "crowding effect." The

NAS-NRC recommended ten optotypes divided into two rows of five; eight letters per row is the minimum accepted. The same number of letters at each size level is required (1).

In individuals with normal vision, visual acuity (VA) increases as a function of the background luminance from mesopic to high photopic conditions until glare is experienced and VA subsequently decreases. VA increases from a luminance of 0.025 cd/m^2 to 60 cd/m^2, but above 80 cd/m^2 the variation is very slight, and above 500 cd/m^2 it becomes negligible (1, 2). Maximal VA is achieved under photopic conditions. It is advisable to avoid VA measurement in a dark room, but ambient background lighting should not exceed one half of the chart background luminance. The ability to identify an optotype is related not only to its angular width but also to the test target contrast. VA is reduced as the contrast between the test target and the background decreases. The maximal VA is achieved when the contrast between optotypes and background is above 80%. The standard chart testing distance should be 4 meters. With this distance, there is easy approximation to infinity by adding algebraically -0.25 D to the refractive correction; easy conversion of the Snellen ratio between 4 meters and 20 feet; and maximal acuity and minimal dispersion of acuity scores at distances close to 4 meters.

1. Distance Charts

The Snellen chart is the most widely used chart for VA testing in all English-speaking countries. It is based on the assumption that a subject with normal recognition acuity can resolve an optotype with a visual angle of 5 and a resolution angle (stroke) of 1 (minute of arc). The VA level is expressed as the ratio between the reading distance and the distance in meters at which the stroke width of the equivalent Landolt ring subtends 1 minute of arc. It has several limitations including a different number of optotypes per row, irregular progression in letter size, differences in the recognition difficulty of the optotypes, and difference in background luminance related to different chart manufacturers. The back-illuminated Snellen visual acuity chart routinely used in a clinic has a luminance of approximately 550 cd/m^2. Snellen is generally credited with inventing letter-chart acuity testing, and although many variants of his original test exist, the Snellen chart has gained universal clinical acceptance.

The basic principle of measuring visual acuity with letter test charts is that the smallest level of letters that can be read satisfactorily provides the index of visual acuity. It is therefore reasonable that each level on the test chart should have an equal degree of difficulty. In 1976, Bailey and Lovie described a chart with the following features: the same number of symbols used on each line; the between-symbol spacing is proportionally the same on each line; the vertical spacing between one line and the next is a constant proportion of symbol size; and the ratio of symbol size on a given line to that on the next line is constant (approximately 1.25) (2,3). The British Standards Institution adopted a series of ten nonserif letters of equal legibility, based on the findings of Coates and Woodruff as reported by Bennett (2). This was the basis for the optotypes selected by Bailey and Lovie to give standard legibility to each row of their acuity chart. Ten 5×5 Sloan letters (S, D, K, H, N, O, C, V, R, and Z) were subsequently adopted by the NAS-NRC Committee. The 5×5 format designates that each optotype is constructed on a square framework 5 units wide by 5 units high and having a stroke width equal to 1 unit (4).

The Bailey–Lovie distance visual acuity chart was developed to overcome the inaccuracies of the Snellen chart and has been widely accepted as an accurate and efficient measure of visual acuity, particularly for assessing patients with low vision (2,5,6). The chart has approximately equally legible letters (British Standards Institution, 1968) on each row, and the separation of letters within rows and between rows is uniform, so that contour interaction is controlled. The visual task at each level of the chart is therefore the same irrespective of acuity or test distance. The Bailey–Lovie chart employs a logarithmic progression of sizes and the logMAR visual acuity notation, which has been shown to represent a good approximation to an equal discriminability scale and has been recognized by many investigators as the most logical measure of visual acuity (4,5,7). LogMAR charts are theoretically superior because interpatient differences and follow-up measurements over time are objectively and consistently evaluated and measured. The LogMAR design also minimizes the crowding phenomenon because of logical spacing of the optotypes. The Bailey–Lovie chart or adaptations of it have been used in notable research projects including the Early Treatment of Diabetic Retinopathy Study, the Macular Photocoagulation Study, and the Prospective Evaluation of Radial Keratotomy Study (7–9), among others.

The Early Treatment Diabetic Retinopathy Study (ETDRS) chart, also known as the Lighthouse Distance Visual Acuity Chart, uses lines of letter combinations determined to be of equal confusability and not containing words or acronyms (7,10). The chart was introduced by Ferris and is a modification of the Bailey and Lovie chart. It utilizes five Sloan optotypes per row with a regular progression of the type size and spacing, following a logarithmic scale in steps of 0.1 logUnits. The reduced number of optotypes may increase the probability of guessing brought about by easier memorization of the few optotypes. The background luminance is about 150 cd/m^2 without any possibility of regulation. (Fig. 5.1.)

2. Near Charts

The near test chart is a 1:10 scaled-down chart that uses a test distance of 40 cm. The range of sizes on these charts extends from 80 point to 2 point print, and the progression of size is essentially logarithmic. The Times Roman font was chosen because it is similar in appearance and legibility to the styles of typefaces customarily used in newspapers and books and because it has already been adopted by the British as the standard typeface for near-vision charts (11).

The Snellen near chart is expressed as the ratio between the test distance in centimeters and the distance in centimeters at which the stroke of the equivalent Landolt ring sub-

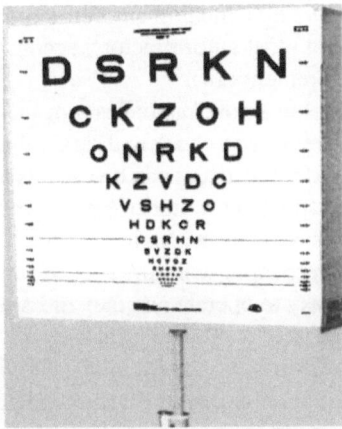

Figure 5.1 ETDRS visual acuity chart. This chart is valuable for LASIK studies, although it may be less convenient than the Snellen chart for routine measurements of visual acuity.

tends 1 minute of arc. With the Sloan M system, a 1-M letter is defined as an optotype whose height subtends a visual angle of 5 at a distance of one meter.

One of the main reasons why near acuity in the consulting room can be misleadingly good is due to the high luminance of the chart and the high contrast of the print.

Furthermore, standardization in near vision tests has not been established with regard to using text-reading or optotypes recognition. Test cards using the "Jaeger system" and the "point system" also vary across different manufacturers, making standardization difficult.

The practical near acuity chart (PNAC) offers a quick but accurate way to measure near acuity and shows a high degree of correlation with distance acuity, contrast sensitivity, and ability to read newsprint (12). The PNAC encompasses print sizes from large (N80, such as newspaper headlines) to small (N5, such as telephone directory entries). It has a regular increasing progression of print size and line spacing (0.1 logMAR). Three words were used on each line; one three letter word, one four letter word, and one five letter word. Thus each line has an equivalent task demand having 12 letters split into 3 words. The words are easy to recognize by children and those with poor language and cognitive skills. The PNAC uses the Times Roman font, as it is a print type commonly used in newspapers and books. Paragraphs of the most commonly used print sizes are located on the reverse side of the chart, so reading a set size of print can be practiced once the near acuity threshold has been established. Although the PNAC only uses three words on each line, it was shown to be as accurate as the Bailey–Lovie near chart. Near acuity threshold was measured in half the time using the PNAC than with the Bailey–Lovie chart. It was found that most people can read newspaper headlines with a near acuity of N48 (1.4 logMAR), large text (such as children's books) with N20 (1.0 logMAR), and normal newspaper text with N6 (0.5 logMAR) or better at 25 cm.

B. AUTOREFRACTORS

It is almost half a century since Collins reported the design and construction of the first objective infrared optometer. However, the first fully automated optometer, the Ophthalmotron, did not appear until 1970 (13). Automated objective refractors that do not require any operator or patient judgment have been available since then. These instruments are easy to use and are much quicker than manual refraction.

An ideal objective refraction technique should be able to determine the "actual" ametropia without dilating with cycloplegic agents. To achieve this, modern autorefractors use fogging techniques to relax accommodation (Fig. 5.2). In most autorefractors, accommodation is relaxed only once prior to the start of the measurement (14).

Ghose believed that the automatic fogging system of some autorefractors cannot sufficiently control accommodation (15). It is therefore still necessary to check and refine the displayed readings by subjective refraction or retinoscopy. Autorefractors can be used as a preliminary refraction or screening method because they provide a starting point for retinoscopy or subjective refraction, but they cannot serve as a substitute for it.

During the 1970s and 1980s, several subjective autorefractors were introduced but were not widely accepted because they were not quick and easy to operate and they did not provide binocular or near point testing. Among the early models were the Humphrey Vision Analyzer and the American Optical SR III Subjective Refraction System (16). The more recent autorefractors are quicker, easier to use, have good reliability and accuracy but still do not provide for binocular balance or nearpoint testing and therefore could not serve as substitutes for conventional refraction. Autorefractors have become an integral part of

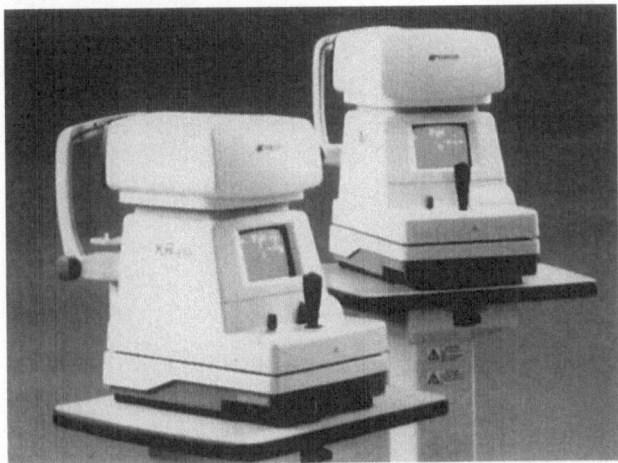

Figure 5.2 Automated refractors are helpful in obtaining a rough idea of the patient's refractive error. They should not be used as the sole basis of LASIK treatments.

ophthalmological practice. They are simple enough to be used by technicians with a moderate degree of training, they save time, and they serve as a complement to subjective refraction.

1. Keratometry, Keratoscopy, and Corneal Topography

The indications for measuring corneal curvature and evaluating corneal topography include contact lens fitting, biometry for determining the power of an intraocular lens, screening for refractive surgery, evaluation of pathologies such as keratoconus, irregular astigmatism, and contact lens warpage, identification of postlaser decentrations, central islands, regressions, and postoperative assessment of astigmatism after penetrating keratoplasty and cataract surgery. Currently, the corneal curvature can be quantified and assessed using the manual keratometer, the automated keratometer, and videokeratoscopes such as the Placido-based topography unit, the rasterphotogrammetry unit, and the scanning slit beam system.

The anterior corneal surface behaves like a convex mirror and reflects light. This property allows the keratometer to measure the size of the reflected image and to determine the radius of curvature of the corneal surface (17,18).

The manual keratometer measures the dimensions of a virtual image from the corneal reflection in two orthogonal meridians simultaneously. Dials indicating the principal curvatures of a toric surface are adjusted with the end result of focusing and aligning reflective mires thereby producing a virtual image with the same dimensions (19). The keratometer has been used as the gold standard to which autokeratometers and corneal topography units have been compared (20). Examples of manual keratometers are the Haag-Streit/Javal Schiotz, the Bausch & Lomb (Fig. 5.3), the Carl Zeiss, and the Marco keratometer.

The limitations of the manual keratometer are that it assumes a spherocylindrical cornea with a major and minor axis separated by 90 degrees; it does not provide information about the cornea outside of a circle 2.8 to 4 mm in diameter where the measurements

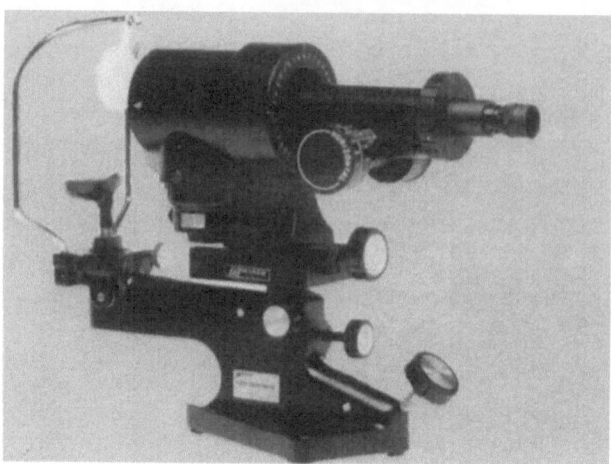

Figure 5.3 Manual keratometer.

are taken, and corneal irregularities can distort the mires making measurements difficult or impossible (17,18).

Autokeratometers utilize the same principles as the manual keratometer but use software that electronically projects light onto the cornea and captures the reflections to produce keratometry readings. The Humphrey automated keratometer (Humphrey Instruments, San Leandro, CA) uses three near-infrared light rays that are reflected off the cornea. Three photodiode receptors receive the images and utilize vector algebra equations to analyze and calculate the keratometry parameters. The Canon automated keratometer projects a single keratoscope ring onto the cornea and analyzes the data in a similar manner.

Several reports have compared the manual and automated keratometer. Tate et al. found no statistical difference in the accuracy of the manual (Haag-Streit) and the automated (Humphrey, Canon) keratometers (21). Lusby et al. concluded that both keratometers have been shown to give reproducible results on repeated measurements of the same eye (22). Binder demonstrated that the Humphrey automated keratometer and the Bausch & Lomb keratometer are comparable in their ability to measure abnormal corneal surfaces following radial keratotomy and corneal transplantation (23). Because it is quick and easy to operate, Nakada et al. recommended that the automated keratometer should be widely used, especially when examining children (24). Automated keratometers have become more popular than manual keratometers because they are accurate and reliable; they can measure a larger range of curvatures and astigmatism, eliminate observer bias, produce a hard copy of the results, and require less skill and less time to operate (25).

In 1993, Sanders et al. stated that videokeratoscopes were becoming invaluable tools and predicted that they will replace keratometers in standard clinical practice (26). Their prediction was based on experience in using keratometers and obtaining misleading keratometric measurements from corneas that had asymmetric astigmatism, asymmetry after radial keratotomy, and unusual variants of keratoconus. With the growing demand for refractive surgery and increased applications in assessment of pathologies and postoperative care, corneal topography units have indeed become indispensable diagnostic tools in ophthalmological practice. Videokeratoscopes offer several advantages over keratometers;

they do not assume that the cornea is spherocylindrical, they allow the assessment of the peripheral cornea, and the images from the systems are digitized, analyzed quantitatively with various softwares, and printed in color-coded images for easy interpretation.

Placido-based topography systems use a transilluminated Placido cone, an imaging system that consists of a lens, a camera, a video grabber, and a computer system (17,18). Illuminated concentric rings are centered and projected radially from the corneal apex. A camera focuses on the image plane of the cornea and captures the image of the rings. Analysis of the size and displacement of the ring segments is used to calculate the slope of the corneal surface. The accuracy of Placido-based units may be affected by intraobserver variability, interobserver variability, centration, alignment, calibration, and software errors. Furthermore, a limitation of Placido systems is that elevation data is generated by fitting the slope to a predefined mathematical model such as spheric, aspheric, or conic, which may not be right for abnormal corneas. Systems currently in use may differ in the number, thickness, and position of the rings, the cone design, the illumination, and the software that they used. Examples of systems using Placido-based topography are the EyeSys, Technomed C-Scan, Topography Modeling System, Alcon EyeMap, and Humphrey Atlas (Fig. 5.4).

Rasterphotogrammetry defines elevation points by projecting a grid of known geometry onto the corneal surface and analyzing the distortion from this pattern (17,18,20,27,28). The PAR Corneal Topography System (CTS, PAR Vision Systems Corp., New Hartford, NY) uses a stereotriangulation technique by utilizing flourescein on the tear film, projecting a grid pattern composed of horizontal and vertical lines spaced about 0.22 mm apart, and viewing the light pattern from an offset angle. A CCD camera collects the reflected images and the x, y, and z coordinates are determined from the geometry of the measured grid position and instrument optics. The PAR CTS determines surface elevation without using the shape assumptions necessary in Placido-based systems. It relies on projection on the flourescein film and therefore does not require a smooth reflective surface nor precise spatial alignment for accurate imaging, making it useful in corneas with scars, epithelial defects, or irregular surfaces.

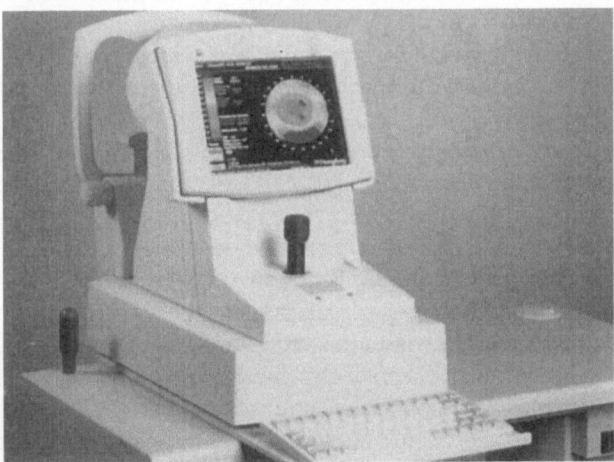

Figure 5.4 Compact placido-based corneal topographical unit.

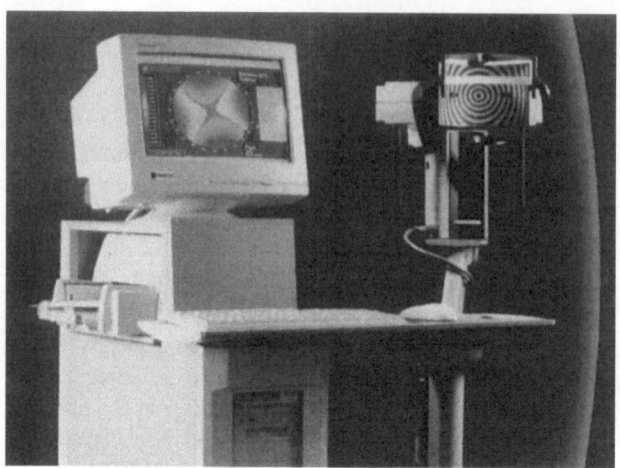

Figure 5.5   An elevation-based topographical unit is useful in detecting substantial changes in the posterior corneal surface and in measuring corneal pachymetry.

The scanning slit beam system is used by the Orbscan (Bausch and Lomb, Rochester, NY; Fig. 5.5) to measure corneal surface elevation using stereotriangulation techniques similar to the PAR CTS system (17,18,20). The examination takes 1.5 seconds wherein two scanning slit lamps project 20 slit beams from the left and 20 slit beams from the right at an angle of 45 degrees covering the whole cornea form limbus to limbus. A tracking system locks on to the eye to minimize errors from involuntary eye movements during the examination. The software analyzes up to 240 data points per slit, enabling it to calculate and produce more data. The Orbscan can provide information on the axial curvature of the anterior and posterior cornea, the elevation of the anterior and posterior corneal surface relative to the best fit sphere, and the corneal thickness on the entire cornea. The system yields more information than Placido or rasterphotogrammetric systems because it takes measurement of the posterior corneal surface as well (29). The Orbscan and the PAR CTS directly measure surface elevation and measure topography regardless of the orientation of the eye, unlike the Placido-based systems.

Previous studies have attempted to determine the most reliable system to use in evaluating corneal curvature by comparing keratometers with corneal topography units and corneal topography units among themselves.

In evaluating normal corneal power measurements, Hannush et al. reported that the manual keratometer was more reproducible than the Corneal Modeling System and the Corneascope (30). Moura et al. compared three computerized videokeratoscopy systems with a manual keratometer and found that the most reproducible was the EyeSys, followed by the manual keratometer, the PAR CTS, and the C-Scan Technomed (31). Jeandervin and Barr, on the other hand, found no statistical differences in repeatability when comparing the Alcon EyeMap, the EyeSys 2000, the Humphrey Mastervue, the Humphrey Atlas, and the Marco manual keratometer (32). However, they observed that the EyeSys had the highest repeatability and that the Humphrey Atlas was the most accurate system tested (32). Wilson et al. reported that the TMS was statistically more accurate in determining the power of calibrated spheres at 1 mm from the apex, while the Corneal Analysis System (CAS, EyeSys Laboratories, Houston, TX) was more accurate at 3 mm from the apex (33). These small differences in accuracy between the EyeSys and the TMS were unlikely to be of clinical significance. Tennen et al. did same-day measurements of the steepest and flattest powers of the central 3 mm of 200 eyes and found no statistical difference in reliability between the Haag Streit, the Marco, the Alcon handheld keratometer, and the Corneal Analysis System (EyeSys Laboratories, Houston, TX) (34). With regard to elevation data, Priest and Munger showed that the PAR CTS presented elevation measurements more accurately than the TMS-1 (Topography Modeling System, Tomey Corp.). Unlike the PAR CTS, which provides a direct measurement of elevation, errors made by the TMS-1 are the result of assumptions made regarding the corneal shape and position (28). Schultze made a similar observation that the PAR CTS accurately provides peripheral elevation data on a model representing an eye after PRK (35).

Numerous studies have presented data on the accuracy and reliability of different systems in evaluating corneal curvature. Perhaps the most significant observation was made by Moura et al. They stated that whenever a particular system is used, it should be used continually for that patient, otherwise errors may be seen when interchanging and interpreting data from one system to another (31).

D. PUPILLOMETRY

Sophisticated pupillometry video equipment, which can determine diameters to hundredths of a millimeter, have been used in neuro-ophthalmic evaluation (36). In refractive surgery, assessment of pupil diameters is important because despite excellent visual acuity, a well-centered ablation zone, a good-looking postoperative topographical map, and the absence of significant corneal haze, widely dilating pupils at low levels of illumination are prone to halos, glare, and reduced night vision when the pupil dilates to a size larger than the ablation zone. These symptoms should be anticipated, considered, and explained to the patient before deciding to proceed with refractive surgery if the pupil size measurements in dim illumination reveal that it can dilate to a size larger than the zone of treatment. Careful measurement of scotopic pupil dilation is therefore an integral part of the preoperative evaluation of the refractive patient.

Comparison pupillometry has been performed using the Rosenbaum card (Cleveland, OH). It contains a series of increasing half-circle diameters denoted by 1.0 mm intervals printed on one edge of the card. The examiner held the card temporal to the patient's eye in the corneal plane and matched the horizontal pupil diameter with the appropriate half-circle. Pupil measurements were made in 1.0 mm steps unless the pupil appeared between two half-circles on the card, and a 0.5 mm measurement interval was then made (37). The Rosenbaum method was found to overestimate consistently the pupil diameter by 0.5 mm, with a standard deviation of 0.6 mm. A conversion factor of subtracting 0.5 mm from the measurement was found to be sufficient to adjust for this overestimation.

Because of the subjective nature of the measurements using the Rosenbaum card, infrared pupillometry is presumed to be more accurate in measuring the pupil, especially in dark conditions. Hippus of the iris and the emotional state of the patient may sometimes affect the pupil diameter and prevent obtaining the largest natural pupil diameter. But the infrared device allows a more objective assessment between examiners.

Infrared pupillometry was previously performed with the Iowa Pupillometer (Henry Louis, Inc., Iowa City, IA) (37). The device consisted of a charged coupling device (CCD) camera tuned for infrared detection and two infrared side lamps for pupil illumination. Using two vertical lines on the video monitor, calibration of the pupillometer was performed for each subject before pupil measurements were made. The center of the monitor was used for measurement because distortions in the peripheral monitor may induce measurement error. This device measured the horizontal pupils to 0.01 mm increments, and analysis was performed rounding to the nearest 0.1 mm.

The Colvard pupillometer (Oasis Medical) is a handheld pupillometer that uses light amplification technology (Fig. 5.6) (38). Low levels of light energy entering the device stimulate a photocathode, which results in electron excitation. The electrons strike a phosphor screen, which intensifies the image. A lens system in the instrument brings the anterior segment into focus, and a bright phosphorescent image of the anterior segment is visualized through the examiner's ocular. A reticle in the device superimposes a millimeter ruler over the enhanced image of the iris and the pupil to measure pupil diameter in a scotopic environment. Using the Colvard pupillometer, pupil dilation at the level of light typically encountered while driving on a suburban street at night, can be reproduced by turning off all the lights in a windowless examining room and opening the door 1 to 2 inches. It was found that mean pupil size at 15 lumens was 5.1 mm (range 2.5 to 8.0 mm) and at 3 lumens was 6.2 mm (range 3.0 to 9.0 mm).

The Video Vision Analyzer (VIVA) pupillometer allows binocular measurement of the dark adapted pupil (39). The subject sits 1 meter in front of and beneath the device and fixates on a red light. Both eyes are focused on a rectangular field on the pupillometer display. Then a button is pressed, and the device automatically takes three images by infrared light. By digital processing, the pupil diameter under scotopic light conditions is calculated. Precise measurements within 0.3 mm at 1 meter are possible.

Several studies using the above-mentioned instruments have measured pupil diameters under scotopic light conditions. Evaluation of the pupil size with the Rosenbaum card detected a mean pupil size of 5.4 ± 1.1 mm, with the IOWA infrared pupillometer 4.95 ± 1.08 mm, and with the Colvard pupillometer 6.2 mm (range 3.0 to 9.0 mm) (37,38). In a recent study by Schnitzler, the mean scotopic pupil diameter was reported to be 6.08 ± 1.16 mm with the Colvard pupillometer and 6.24 ± 1.28 mm with the VIVA pupillometer. She concluded that measurements with the VIVA pupillometer seem slightly overestimated,

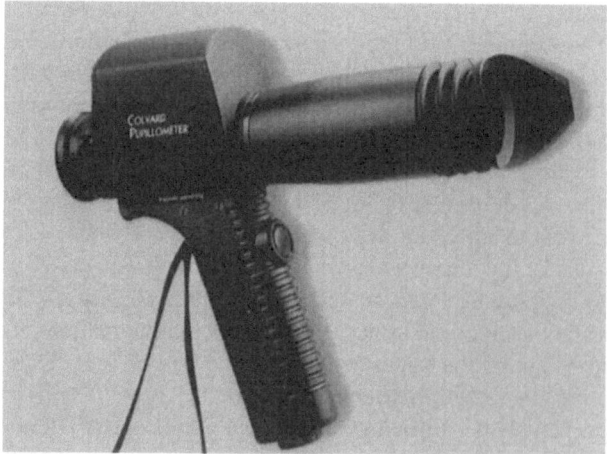

Figure 5.6 Colvard pupillometer. Measurement can be optimized by controlling ambient illumination during pupil measurements.

whereas measurements with the Colvard delivered more similar data on scotopic pupil size, indicating that measurements with the Colvard are more reliable and precise (39).

Pupil diameters have also been measured using topography devices including the Technomed C-Scan, the Humphrey Masterview, and the Alcon EyeMap. The measurements obtained were 3.35 mm (C-Scan), 2.96 mm (Masterview), 2.34 m (EyeMap), and 5.94 mm (mesopic condition). It was concluded that topography devices gave significantly smaller pupil measurements than mesopic conditions because of the bright luminance of the Placido rings. These instruments are not recommended in the determination of pupil diameters prior to refractive surgery (37).

E. PACHYMETRY

Pachymetry is the measure of corneal thickness. It is essential to measure central corneal thickness in myopic eyes before scheduling for LASIK surgery to ensure that the central thickness is sufficient to prevent leaving the corneal bed too thin after treatment and prone to ectasia. The residual bed depth is dependent on both the thickness of the flap and the depth of laser ablation. The U.S. Food and Drug Administration (FDA) has recommended that the residual thickness in the bed not be less than 250 μm to avoid corneal ectasia (40). Because of the variability of resection depths of different microkeratomes, calculations by the surgeon should consider leaving a generous residual bed after resection and planned ablation.

The electronic digital optical pachymeter used a depth measuring attachment for the 900 Haag Streit slit lamp and the 6090 package by Diagnostic Concept. It was calibrated on PMMA lenses according to the method described by Mandell and Polse (41–43). The angle between the measuring eyepiece (right) and the illumination system of the optical pachometer was set at 47.5°. The Haag Streit optical pachymeter emphasized keeping the slit beam of light perpendicular to the surface of the central cornea. Care was taken to ensure that the slit of light that passed through the cornea bisected the pupil, both vertically and horizontally, as seen by the split image during alignment. Ideally, the pupillary axis should coincide with the pachometric one. Fluorescein was instilled in the eye and the measurement done in darkness to increase contrast and facilitate alignment. Appropriate alignment was attained when the internal boundary of the endothelium was continuous with the epithelium seen in the lower field of the pachometer (touch criterion). Alignment was achieved when the reflecting images of the centration lights were aligned at the projected slit and in front of the pupil center; 10 readings were then recorded on each eye (44,45). The Mishima–Hedbys attachment could be utilized to improve the accuracy of the optical method (46). The disadvantages of the optical pachymeter with the Haag Streit device are that it is a subjective measurement wherein the examiner must make sure the slit of light is perpendicular to the cornea when making the reading and that it requires the cooperation of the patient in holding fixation during the duration of the measurement.

Ultrasonic pachymetry eliminates the disadvantages of the optical pachymeter since it can take rapid measurements without asking the patient to hold still for a long time (Fig. 5.7). There is no examiner variability since the machine takes readings upon contact with the cornea. It is easy to use and allows mapping of corneal thickness. In addition, the ultrasonic units are portable with small probe tips making possible intraoperative measurements before proceeding with laser ablation.

The Humphrey ultrasonic pachometer model 8050 uses pulsed ultrasound to evaluate corneal thickness. Although the location of the measurement is arbitrary, it is possible

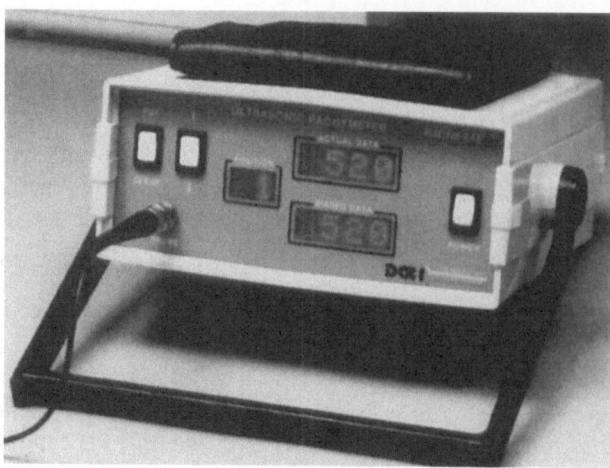

Figure 5.7   Ultrasonic pachymetry. To be able to measure intraoperative corneal pachymetry, the machine may require standardization in the range of 200 μm.

to take peripheral measurements by direct touch of the probe to the cornea. The instrument has automatic alignment properties so that the probe has to be within 3° from normal to the posterior corneal surface for a thickness to be recorded. Other models (DGH Technology, Inc., Exton, PA) have since been manufactured with variable features. The probe diameters range from 1.6 to 3.0 mm. The probes emit and receive pulses with frequencies of 12–20 MHz. Most instruments use a calibration speed of 1640 m/s. Some manufacturers suggested 1550 as the correct sound velocity, although it has been reported that 1639 is the velocity of sound through the human cornea at 37°C (47). The probe has to be aligned as perpendicularly as possible to the cornea. Some pachymeters provide a tone or beep when proper alignment or a measurement is obtained.

In a study by Salz et al., it was found that the optical pachymeter had two to three times as much intrasession variation as that of the ultrasound pachymeters, significant interobserver variation ($P = 0.015$), and significant differences between left and right eye thickness determinations ($P \leqq 0.005$). On the other hand, ultrasonic pachymeters showed superiority by demonstrating high reproducibility, no interobserver variation, and no left/right variation, in addition to its user- and patient-friendly features (45).

The Obscan Topography System (Orbtek, Inc.) is an optical scanning slit instrument that provides both topographic analysis and pachymetric measurements in the same examination (Fig. 5.5) (48). This instrument is capable of measuring corneal thickness at any point on the cornea with one procedure. Its sampling method takes into account a broader area of the cornea than does the ultrasonic pachymeter. A calibrated video and scanning slit beam system measures the position of several thousand points throughout the thickness of the cornea. Computer analysis then converts these data into a topographic map of the corneal surface and provides measurements of corneal thickness over the entire corneal surface, as well as keratometric measurements and corneal power and elevation maps.

The Orbscan system is noninvasive, requiring no contact for data acquisition, but it does require the patient to be able to sit at a chin rest while fixating for 1 to 3 seconds. Ultrasonic pachymetry, on the other hand, is associated with problems and limitations that the

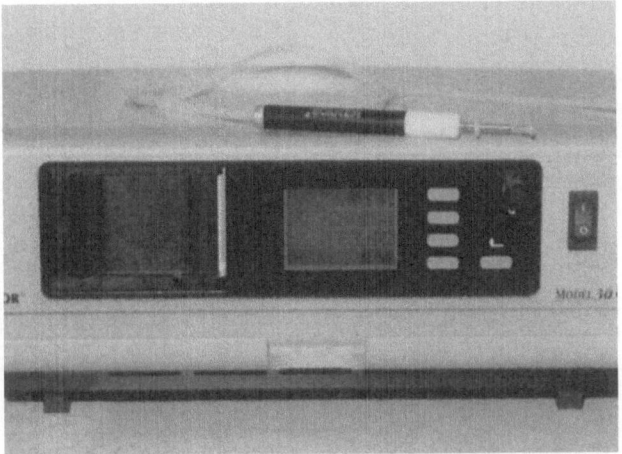

Figure 5.8 A pneumatonometer is used to check the intraocular pressure after application of the suction ring.

Orbscan system avoids. The ultrasonic pachymeter lacks fixation lights for precise control of patient gaze during repeated measurements, so probe placement in a reproducible manner is difficult and is markedly affected by the person performing the evaluation. Also, the speed of sound may vary in edematous tissue compared with that in normally hydrated tissue.

In a study by Yaylali, it was found that the two devices were quite comparable in their measurements in the same subjects, with the difference in corneal thickness between the two devices ranging from 23 to 28 μm (48).

Corneal pachymetry can also influence Goldmann tonometry. Use of a pneumatonometer (Fig. 5.8) may yield more accurate IOP measurements. See Chapter 27 for more details.

F. INSTRUMENTATION

1. Eyelid Drape

Plastic disposable eyelid drapes are used to maintain sterility of the surgical field during LASIK (Fig. 5.9A). The drape is applied after sterilizing the periocular area with a betadine solution. Aside from sterility, the eyelashes can be moved out of the way and secured when applying the adhesive on the eyelid. Retracting the adhesive along with the eyelid can aid the speculum in providing adequate exposure to the globe. Patient comfort is not compromised when breathing under the disposable drape. We have had good experience in using the 15 inch × 15 inch Steri-Drape (3M Healthcare, St. Paul, MN).

2. Speculum

Stable retraction of the eyelids and adequate exposure of the cornea are necessary in refractive surgery. This is even more critical in laser in situ keratomileusis (LASIK) because a pneumatic suction ring is applied on the globe during construction of the corneal flap. The ideal speculum should provide maximal access to the globe, accommodate the pneumatic suction

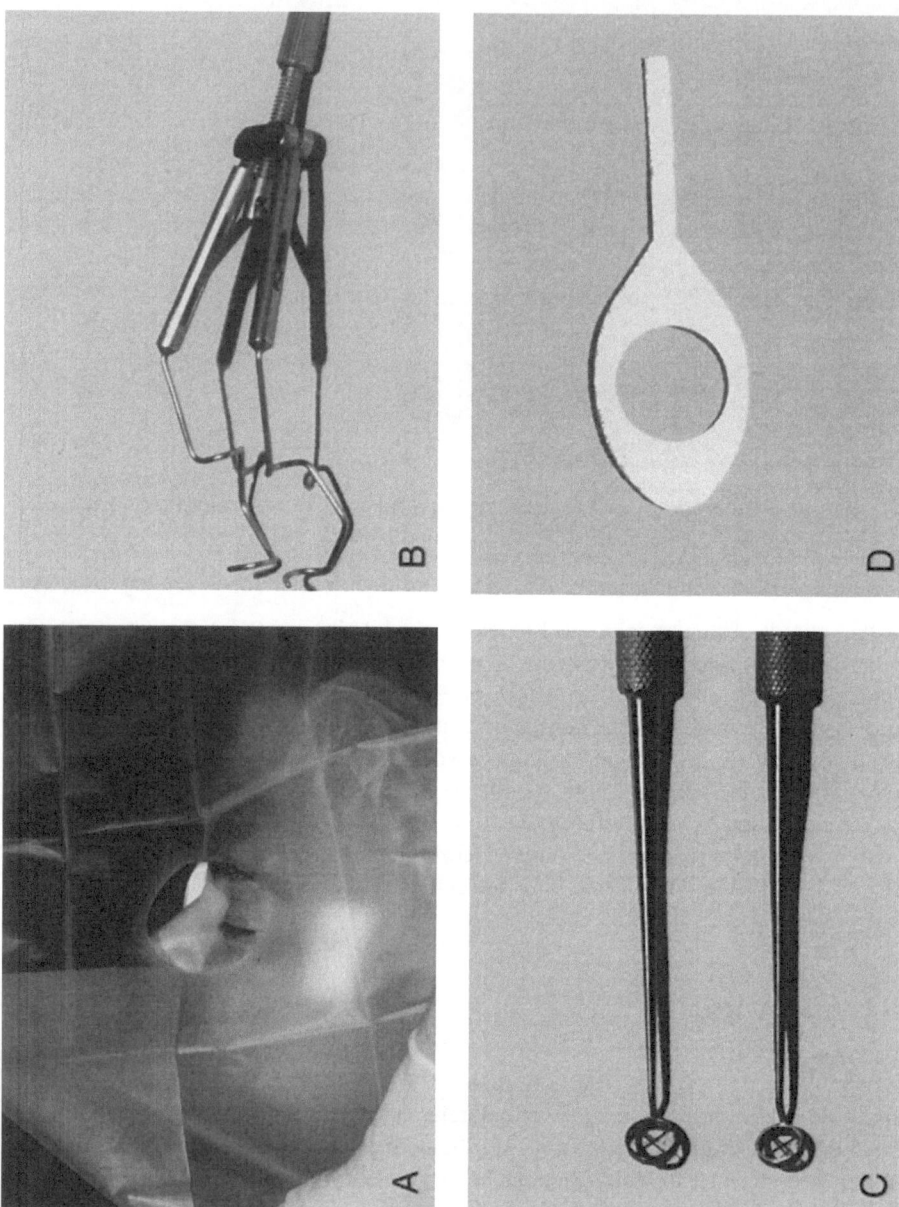

Figure 5.9 Intraoperative adjunctive instrumentation. (A) An eyelid drape is applied to ensure sterility and move the eyelashes out of the surgical field. (B) A wire speculum is used to provide maximal exposure of the globe for accommodating the suction ring. (C) An RK marker may be used to place asymmetric peripheral corneal marks. The Chayet ring (D) is helpful in minimizing deposition of debris into the flap interface.

ring within the palpebral opening, allow for temporal and superior surgical approaches, and provide maximum comfort when fully opened (49). Wire speculums are preferred over solid blade speculums because they provide more space for applying the suction ring.

After applying the wire speculum, a few minutes are allowed to pass for the eyelids to adjust to the pressure of the speculum. We have found it helpful to instill one or two additional drops of topical anesthesia before completely opening the speculum. These maneuvers minimize patient discomfort and enable the surgeon to maximize the capability of the speculum in providing adequate exposure. If exposure is still inadequate, the globe can be proptosed by exerting downward pressure on the arms of the speculum while applying the suction ring.

Innovations in speculum design have been made to aid in providing better exposure and added comfort to the patient. Among these are increased angulations in the arms of the speculum to maximize globe exposure, heavy duty wire bases strong enough to resist powerful eyelid squeezing, and suction attachments to remove tears and debris from the surgical area. Popular designs available are the Barraquer wire speculum, the Liebermann Adjustable wire speculum (Fig. 9B), the Machat adjustable speculum (ASICO, Westmont, IL), the Slade speculum (ASICO), and the Lindstrom-Chu Aspirating speculum (Rhein).

3. Nonfragmenting Merocel Sponges and Rings

The Chayet ring is an oval sponge with a 10 mm circular opening in the center and a tail in one of its long ends (Fig. 5.9D). It is placed on the eye after construction of the LASIK flap with the tail oriented on the opposite meridian across the flap hinge. It has three main uses. First, it serves as a soft, lint-free bed where the epithelial side of the LASIK flap rests during laser ablation. Second, it prevents fluid and debris outside the sponge area from gaining access to the interface during the ablation and flap repositioning steps. Third, it sucks excess fluid during interface irrigation and floating, preventing flooding of the flap area. Some surgeons prefer to use a semicircular sponge, which they position in the hinge region to rest the flap during ablation. The Chayet LASIK drainage rings are manufactured by Visitec (Becton Dickinson and Company, Franklin Lakes, NJ) and Solan (Medtronic, Jacksonville, FL).

It is essential to use a nonfragmenting sponge (Merocel, Xomed Surgical Products, Jacksonville, FL; Fig. 5.10A) throughout the LASIK surgery to avoid any lint fiber from being left on the flap interface. The Merocel sponge can be used to wipe off any debris, blood, or fluid on the exposed stroma prior to laser ablation, aspirate excess fluid within the Chayet ring, and iron the flap during flap repositioning.

4. Markers and Marking Pens

Corneal epithelial marks are placed in the paracentral area of the cornea prior to creation of the flap with the microkeratome. These marks serve as a guide in realigning the flap after laser ablation. In the event of a free flap, the marks will help in replacing and repositioning the flap and aid in orienting which side is epithelial and stromal. The design of optical zone markers and the marks they create can be circular (Fig. 5.9C), radial, or a combination of both shapes. Among the popular markers are those designed by Machat, Chayet, Burrato, and Slade. It is important that the marks be still visible upon flap repositioning but slowly fade a few hours after the surgery. The marker can be dipped in a gentian violet inkpad (Visitec, Becton Dickinson and Co., Franklin Lakes, NJ) or painted with a gentian violet marking pen

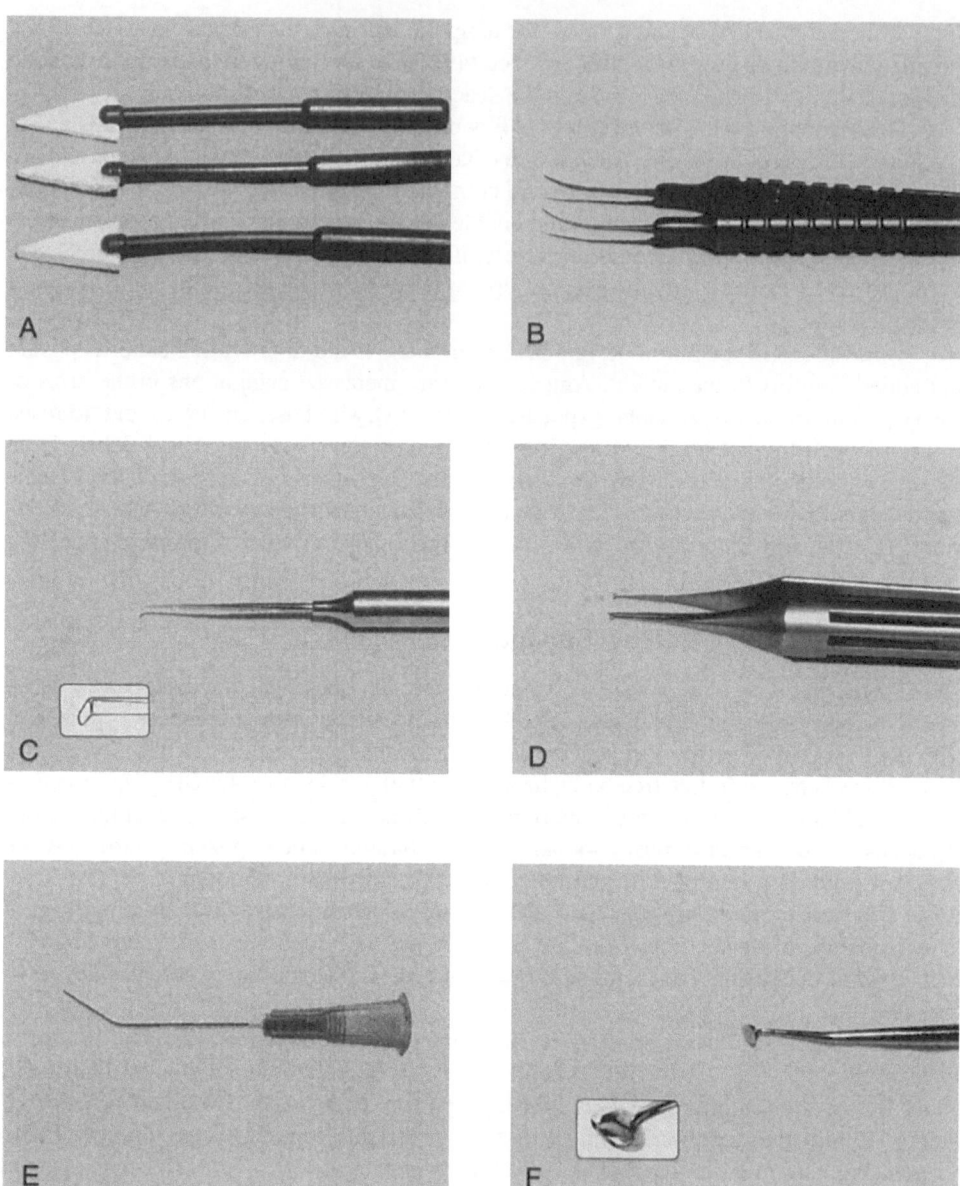

Figure 5.10 (A) A Merocel sponge is used to wipe off any blood from the exposed stromal bed and to sweep the flap during repositioning. (B) A nontoothed forceps is used to lift the flap. (C) A Machat retreatment spatula and a jeweler's forceps are used to locate the interface plane and dissect the flap edge. (D) A Fechtner conjunctival ring forcep is used to grasp the flap edge and lift the flap. The same nontoothed forceps can be used to reposition the flap. (E) An irrigating cannula is used to hydrate the stroma after ablation and to float the flap and avoid wrinkles. Illustrated is a straight disposable cannula. Several surgeons prefer curved cannulae (to conform to the curvature of the corneal stromal bed). (F) A Pineda iron is helpful to iron flap wrinkles especially during LASIK retreatment procedures.

(Devon Skin Markers, Graphic Controls, Buffalo, NY). The marking pen is also useful when placing marks on the flap edge prior to lifting during retreatments.

5. Flap Forceps and Spatulae

Forceps are used to elevate and flip over the flap before and after laser ablation. This can be achieved without grasping the flap, thereby avoiding any unnecessary trauma (Fig. 5.10B). Virtually any design, whether angled or curved, with or without a tying platform, can be used, since the ends preferably remain apposed during flap manipulation. Spatulas are as efficient as forceps in lifting and manipulating the LASIK flap with minimal trauma.

For retreatment purposes, the Machat LASIK retreatment spatula (ASICO) has a semisharp angulated tip at one end to lift the LASIK flap edge (Fig. 5.10C). The short, fine tip on the other end can be used for dissection along the Bowman's layer without excessive insertion of the instrument underneath the flap. We have found that an ordinary jeweler's forcep can be as effective in dissecting the flap edge and locating the interface plane. For peeling and lifting the flap, we use a Fechtner conjunctival ring forcep (Moria), which gives the surgeon a firm grasp of the flap during this maneuver but does not cause perforation or tearing of tissue even when a gentle pulling force is exerted (Fig. 5.10D).

6. Irrigating Cannulae

An irrigating cannula is used to irrigate under the flap, wash out any interface debris, and float the flap into the correct position. The diameter of the cannula can range from gauge 26 to 30 and the length and angulation can be variable depending on the designer and manufacturer (Fig. 5.10E). Some cannulas have spatulated or flattened tips to allow for easy insertion underneath the LASIK flap. Other innovations are side ports or multiple openings for diffuse irrigation and effective floating of the flap. Examples of specialized cannulas are the 26 gauge Slade cannula (ASICO) with a spatulated tip, the 25 gauge Buratto cannula (ASICO), and the Kritzinger needle (Storz). Our preference is a 22 mm 30 gauge Rycroft anterior chamber cannula (Becton Dickinson and Co., Franklin Lakes, NJ), which provides easy insertion into the flap interface and gentle controlled irrigation (Fig. 5.10E). Excessive irrigation should be avoided because it can cause delayed flap adherence and stromal hydration.

7. Intraoperative Tonometry and Pachymetry

To create a smooth flap with suitable thickness, it is believed that the suction ring should increase the intraocular pressure to at least 65 mmHg. To ensure that this is consistently achieved, the pressure needs to be checked prior to advancing the microkeratome to resect the flap. The Barraquer applanation tonometer is a popular instrument that has been used to evaluate the intraocular pressure (50). The design of this instrument is an inverted methacrylate cone. It weighs approximately 10 grams and is calibrated according to Maklakov's principle with the Posner scale. The superior surface is convex, with a radius of 22.15 mm to magnify the image obtained on the lower portion, which is flat and has a thin circular sulcus. When the eye pressure reaches 65 mmHg, the 10 gram tonometer flattens a circular area 3.8 mm in diameter corresponding to the diameter of the circular mire engraved on the applanation surface. An applanated area smaller than the mire on the tonometer indicates a pressure of at least 65 mmHg, which is adequate for flap resection. If the applanated area is larger than the mire, reflecting an intraocular pressure of less than 65 mmHg, the suction should be discontinued, the tonometer checked to ensure dryness to avoid false readings, and the ring reapplied. If the readings are still inadequate, the procedure should be aborted and all the instruments checked.

The pneumatonometer (Model 30 Classic, Medtronic, Jacksonville, FL) is an alternative, easy-to-use instrument with tonometry functions (Fig. 5.8; also see Fig 12.3.C). It utilizes a pneumatic sensor, consisting of a piston floating on an air bearing, that is touched to the anesthetized cornea. A precisely regulated flow of filtered air from an internal pump enters the piston. A small 5 mm fenestrated membrane (soft silicone tip) at the end of the piston reacts both to the force of the air blowing through it and to the force represented by the pressure behind the cornea, against which it is pressed. The balance between these two forces represents the intraocular pressure, and it is displayed on the screen. The system records pressures in the range of 5 to 80 mmHg. The pneumatonometer allows us to evaluate the adequacy of suction by displaying real-time readings of the progressive rise in intraocular pressure. Should the steady rise of pressure falter, the suction can be discontinued and reapplied right away. There is also no added variable of maintaining a dry cornea, which could give false readings.

In order to avoid excessive laser ablation and subsequent corneal ectasia, the use of intraoperative ultrasound or optical pachymetry is increasing in patients with high myopia or thin corneas (Fig. 5.7). See chapter 10 for details.

8. Iron and Scrapers

Irons are used to exert localized pressure on the corneal surface and flatten folds or wrinkles on the flap interface. The basic design consists of a smooth metallic stump with a flat surface and rounded edges. A scraper is an instrument with sharpened edges developed to remove corneal epithelium mechanically. It is used in conjunction with an iron, since it is believed that if the epithelium above the wrinkle is not scraped and removed, it will not allow horizontal expansion and flattening of the area where the wrinkle is localized. Examples of irons are the Pineda LASIK Iron (Fig. 5.10F) and the Herzig LASIK Depressor (ASICO).

REFERENCES

1. F Ricci, C Cedrone, L Cerulli. Standardized measurement of visual acuity. Ophthalmic Epid 1998;5:41–53.
2. IL Bailey, JE Lovie. New design principles for visual acuity letter charts. Am J Optom Phys Opt 1976;53:740–744.
3. JB Sprague, LA Stock, J Connett, J Bromberg. Study of chart designs and optotypes for preschool vision screening—I. Comparability of chart designs. J Pedia Ophthalmol Strab 1989;26:189–197.
4. G Strong, GC Woo. A distance visual acuity chart incorporating some new design features. Arch Ophthalmol 1985;103:44–46.
5. LL Sloan. Needs for precise measurements of acuity. Arch Ophthalmol 1980;98:286–290.
6. B McAllister. Two distance acuity charts for the partially sighted. J Vis Rehab 1987;1:27–32.
7. FL Ferris III, A Kassoff, GH Bresnick, I Bailey. New visual acuity charts for clinical research. Am J Ophthalmol 1982;94:91–96.
8. Macular Photocoagulation Study Group. Argon laser photocoagulation for neovascular maculopathy: three year results from randomized clinical trials. Arch Ophthalmol 1986;104: 694–701.

9. GO Waring, SD Moffitt, H Gelender. Rationale for a new design of the National Eye Institute Prospective Evaluation of Radial Keratotomy (PERK) study. Ophthalmology 1983;90:40–58.

10. A Arditi, R Cagenello. On the statistical reliability of letter-chart visual acuity measurements. Invest Ophthalmol Vis Sci 1993;34:120–129.

11. IL Bailey, JE Lovie. The design and use of a new near-vision chart. Am J Optom Phys Opt 1980;57:378–387.

12. JS Wolffsohn, AL Cochrane. The practical near acuity chart (PNAC) and prediction of visual ability at near. Ophthal Physiol Opt 2000;20:90–97.

13. ICJ Wood. A review of autorefractors. Eye 1987;1:529–535.

14. W Wesemann, B Dick. Accuracy and accommodation capability of a handheld autorefractor. J Cataract Refract Surg 2000;26:62–70.

15. S Ghose, BK Nayak, JP Singh. Critical evaluation of the NR-1000F autorefractometer. Br J Ophthalmol 1986;70:221–226.

16. DA Goss, T Grosvenor. Reliability of refraction—a literature review. J Am Optom Assoc 1996; 67:619–630.

17. EJ Cohen, MW Belin, MJ Mannis. Corneal topography. Ophthalmology 1999;106:1628–1638.

18. DT Azar, M Salvat, A Benson. Curr Opin Ophthalmol 1996;7:83–93.

19. PS Binder. Videokeratography. CLAO J 1995;21:133–144.

20. B Seitz, A Behrens, A Langenbucher. Corneal topography. Curr Opin Ophthalmol 1997;8:8–24.

21. GW Tate, A Safir, CZ Mills, JE Bowling, JL McDonald, MR Craig. Accuracy and reproducibility of keratometry readings. CLAO J 1987;13:50–58.

22. FW Lusby, JW Franke, JM McCaffery. Clinical comparison of manual and automated keratometry in a geriatric population. CLAO J 1987;13:119–121.

23. PS Binder. Measurement of corneal curvature after corneal transplantation and radial keratotomy using standard and automated keratometry. CLAO J 1989;15:201–205.

24. S Nakada, M Tanaka, A Nakajima. Comparison of automated and conventional keratometers. Am J Ophthalmol 1984;97:776–778.

25. VN Jarvis, R Levine, PA Asbell. Manual vs. automated keratometry: a comparison. CLAO J 1987;13:235–237.

26. DR Sanders, JP Gills, RG Martin. When keratometric measurements do not accurately reflect corneal topography. J Cataract Refract Surg 1993;19:131–135.

27. MW Belin, JL Cambier, JR Nabors, CD Ratcliff. PAR corneal topography system (PAR CTS): the clinical application of close range photogrammetry. Optom Vis Sci 1995;72:828–837.

28. D Priest, R Munger. Comparative study of the elevation topography of complex shapes. J Cataract Refract Surg 1998;24:741–750.

29. Z Liu, AJ Huang, SC Pflugfelder. Evaluation of corneal thickness and topography in normal eyes using the Orbscan corneal topography system. Br J Ophthalmol 1999;83:774–778.

30. SB Hannush, SL Crawford, GO Waring III, MC Gemmill, MJ Lynn, A Nizam. Reproducibility of normal corneal power measurements with a keratometer, photokeratoscope, and video imaging system. Arch Ophthalmol 1990;108:539–544.

31. RC Moura, BL Bowyer, S Stevens, JJ Rowsey. Comparison of three computerized videokeratoscopy systems with keratometry. Cornea 1998;17:522–528.

32. M Jeandervin, J Barr. Comparison of repeat videokeratography: repeatability and accuracy. Optom Vis Sci 1998;75:663–669.

33. SE Wilson, SM Verity, DL Conger. Accuracy and precision of the Corneal Analysis System and the Topographic Modeling System. Cornea 1992;11:28–35.

34. DG Tennen, RH Keates, C Montoya. Comparison of three keratometry instruments. J Cataract Refract Surg 1995;21:407–408.

35. RL Schultze. Accuracy of corneal elevation with four corneal topography systems. J Refract Surg 1998;12:100–104.

36. PA Bloom, D Papakostopoulos, Y Gogolitsyn, JA Leenderz, S Papakostopoulos, RH Grey. Clinical and infrared pupillometry in central retinal vein occlusion. Br J Ophthalmol 1993; 77:75–80.

37. BS Wachler, RR Krueger. Agreement and repeatability of infrared pupillometry and the comparison method. Ophthalmology 1999;106:319–323.

38. M Colvard. Preoperative measurement of scotopic pupil dilation using an office pupillometer. J Cataract Refract Surg 1998;24:1594–1597.

39. EM Schnitzler, M Baumeister, T Kohnen. Scotopic measurement of normal pupils: Colvard versus Video Vision Analyzer infrared pupillometer. J Cataract Refract Surg 2000;26:859–866.

40. FW Price, DL Koller, MO Price. Central corneal pachymetry in patients undergoing laser in situ keratomileusis. Ophthalmology 1999;106:2216–2220.

41. AC Snyder. Optical pachometry measurements: reliability and variability. Am J Optom Physiol Opt 1984;61:408–413.

42. RB Mandell, KA Polse. Keratoconus: spatial variation of corneal thickness as a diagnostic test. Arch Ophthalmol 1969;82:182–188.

43. PS Binder, JA Kohler, DA Rorabaugh. Evaluation of an electronic pachometer. Invest Ophthalmol Vis Sci 1977;16:855–858.

44. C Giasson, D Forthomme. Comparison of central corneal thickness measurements between optical and ultrasound pachymeters. Optom Vis Sci 1992;69:236–241.

45. JJ Salz, SP Azen, J Berstein, P Caroline, RA Villasenor, DJ Schanzlin. Evaluation and comparison of sources of variability in the measurement of corneal thickness with ultrasonic and optical pachymeters. Ophthalmic Surg 1983;14:750–754.

46. S Mishima, BO Hebdys. Measurement of corneal thickness with the Haag Streit pachymeter. Arch Ophthalmol 1981;80:710–713.

47. DZ Coleman, FL Lizzi, RL Jack. Ultrasonography of the eye and orbit. Philadelphia: Lea and Febiger, 1977, pp 113–114.

48. V Yaylali, SC Kaufman, HW Thompson. Corneal thickness measurements with the Orbscan Topography System and ultrasonic pachymetry. J Cataract Refract Surg 1997;23:1345–1350.

49. LE Probst. LASIK instrumentation. In: J Machat, S Glade, L Probst, eds. The Art of LASIK. Thorofare, NJ: Slack, 1999, pp 73–78.

50. L Buratto, S Brint, M Ferrari. Surgical instruments. In: L Buratto, SF Brint, eds. LASIK principles and techniques. Thorofare, NJ: Slack, 1998, pp 35–68.

6

LASIK Indications, Contraindications, and Preoperative Evaluation

RICHARD E. BRAUNSTEIN and MARC WINNICK

*Columbia University College of Physicians and Surgeons,
Harkness Eye Institute, New York, New York, U.S.A.*

KENNETH A. GREENBERG

*Columbia University College of Physicians and Surgeons, New York,
New York, U.S.A.*

A. INTRODUCTION

Corneal refractive procedures are currently widely applied to correct ametropia. A successful refractive procedure is gauged by many criteria: safety, efficacy, predictability, and long-term stability. Laser-assisted in-situ keratomileusis (LASIK) is presently the most widely performed refractive procedure, but it is not appropriate for all patients. Optimal results are achieved through proper patient selection, education, examination, and consent. A complete understanding of the risks of the procedure and the effects of pre-existing ocular conditions are critical in selecting patients for surgery. The ability to recognize subtle ocular conditions through careful patient examination will reduce the likelihood of complications. Finally, helping patients have realistic expectations and the ability to say no to patients who clearly are poor surgical candidates are the keys to building a successful LASIK practice. This chapter will outline the present refractive indications for LASIK with special attention given to the preoperative evaluation and patient preparation prior to refractive surgery. Clinical tips for maximizing refractive outcomes and contraindications to LASIK will be discussed.

B. INDICATIONS

Laser in situ keratomilieusis may be considered for patients who are dependent on optical correction of various refractive errors who desire to reduce or eliminate their dependence on glasses or contact lenses. In the United States, FDA approval for LASIK is a confusing issue for surgeons and patients alike. The FDA does not approve procedures, it only approves drugs and devices. How those drugs and devices are used after approval is up to physicians under a provision known as the practice of medicine. The FDA labels the devices and drugs according to the information provided by the developers and serves as a guide for their use. The specific approval guidelines for LASIK are different for each excimer laser manufacturer based on data from FDA clinical trials. The approval range of refractive errors is only one criterion of judging a prospective candidate, as patients who fall within the guidelines may not qualify for surgery owing to other conditions (e.g., thin cornea or flat cornea).

The excimer laser is currently approved for a wide range of myopia, myopic astigmatism, and hyperopia. Many studies indicate that the predictability of LASIK decreases with increasing preoperative myopia and astigmatism (1). Hyperopia ranging up to 6 diopters is correctible, but at higher levels of attempted correction, predictability is again reduced (2). For hyperopia greater than 6 diopters, loss of spectacle-corrected visual acuity occurred in a significant number of eyes in some studies, and accuracy was sufficiently poor to advise against LASIK in these eyes (3). Approval for treatment of hyperopic astigmatism and mixed astigmatism is expected in the near future.

C. CONTRAINDICATIONS

Contraindications for LASIK include patients with systemic collagen vascular disease, immunodeficiency, autoimmune disease, severe atopy, and diabetes mellitus, diseases all likely to affect corneal wound healing. Patients who have unstable refractive errors or significant pre-existing ocular pathology of the cornea or anterior segment including but not limited to scarring, severe dry eye syndrome, uncontrolled blepharitis, uveitis, or early cataract should also not have laser vision correction. Surgery should not be performed on women who are pregnant or nursing or on patients taking Amiodarone or Acutane. LASIK is contraindicated in eyes with a history of herpes simplex keratitis or herpes zoster ophthalmicus. Special concern should be given to eyes with corneal neovascularization within 1 mm of the ablation zone and those patients with difficult anatomy including small orbital aperture, narrow interpalpebral fissure or deep-set eyes. Patients with keratoconus or keratoconus suspects should not have LASIK surgery. Finally, patients with signs of anterior basement membrane dystrophy may be better served with photorefractive keratectomy (surface ablation) rather than LASIK, as the likelihood of an intraoperative epithelial defect may create numerous postoperative management difficulties.

The cornea should not be flattened to less than 33 D or steepened to greater than 52 D, as refractive outcomes in this range are less predictable (4). To determine the postoperative corneal curvature, the preoperative keratometry is reduced or increased by the amount of desired correction at the corneal plane. All candidates for LASIK procedures should have a stable refraction for at least 12 months prior to the procedure differing by no more than 0.50 diopter in manifest sphere or manifest cylinder. For hyperopic patients, manifest and cycloplegic refraction should not differ more than 0.75 diopter.

D. IATROGENIC KERATECTASIA

LASIK alters both the shape and the structural integrity of the cornea. Preoperative evaluation involves determining what the resultant corneal curvature and residual stromal thickness will be, prior to proceeding with surgery. Preoperative corneal thickness is of particular concern in preventing iatrogenic keratectasia. Post LASIK keratectasia results in a progressive central corneal steepening and myopic shift causing irreversible damage by one year. It occurs in approximately 1 in 1000 eyes (5). Preoperative assessment of corneal thickness, flap and resultant stromal bed thickness, and amount of desired ablation are essential to prevent such ectasias. The average thickness of the human cornea is 520 microns, and an average flap created by a microkeratome is from 130 to 160 microns. The keratectomy depth of the excimer laser ablation on average must not exceed 45 to 120 microns with 325 (conservative case) to 250 microns, respectively, left in the stromal bed (6). This sparks questions regarding the minimal thickness of residual stroma, which needs to be maintained to prevent keratectasia. Many LASIK surgeons currently employ a 250 micron limit to the residual stromal bed following LASIK, but this is only an average value, and the biomechanical constants of the human cornea vary over a wide range, so that the range of residual corneal thickness that would prevent keratectasia is unknown. Some advocate using a percentage of the corneal thickness as a minimal residual stromal thickness rather than an absolute number, given ultrasound pachymetry measurement errors and biomechanical considerations, such as the deeper stroma having less tensile strength compared to the anterior layers (6). This dilemma can ultimately be resolved when we are better equipped to measure the biomechanical constants of the cornea in vivo. Promising approaches such as mechanical spectroscopy and measurement of birefringence of the cornea can assist in future determination of preoperative stromal bed thickness, which would be necessary to avoid iatrogenic keratectasia. The residual stromal bed following a LASIK procedure should be calculated prior to surgery based on a nonnomogram adjusted treatment of the refractive error to be corrected.

E. THE CONSULTATION VISIT

Preoperatively, each patient must have a complete evaluation including a medical, surgical, and ocular history as well as an ocular examination. A general medical history with emphasis on the above-mentioned systemic diseases should be discussed and a medication list obtained. Past ocular surgery and any previous or existing ophthalmic conditions, such as glaucoma, dry eye, amblyopia, and past contact lens use, should be reviewed.

An initial preoperative evaluation for LASIK in contact lens wearers should be performed at least two weeks after discontinuation of soft contact lenses or at least three weeks after discontinuation of soft toric, hard, or rigid gas permeable lenses. Patients wearing rigid lenses must demonstrate keratometric and refractive stability prior to treatment. It may be necessary to discontinue contact lenses in these patients at least one month for every decade of contact lens use. Previous glasses and contact lens prescriptions should be compared to the manifest refraction.

F. VISUAL ACUITY AND REFRACTION

Uncorrected and best corrected visual acuity should be assessed. A careful refraction is critical to maximizing refractive surgery outcomes. Different refraction techniques are applicable to different refractive errors. When refracting the myope, a resolution-based refraction should be performed to avoid overcorrections. A resolution-based end point involves using the least minus lens to visualize the most letters. The refraction is not terminated at 20/20 if an additional 0.25 diopters yields several letters on the 20/15 line. The Jackson Cross cylinder is used to determine the maximal amount of cylinder. The correct axis of the cylinder is easier to determine in eyes with higher degrees of astigmatism. Occasionally, autorefraction may be helpful in finding the astigmatic axis. Care should be taken to ensure that the trial lens frame or phoropter is appropriately positioned and level to define the axis most accurately.

Hyperopic manifest refraction should emphasize a "push plus" technique. Patients are encouraged to accept the most plus sphere to see the most letters. Cycloplegic refraction with 1% cyclopentolate should be performed on all patients because it eliminates accommodation. This is essential to identify the overminused myope and to uncover latent hyperopia. For patients with hyperopia, manifest and cycloplegic examination should differ by 0.75 diopter or less. If a large amount of latent hyperopia is identified or if there is a significant discrepancy between the manifest and cycloplegic refraction in a myope, a post cycloplegic manifest refraction should be performed with an emphasis on pushing additional plus power. Occasionally, glasses may be prescribed temporarily to help the patient accept the additional plus power prior to performing surgical correction.

A clinical workup should include manual keratometry, a pupillary examination, and a slit lamp examination with emphasis on any lid margin inflammation, corneal epithelial disease, basement membrane dystrophy, or stromal scars consistent with prior keratitis. Tonometry should be performed on all patients and gonioscopic examination on all hyperopes. Central corneal pachymetry readings should be performed on all patients. A careful, dilated fundus examination is performed to analyze the optic nerve and retina for any pathology with careful attention to the peripheral retina in highly myopic eyes that may be at risk for lattice degeneration. Identified retinal tears or large areas of lattice may require laser photocoagulation prior to performing LASIK (7).

Special attention should be given to the pupillary examination in myopic and particularly astigmatic patients. Pupil size should be measured in dim and in bright lighting conditions and recorded. Measurement can be made with a pupil gauge or with an infrared pupillometer. Patients with higher degrees of refractive error and larger pupils may be at greater risk for postoperative night vision disturbances, although this remains a subject of great controversy (3).

G. CORNEAL TOPOGRAPHY

Corneal topography is essential in all patients prior to refractive surgery. Topography is used to identify patients with corneal curvature abnormalities that are not apparent on slit lamp examination. True keratoconus is often easy to detect by clinical history and examination, but subclinical cases may only be apparent by corneal topography. Corneal topography is necessary to determine whether patients have contact lens related warpage and to help determine when a cornea is stable following contact lens discontinuation. We recommend that any patient who wears contact lenses have corneal topography repeated 1 week apart to ascertain stability prior to surgery. Topography is also used to verify postoperative results and complications such as decentrations, central islands, and irregular astigmatism.

H. DISCUSSION OF SPECIFIC CONDITIONS

1. The Keratoconus Suspect

Keratoconus is a noninflammatory bilateral corneal ectasia that produces irregular astigmatism and leads to marked refractive error. Clinical signs differ depending on the severity of the disease. External signs include Munson's sign and the Rizzuti phenomenon. Slit lamp findings include a Fleischer's ring, Vogt's striae, stromal thinning and scarring, prominent corneal nerves, and epithelial nebulae. Retroillumination signs include scissoring on retinoscopy, which is often the first evidence of early keratoconus, and an oil droplet sign. Early in the disease, many corneas appear normal on slip lamp biomicroscopy. Several devices are currently available for detecting early keratoconus. Simple, inexpensive devices such as a handheld keratoscope can show egg-shaped or inferocentral compression of mires, which may be indicative of early keratoconus. Ultrasonic pachymetry to demonstrate central and peripheral corneal thickness has been studied, and although it is highly accurate and reproducible for measuring corneal thickness, its use has failed to identify a large percentage of patients with clinically obvious keratoconus, and it should only be used as corroborative evidence for the diagnosis of keratoconus (8).

Computer-assisted videokeratoscopes, which generate color-coded maps and topographic indices, are an excellent tool for the diagnosis of keratoconus even when signs of the disease are not obviously apparent at the slit lamp. Three features of keratoconus are common to video keratography; a localized area of increased surface power, inferior–superior power asymmetry, and skewed steep radial axes above and below the horizontal meridian depicting irregular astigmatism. Much work has been done to quantify the minimal topographic criteria for diagnosing keratoconus. One method is pattern recognition and one specific topographic pattern, asymmetic bow tie with skewing of the radial axis above and below the horizontal meridian, was found by Rabinowitz in virtually 100% of patients with clinical keratoconus. This pattern could represent the earliest sign of irregular astigmatism and might be a reasonable cutoff point in the transition from normal topography to keratoconus (9). The second method, the use of quantitative videokeratography derived indices, may represent a more reproducible way to quantify keratoconus and its early phenotypes. Maeda and coauthors devised an expert system classifier, utilizing an analysis of eight topographic indices derived from the TMS videokeratoscope. A linear determinant function is used to determine a composite discriminant value for each map: the KPI. A KPI value greater than the optimum cutoff is classified as keratoconus (10). Rabinowitz described a KISA% index, a quantitative videokeratographic algorithm embodying minimal topographic criteria for diagnosing keratoconus. Using a combination of four indices: central K, an expression of central corneal steepening; the I-S value, an expression of inferior–superior dioptric asymmetry; the AST index, which quantifies the degree of regular corneal astigmatism; and the SRAX index, the skewed radial axial index, the KISA index is derived. Kisa% = K × I-S × AST × SRAX × 100 (11). This has been shown to have excellent preliminary clinical correlation and can be used by surgeons to determine a patient's chance of having early keratoconus. A single index with excellent clinical correlation would be optimal to depict early keratoconus and warn a refractive surgeon of potential intra- and postoperative risks and complications. The formulation of these indices are still being altered to improve accuracy and at present should be used with appropriate clinical correlation including slit lamp biomicroscopy, pachymetry, retinoscopy, and keratometry to determine the relative risk of laser refractive surgery. Patients with keratoconus or those who are likely keratoconus suspects are not candidates for LASIK using present algorithms and treatment profiles and should be considered to have a progressive corneal disease. Patients with asymmetric bow tie astigmatism and inferior steepening who do not appear to have keratoconus may be treated surgically with appropriate informed consent.

2. The Incipient Cataract

The incipient cataract patient requires special consideration. Cataract extraction should be viewed as both a media clearing surgery and a refractive surgery. Progression of central visual axis opacity will decrease the best corrected visual acuity post laser and result in a patient unhappy with LASIK and in need of a second surgical procedure. It is therefore recommended that the best corrected visual acuity be assessed preoperatively and the effect of the incipient cataract on visual acuity be determined. If it is believed that the cataract is significant or is progressing rapidly, laser vision correction should not be performed, and consideration may be given to cataract surgery, if appropriate. Although phacoemulsification can be performed on an eye that has had LASIK, the intraocular lens power calculation can be problematic, and a more reliable refractive outcome may be achieved with lens extraction and intraocular lens implantation (12).

3. The Dry Eye Patient

Patients with a history of dry eye symptoms and contact lens intolerance frequently seek laser vision correction. Dry eye symptoms and corneal epithelial staining are common problems following LASIK. The mechanism of this disorder following surgery is not well understood, although alteration of corneal innervation following LASIK is the most likely cause. Evaluation of these patients includes assessment of tear film quality and breakup as well as corneal epithelial integrity. Patients with evidence of corneal staining should be treated preoperatively. Management may include topical lubricants, punctal occlusion, and occasionally oral doxycycline if the patient has evidence of meibomian gland dysfunction. Schirmers' testing has not been shown to be predictive of postoperative dry eye problems following LASIK.

4. The Glaucoma Suspect

If preoperative screening identifies a patient with elevated intraocular pressure or optic nerve head cupping, focal ischemia, or hemorrhage, a 24-2 Humphrey visual field is recommended, and further testing or consultation is necessary to determine if indeed the patient has glaucoma. If the patient has glaucoma, LASIK should not be performed. Patients who are glaucoma suspects by family history, borderline elevated intraocular pressure, or mild disc asymmetry must be treated cautiously. If the patient does not have glaucomatous optic neuropathy, and a diagnosis of glaucoma is considered unlikely, they may be considered for laser vision correction. However, informed consent discussing the potential reduced value to tonometry measurement must be discussed with the patient.

In general, the validity of applanation tonometry following laser vision correction is less accurate and ultimately may limit the ability to treat glaucoma in selected patients. Falsely low intraocular pressure measurements are obtained by applanation due to easy compressibility of the fluid-filled space between the corneal flap and the stromal bed and the direct relationship between corneal thickness and Goldman applanation tonometry (13). In addition, the intraoperative increase in intraocular pressure following application of the suction ring during LASIK will further decrease optic nerve head perfusion pressure and can cause additional damage to an already susceptible glaucomatous optic nerve.

5. The Presbyope

Many LASIK patients are presbyopes. Patients who already wear some reading correction are easier to counsel than patients who simply remove their glasses to read. Patients need to be informed that the procedure will not correct distance and near vision completely. An informed patient can help determine what would be best for them. Patients should be offered various options including distance vision in both eyes, monovision, or slight undercorrection of both eyes. If the patient is a successful contact lens wearer with monovision, this is likely to be the best route. If the patient does not wear lenses, a preoperative monovision contact lens trial can be used to demonstrate the effects of monovision to the candidate for refractive surgery (14). The add power and selection of the distance and near eye can also be determined with a contact lens trial.

6. The Low Myope

For peripresbyopic and presbyopic lower myopes (−1.00 through −3.50 diopters), we frequently treat the dominant eye first and postoperatively determine the correction for the nondominant eye, if any. Some patients happily tolerate large amounts of anisometropia, while others are intolerant of as little as 0.50 diopters. The refractive goal needs to be tailored to the requirements of the individual patient. Patients who spend most of their time doing near work without glasses preoperatively need to understand that correcting their distance vision will necessitate the use of reading glasses. Often, patients have a preconceived notion that surgery will allow them to throw away their glasses. Occasionally, patients misunderstand or are misinformed and are disappointed in their postoperative spectacle dependence for near work when they did not require glasses preoperatively.

7. The Very High Myope

Patients with high degrees of myopia are usually very motivated as they have greater visual disability. A preoperative evaluation in high myopes must include a careful dilated retinal examination using indirect ophthalmoscopy to search for peripheral retinal pathology as well as a careful macular exam. Preoperative retinal consultation is of value to determine if existing retinal pathology requires any treatment prior to surgery. Additionally, with higher degrees of myopia, there is an increase in the loss of BSCVA as well as reduced accuracy. Patients need appropriate preoperative counseling to help understand these risks.

8. The Hyperope

LASIK, at present, shows great promise for effective and stable correction for mild to moderate hyperopia. A gonioscopic examination should be performed prior to LASIK in all hyperopic patients and a prophylactic peripheral iridotomy may be indicated for an occludable angle. Although there is no cause and effect relation between hyperopic LASIK and acute angle closure glaucoma, patients with hyperopia and narrow angles should be followed for the possibility of angle closure at a later time (15). The ablation profile for hyperopia extends out to 9 mm requiring a large corneal flap. Patients with a history of contact lens wear and corneal neovascularization may have significant bleeding with LASIK surgery, and potential complications of bleeding should be discussed and included in the consent prior to surgery.

9. The Astigmat

A preoperative evaluation of the astigmat is essential for successful refractive surgery. Astigmatism has a directional component and a magnitude, and sources of astigmatism can be corneal or lenticular. As the magnitude of cylinder decreases, the ability to measure precisely the cylinder axis also decreases. Refractive, keratometric, and topographic cylinder occasionally do not match in axis or magnitude, but treatment is based on refractive cylinder. When disparity occurs, proceed cautiously and ascertain stability by repeating measurements over time.

I. PATIENT SELECTION

Selecting the appropriate candidate for refractive surgery requires an understanding of the patient's expectations, desires, and disposition in addition to a clinical ocular examination. A candidate must have the ability to understand the risks and benefits of LASIK and be able to give informed consent. The patient must be able to tolerate the procedure and have the ability to lie flat without difficulty, to tolerate topical anesthesia, and to fixate steadily and accurately for the duration of the procedure. Patients must be targeted toward their differing visual needs. A myope prior to laser vision correction enjoyed close and clear visual space and will be disappointed if overcorrected postoperatively. Some presbyopes desire monovision, while others would rather wear spectacle correction. Patients who demand spectacle independence all the time and have unrealistic expectations of laser vision correction should be avoided in addition to all patients with the above-mentioned systemic diseases or ocular pathology that otherwise jeopardize the efficacy, safety, and stability of LASIK.

J. LASIK CONSENT

A patient's understanding of the possible postoperative complications and adverse symptomatology is an essential component of an informed consent. Patients should be given a copy of the FDA brochure provided from the excimer laser manufacturer citing the results of clinical trials using the specific laser. Additional statistics may be provided regarding the doctor's own data and experience.

A detailed informed consent document is often helpful in highlighting many of the known side effects and complications of LASIK surgery. Undercorrection, overcorrection, and induced astigmatism and the possibility of additional surgery should be discussed. Complications that could lead to a loss of best corrected visual acuity include but are not limited to irregular flaps, irregular astigmatism, haze, scarring, infection, central islands, striae, and epithelial ingrowth; these must be explained to the patient in a manner that they can understand. Many patients do not appreciate that they do risk a loss in best corrected visual acuity and possibly blindness due to an infection or retinal vascular event. Patients who require excellent night vision (e.g., truck drivers) should be cautioned prior to LASIK surgery regarding their risk of night vision impairment. Night vision impairment has been reported by Guell and Muller in 23% of patients at 6 months postoperatively, and other reports of night halos occurred in up to 30% of eyes at 6 months (16). Halos around lights and night vision impairment appear to decrease with larger ablation zones and smaller pupil size and often improve with time (17). Finally, patients should be advised of the possibility of dry eye symptoms, which may affect vision following laser vision correction. Prior to surgery, the patient should be given an opportunity to read all of the materials provided and to have all of their questions answered by their surgeon.

REFERENCES

1. T Salah, GO Waring III, A El-Maghraby, K Moadel, SB Grimm. Excimer laser in situ keratomileusis under a corneal flap for myopia of 2 to 20 diopters. Am J Ophthalmol 1996;121: 143–155.
2. S Esquenazi, A Mendoza. Two year follow-up of laser in situ keratomileusis for hyperopia. J Refract Surg 1999;15:648–652.
3. MC Arbelaez, MC Knorz. Laser in situ keratomileusis for hyperopia and hyperopic astigmatism. J Refract Surg 1999;15:406–414.
4. DJ Salchow, ME Zirm, C Stieldorf, A Parisi. Comparison of objective and subjective refraction before and after laser in situ keratomileusis. J Cataract Refract Surg 1999;25:827–835.
5. T Seiler. Iatrogenic keratectasia: academic anxiety or serious risk? J Cataract Refract Surg 1999;25:1307–1308.
6. T Seiler, K Koufala, G Richter. Iatrogenic keratectasia after laser in situ keratomileusis. J Refract Surg 1998;14:312–317.
7. TP Werblin. Barraquer Lecture 1998. Why should refractive surgeons be looking beyond the cornea? J Refract Surg 1999;15:357–376.
8. YS Rabinowitz, K Rasheed, H Yang, J Elashoff. Accuracy of ultrasonic pachymetry and videokeratography in detecting keratoconus. J Cataract Refract Surg 1998;24:196–201.
9. YS Rabinowitz. Keratoconus. Surv Ophthalmol 1998;42:297–319.
10. N Maeda, SD Klyce, MK Smolek. Comparison of methods for detecting keratoconus using videokeratography. Arch Ophthalmol 1995;113(7):870–874.
11. YS Rabinowitz, K Rasheed. KISA% index: a quantitative videokeratography algorithm embodying minimal topographic criteria for diagnosing keratoconus. J Cataract Refract Surg 1999;25:1327–1335.
12. B Seitz, A Langenbucher. Intraocular lens calculations status after corneal refractive surgery. Curr Opin Ophthalmol 2000;11:35–46.
13. J Najman-Vainer, RJ Smith, RK Maloney. Interface fluid after LASIK: misleading tonometry can lead to end-stage glaucoma. J Cataract Refract Surg 2000;26:471–472.
14. MM Hom. Monovision and LASIK. J Am Optom Assoc 1999;70:117–122.
15. M Paciuc, CF Velasco, R Naranjo. Acute angle closure glaucoma after hyperopic laser in situ keratomileusis. J Cataract Refract Surg 2000;26:620–623.
16. JL Guell, A Muller. Laser in situ keratomileusis (LASIK) for myopia from −7 to −18 diopters. J Refract Surg 1996;12:222–228.
17. SG Farah, DT Azar, C Gurdal, J Wong. Laser in situ keratomileusis: literature review of a developing technique. J Cataract Refract Surg 1998;24:989–1006.

Preoperative Optical Considerations in LASIK

Refractive Errors, Monovision, and Contrast Sensitivity

BALAMURALI K. AMBATI

Massachusetts Eye and Ear Infirmary and Harvard Medical School, Boston, Massachusetts, U.S.A.

LEON STRAUSS

The Wilmer Eye Institute, Johns Hopkins University School of Medicine, Baltimore, Maryland, U.S.A.

DIMITRI T. AZAR

Massachusetts Eye and Ear Infirmary, Schepens Eye Research Institute, and Harvard Medical School, Boston, Massachusetts, U.S.A.

Preoperative optical considerations in LASIK have gained increased importance, for they allow interpretation and anticipation of postoperative aberrations and provide a basis for patient education prior to surgery. This chapter will focus on refractive error evaluation, monovision, and contrast sensitivity. Subsequent chapters will cover the topics of corneal topography, wavefront analysis, and corneal biomechanics.

A. REFRACTIVE ERRORS

Emmetropic eyes focus parallel rays from an object point at optical infinity to a point on the retina. The secondary focal point of such an eye is on the retina, and the far point plane is at optical infinity. Myopic eyes focus parallel rays anterior to the retina. Thus the focal point of the eye is in the vitreous, and the far point of the eye is located between the eye and optical infinity (1). Hyperopic eyes have insufficient power without accommodation to focus parallel rays of light on the retina; accommodation may produce enough plus power to bring parallel or even diverging rays to focus on the retina. Astigmatism is due to asymmetry usually of the cornea and sometimes of the lens. Regular astigmatism is correctable with a spherocylindrical lens, whereas irregular astigmatism is not correctable with such a lens. Regular astigmatism is called with the rule when the steepest (most refracting) meridian lies near 90 degrees. It is termed against the rule when the steepest meridian lies near 180 degrees. When regular astigmatism is neither with nor against the rule, it is termed oblique.

1. Spectacle-Correction of Ametropias

Spectacle lenses placed in front of the eye must have their focal point coinciding with the far point of the eye, so that parallel rays are focused onto the retina. Drawbacks of this system include image distortion, prism effects, anisometropic effects, and field tilt. Minus lenses minify images by approximately 2% per diopter, while plus lenses magnify the image but create a peripheral scotoma between what is viewed inside and outside the spectacle frame. Astigmatic correction produces meridional minification or magnification, distorting the image. Off-axis viewing and lens tilt alter the effective spherocylindrical power of the lens, while viewing away from the center of the lens produces prism, leading to the well-known pincushion and barrel distortions of hyperopic and myopic lenses, respectively. Disparity between astigmatic correction of the two eyes produces a perceived tilt of the object. This can be minimized by decreasing the cylinder power and/or rotating the axis of the cylinder, albeit at the expense of clarity. All of these effects are heightened in higher power lenses.

B. PREOPERATIVE CONSIDERATIONS

What should the refractive surgeon aim for in patients whose spectacle usage has entailed such compromises? The surgeon should still aim for full correction of astigmatism, as correction at the cornea minimizes distortion effects. Further, surgery may relieve distortion due to anisometropia. Indeed, patients who are undercorrected with surgery often report double images not eliminated by monocular patching and other distortion effects not due to meridional magnification. Some patients who have adapted to spectacle distortion and tilt may take some time to readapt their binocular spatial sense and appreciate the lack of optical distortion. Refractive surgery in the myope, by removing the minification of the spectacle lens, produces a larger retinal image of objects, improving visual acuity even when clarity, i.e., optic resolving power, is the same or decreased.

For the same reason that a presbyopic myope has a more remote near point when wearing contact lenses than when wearing glasses, refractive surgery giving full correction of myopia may make reading without reading glasses more difficult than it was with glasses before surgery.

1. Contact Lens Wear

Preoperative evaluation for refractive surgery is influenced by several considerations. Contact lens wearers should discontinue soft contacts for at least 3 days and rigid lenses for at least 3 weeks so that the cornea can assume its natural shape prior to evaluation. Vertex distance considerations become significant for refractive error over approximately 5 D; vertex distance should be measured from the rear surface of a corrective lens to calculate the refractive power at the cornea.

2. High Myopia

In patients with unilateral high myopia, placement of a corrective contact lens allows a pre-operative prediction of the degree of aniseikonia they may experience after refractive surgery. Patients with bilateral high myopia should be appraised of the possibility of disturbing aniseikonia after one eye has undergone surgery before the other eye: the possibility of unequal photoreceptor spacing is considered in cases of high refractive errors, in which case aniseikonia testing should be performed.

3. Cycloplegic Refraction

Cycloplegic refraction allows the examiner to discern the degree of myopia in the manifest refraction due to accommodative tone; however, pupil dilation leads to a mild myopic shift due to spherical aberration of the lens. Cycloplegic refractions of hyperopes enables the determination of latent, manifest, and therefore total hyperopia; the surgeon must consider that the latent portion will gradually become manifest as the patient ages.

4. Diabetes

Diabetic fluctuations in blood sugar can change lens size and curvature. Stability of refractive error is essential prior to refractive surgery. Further, diabetes is a relative contraindication to elective corneal surgery, as diabetic corneal epithelium is more prone to persistent epithelial defects, duplication of basement membrane, and recurrent erosions.

5. Pupil Size

Larger pupils allow light rays peripheral to the optical zone to be transmitted to the fovea. The Styles–Crawford effect dampens this somewhat, as photoreceptors are oriented towards reception of light passing through the central cornea.

6. Ocular Motility

Motility examination with measurements of convergence and divergence amplitudes is part of the preoperative evaluation for refractive surgery, which can increase or decrease accommodative requirements in various circumstances. As mentioned above, the myope previously corrected with spectacles will lose the near effectivity of distance-corrective minus lenses. Undercorrection of myopia with surgery relieves the demand for accommodation at near but increases the need for nonaccommodative convergence at near. Patients with low reserves of fusional divergence may become symptomatic if surgery overcorrects myopia, as the resultant hyperopia increases the demand for accommodation and attendant accomodative convergence. Thus measuring with prisms the amplitudes of convergence and divergence (far and near, and with or without accomodation) helps predict whether a change of accomodative demand may create problems of convergence or divergence insufficiency.

7. Accomodation

Accomodative amplitude with the correction mode at the cornea should be measured before surgery to plan targeting for near vision, i.e., equal correction vs. monovision, full correction vs. partial. The amplitude of accomodation can be measured several ways, e.g., the difference in diopters between the least and most spheres accepted with clear vision while gazing at a distant target. Low amplitudes may be due to medication, oculomotor nerve paresis, trauma, lack of effort, incorrect distance refraction, or accomodative spasm. Measurement of the near point while wearing myopic spectacles will overestimate the amplitude of accomodation amplitude, because of the so-called near-effectivity of the myopic spectacle lens. Correcting the same eye for emmetropia by contact lens or refractive surgery will yield a more remote near point and smaller amplitude of accomodation.

Myopes who have been "overminused" with presbyopic symptoms may become less symptomatic once the extra minus is eliminated. Determination that a patient is overminused can be performed with cycloplegia or possibly with prolonged fogging with plus lenses. If the cycloplegic manifest refraction is accepted in new glasses, surgery should be based on those values. However, it should be borne in mind that some patients who have had overcorrected myopia for years will not be able to relax completely their accomodative tone soon after surgery. The surgeon and patient must then be aware of the prospect of blurred vision in either the short or the long term.

C.   REFRACTIVE EVALUATION

Making the central cornea flatter and the peripheral cornea steeper with LASIK produces blur, which is more pronounced when the pupil is large, as it is in dim light. When the pupil dilates, the peripheral lens is also more exposed; this part of the lens has greater plus power. The clinical relevance of peripheral corneal irregularity, scars, decentration, and central corneal haze are topics of active investigation. The impact of postoperative irregular astigmatism of the central cornea on uncorrected and spectacle-corrected vision is unclear. Predictive factors for good spectacle correction remain to be identified.

1.   Astigmatism

An objective for surgical correction of astigmatism is a relatively spherical central corneal zone. The outline of this region is oval, the narrower aspect being the meridian with the maximum difference in curvature between central and peripheral cornea. When the pupil dilates, the peripheral cornea becomes more relevant, resulting in blur or monocular diplopia, especially noticeable when details vary with torsion of the eye or observed object. As these patients have a clear image from the central zone, the blurred regions of an object stand in contrast to the sharper portions: this can be more disturbing than preoperative diffuse blur.

2.   Retinoscopy

Streak retinoscopy is performed in the standard fashion with attention to the central reflex. Retinoscopy after refractive surgery may be more easily performed using minus cylinder techniques to neutralize against motion. The endpoint of retinoscopy is less influenced by the steeper peripheral cornea if the target is neutralization of any part of the against motion, generally seen first in the flattest central cornea. A novice depending on complete neutralization of against motion or any part of with motion may overcorrect patients significantly. Further, when against motion is observed, the patient is fogged and thus less likely to accomodate during retinoscopy.

During retinoscopy, skew, break, and straddling are useful to refine the axis of corrective cylinder. Skew is streak motion not paralleling the motion of the retinoscope and is helpful in patients with postoperative irregular astigmatism, when break (when the streak falls on iris, indicating imperfect alignment of the retinoscopic reflex) is not easily observed. Straddling involves observing reflexes 45 degrees on either side of the presumed axis. With motion should be observed with this technique and can be produced by adding minus sphere or moving closer to the eye.

When using plus cylinders, the correct axis is approached turning towards the thinner, brighter reflex. When using minus cylinders, the correct axis is approached by turning away from the thinner, brighter reflex. Retinoscopy after dilation may be confused due to scissoring of the reflex; this is commonly seen after refractive surgery. In this situation, one should focus on the reflex of the central three millimeters. Further, it should be remembered that off-axis retinoscopy will give a false measurement of astigmatism.

3. Confirmation of Retinoscopic Findings

Other tools used in refraction include automated refractors, wavefront analyzers, topographic maps, astigmatic dials, and stenopeic slits. In the final analysis, subjective refraction, based on these objective methods, is the most important test used for planning refractive surgery. Automated refractors have little utility after refractive surgery. Topography may be of use in detecting lenticular astigmatism, as it can be detected preoperatively by a disagreement between the axis of astigmatism found in topography and manifest refraction. The astigmatic dial is useful to determine axis and power of cylinder when retinoscopy and the Jackson cross-cylinder fail. With fogging to 20/40 acuity, the patient is asked to identify the lines that appear blackest and sharpest. The minus cylinder axis is determined by multiplying the smaller "hour" number by 30. Minus cylinder is then added until the lines are equally blurred. The stenopeic slit, essentially an elongated pinhole, can be used in manifest refraction of patients with irregular astigmatism with unhelpful retinoscopy. The patient is first refracted with spheres. The stenopeic slit is then placed in front of the eye and rotated to the position with best acuity. Sphere is again adjusted, indicating the power needed at the axis parallel to the slit. The slit is rotated 90 degrees away, and the sphere once again adjusted, providing an estimate of the power of cylindrical correction. At the conclusion of these objective methods of refraction, subjective refraction should be performed with relaxed accomodation and/or cycloplegia.

When patients still need spectacles after refractive surgery, the spectacle prescription of young patients may be overminused 0.25 or 0.40 D to blunt postoperative diurnal fluctuation and aid the patient in tasks requiring sharpest acuity. Cycloplegic refraction can be done with an aperture blocking peripheral light rays, for reasons noted above.

4. Anisometropia

During the preoperative evaluation, a discussion of the possibility of anisometropia encountered postoperatively is valuable. The management of these cases is similar to that of anisometropes in general, depending on what sensorimotor adaptations the patient has developed, the presence of amblyopia, etc. A contact lens worn in the unoperated eye can alleviate aniseikonia and spectacle-induced vertical prism effects on up and downgaze. Partial correction or a balance lens can be used in spectacle correction in cases where deep amblyopia is present or symptoms of aniseikonia and anisophoria are severe. Spectacles may be attempted in the postoperative period to protect a dominant eye when the other eye is amblyopic.

Monovision (one eye targeted for distance, the other for near) may be given without compromise when there is good vision but little stereopsis in both eyes. A preoperative trial with contact lenses can be used to predict whether significant anisophoria or aniseikonia would occur in patients after correction for monovision. In patients with high myopia, pre-existing strabismus and suppression may be present. Surgical overcorrection may lead to accommodative spasm and esodeviations. In this situation, contact lenses or enhancement surgery may correct the consecutive hyperopia.

5. Spasm of Accommodation

Convergence and accommodation issues are also encountered postoperatively. Uncorrected hyperopes, astigmatics, and overcorrected myopes can develop spasm of accommodation, causing asthenopia, headache, or blurred vision. Exophoria, stress, convergence insufficiency, iridocyclitis, and certain medications (especially anticholinesterase agents) can worsen this phenomenon. Accommodative spasm can be addressed with reading glasses, adding plus to spectacles, bifocals, or chronic cycloplegia. Subclinical convergence insufficiency may be unmasked after refractive surgery for hyperopia, as accommodation-related convergence is lessened. Spectacle-induced hyperopia usually solves this problem.

6. Optical Requirements for Near Vision

As noted above, the borderline presbyopic myope may lose the near effectivity of minus spectacles and have increased difficulty at near after refractive surgery. In general, patients are better served by choosing a lesser add to give a larger range of accommodation and to not blur middle distances. High-riding progressive adds can be useful in patients with diurnal fluctuations in refractive error. Very anisometropic patients may have unequal amplitudes of accommodation, and may need unequal adds. The more myopic eye will need less plus in its bifocal segment. Horizontal phorias can be aggravated by reading adds; trial frame evaluation is very useful in this circumstance to judge comfort of focusing and fusion. Stronger adds will minimize accommodative convergence in esophoric patients, while weaker adds will stimulate it in exophoric patients. Those with large cylindrical errors may need cross-cylinder refraction at near, as torsion of the globe can occur with convergence and downgaze. When prescribing bifocals, surgically undercorrected myopes benefit from flattop bifocal segments, which minimize image jump (as the optical center of the add is close to that of the far correction segment) and prism displacement (counterbalanced by the opposite effect of the underlying minus lens). The overcorrected myope must choose between the greater image displacement of flattop segments and the greater image jump of roundtop segments. Vertical prism effects can be minimized by slabbing off prism from the more myopic lens, lowering the optical centers of the distance correction, or using different segment types for the two eyes. These problems of off-axis viewing can be avoided by single-vision reading glasses. Options for patients with minimal amplitudes of accommodation include trifocals, progressive-add bifocals, and separate intermediate-zone glasses.

D. MONOVISION REFRACTIVE SURGERY

An often successful strategy for presbyopia is monovision, which is refractive correction of one eye for distance and the other for near. In myopes, the dominant eye is generally corrected for distance and the nondominant eye is undercorrected (2). Ideally, such a patient should see clearly at all distances, without significant functional impairment. Monovision acceptance rates for contact lens wearers usually range from 60 to 80%.

Definitions of monovision success vary. One commonly used set of criteria is adequate adaptation to 1 to 2 diopters of monocular blur after 3 weeks. The mean success rate of patients reported in 19 articles was 76% (434 out of 573 patients). Failure was due to contact lens intolerance or poor visual adaptation. If previously contact-lens intolerant patients are excluded, monovision success rates are approximately 86% (2).

There are several factors determining monovision success: ocular dominance, sighting preference, interocular blur suppression, stereo acuity, and phorias. When the dominant eye was corrected for distance, overall monovision success rate was 75% (3). These patients performed better at visual locomotor tasks requiring directional prediction (walking, driving) and also had lesser esophoric shifts at distance. Patients with alternating dominance (no sighting preference) have interocular blur suppression, another factor predictive of monovision success. Those with strong sighting preferences had reduced blur suppression, decreased binocular depth of focus (relative to others), and higher monovision failure rates; they frequently reported ghosting at near or distance (secondary images that can be distracting and sometimes affect balance) (4). After monovision correction, unsuccessful monovision patients had a mean of 50 to 62 seconds of arc less in stereopsis than successful patients (5–6). Postoperative esophoric shifts were less in successful monovision patients than in unsuccessful patients, but no differences in fusional vergence ranges have been documented. Age has yet to be shown to be a factor affecting monovision success.

Monovision affects several visual functions (7–13). Monovision correction generally produces a small reduction in high and low-contrast visual acuity, especially in conditions of low lighting (11). The average visual acuity reduction was 0.05 ± 0.02 logMAR units. The decrease in high-contrast binocular visual acuity is quite variable and worsens with larger pupils and greater astigmatic errors. Monovision has no significant effect on binocular peripheral visual acuity or visual field width (6). Contrast sensitivity is 42% less with monovision than with binocular vision (12). Thus monovision is not preferable in those whose occupations require fine, detailed work. Task performance is reduced by less than 6% in activities requiring moderate stereopsis, e.g., card-filing (13). In those with alternating dominance (no sighting preference), the binocular depth of focus is almost equal to the sum of monocular depths of focus (9). In those with strong sighting preferences, the binocular image becomes blurred as the object moves from the dominant eye's clear range to the nondominant eye's clear range, and thus the binocular depth of focus in these patients is much less than the sum of the monocular depths of focus. After 3 weeks of monovision adaptation, a significant recovery of stereo acuity occurs (8). Increasing the ocular blur increases the stereoscopic threshold. In presbyopes, the stereo acuity decreased greatly when the blur was more than $+1.75$ D. Monovision reduced secondary fusion in 10 to 20% of patients but did not affect simultaneous perception or gross stereopsis. The binocular visual stress created by monovision is thought to cause esophoric shifts. These shifts are greater when the nondominant eye is corrected for distance. Divergence and convergence ranges at distance are reduced with monovision, but reductions in fusional vergence ranges are significant only when the nondominant eye is corrected for distance. Monovision reduces the typical exophoria seen in presbyopes at near by 2.5 to 5.2 prism diopters (6). The divergence range is significantly less with monovision at near viewing, but not the convergence range.

Monovision should be avoided in patients with strong sighting preference, significant loss of stereoacuity with monocular correction, large esophoric shifts, minimal interocular suppression, or occupations requiring fine work. Patients must be informed of the reduction in visual acuity and stereopsis. Spectacle lenses may need to be prescribed for tasks requiring sharp distance vision (aniseikonia is generally acceptable in these circumstances). Monovision is clearly not a panacea for presbyopia and should be used only in patients who have been carefully screened and who are willing to tolerate its attendant visual compromises. Preoperative use of monovision contact lenses may identify those who are likely to do well with monovision refractive surgery; these should be conducted for at least 3 weeks. If patients do not improve significantly in their adaptation to monovision over that time period, they may not be good candidates. Lastly, it should be noted that there are presently no published reports of LASIK being used to produce monovision.

E. CONTRAST SENSITIVITY AND GLARE TESTING

Contrast and glare sensitivity are two important parameters of visual function that can be affected by LASIK (14). Refractive surgery can cause light scatter (due to corneal haze) and aberrations of the corneal curvature, both of which can affect contrast and glare sensitivity. Light scatter can cause starburst phenomena, while spherical aberration can cause haloes to appear around bright objects. Pupil size and the size of the treated area are important factors in the prominence of the starburst and halo effects.

Contrast measures of sensitivity assess how much a pattern must vary in luminance to be seen; this generally parallels visual acuity in normal, healthy eyes. In various disorders, including cataracts, amblyopia, glaucoma, optic neuritis, cerebral lesions, and diabetic retinopathy, the two may not correlate well. Loss of contrast sensitivity can make the world appear hazy. Loss of low spatial frequency contrast sensitivity hampers face recognition, navigation in unfamiliar environments, and reading of low-contrast text (15).

Contrast sensitivity is traditionally measured by using sine wave gratings that vary in spatial frequency (bar width) and contrast; a contrast sensitivity function is generated by measuring the lowest detectable contrast across a range of spatial frequencies. Rubin and Legge (17) have shown that global changes in contrast sensitivity and changes near the peak of the function curve are more clinically relevant than subtle variations in the curve. The Pelli-Robson Letter Sensitivity Chart is a commercially available test that provides a single, global measure of contrast sensitivity (16). Letters consisting of contrasting lighter and darker bars are arranged in triplets of decreasing contrast and are equivalent to a 20/720 letter with respect to visual angle subtended. They reliably measure contrast sensitivity for patients with visual acuity of 20/400 or better.

One of the most common visual side effects of refractive surgery is glare. Disability glare occurs when light sources in the visual field reduce visibility of a target, and it occurs when light from the glare source is scattered by the ocular media, forming a veiling illuminance that dampens the contrast and thus the visibility of the target (17). Glare testing uses contrast or acuity tests in the presence of a glare source (18). The most commonly available glare test is the Brightness Acuity Test (BAT), a brightly illuminated dome held in front of the eye through which a standard eye chart is viewed (19).

There have been few studies of the effects of LASIK on contrast and glare sensitivity. Holladay et al. found that contrast threshold worsened the first postoperative day by a mean of 0.6 ± 1.0 lines in darkness and 0.8 ± 0.7 lines at high BAT (20). Contrast sensitivity in light conditions recovered by 1 week, but contrast threshold in darkness did not return to baseline through 6 months. Larger pupil sizes were associated with worse contrast outcomes. This study speculated that the conversion by LASIK of corneal asphericity to an oblate shape accounted for this result. El Danasoury compared night glare after using LASIK in two different ways: a single ablation zone of 5.5 mm in one eye, and an ablation zone of 5.5 mm with a transition zone of 1.0 mm diameter larger on the other eye (21). Use of the transition zone significantly decreased night glare in this study. Carr et al. compared single-zone vs. multizone LASIK (22). Multizone eyes were found to have a greater decrease in log contrast sensitivity at 12 cycles/degree under undilated conditions. Perez-Santonja et al. found that contrast sensitivity 1 month after LASIK decreased significantly only at low and intermediate spatial frequencies (3 and 6 cycles/degree) (23). By 3 months, there were no significant differences in contrast sensitivity at all spatial frequencies compared to baseline. Wang et al. found that LASIK eyes recovered contrast sensitivity by 3 months as well, a significant difference from their control group, PRK eyes, in whom recovery took 6 to 12 months (24).

F. CONCLUSION

Several preoperative optical considerations are important when evaluating a patient considering LASIK surgery. In addition to understanding the basics of refractive error evaluation, anticipation of postoperative outcomes and of optical aberrations after surgery are essential for patient education prior to surgery. The use of corneal topography and wavefront analysis is valuable to achieve this goal. An understanding of certain fundamental principles of optics will facilitate and optimize clinical application of LASIK. Refractive surgeons must be aware of more than spherocylindrical thin-lens first-order optics in order to make informed decisions. The following chapters will cover additional preoperative considerations that are necessary to optimize LASIK outcomes and improve patient satisfaction.

REFERENCES

1. American Academy of Ophthalmology. Ophthalmology, Optics, Refraction, and Contact Lenses: Basic and Clinical Science Course. San Francisco, 1998.
2. S Jain, I Arora, DT Azar. Success of monovision in presbyopes: review of the literature and potential applications to refractive surgery. Surv Ophthalmol 1996;40:491–499.
3. EC McGill, P Erickson. Sighting dominance and monovision distance binocular fusional ranges. J Am Optom Assoc 1991;62:738–742.
4. C Schor, M Carson, G Peterson, J Suzuki, P Erickson. Effects of interocular blur suppression ability on monovision task performance. J Am Optom Assoc 1989;60:188–192.
5. P Erickson, EC McGill. Role of visual acuity, stereo acuity, and ocular dominance in monovision patient success. Optom Vis Sci 1992;69:761–764.
6. MJ Collins, B Brown, SJ Verne, M Makras, KJ Bowman. Peripheral visual acuity with monovision and other contact lens corrections for presbyopia. Optom Vis Sci 1989;66:370–374.
7. JE Sheedy, MG Harris, L Busby, E Chan, I Koga. Monovision contact lens wear and occupational task performance. Am J Optom Physiol Opt 1988;65:14–18.
8. JH McLendon, JL Burcham, CH Pheiffer. Presbyopic patterns and single vision contact lenes. South J Optom 1968;10:7–10.
9. A Back, T Grant, N Hine. Comparative visual performance of three presbyopic contact lens corrections. Optom Vis Sci 1992;69:474–480.
10. M Collins, A Good, B Brown. Distance visual acuity and monovision. Optom Visc Sci 1989; 66:370–374.
11. S Pradhan, J Gilchrist. The effect of monocular defocus on binocular contrast sensitivity. Ophthal Physiol Opt 1990;10:33–36.
12. MJ Collins, B Brown, KJ Bowman. Contrast sensitivity with contact lens corrections for presbyopia. Ophthal Physiol Opt 1989;9:133–138.
13. KA Lebow, JB Goldberg. Characteristics of binocular vision found for presbyopic patients wearing single vision contact lenses. J Am Optom Assoc 1975;46:1116–1123.

14. GS Rubin. Contrast sensitivity and glare testing in keratorefractive surgery. In: D Azar, ed. Refractive Surgery. Stamford, CT: Appleton & Lange, 1997, pp 143–151.

15. JA Marron, IL Bailey. Visual factors and orientation-mobility performance. Am J Optom Physiol Opt 1982;59:413–426.

16. DG Pelli, JG Robson, AJ Wilkins. The design of a new letter chart for measuring contrast sensitivity. Clin Vis Sci. 1988;2:169–177.

17. GS Rubin, GE Legge. Psychophysics of reading—the role of contrast in low vision. Vis Res 1989;29:79–91.

18. DB Elliott, MA Bullimore. Assessing the reliability, discriminative ability, and validity of disability glare tests. Inv Ophthalmol Vis Sci 1993;34:108–119.

19. JT Holladay, TC Prager, J Trujillo, RS Ruis. Brightness acuity test and outdoor visual acuity in cataract patients. J Cataract Refract Surg 1987;13:67–69.

20. JT Holladay, DR Dudeja, J Chang. Functional vision and corneal changes after laser in situ keratomileusis determined by contrast sensitivity, glare testing, and corneal topography. J Cataract Refract Surg 1999;25:663–669.

21. MA El Danasoury. Prospective bilateral study of night glare after laser in situ keratomileusis with single zone and transition zone ablation. J Refract Surg 1998;14:512–516.

22. JD Carr, RD Stulting, Y Sano, KP Thompson, W Wiley, GO Waring III. Prospective comparison of single zone and multizone laser in situ keratomileusis for the correction of low myopia. Ophthalmology 1998;105:1504–1511.

23. JJ Perez-Santonja, HF Sakla, JL Alio. Contrast sensitivity after laser in situ keratomileusis. J Cataract Refract Surg 1998;24:183–189.

24. Z Wang, J Chen, B Yang. Comparison of laser in situ keratomileusis and photorefraactive keratectomy to correct myopia from −1.25 to −6.00 diopters. J Refract Surg 1997;13:528–534.

8

Corneal Topography and LASIK Applications

LI WANG and DOUGLAS D. KOCH

Cullen Eye Institute, Baylor College of Medicine, Houston, Texas, U.S.A.

DIMITRI T. AZAR

*Massachusetts Eye and Ear Infirmary, Schepens Eye Research Institute,
and Harvard Medical School, Boston, Massachusetts, U.S.A.*

ROBERT T. ANG

*Massachusetts Eye and Ear Infirmary and Harvard Medical School, Boston,
Massachusetts, U.S.A., and Asian Eye Institute, Makati, The Philippines*

RENGIN YILDIRIM

Cerrahpasa Medical School, University of Istanbul, Istanbul, Turkey

The use of computerized videokeratography (CVK) for the evaluation of the corneal surface has become widespread. CVK is an indispensable tool for refractive surgeons for preoperative screening, surgical planning, assessment of surgical outcomes, detection and management of complications, and refinement and development of surgical techniques. This chapter reviews the basic principles of CVK, the recognition of corneal topographic patterns, and the role of corneal topography in refractive surgery.

A. PRINCIPLES OF CORNEAL TOPOGRAPHY

1. Terminology

It is important to introduce some terminology first. The corneal light reflex is in fact an image reflected off the tear film and is the basis for placido-based topographic measurements.

The tear film of the anterior corneal surface acts like a convex mirror to form a virtual, erect image of reflected light. This image is called the corneal light reflex or the first Purkinje image.

The line of sight is a line connecting a fixation point at optical infinity with the center of the entrance pupil (1). The pupillary axis is a line normal to the corneal surface passing through the center of the entrance pupil, which is usually temporal to the line of sight, and the angle between them is known as angle lambda and is in the range of 3° to 6°.

The topography of the cornea can be arbitrarily broken down into four zones. The central zone generally refers to the central 3 to 4 mm of the cornea. The paracentral zone is an annulus with inner and outer diameters of 4 and 7 mm, respectively. The peripheral zone is an annular region with inner and outer diameters of 7 and 11 mm, respectively. The limbal zone is the border, about 0.5 mm wide, between the cornea and sclera.

A meridian is a line that spans the diameter of the cornea from one point on the limbus to a point on the opposing limbus. Meridians are located by their angular position, increasing counterclockwise from 0° at the 3 o'clock position to 180° at the 9 o'clock position for both the right and left eyes (2). A semimeridian is a radial line on the corneal surface from its center, and it is located by its angular position from 0° at the 3 o'clock position, increasing counterclockwise around the full 360° for both the right and the left eyes.

In the literature, there is confusion over the terms apex and vertex as applied to the cornea. Waring defined the apex as the high spot of the corneal (2). Maloney suggested denoting the high point of the cornea as the corneal vertex and the apex as the region of greatest curvature (3). According to Webster, however, both terms refer to a point on a shape furthest from its base (4). A vertex sometimes also refers to the point where the axis of a curve intersects the curve itself. It is important to understand that the high point and the region of greatest curvature often do not coincide. In this chapter, we will use Maloney's definitions, referring to the vertex as the high point on the cornea relative to the imaging system (and hence the center of the placido disk rings), apex referring to the region of steepest curvature.

2. Placido Disk System

a. Data Acquisition

Placido disk technology has been most widely accepted, used, and understood. The different units share certain components but can differ in data acquisition, processing, and performance (5). All systems contain a transilluminated disc or cone (modified Placido disc), an imaging system consisting of an objective lens, a black and white (B&W) camera (TechnoMed utilizes a color camera and color ring system), a video frame grabber, and a computer system. The number, thickness, color, and position of the rings relative to each other vary from system to system. Most systems can be divided into "near design" (Tomey TMS, TechnoMed C-Scan, and Keratron) and "distant design" (EyeSys Corneal Analysis System-2000, Humphrey Atlas, Alcon EyeMap EH-290, and Dicon CT-200). The near design units typically image a greater portion of the cornea and require lower levels of illumination, but they may be more susceptible to focusing error (unless they are software corrected), and at times the patient's brow may interfere with the positioning of the cone. The distant design systems are less susceptible to focusing error and typically are not affected by the patient's anatomy, but they require brighter illumination and have less corneal coverage. Recently, the additions of new cone designs, more sensitive video cameras, and correcting algorithms have decreased the clinical distinction between near and distant units.

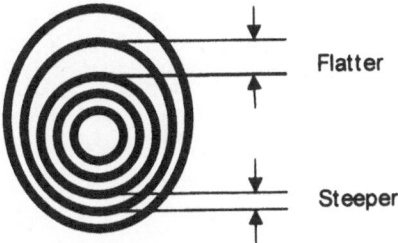

Flatter

Steeper

Figure 8.1 The principles of Placido disk technology. The larger the distances between the rings, the flatter the cornea, and the less dioptric power it has. The reverse is true with a steeper cornea, which shows smaller distances between the rings and a higher corneal power.

The placido target is projected onto the cornea and reflected off the tear film to form a smaller upright image that is in focus near the iris plane. This two-dimensional digital image is captured by a CCD camera and analyzed to reconstruct three-dimensional corneal shapes, using the distances between rings or ring edges as the basis for calculating the radius of curvature or refractive power. A larger spacing between ring edges indicates a flatter cornea with a greater radius of curvature (Fig. 8.1).

b. Data Processing and Map Display

Three basic formulas exist for calculating corneal power: axial radius of curvature, instantaneous (or tangential) radius of curvature, and refractive. Clinically significant differences exist in the corneal power values calculated by the three formulas (6). The topographic data may then be represented in a variety of ways. Clinically, the most useful representation to the clinician is the color-coded map. The warm colors, red and orange, represent relatively higher powers (steeper curvatures), green and yellow are used for powers associated with normal corneas, and cool colors, hues of blue, denote relatively lower powers (flatter curvatures). Types of topographic displays include

1. *Axial radius of curvature maps.* The axial radius of curvature maps are the original and most commonly used CVK maps and are derived from the axial radius of curvature. This formula is used by the keratometer and is based on the distance from the corneal vertex to the center or edge of the ring. This distance is then used to calculate the length of the radial line connecting this point to the optical (or sagittal) axis. This approach simplifies the optical principles of the cornea by assuming that the rays of light striking the cornea are paraxial, i.e., the angles of incidence are small. The simplified paraxial formula is

$$P_{\text{axial}} = \frac{n' - 1}{r_{\text{axial}}} \tag{1}$$

where $n' = 1.3375$ (standardized value for keratometric index of refraction) and r_{axial} the distance from the corneal surface to a point of intersection on the optical axis (Fig. 8.2A). The standardized value for keratometric index of refraction, n', is not the true refractive index of the cornea but an approximated index to yield the total corneal power as a single refracting surface by compensating for the negative power of the posterior surface. Axial power tends to have a spherical bias because each curvature measured is referred to the optical axis. For aspherical surfaces, this bias gives an accuracy of 0.25 D in the central cornea, but errors of 3 D or more can be found in the periphery (7).

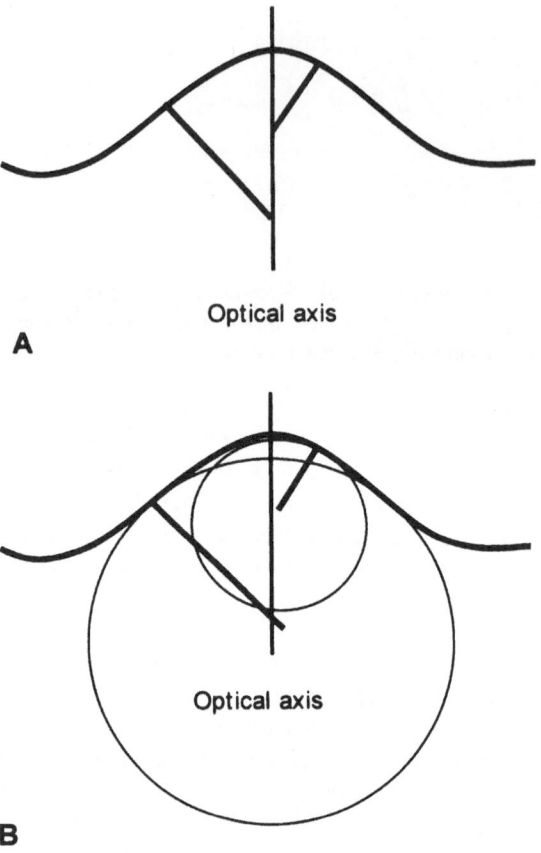

Optical axis

A

Optical axis

B

Figure 8.2 Two approaches for the calculation of the corneal radius of the curvature: (A) axial radius, (B) instantaneous radius.

The axial radius of curvature map is the standard that may be used by most clinicians. However, it is less accurate than instantaneous radius of curvature maps in providing detail regarding corneal curvature, and it is less accurate than refractive maps in portraying the refractive power of the anterior corneal surface. As a result, it may be less valid than these other two maps, despite its popularity.

2. *Instantaneous radius of curvature maps.* The instantaneous radius of curvature varies from the axial radius of curvature in that it calculates a true radius of curvature independent of the sagittal axis (Fig. 8.2B):

$$P_{inst} = \frac{n' - 1}{r_{inst}} \tag{2}$$

where r_{inst} is the radius of curvature for any given point on the cornea. The difference between axial radius of curvature and instantaneous radius of curvature maps can be dramatic. Axial radius of curvature maps tend to appear more uniform because abrupt changes in local curvature are underestimated because the calculated radius of curvature must terminate at the sagittal axis. Instantaneous radius of curvature maps typically show more marked changes in dioptric power over smaller regions and provide more accurate measurements of corneal curvature and certainly better representation of local irregularity (7).

Both of these maps, however, have marked limitations in predicting corneal refractive power. For the central paraxial rays, these formulas can be used to estimate corneal refractive power. Outside of the central region, however, the assumptions and their equations are not necessarily valid, and in particular they ignore the incident angle of the incoming light, thereby underestimating the refractive effect of peripheral rays (spherical aberration) (8).

3. *Refractive maps.* The appropriate equation for the refractive power (secondary focal point power) for the incoming parallel rays was first described by Gullstrand (9) and modified by Klein (10) as

$$P = \frac{n}{f} = \frac{n}{x/\tan(\theta i - \theta r)} \tag{3}$$

where f is the focal length, defined as the distance from the corneal vertex to the intersection of the refracted ray with the optical axis, x the corneal zone, θi the angle of incidence, and θr the angle of refraction. Maps calculated using this formula attempt to estimate the refractive power of the anterior corneal surface.

This map best characterizes the image-forming properties of the anterior corneal surface.

4. *Elevation maps.* Elevation data, which describe the difference between the height of the cornea and a reference surface, are provided by many of the Placido-based units. These elevation data are derived from the placido ring measurements, which is an approach that obviously differs from the projection principle used by elevation-based systems to obtain direct height measurements (see below).

As will be described below, elevation maps have particular value in assessing postoperative visual problems, such as central islands.

5. *Difference maps.* These are typically calculated using axial radius of curvature maps. They are useful in characterizing the change that has occurred during any interval. As with any color-coded map, it is important to note the scale for the difference map. In the authors' view, a 0.5 D and 0.25 D interval is often most useful.

6. *Other comparative maps.* Different devices have a number of color-coded maps that compare corneal curvature or refractive power to some standard surface. An irregularity map may compare local changes in curvature to an idealized spherical cylindrical surface. A profile map may compare corneal curvature to a standard aspheric corneal surface as a way of evaluating the asphericity of the cornea. Corneal acuity maps display the estimated visual acuity potential for any given region of the cornea and for the cornea as a whole.

In viewing a color-coded dioptric map, it is critical first to ascertain the dioptric scale. A number of different dioptric intervals have been recommended for standardized scales, but the authors prefer a 0.5 D scale. Scales with intervals greater than 0.5 D are useful for corneas with large dioptric ranges, such as advanced keratoconus. However, for refractive surgery, a 0.5 D scale is required to obtain sufficient detail regarding nuances that affect visual performance. Fortunately, most topographers now offer some type of standardized absolute scale and adjustable scales that allow the clinician to customize the information for maximal clinical value.

c. Indices

CVK devices provide a number of quantitative indices that can tremendously enhance analysis of topographic maps. Simulated Keratometry (Sim K), which is provided by all devices, is a value that attempts to mimic conventional keratometry readings. However, there are differences between Sim K values and standard keratometry. Whereas Sim K values represent orthogonal curvatures at the 3 mm zone, for the keratometer, the diameter of the measured zone varies according to corneal curvature: the flatter the cornea the larger the diameter of the zone that is measured (11). In addition, different devices presumably use different formulas for calculating Sim K, depending upon the number of points that are sampled in order to make this calculation.

Many devices offer a number of specialized indices. The Tomey unit (Tomey Corporation USA, Waltham, MA) provides several indices, including the surface regularity index (SRI) and the surface asymmetry index (SAI) (12). The SRI is a measure of the local regularity of the corneal surface within the central 4.5 mm diameter. SRI values increase with increasing irregular astigmatism and approach zero for a smooth corneal surface. Studies have demonstrated that the SRI is highly correlated with best spectacle-corrected visual acuity (12–15). SAI measures the difference in corneal powers at each ring 180 degrees apart as a measure of symmetry. Theoretically, the SAI value would be zero for a perfect sphere, a surface with perfectly spherocylindrical regular astigmatism, and for any surface with a power that is radially symmetrical. The potential visual acuity (PVA) is an estimation of predicted visual acuity based on surface regularity index. Other Tomey indices include those that can be used to estimate the likelihood of the presence of keratoconus (see below).

The EyeSys Corneal Analysis System (EyeSys Technologies, Houston, TX) also provides several numeric indexes in its Holladay Diagnostic Summary Display (16). Effective refractive power (EffRP) is the calculated mean refractive power of the cornea over the central 3 mm, including the role of the Stiles Crawford effect. Corneal uniformity index (CUI) is a measure of the uniformity of the distortion of the corneal surface within the 3 mm pupil, expressed as a percentage. A CUI of 100% indicates that the optical quality of the cornea is perfectly uniform over the 3 mm pupil, and a CUI of 0% indicates the nonuniform optical quality of the cornea. It is important to note that a CUI of 100% does not indicate that the cornea has good optical quality, simply that it is uniform; it could be uniformly bad or good. Predicted corneal acuity (PCA) measures the extent of corneal microirregularity by comparing the video-captured image with a best-fit ellipse (17). It is the estimated range of visual acuity that could be expected if the cornea were the only factor limiting vision. Weiss and Oplinger found that the PCA appears to be most useful in predicting the BCVA in patients with normal corneas but is less precise in patients with corneal abnormalities (18).

In the Humphrey Atlas, the irregularity map displays wavefront error to characterize the irregularity of anterior corneal surface. Wavefront error is the difference between the corneal surface and a best fitted toric surface. It describes the condition of the light rays as they pass through the corneal surface and are refracted onto the retina through the clear media of the eye. Wavefront error, which closely measures a toric surface, will be displayed as green, with red and blue representing positive and negative wavefront errors, respectively.

Early Placido-based systems were susceptible to errors induced by focusing and alignment (centration) (19). To minimize these sources of errors, most current units use special methods, such as correcting algorithms (Tomey, Humphrey, and TechnoMed) or employing three cameras to measure precisely the distance from the Placido surface to the cornea (EyeSys). However, the Placido-based topography systems still have some limitations:

1. Missed central zone data have to be interpolated.
2. Calculations are based on assumption that the cornea has sufficient smoothness in the radial direction; therefore, these systems lose accuracy when used to map nonspherical and irregular surfaces (20–21).
3. Information regarding the corneal contour is only gained through the reflection of light rays from the tear film; abnormalities of the tear film and corneal surface, e.g., epithelial irregularities, may result in poor quality mires and misleading results.

3. Elevation-Based Systems

Elevation-based systems utilize the principle of projection to measure directly corneal elevation. Curvature values are derived from the elevation data.

a. Scanning Slit Imaging System

The Orbtek ORBSCAN (Bausch & Lomb) uses a scanning slit beam and direct stereotriangulation to measure the anterior corneal surface, the posterior corneal surface, and the anterior iris and anterior lens surfaces (Fig. 8.3). It employs a calibrated video and a forty scanning slit beam system (20 from the left and 20 from the right) to measure independently the x, y, and z locations of several thousand points on each surface with a resolution of 2 μm. Figure 8.4 illustrates the data acquisition by the slit beam system. The cornea is scanned limbus to limbus, and the images are accessed by a calibrated video camera with 240 data points per slit. These directly measured points are used to construct topographic maps.

Orbscan displays color maps as 3-D, profile, and traditional for elevation, curvature, and pachymetry. The elevation map shows the difference between the best fit sphere (BFS)

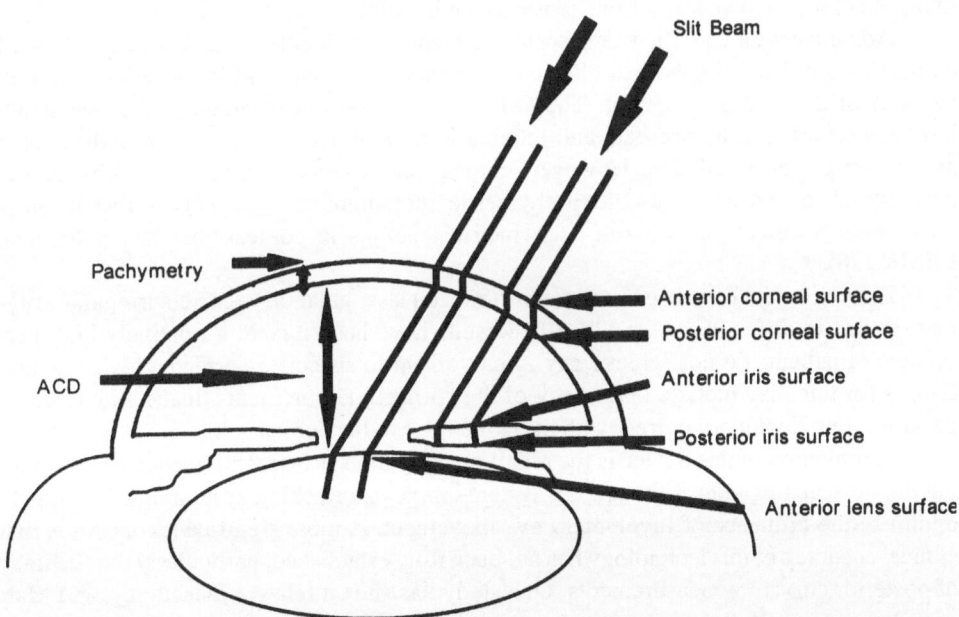

Figure 8.3 Series of surface planes measured with the Orbscan system from anterior corneal surface to anterior lens surface.

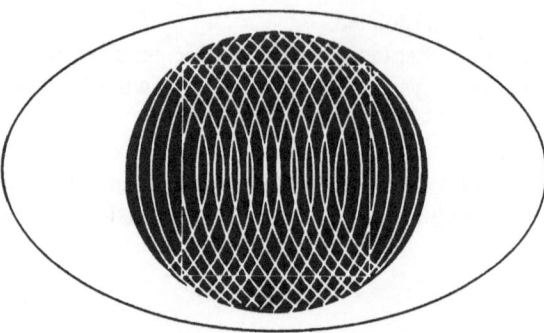

Figure 8.4 Data acquisition by the slit beam system. Forty single images are captured by a calibrated video camera (240 data points/slit). Resolution and accuracy of the central area (3–5 mm) are improved by the overlapped images.

and the eye surface in mm, expressed in distance radially from the center of the sphere (by default) or sagittal height between the two surfaces. The BFS is used to match best the anterior or posterior corneal surfaces, and this match is determined using a least squares method. Positive elevation measurements indicate that the corneal surface falls above the BFS and are represented as warm colors, while negative values indicate that the corneal surface falls below the BFS and are represented as cool colors on the elevation maps. It should be noted, however, that the elevation display depends on reference surface size, shape, alignment, fitting zone, and elevation direction (normal or axial) (22–23).

Corneal pachymetry is calculated at more than 5000 points from the elevation difference of the anterior and posterior surfaces. The pachymetry map displays thickness at the thinnest point and in an array from center to the limbus.

Advantages of the slit beam scanning technology include direct measurement of corneal height, lack of spherical bias, entire corneal coverage, and information about all surfaces of the anterior segment. The Orbscan measurement of anterior chamber depth has been reported to be accurate and reliable in normal eyes, as well as in high myopic and hyperopic eyes (24–25). However, corneal pachymetry measured by Orbscan has been found to exceed ultrasonic pachymetric measurements (26–27). A recent study found poor accuracy of Orbscan pachymetric readings in corneas that had undergone LASIK (28).

Elevation data have been used for customized laser ablation to correct irregular astigmatism due to different causes (29–30). Results have been mixed, a relatively high percentage of patients do not achieve any improvement in spectacle-corrected visual acuity. Causes for this may include inaccuracy of the corneal measurements, inaccurate laser algorithms, or difficulty in correctly aligning the laser to the cornea.

A limitation of this device is the relatively long time (1.5 seconds) required for imaging the 40 scanning slits, although the system employs a tracking system that attempts to minimize the influence of involuntary eye movement. A more significant concern is that clinical accuracy of this technology has not been fully established, particularly the accuracy of posterior curvature measurements. One study has shown relative inaccuracy, and Maloney has suggested that measuring the test–retest variability is an appropriate method of controlling the accuracy of posterior curvature measurements(31).

b. Rasterphotogrammetry

The PAR Corneal Topography System (PAR CTS, PAR Vision System Corp., New Hartford, NY) was the first topography system to produce an elevation map of the corneal surface. The system projects onto the corneal surface a grid composed of horizontal and vertical lines spaced about 0.2 mm (200 microns) apart and computes elevation data based on the distortion of the grid. The PAR system requires that a small amount of fluorescein be placed in the tear film, and the images are collected using standard fluorescence-based photography. Image acquisition is rapid and relatively insensitive to focusing. From the known geometry of the grid projection and imaging system paths, rays can be intersected in three-dimensional space to compute the x, y, and z coordinates of the surface (32).

Studies showed that the PAR system was both accurate and reproducible and had the ability to image irregular, deepithelialized, and keratectomized corneas (33–36). On the other hand, the use of fluorescein staining and limited measurement points (1400) are among the major drawbacks of this system. Although this technology is intriguing, it is no longer commercially available.

c. Interferometric System

The KeraMetrics Corneal Laser Analysis System 1000 (CLAS 1000; Kera Metrics Inc., Solana Beach, CA) utilizes laser holographic interferometry fringe patterns to depict deviation of the corneal surface. Interferometry records the interference pattern generated on the corneal surface by two coherent wave fronts (37). Although high accuracy is theoretically possible here, there have been no detailed studies on the accuracy of topographic measurement using this technology or on specific clinical applications. This device is not commercially available.

d. Moiré Interference System

Moiré interference occurs when two sets of parallel lines are superimposed at different orientation (38). There are few peer-reviewed data available validating the system.

B. CORNEAL TOPOGRAPHIC PATTERN IN MYOPIA, HYPEROPIA, AND ASTIGMATISM

1. Myopia

Although myopia is predominantly caused by increased length, a weak but statistically significant relation has been shown to exist between the corneal power and refractive error, i.e., corneal power increases (corneal radius decreases) with increasing myopia (39–45). Two studies have noted that the cornea flattens less rapidly in the periphery with increasing myopia (more negative Q values, see below) (45–46).

Using the EyeSys Corneal Analysis System™, Budak and colleagues provided a corneal topographic classification of myopic eyes based on axial, instantaneous, refractive, and profile difference maps (47). They defined six types of patterns for axial, instantaneous, and refractive maps: circular, circular with central bow tie, circular with central irregularity, symmetric bow tie, asymmetric bow tie, and irregular pattern (Fig. 8.5A–F)

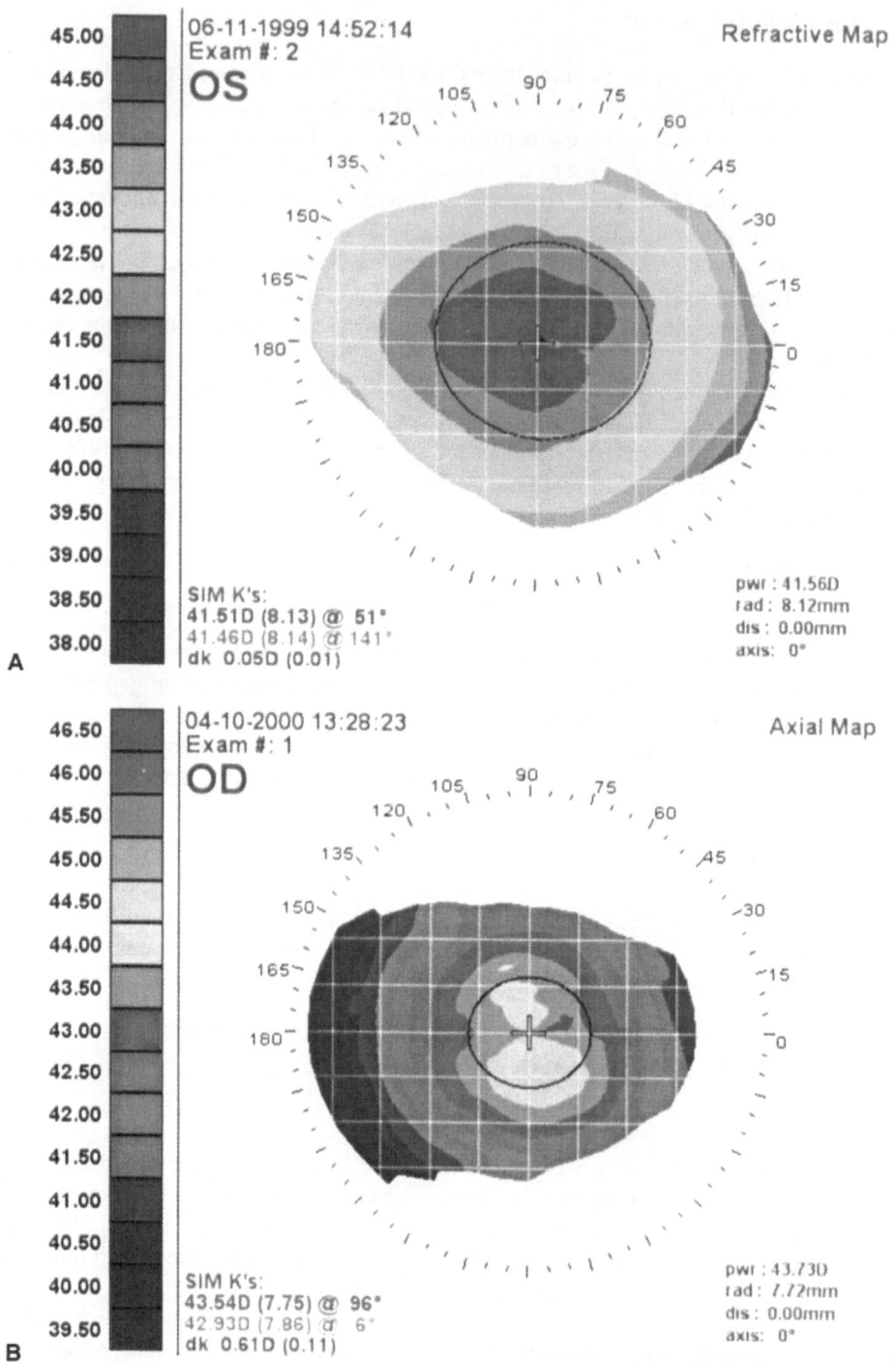

Figure 8.5 Six types of myopic patterns for axial, instantaneous, and refractive maps: (A) circular, (B) circular with central bow tie, (C) circular with central irregularity, (D) symmetric bow tie, (E) asymmetric bow tie, and (F) irregular pattern.

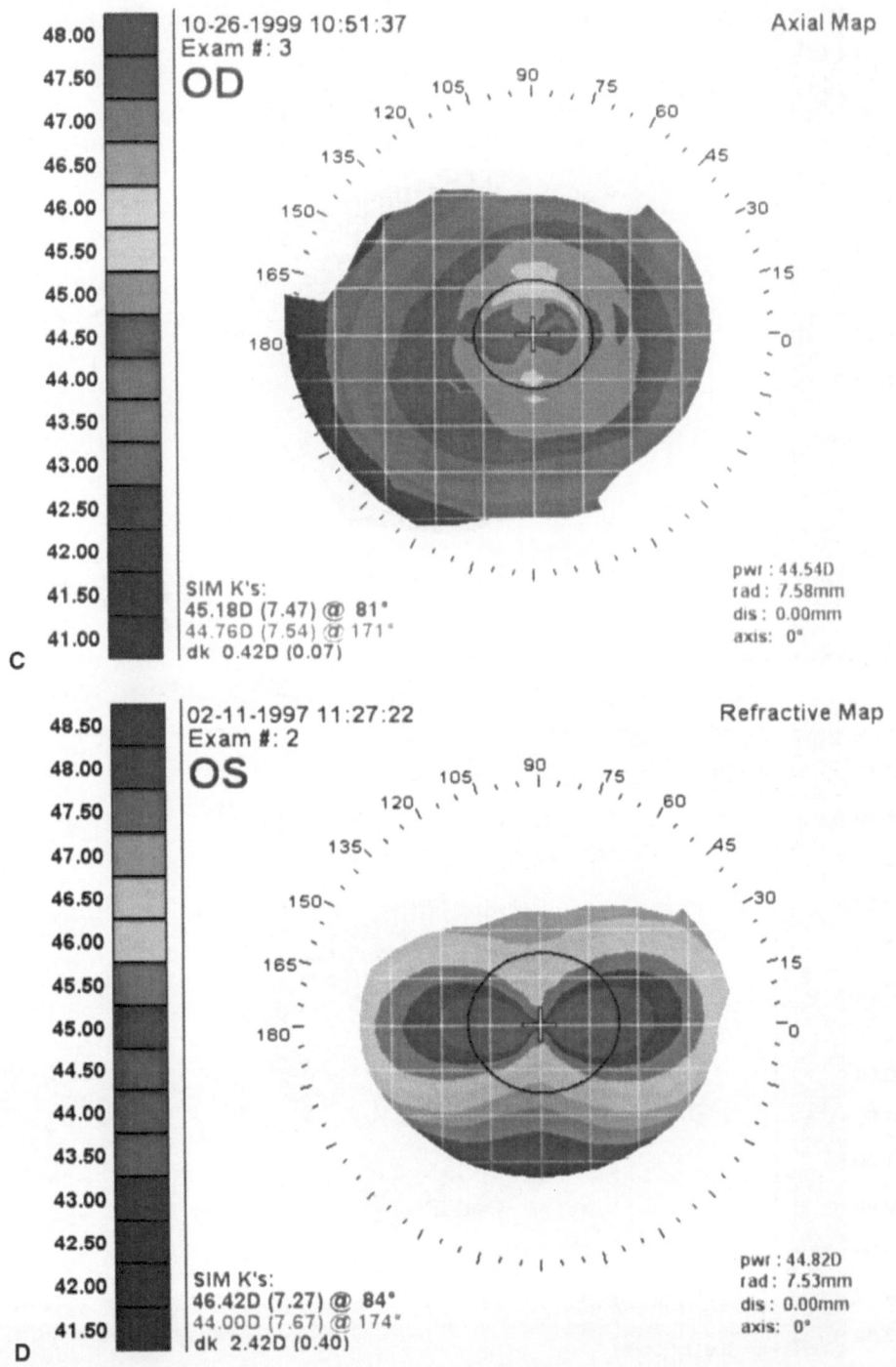

Figure 8.5 *Continued*

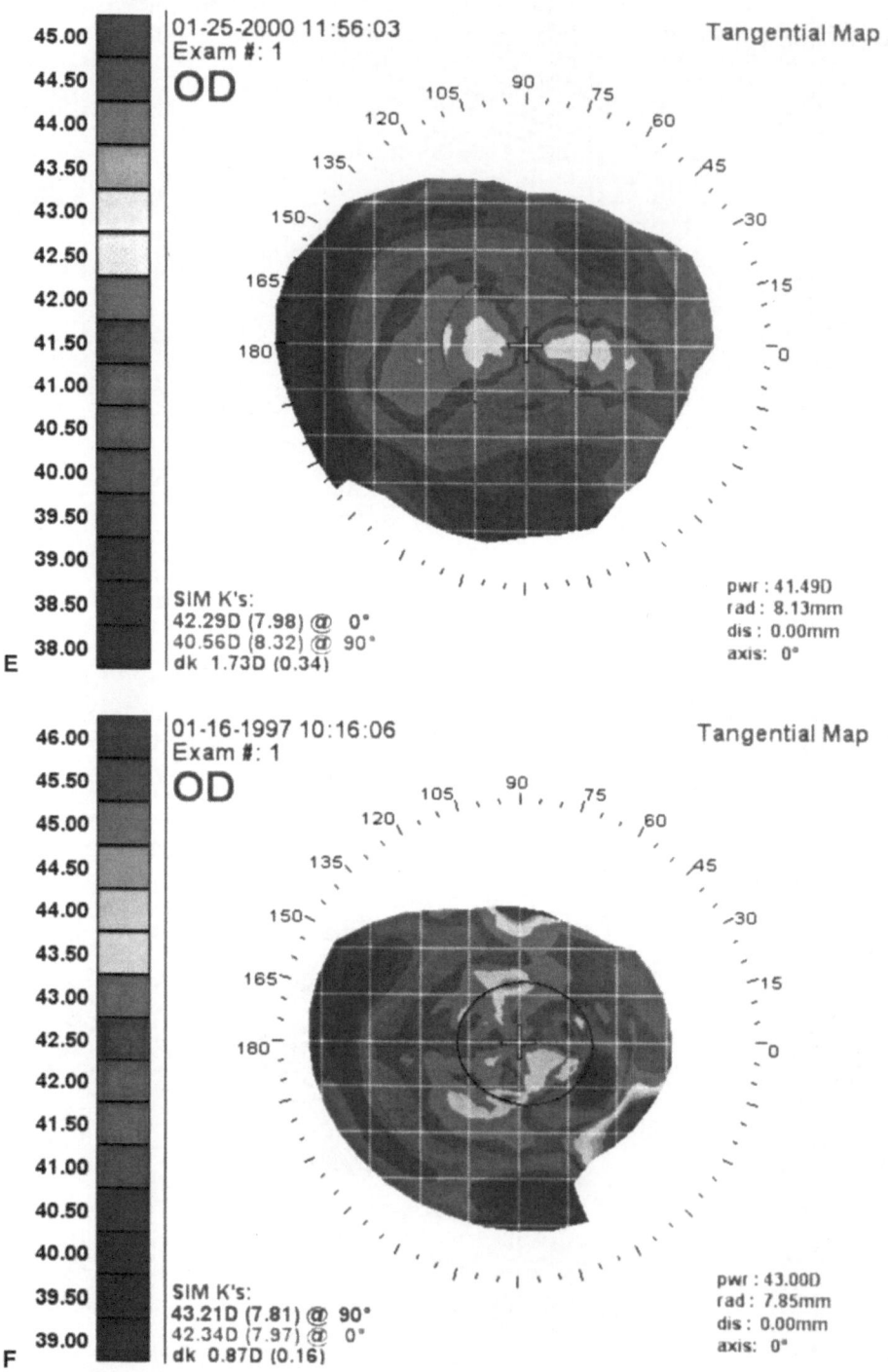

Figure 8.5 *Continued*

(Table 1). The circular with central irregularity and irregular patterns were associated with lower values for Predicted Corneal Acuity and Corneal Uniformity Index.

2. Hyperopia

A study by Strang and coauthors found that hyperopia, like myopia, is predominantly axial in nature, although in some hyperopes the cornea is abnormally flat and either contributes to or accounts for the hyperopic refractive error (48). No study has yet been done to classify the patterns on topographic maps using computerized videokeratography (CVK).

3. Astigmatism

In patients with regular astigmatism, the astigmatic patterns in curvature maps are often represented as a bow tie or figure eight, with the steepest and flattest axes of curvature of the cornea lying at right angles to one another (orthogonal) (Fig. 8.6A). On the elevation map, the astigmatic cornea may appear as a regular, irregular, or incomplete ridge pattern, with the elevated portion or ridge representing the flatter astigmatic cylinder of the cornea (Fig. 8.6B).

In patients with irregular astigmatism, corneal topographic patterns include circular with central irregularity, asymmetric bow tie (characterized by asymmetric powers in orthogonal steep and/or flat semimeridians or by nonorthogonal semi-meridians), and irregular pattern as defined by Budak et al. (47) (Fig. 8.5). In elevation maps, the pattern may be an irregular ridge, an incomplete ridge, or an unclassified pattern.

C. CORNEAL ASPHERICITY

The anterior corneal surface is asymmetrically aspheric, as the radius of curvature changes from the center to the limbus and does so at different rates along different semimeridians (49–50). Many authors have tried to describe the complex aspheric asymmetric shape of the cornea, either mathematically or graphically (49, 51–54).

The ellipse is perhaps the most useful shape for describing corneal curvature, and the profile of the cornea along any meridian can be considered as part of an ellipse. The normal cornea has a prolate shape, which means that the central zone is steeper than the paracentral and peripheral zones; this is the shape of a section across the steep end of an ellipse

Table 1 Distribution of Topographic Patterns in Axial, Instantaneous, and Auto-Scale Refractive Maps

Pattern	Axial map (%)	Instantaneous map (%)	Auto-scale refractive map (%)
Circular	21.6	8.5	31.4
Circular with central bow tie	28.1	24.2	49.7
Circular with central irregularity	5.2	13.7	2.6
Symmetric bow tie	23.5	14.4	14.4
Asymmetric bow tie	15.0	17.6	1.3
Irregular	6.5	21.6	0.7

Source: Modified from Ref. 47.

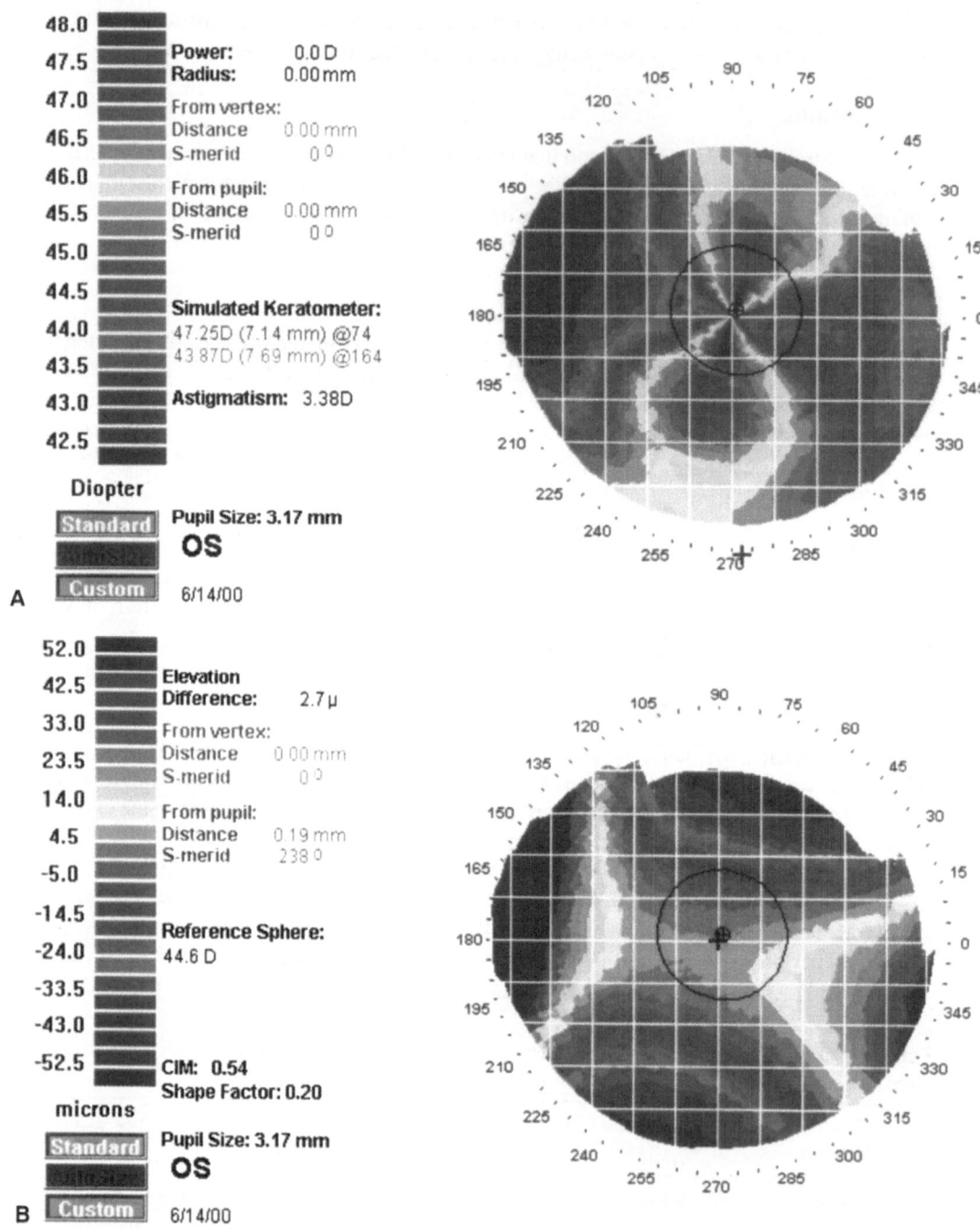

Figure 8.6 Patient with regular astigmatism: (A) bow tie pattern on curvature map, (B) irregular ridge pattern on elevation map.

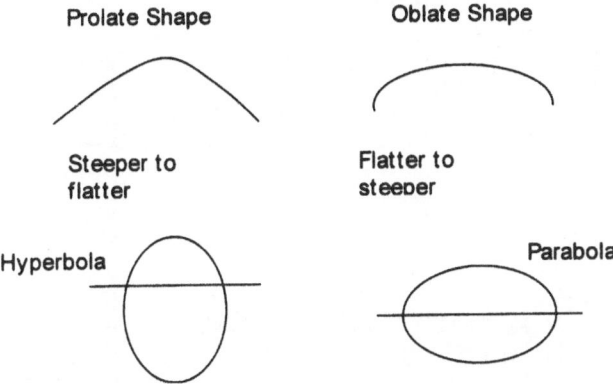

Figure 8.7   Aspherical corneal shapes.

(Fig. 8.7). The reverse shape is oblate, in which the central zone is flatter than the peripheral zone; this corresponds to the flat side of an ellipse and is often seen in corneas that have undergone myopic refractive surgery.

Usually corneal asphericity is quantitatively described by the Q value. For a sphere, $Q = 0$. For prolate surfaces, $Q < 0$, and for oblate surfaces, $Q > 0$ (55). For example, a corneal asphericity with $Q = -0.26$ indicates that, at a distance of 5 mm from the center, the cornea flattens by about 7% as radius of curvature compared to a sphere. Mean reported Q values have ranged from -0.15 to -0.30 (56–60). Related parameters include eccentricity of the equivalent conic section (e) and shape factor (P), where $Q = -e^2$, and $P = Q + 1$, respectively.

D.   VALUE OF COMPUTERIZED VIDEOKERATOGRAPHY IN REFRACTIVE SURGERY

CVK plays a critical role in the ongoing evaluation of potential and in all phases of the care of the refractive surgical patient, including preoperative screening, postoperative monitoring of results, and postoperative planning for retreatment procedures.

1.   Preoperative Screening

CVK plays several roles in the preoperative evaluation of refractive surgical patients.

a.   Determining Topographic Stabilization Following Discontinuation of Contact Lens Wear

Contact lens wear can alter the shape of the cornea by a process termed warpage, which results from direct mechanical pressure of the lens and possibly from metabolic factors, such as low oxygen tension. Corneal topographic patterns of warpage are characterized by the presence of central irregular astigmatism, loss of radial symmetry, and frequent reversal of the normal topographic pattern of progressive flattening of corneal contour from the center to the periphery (61). Superior-riding lenses produced flattening superiorly and result in a relatively steeper contour inferiorly that simulates the topography of early keratoconus. Using the Orbscan topography system, Liu and Pflugfelder found that long-term contact lens

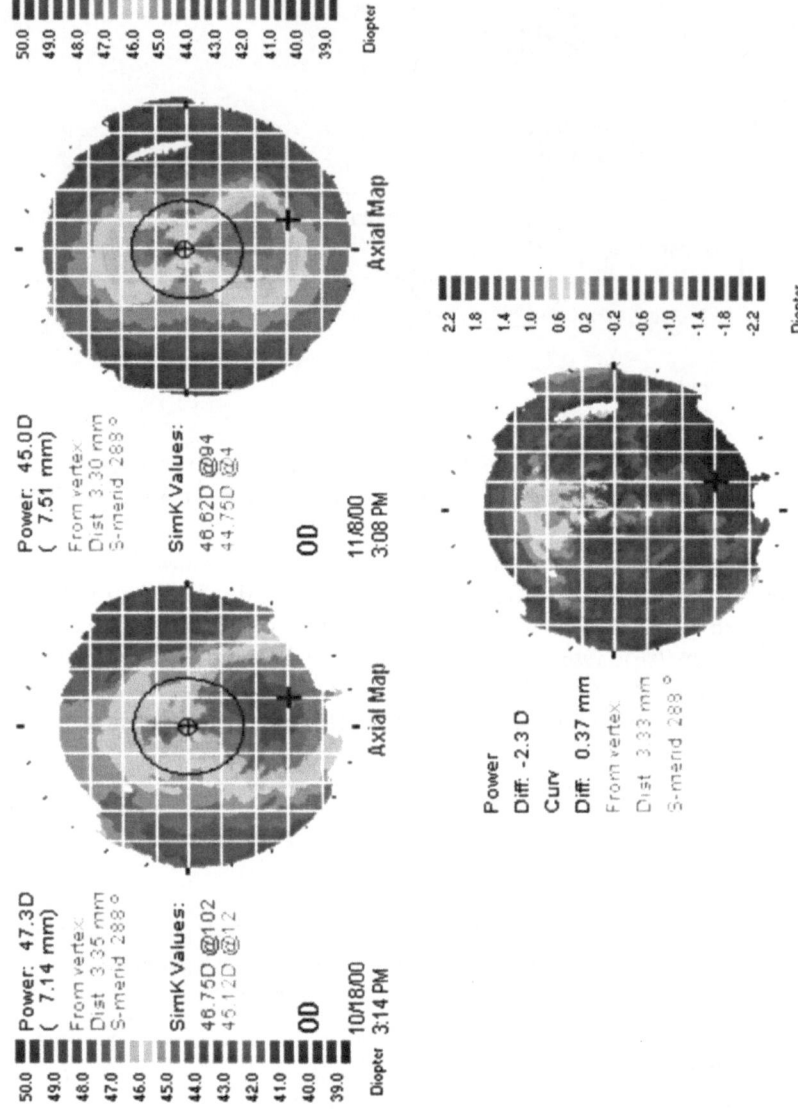

Figure 8.8   Contact lens–induced corneal warpage reversed in 1 month after discontinuation of contact lens wear.

wear ($\geq$ 5 years) appeared to decrease the entire corneal thickness and increase the corneal curvature and surface irregularity (62).

Following discontinuation of contact lens wear, it is important to monitor corneal topographic changes and defer obtaining final refractive measurements until corneal topography stabilizes (Fig. 8.8). Using the CVK (EyeSys Corneal Analysis System), Budak and colleagues evaluated corneal stability after discontinuation of contact lens wear in preoperative refractive surgery candidates (63). They found that, if the manifest refraction and CVK maps were within 0.5 diopters of values obtained 2 weeks earlier, topographic indices were normal, suggesting return of the cornea to its baseline topographic state. In their study this was noted after discontinuation of soft contact lenses wear for 2 weeks and of rigid gas-permeable contact lenses wear for 5 weeks.

b. Detecting Ectatic Corneal Disorders or Other Topographic Abnormalities

Keratoconus

The detection of keratoconus and keratoconus suspects has assumed greater significance in light of the development and expansion of refractive surgery over recent years. Patients with keratoconus do not achieve high-quality vision with either glasses or contact lenses, and they tend to seek out refractive surgery. The percentage of candidates who were found to have keratoconus or subclinical keratoconus during the preoperative screening for refractive surgery has been reported to be as high as 33% (64).

Patients with moderate to advanced keratoconus are readily recognizable on the topographic maps and easily diagnosed clinically (Fig. 8.9). The difficulty is to detect the

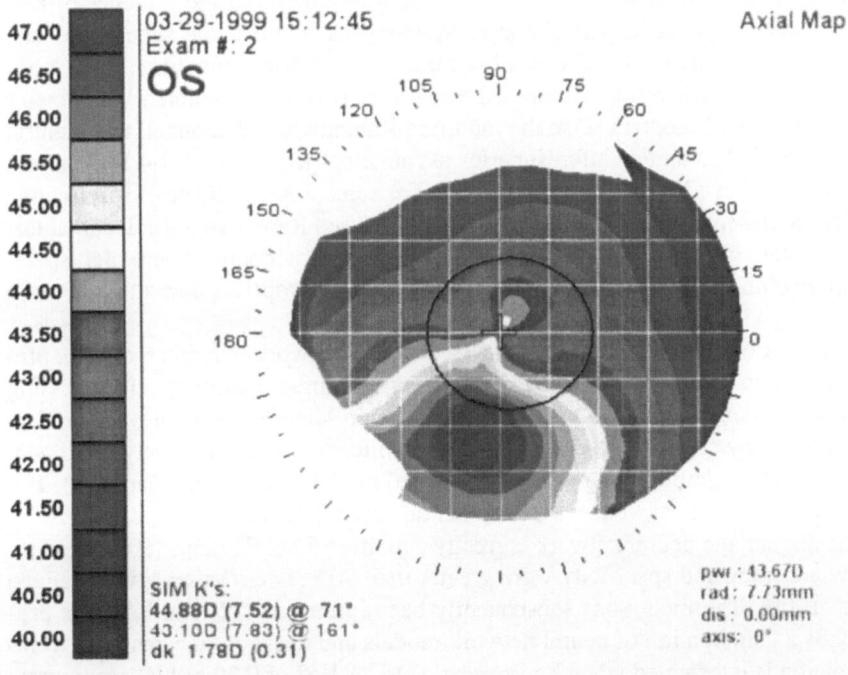

Figure 8.9 Topographic map of keratoconus on curvature map.

keratoconus in its early stages before obvious topographic and clinical signs are present. These corneas are sometimes referred to as forme fruste keratoconus or keratoconus suspects, because of the subtle topographic abnormalities that are present. Several quantitative specific corneal indices and detection programs designed to aid the topographic diagnosis of keratoconus have been developed.

1. RABINOWITZ–MCDONNELL INDICES.   These investigators described two criteria for detected keratoconus. The first is the *inferior–superior value (IS)*, which is defined as an average refractive power difference between five inferior points and five superior points 3 mm from the center at 30° intervals (65); it is designed to detect clinically significant inferior corneal steepening. When used alone, an IS value greater than 1.4 D is suggestive of keratoconus. A disadvantage of the I-S value is that the steepening in keratoconus is not always limited to the inferior periphery (66–67). The second criterion, which is designed to detect central cones, is central corneal power > 47.2 D. Because of the variability of the location of the cone, these two diagnostic features should be used in concert, and subjective interpretation is necessary (68).

2. KERATOCONUS PREDICTABILITY INDEX (**KPI**).   Maeda and colleagues developed the KPI, which is a single value derived by linear discriminant analysis of eight quantitative topographic indices (69). A KPI value greater than 0.23 is indicative of keratoconus.

3. KERATOCONUS INDEX (**KCI**).   In addition to the discriminant analysis classifier, the authors (69) developed an expert system classifier. An expert system is a form of artificial intelligence that comprises an extensive set of decision rules. Decisions by the expert system are made deductively with step-by-step logical operation. In addition to the KPI, four indices were used in the binary decision tree. The degree of the keratoconus-like pattern is determined and expressed as a percentage, KCI%. A value of zero is normal, with greater values describing an increasing likelihood of the presence of keratoconus. In their study, the expert classifier system was found to be superior to discriminate analysis in sensitivity and overall accuracy. In a subsequent study, three keratoconus detection schemes were compared: keratometry (average simulated keratometry [SimK] readings > 45.7 diopters [D]); the modified Rabinowitz–McDonnell test (central corneal power > 47.2 D and/or inferosuperior asymmetry [IS] value > 1.4 D); and the expert system classifier (70). Results showed that for screening candidates for refractive surgery, where high sensitivity is needed, either the modified Rabinowitz–McDonnell test or the expert system classifier is suitable. For diagnosing keratoconus, where high specificity is more useful, the expert system classifier is more appropriate than the other two methods.

4. KERATOCONUS SEVERITY INDEX (**KSI**).   Neural networks can interpolate or predict complicated data through "learning," by simulating human neurological processing abilities, and have been attracting considerable attention in science, economics, and industry, as well as in many areas of medicine. The first application of a neural network model to classify corneal topography was reported and tested in 183 topographic maps (71). The correct classification was achieved by a trained neural network for all 108 maps in the training set. In the test set, the neural network correctly classified 60 of 75 maps (80%). For every category, accuracy and specificity were greater than 90%, whereas sensitivity ranged from 44% to 100%. The model has subsequently been improved (72) and KSI was proposed, which is a combination of neural network models and decision tree analysis. Keratoconus suspicion is interpreted when KSI reaches 0.15. A KSI of 0.30 or higher indicates clinical keratoconus.

5. KISA% INDEX. The KISA% index is derived from the product of four indices: K value, IS value, AST index, and skewed radial axis (SRAX) index (73). At a cutoff point for KISA% of 100, 280 of 281 participants (99.6%) were correctly classified. The KISA% index set at 100 is highly sensitive and specific for diagnosing keratoconus, and a range of 60% to 100% can be used to designate or label patients as keratoconus suspects with minimal fear of significant overlap with the normal population (<0.5%).

6. OTHER INDICES. The highest rate of steepening (HRS) is the highest rate of corneal power changes (in diopters per millimeter) away from the apex (the point of maximum curvature) to the periphery measured along its semimeridian (74). The authors found that a cutoff value of HRS of 1.40 D/mm has a sensitivity of 95.7% (67/70), a specificity of 96.4% (16 false positive cases), and an accuracy of 96.3% for detection of keratoconus.

Langenbucher and colleagues developed a keratoconus detection scheme with wavefront parameters based on topography height data (75). A decomposition of corneal topography height data into orthogonal Zernike polynomials was performed using the corneal topographer TMS-1. This index was found to perform at least as well (sensitivity in mild/severe keratoconus 93.4%/100%, with a specificity of 100%) as keratoconus detection schemes based on the Klyce–Maeda and the Rabinowitz–McDonnell indices.

Clinical approach. The authors use two approaches to screen patients for keratoconus. First, patients are graded according to the keratoconus-screening chart proposed by Azar, which accounts for both topographic features and slit lamp findings (for details see Chap. 10). As a second step, corneas are measured using the Tomey topographer, and values for the KCI and KSI are obtained; any patient with any likelihood of the presence of keratoconus by either index is rejected for LASIK surgery.

Other Corneal Ectasias

Pellucid marginal degeneration and keratoglobus may represent variants of keratoconus, as there is considerable overlap among their clinical and topographic features, and they may coexist in an individual or in the same family.

In pellucid marginal degeneration, the topographic pattern has a classical butterfly appearance, demonstrating large amounts of against-the-rule astigmatism (Fig. 8.10) and inferior corneal steepening (76–78). Rare cases of superior corneal thinning in pellucid marginal degeneration have been reported (79–81).

Keratoglobus is a rare disorder characterized by limbus-to-limbus corneal thinning and a globular protrusion of the cornea evident on profile examination (82,83). The topographic appearance is diffuse corneal steepening with irregular astigmatism.

Corneal Scarring

The topographic pattern produced by corneal scars depends on the site and size of the scar. Typically, there is corneal flattening overlying the scar with adjacent corneal steepening. With larger scars, particularly if they are located in the anterior cornea, the videokeratoscopic rings may merge into one another and cannot be distinguished well enough for the topography to be reconstructed accurately, resulting in misleading or absent data (Fig. 8.11A, B).

c. Selecting the optimal surgical procedure

In some patients, the preoperative corneal topographic findings can be used to select the appropriate surgical procedure. For example, one might recommend PRK if there is suspicion of forme fruste keratoconus. This is certainly an area of controversy, because one could ar-

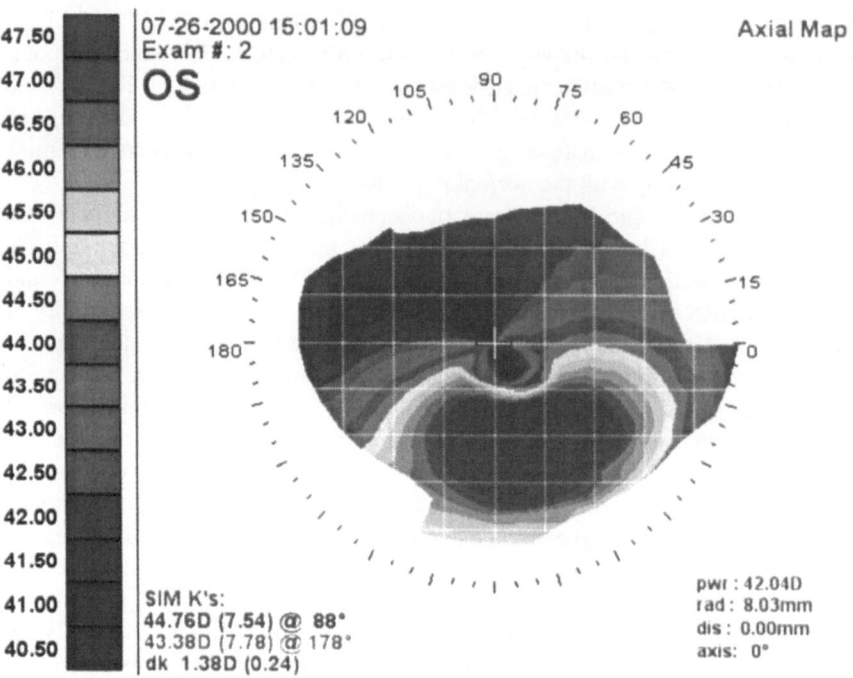

Figure 8.10   Topographic map of pellucid marginal degeneration.

gue that patients with any form of topographic irregularity should be excluded from undergoing corneal refractive surgery. However, there is growing evidence that patients with asymmetric inferior steepening may be at risk for developing keratectasia following LASIK (84), whereas PRK may be a safe option in these instances. Another option in these patients might be Intacs, assuming that the refractive error is low and there is little pre-existing refractive astigmatism. Finally, detection of forme fruste keratoconus or other sight-threatening disorders may not preclude patients from undergoing a noncorneal procedure, such as implantation of a phakic intraocular lens.

d.   Topographically Driven Corneal Ablation

Several studies have addressed the potential role of CVK in determining the ablation pattern to be employed. Tamayo and Serrano reported promising results performing customized excimer laser ablation based on the Contoured Ablation Patterns (CAP) software (VISX, Inc.), which enables the surgeon to control the size, pattern, depth, and location of the ablation based on the elevation data (85). Alessio and colleagues reported promising results in correcting irregular astigmatism using Corneal Interactive Programmed Topographic Ablation (CIPTA) (LIGI, Taranto, Italy), which provides customized laser ablation by transferring programmed ablation from the corneal topography to a flying-spot excimer laser (30).

2.   Monitoring Postoperative Outcomes

CVK plays a crucial role in assessing patients' postoperative outcome, particularly when complications occur. Hersh (86) have identified eight postoperative topographic patterns in eyes that have undergone laser refractive surgery. Unfortunately, there is no strict correlation between postoperative symptoms and topographic findings.

In evaluating postoperative CVK, the authors find it useful to examine several different kinds of maps, depending upon the circumstances. The axial radius of curvature map is useful because the patterns are familiar and abnormal patterns are therefore readily detected. To evaluate more precisely local irregularities, the instantaneous radius of curvature map provides the requisite detail. Refractive maps best correlate with quality of vision and are therefore useful to supplement the curvature data. Finally, elevation maps can sometimes provide detail that is not as obvious in examining the other maps. In

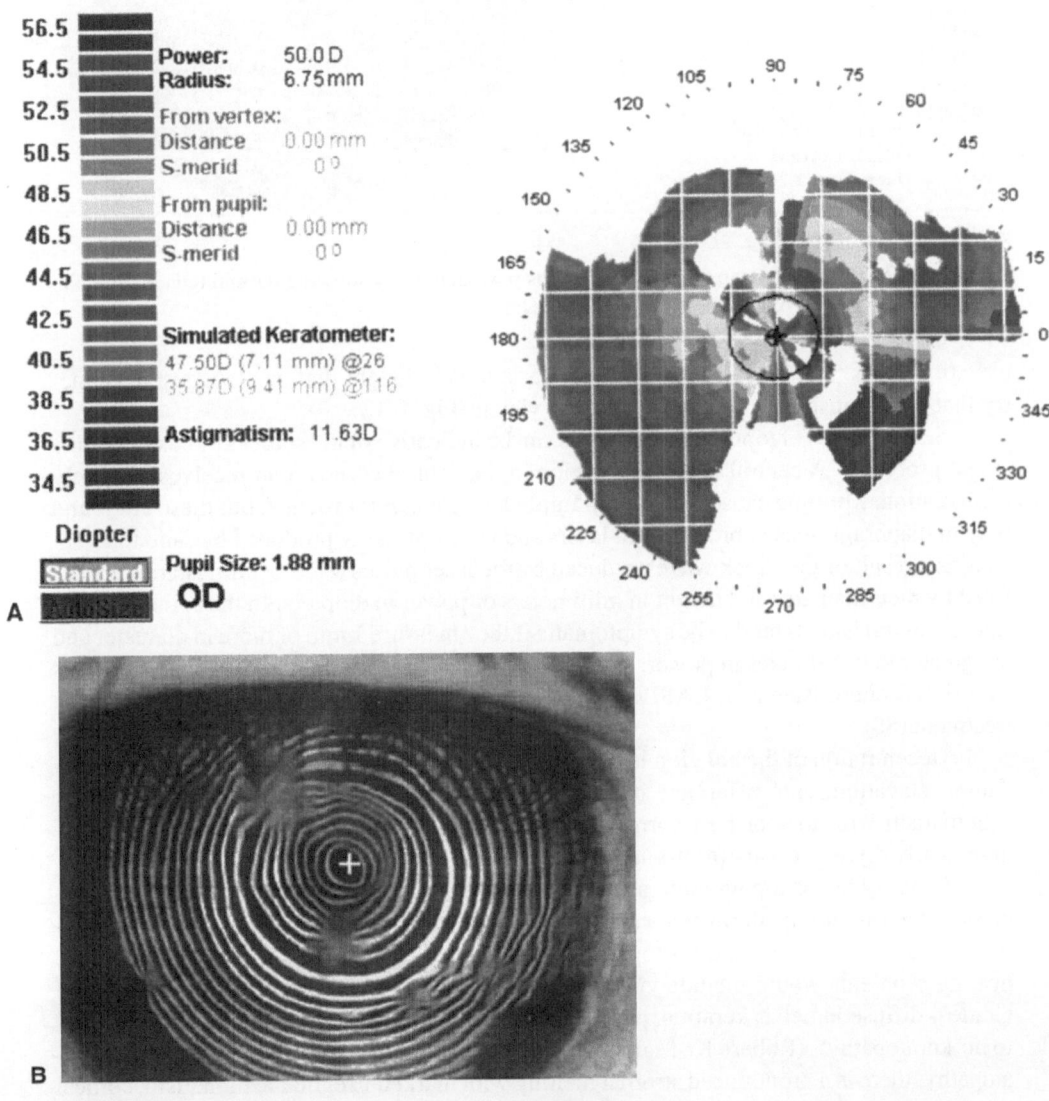

Figure 8.11 Corneal scarring: (A) power map, (B) ring image.

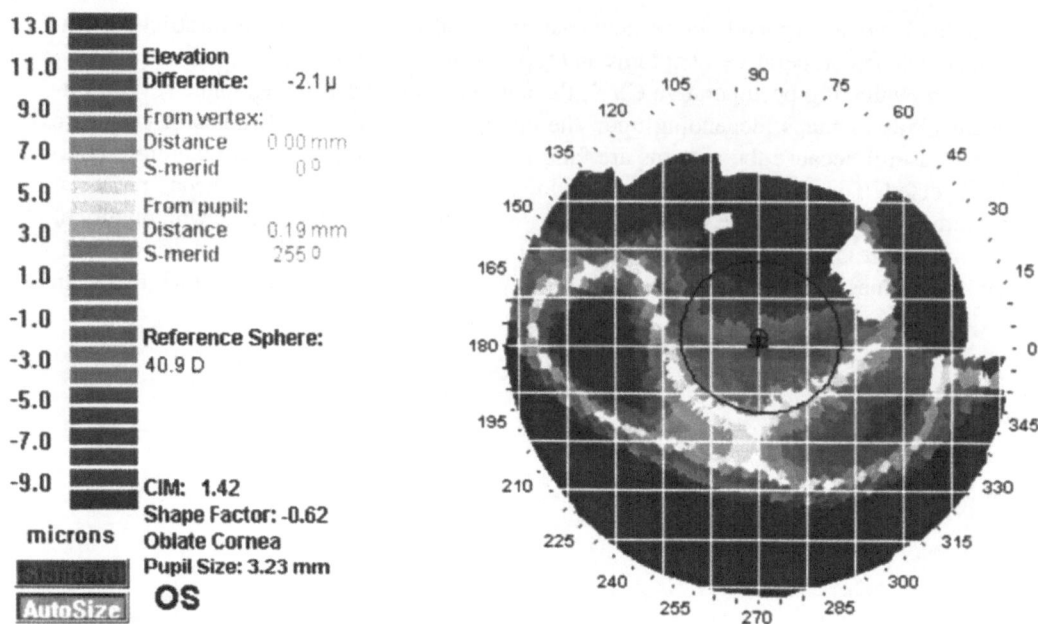

Figure 8.12 Elevation map on an eye 3 months postoperatively showing decentered ablation. Patient has lost two lines of spectacle-corrected visual acuity.

elevation maps, the authors look for local variations in height that may suggest asymmetry that can contribute to loss of quality of vision (Fig. 8.12).

Several types of topographic patterns can be indicative of the sources of postoperative visual problems. A central island is a region in the central corneal that receives relatively less ablation. Multiple causes have been implicated for central islands, but these are found only in diaphragm-based broad-beam lasers and are most likely produced by fluid that collects as a result of the shock wave produced by the laser pulses (87). Central islands are defined by their diameter and height in millimeters or power in diopters. In the authors' experience, central islands tend to be symptomatic if they measure 1 mm or more in diameter and are greater than 1 diopter in power. Whereas central islands following PRK tend to regress over time, central islands of LASIK eyes tend to be more stable and therefore may require treatment (88).

Decentration of the ablation is usually best seen with the instantaneous radius of curvature, elevation, and difference maps. Decentration can produce regular and irregular astigmatism with loss of best-correct acuity, glare, and halos. Treatment requires topographically driven or wavefront-guided ablation.

Other types of topographic abnormalities that can be seen include a variety of unclassifiable irregular patterns that can have multiple etiologies, including epithelial irregularity, irregular ablation, and postoperative wound healing problems. Examples of wound healing problems would include visually significant haze or scarring following PRK and Grade 4 diffuse lamellar keratitis, particularly the variant that has alsobeen called "central toxic keratopathy" (Robert K. Maloney, personal communication). In central toxic keratopathy, there is a pronounced stromal melting with marked irregular astigmatism, corneal thinning, and striae (Fig. 8.13). Spectacle-corrected acuity can be reduced to as low as 20/200 and may require corneal transplantation.

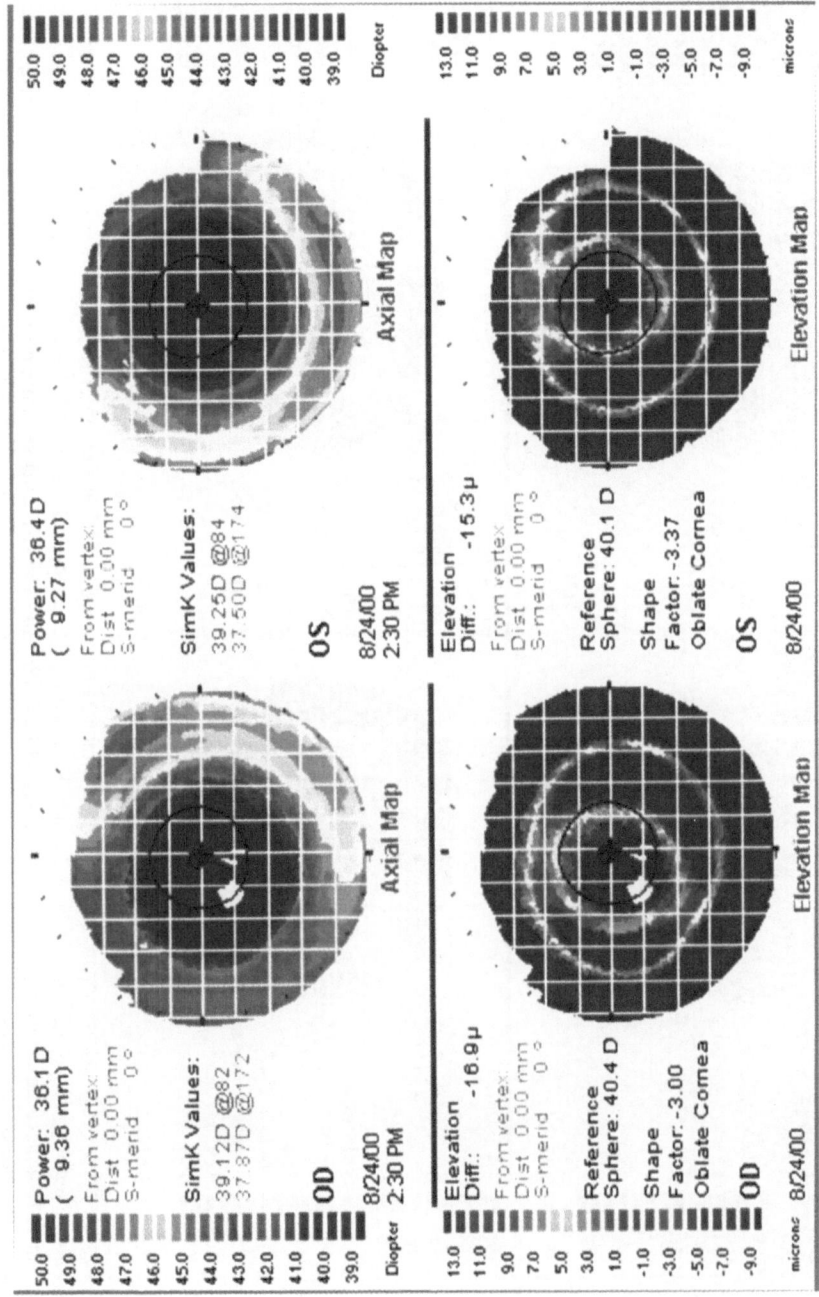

Figure 8.13 An example of central toxic keratopathy (both eyes), with pronounced stromal melting, corneal thinning, and striae. Spectacle-corrected visual acuity reducted to 20/32 (right eye) and 20/25 (left eye), respectively.

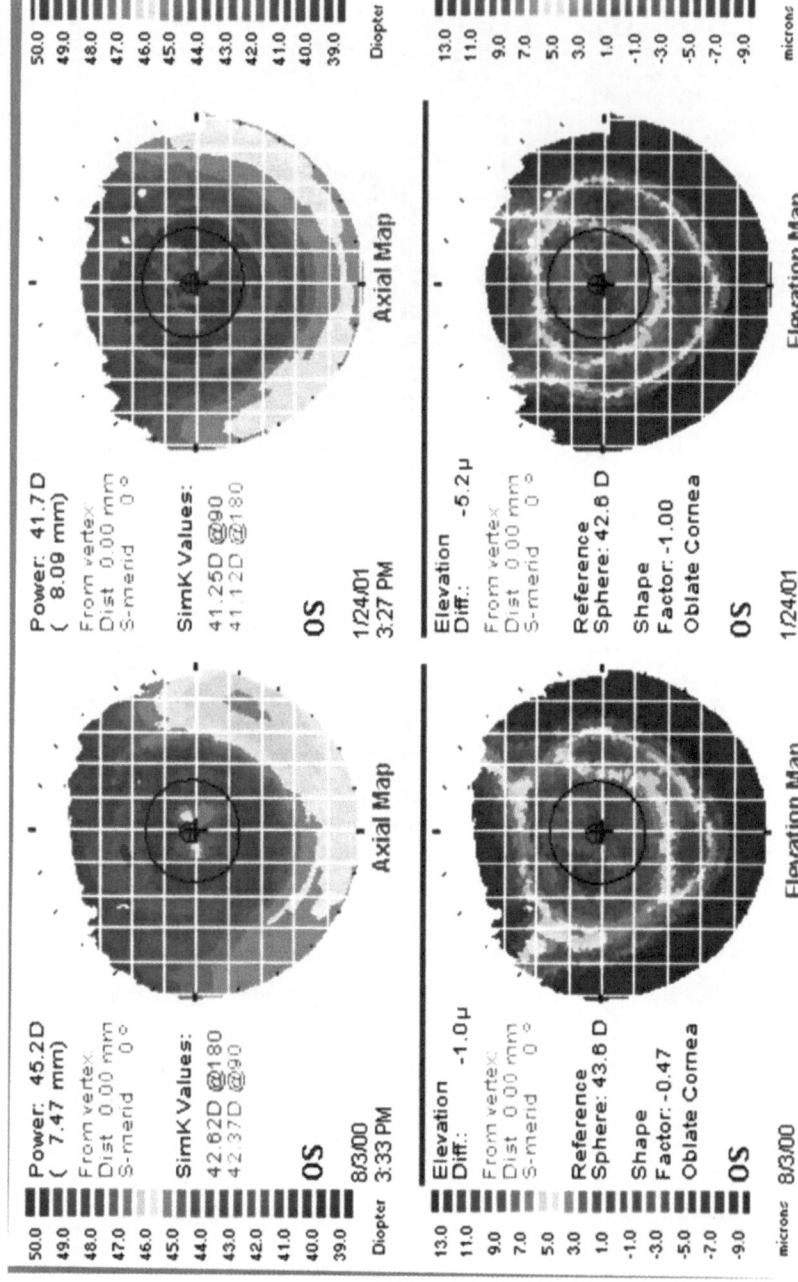

Figure 8.14 Patient with apparent central island 4 months following LASIK (upper left). Elevation (lower left) shows higher elevation inferiorly in shape of a peninsula. A 7 μm PTK measuring 2.2 mm optical zone with 0.5 mm transition zone was performed decentered 0.4 mm inferiorly; this was calculated using VISX CAP™ software. Note marked improvement in curvature (upper right) and elevation (lower right) maps.

3. Planning for Reoperation

CVK is important for determining when the cornea has stabilized following the initial refractive surgical procedure. CVK can also be used to assist in planning the next surgical
procedure. This is particularly relevant if there is a topographic abnormality such as a central island or decentration. Certainly, topographic data are essential in planning treatment
of central islands, and outcomes may be enhanced if the ablation can be customized using
special software such as CAP (Fig. 8.14). In the near future, software and hardware developments, including wavefront-guided ablation, will permit more precise planning and treatment of a range of pre-existing and surgically induced topographic abnormalities.

REFERENCES

1. H Uozato, DL Guyton. Centering corneal surgical procedures. Am J Ophthalmol 1987;103:
   264–275.
2. GO Waring. Making sense of keratospeak II: proposed conventional terminology for corneal topography. Refract Corneal Surg 1989;5:362–367.
3. RK Maloney. Corneal topography and optical zone location in photorefractive keratomy. Refract Corneal Surg 1990;6:363–371.
4. FC Mish, ed. Webster's Ninth New Collegiate Dictionary. Springfield, MA: Merriam-Webster,
   1984.
5. MW Belin, CD Ratliff. Evaluating data acquisition and smoothing functions of currently available videokeratoscopes. J Cataract Refract Surg 1996;22:421–426.
6. S Bafna, T Kohnen, DD Koch. Axial, instantaneous, and refractive formulas in computerized
   videokeratography of normal corneas. J Cataract Refract Surg 1998;24:1184–1190.
7. C Roberts. Characterization of the inherent error in a spherically-biased corneal topography
   system in mapping a radially aspheric surface. J Refract Corneal Surg 1994;10:103–111.
8. C Roberts. The accuracy of power maps to display curvature data in corneal topography systems. Invest Ophthalmol Vis Sci 1994;35:3525–3532.
9. A Gullstrand. Appendices to part I. II. Procedure of the rays in the eye; imagery-laws of the first
   order. In: JPC Southall, ed. Helmholtz's Treatise of Physiological Optics; translated from the
   third German edition. New York: Optical Society of America, 1924.
10. SA Klein. A corneal topography algorithm that produces continuous curvature. Optom Vis Sci
    1992;69:829–834.
11. DD Koch, EA Haft. Introduction to corneal topography. In: JP Gills et al., eds. Corneal topog-
    raphy: the state of the art. Thorofare, NJ: Slack Incorporated, 1995, pp 3–15.
12. SE Wilson, SD Klyce. Quantitative descriptors of corneal topography. A clinical study. Arch
    Ophthalmol 1991;109:349–353.
13. DT Lin. Corneal topographic analysis after excimer photorefractive keratectomy. Ophthalmol-
    ogy 1994;101:1432–1439.
14. MK Smolek, T Oshika, SD Klyce, N Maeda, DH Haight, MB McDonald. Topographic assess-
    ment of irregular astigmatism after photorefractive keratectomy. J Cataract Refract Surg
    1998;24:1079–1086.
15. Y Shiotani, N Maeda, T Inoue, H Watanabe, Y Inoue, Y Shimomura, Y Tano. Comparison of
    topographic indices that correlate with visual acuity in videokeratography. Ophthalmology
    2000;107:559–564.
16. JT Holladay. Corneal topography using the Holladay diagnostic summary. J Cataract Refract
    Surg 1997;23:209–221.
17. PS Hersh, SI Shah, D Geiger, JT Holladay. Corneal optical irregularity after excimer laser pho-
    torefractive keratectomy. J Cataract Refract Surg 1996;22:197–204.
18. JS Weiss, NL Oplinger. An analysis of the accuracy of predicted corneal acuity in the Holladay
    diagnostic summary program. CLAO J 1998;24:141–144.

19. RE Hubbe, GN Foulks. The effect of poor fixation on computer-assisted topographic corneal analysis. Ophthalmology 1994;101:1745–1748.

20. C Roberts. Analysis of the inherent error of the TMS-1 topographic modeling system in mapping a radially aspheric surface. Cornea 1995;14:258–265.

21. MW Belin, CD Ratliff. Evaluating data acquisition and smoothing functions of currently available videokeratoscopes. J Cataract Refract Surg 1996;22:421–426.

22. SE Wilson, SD Klyce. Background of corneal topography. In: HK Wu, VM Thompson, RF Steinert, PS Hersh, SG Slade, eds. Refractive Surgery. New York: Thieme, 1999, pp 53–62.

23. L Wang. Keratoconus evaluation using the Orbscan Topography System. Medical doctoral dissertation, 1999, Ruprecht-Karls-University of Heidelberg, Heidelberg, Germany.

24. GU Auffarth, MR Tetz, Y Biazid, HE Volcker, Measuring anterior chamber depth with Orbscan Topography System. J Cataract Refract Surg 1997;23:1351–1355.

25. M Vetrugno, N Cardascia, L Cardia. Anterior chamber depth measured by two methods in myopic and hyperopic phakic IOL implant. Br J Ophthalmol 2000;84:1113–1116.

26. V Yaylali, SC Kaufman, HW Thompson. Corneal thickness measurements with the Orbscan Topography System and ultrasonic pachymetry. J Cataract Refract Surg 1997;23:1345–1350.

27. MW Marsich, MA Bullimore. The repeatability of corneal thickness measures. Cornea 2000;19:792–795.

28. NG Iskander, EA Penno, NT Peters, HV Gimble, M Ferensowicz. Accuracy of Orbscan pachymetry measurements compared to DGH ultrasound pachymetry in primary LASIK and LASIK enhancement procedures. J Cataract Refract Surg. In press.

29. MC Knorz, T Neuhann. Treatment of myopia and myopic astigmatism by customized laser in situ keratomileusis based on corneal topography. Ophthalmology 2000;107:2072–2076.

30. G Alessio, F Boscia, MG La Tegola, C Sborgia. Topography-driven photorefractive keratectomy: results of corneal interactive programmed topographic ablation software. Ophthalmology 2000;107:1578–1587.

31. Z Wang, J Chen, B Yang. Posterior corneal surface topographic changes after laser in situ keratomileusis are related to residual corneal bed thickness. Ophthalmology 1999;106:406–409; discussion 409–410.

32. MW Belin, D Litoff, SJ Strods, SS Winn, RS Smith. The PAR technology corneal topography system. Refract Corneal Surg 1992;8:88–96.

33. MW Belin, P Zloty. Accuracy of the PAR corneal topography system with spatial misalignment. CLAO J 1993;19:64–68.

34. OO Ucakhan, G Sternberg, C Bodian, K Kelliher, PA Asbell. Intraoperative PAR corneal topography system (CTS): comparison of its keratometric readings to manual keratometer, autokeratometer, EyeSys Corneal Analysis system, and slit lamp PAR CTS in healthy eyes. CLAO J 2000;26:151–158.

35. D Priest, R Munger. Comparative study of the elevation topography of complex shapes. J Cataract Refract Surg 1998;24:741–750.

36. RL Schultze. Accuracy of corneal elevation with four corneal topography systems. J Refract Surg 1998;14:100–104.

37. PC Baker. Holographic contour analysis of the cornea. In: BR Masters, ed.: Noninvative diagnostic techniques in ophthalmology. New York: Springer-Verlag, 1990.

38. MC Corbett, DP O'Brart, BATh Stultiens, FHM Jongsma, J Marshall. Corneal topography using a new moiré image-based system. Eur J Implant Ref Surg 1995;7:353–370.

39. GWHM Van Alphen. On emmetropia and ametropia. Ophthalmologica 1961;142(suppl):1–92.

40. LF Garner, CK Meng, TP Grosvenor, N Mohidin. Ocular dimensions and refractive power in Malay and Melanesian children. Ophthalmic Physiol Opt 1990;10:234–238.

41. DA Goss, VD Cox, GA Herrin-Lawson, ED Nielsen, WA Dolton. Refractive error, axial length, and height as a function of age in young myopes. Optom Vis Sci 1990;67:332–338.

42. T Grosvenor, R Scott. Role of the axial length/corneal radius ratio in determining the refractive state of the eye. Optom Vis Sci 1994;71:573–579.

43. WSH Goh, CSY Lam. Changes in refractive trends and optical components of Hong Kong Chinese aged 19–39 years. Ophthalmic Physiol Opt 1994;14:378–382.

44. Z Liu, J Chen, S Li. The differences in corneal shape between myopic and normal eyes. Chung Hua Yen Ko Tsa Chih 1995;31:282–284.

45. K Budak, TT Khater, NJ Friedman, JT Holladay, DD Koch. Evaluation of relationships among refractive and topographic parameters. J Cataract Refract Surg 1999;25:814–820.

46. LG Carney, JC Mainstone, BA Henderson. Corneal topography and myopia: a cross-section study. Invest Ophthalmol Vis Sci 1997;38:311–320.

47. K Budak, AM Hamed, NJ Friedman, DD Koch. Corneal topography classification in myopic eyes based on axial, instantaneous, refractive, and profile difference maps. J Cataract Refract Surg 1999;25:1069–1079.

48. NC Strang, KL Schmid, LG Carney. Hyperopia is predominantly axial in nature. Curr Eye Res 1998;17:380–383.

49. RB Mandell, R St. Helen. Mathematical model of the corneal contour. Br J Physiol Opt 1971;26:183–197.

50. DM Maurice. The cornea and sclera. In: H Davson, ed. The Eye. New York: Academic Press, 1984.

51. RH Webb. Zernike polynomial description of ophthalmic surfaces. In: Ophthalmic and Visual Optics Technical Digest. Washington, DC: Optical Society of America, 1992, pp 38–41.

52. HC Howland, A Glasser, R Applegate. Polynomial approximations of corneal surfaces and corneal curvature topography. In: Ophthalmic and Visual Optics Technical Digest. Washington, DC: Optical Society of America, 1992, pp 34–37.

53. C Edmund, E Sjontoft. The central-peripheral radius of the normal corneal curvature: a photokeratoscopic study. Acta Ophthalmol 1985;63:670–677.

54. J Wang, DA Rice, SD Klyce. A new reconstruction algorithm for improvement of corneal topographic analysis. Refract Corneal Surg 1989;5:379–387.

55. PS Hersh, SI Shah, JT Holladay. Corneal asphericity following excimer laser photorefractive keratectomy. Summit PRK Topography Study Group. Ophthalmic Surg Lasers 1996;27(suppl): S421–S428.

56. W Lotmar. Theoretical eye model with aspherics. J Opt Sci Am 1971;61:1522–1529.

57. PM Kiely, G Smith, LG Carney. The mean shape of the human cornea. Optica Acta 1982; 29:1027–1040.

58. SG El Hage, B Berney. Contribution of the crystalline lens to the spherical aberration of the eye. J Opt Sci Am 1973;63:205–211.

59. M Townsley. New knowledge of the cornea contour. Contacto 1970;14:38–43.

60. M Guillon, DPM Lydon, C Wilson. Corneal topography: a clinical model. Ophth Physiol Opt 1986;6:47–56.

61. SE Wilson, DT Lin, SD Klyce, JJ Reidy, MS Insler. Topographic changes in contact lens-induced corneal warpage. Ophthalmology 1990;97:734–744.

62. Z Liu, SC Pflugfelder. The effects of long-term contact lens wear on corneal thickness, curvature, and surface regularity. Ophthalmology 2000;107:105–111.

63. K Budak, AM Hamed, NJ Friedman, DD Koch. Preoperative screening of contact lens wearers before refractive surgery. J Cataract Refract Surg 1999;25:1080–1086.

64. SE Wilson, SD Klyce. Screening for corneal topographic abnormalities before refractive surgery. Ophthalmology 1994;101:147–152.

65. YS Rabinowitz, PJ McDonnell. Computer-assisted corneal topography in keratoconus. Refractive Corneal Surg 1989;5:400–406.

66. GU Auffarth, L Wang, HE Volcker. Keratoconus evaluation using the Orbscan topography system. J Cataract Refract Surg 2000;26:222–228.

67. RA Eiferman, L Lane, M Law, Y Fields. Superior keratoconus (letter). Refract Corneal Surg 1993;9:394–395.

68. DD Koch, SE Husain. Corneal topography to detect and characterize corneal pathology. In: JP Gills et al., eds. Corneal topography: the state of the art. Thorofare, NJ: Slack Incorporated, 1995, pp 159–169.

69. N Maeda, SD Klyce, MK Smolek, HW Thompson. Automated keratoconus screening with corneal topography analysis. Invest Ophthalmol Vis Sci 1994;35:2749–2757.
70. N Maeda, SD Klyce, MK Smolek. Comparison of methods for detecting keratoconus using videokeratography. Arch Ophthalmol 1995;113:870–874.
71. N Maeda, SD Klyce, MK Smolek. Neural network classification of corneal topography. Preliminary demonstration. Invest Ophthalmol Vis Sci 1995;36:1327–1335.
72. MK Smolek, SD Klyce. Current keratoconus detection methods compared with a neural network approach. Invest Ophthalmol Vis Sci 1997;38:2290–2299.
73. YS Rabinowitz, K Rasheed. KISA% index: a quantitative videokeratography algorithm embodying minimal topographic criteria for diagnosing keratoconus. J Cataract Refract Surg 1999;25:1327–1335.
74. MH Dastjerdi, H Hashemi. A quantitative corneal topography index for detection of keratoconus. J Refract Surg 1998;14:427–436.
75. A Langenbucher, GC Gusek-Schneider, MM Kus, D Huber, B Seitz. Keratoconus screening with wave-front parameters based on topography height data. Klin Monatsbl Augenheilkd 1999;214:217–223.
76. JH Krachmer. Pellucid marginal corneal degeneration. Arch Ophthalmol 1978;96:1217–1221.
77. LJ Maguire, SD Klyce, MB McDonald, HE Kaufman. Corneal topography of pellucid marginal degeneration. Ophthalmology 1987;94:519–524.
78. CH Karabatsas, SD Cook. Topographic analysis in pellucid marginal corneal degeneration and keratoglobus. Eye 1996;10(pt 4):451–455.
79. JA Cameron, MA Mahmood. Superior corneal thinning with pellucid marginal corneal degeneration. Am J Ophthalmol 1990;109:486–487.
80. KS Bower, DK Dhaliwal, DA Barnhorst Jr, J Warnicke. Pellucid marginal degeneration with superior corneal thinning. Cornea 1997;16:483–485.
81. DP Taglia, J Sugar. Superior pellucid marginal corneal degeneration with hydrops. Arch Ophthalmol 1997;115:274–275.
82. F Verrey. Kératoglobe aigu. Ophthalmologica 1947;114:284–288.
83. V Cavara. Keratoglobus and keratoconus: a contribution to the nosological interpretation of keratoglobus. Br J Ophthalmol 1950;34:621–626.
84. SP Amoils, MB Deist, P Gous, PM Amoils. Iatrogenic keratectasia after laser in situ keratomileusis for less than −4.0 to −7.0 diopters of myopia. J Cataract Refract Surg 2000;26:967–977.
85. GE Tamayo Fernandez, MG Serrano. Early clinical experience using custom excimer laser ablations to treat irregular astigmatism (1). J Cataract Refract Surg 2000;26:1442–1450.
86. PS Hersh. A standardized classification of corneal topography after laser refractive surgery. J Refract Surg 1997;13:571–575; discussion 575–578.
87. T Oshika, SD Klyce, MK Smolek, MB McDonald. Corneal hydration and central islands after excimer laser photorefractive keratectomy. J Cataract Refract Surg 1998;24:1575–1580.
88. SW Kang, ES Chung, WJ Kim. Clinical analysis of central islands after laser in situ keratomileusis. J Cataract Refract Surg 2000;26:536–542.

9

Wavefront Technology and LASIK Applications

NAOYUKI MAEDA

Osaka University Medical School, Osaka, Japan

A. INTRODUCTION

Spherical and cylinder corrections with spectacles for the refractive errors of the eyes have been performed since the thirteenth and nineteenth centuries. From the latter time, refractive errors have been measured for sphere and cylinder components in the general ophthalmic practice. Although corneal topographic analysis can be performed to evaluate the corneal irregular astigmatism, and rigid contact lenses can be used to correct corneal irregular astigmatism, it is still difficult to evaluate the irregular astigmatism components in refraction and to correct for irregular astigmatism with any optical device until recently.

Nevertheless, we will eventually have the means of determining the complete refractive status including higher-order irregular astigmatism by wavefront sensing and to obtain "supernormal vision" (1) with refractive surgery by applying the principle of adaptive optics. In this chapter, the concepts of wavefront analysis and adaptive optics, (2) and the application of these to the LASIK procedure, will be presented from an ophthalmologist's point of view.

B. PRINCIPLES OF WAVEFRONT SENSING

1. What Is the Wavefront?

We first need to know what is meant by a wavefront. Figure 9.1 shows how light is expressed differently in geometrical and physical optics. The rays from a point source of light radiate out in all directions in geometrical optics. However, in physical optics, light is considered as a wave and the light wave spreads in all directions as in the widening rings on a still pond when a stone is thrown into it. The wavefront is a ripple that is in phase.

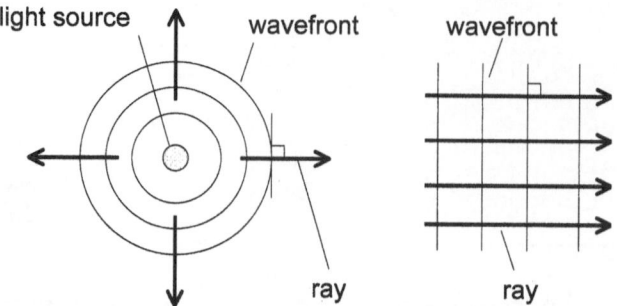

Figure 9.1 Ray and wavefront.

Similarly, light coming from infinity is considered to be linear bundles of rays in geometrical optics. In physical optics, the wave from infinity has a plane wavefront, and the plane of the wavefront is always perpendicular to the direction of the rays.

Although an optical system or lens is usually defined as one that refracts light rays, it can also be defined as one that transforms the shape of wavefront (Fig. 9.2). If we think of light emitted from the fovea passing through the lens and cornea towards the outside, the refractive status, such as myopia, hyperopia, supernormal eyes, and eyes with higher-order aberrations (irregular astigmatism), can be displayed using wavefronts as shown in Fig. 9.3. The wavefront of the supernormal eye, that is, an emmetropic eye without any aberrations, is shown as a perfect plane that is perpendicular to the line of sight. In myopic eyes, the wavefront has a bowllike shape with the peripheral wavefront more advanced than the central wavefront. As the wavefront is perpendicular to the ray, it is easy to imagine that the peripheral rays go to the primary line of sight and bundles of ray converge on the axis.

The wavefront exiting the hyperopic eye, on the other hand, has a hill shape with the central wavefront more advanced than the peripheral wavefront. Therefore the rays of a hill shaped wavefront will diverge. If the measured eye has irregular astigmatism or higher-order aberrations, the wavefront of the eye will have an irregular shape.

2. Wavefront Analysis

The purpose of wavefront analysis is to evaluate the optical quality of the eye by evaluating the shape of its wavefront. The optical quality of a wavefront is usually expressed as wavefront aberrations, where wavefront aberration is defined as the deviation between the wavefront that comes from an ideal optic system and the wavefront that originates from an

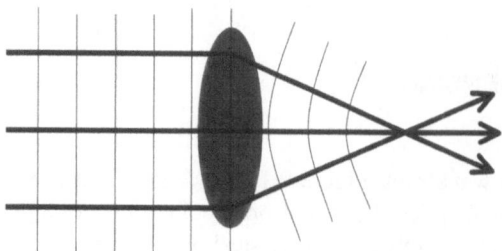

Figure 9.2 Optical system and wavefront.

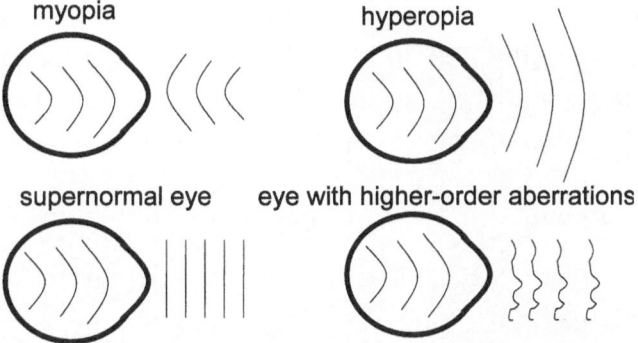

Figure 9.3 Refractive errors and diagram using wavefront.

actual optical system. The unit used for wavefront analysis is not diopters but microns or fractions of wavelength, because wavefront expresses the deformity of wavefront shape in three-dimensional space. It is usually expressed as the root mean square or RMS.

The instruments used for wavefront analysis are called wavefront sensors, and these instruments are classified into two categories based on their method of measurement, the ray tracing method and the laser interferometry method. Examples of wavefront sensors that use ray tracing are the Tscherning aberroscope, the Hartmann–Shack sensor, the cross cylinder aberroscope, optical path difference, and subjective ray tracing.

Higher-order aberrations in the human eye were measured first by Smirnov (3) in 1961 by a psychophysical method, and he predicted that custom lenses will be made to compensate for the higher-order aberrations of individual eyes. A modified aberroscope technique was developed by Howland (4), and Liang and Bille (5) measured the wavefront aberration of the human eye objectively using the Hartmann–Shack sensor in 1994.

The principle of the Hartmann–Shack sensor is shown in Fig. 9.4. A very narrow beam of light is projected onto the retina, and the light reflected from the fovea passes through the lens and cornea and exits from the eye. The Hartmann–Shack sensor has an ar-

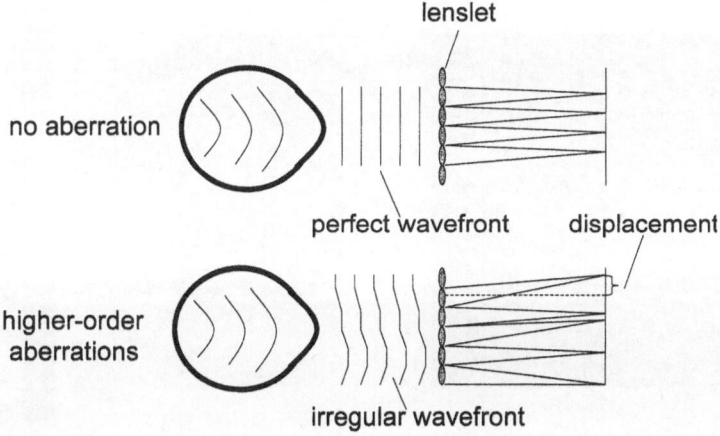

Figure 9.4 Principles of Hartmann–Shack sensor.

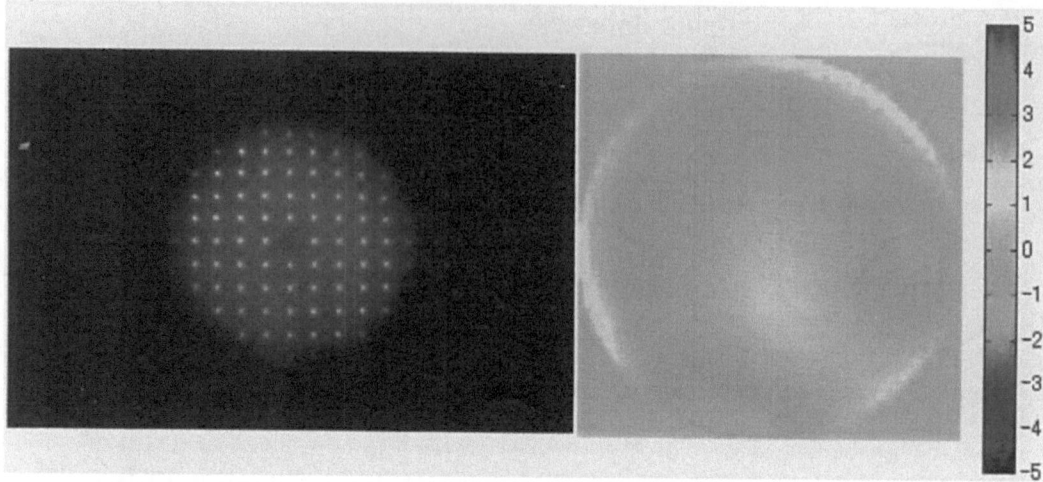

Figure 9.5   Spot patterns in normal subject.

ray of lenslets that consist of a matrix of small lenses (2,6). The light emerging from the eye is focused on a CCD camera by each lenslet to form a spot pattern. The spot pattern of an ideal subject with a perfect wavefront will be exactly the same pattern as the reference grid. The spot pattern of a subject with a distorted wavefront will create an irregular spot pattern. Displacements of lenslet images from their reference position are used to calculate the shape of the wavefront.

Figures 9.5 and 9.6 show examples of spot patterns from a normal and a keratoconic subject with the Topcon Hartmann–Shack sensor. Although the spot pattern in the normal subject is regular, the spot pattern in the patient with keratoconus is markedly distorted. As the wavefront of each lenslet is perpendicular to the direction of the ray, i.e., displacement

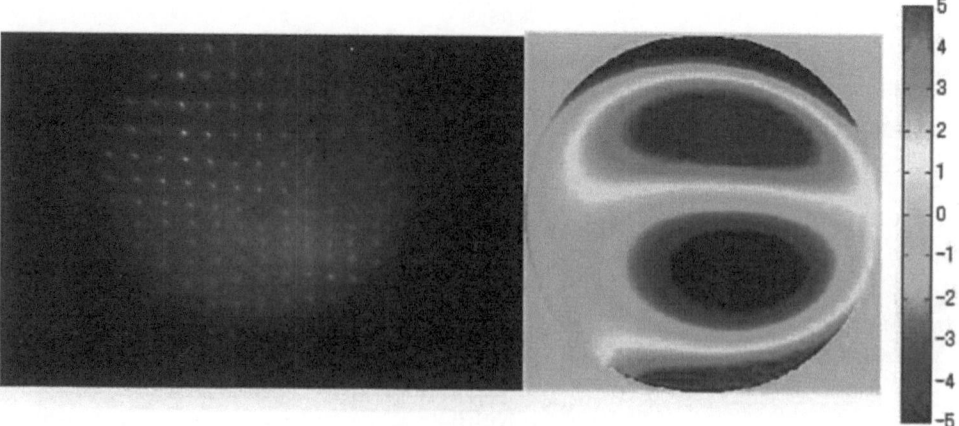

Figure 9.6   Spot patterns in keratoconus.

$$Y = Z_{nm} = R_n^{n-2m}(r) X(n-2m)\,\theta$$

$$X: \sin \text{ (when } n-2m>0)$$
$$\cos \text{ (when } n-2m<0)$$

$$R_n^{n-2m}(r) = \sum_{S=0}^{m} (-1)^s \frac{(n-s)!}{s!(m-s)!(n-m-s)!} r^{n-2s}$$

Figure 9.7 Equation of Zernike polynomials.

of their focusing spots, the wavefront of the measured subjects can be reconstructed from these spot patterns.

Wavefront aberrations, the quantitative measure of wavefront distortions, are usually calculated using Zernike polynomials. The wavefront is expanded into sets of Zernike polynomials to extract the characteristic components of the wavefront. The Zernike polynomials are the combination of trigonometric functions and radial functions, and the terms of the Zernike polynomials, represented as Z (Fig. 9.7), are useful to show the wavefront aberrations because of their orthogonality (2).

Examples of Zernike polynomials up to the fourth order are shown in Fig. 9.8. The zero order has one term that represents a constant. The first order represents tilt (two terms, one for the X axis and another for the Y axis). The second order includes three terms that represent defocus and astigmatism in the two directions. The third order has four terms that represent coma and trefoil aberrations. The polynomials can be expanded up to any arbitrary order unless there are enough numbers of measurements of points for calculations. Spectacles can correct only second-order aberrations, not the third and higher orders that represent irregular astigmatism. Using the Zernike coefficients of each term, monochromatic aberrations can be evaluated quantitatively (7).

The wavefront can also be displayed as color-coded maps as shown in Figs. 9.5 and 9.6. The advancing part of a wavefront is shown by warmer colors and the trailing part of the wavefront is shown by cooler colors.

3. Adaptive Optics

In general, optical systems, such as cameras, telescopes, fundus cameras, or spectacles, with lower aberrations have better optical properties. However, even if we minimize the aberrations in an optical system such as an astronomical telescope or a fundus camera, the aberrations induced by the atmosphere or the aberrations of normal human eyes are usually larger than the aberrations in the optic devices, and thus the final resolution of the images is reduced, i.e., the optical quality is limited by the higher-order aberrations of the subjects.

Adaptive optics is the concept of intentionally designing the optics of the observatory system to compensate for the measured aberrations of the subject. As a result, the total aberrations of the subject and observatory system are reduced, and one can observe with minimal aberrations.

An example of an adaptive optical system is shown in Fig. 9.9. The wavefront sensor measures the aberrations of the subject, and this information is processed and sent to actuators. The shape of the deformable mirror is controlled by actuators to reshape the surface of the thin mirror to compensate for the aberration of the subject.

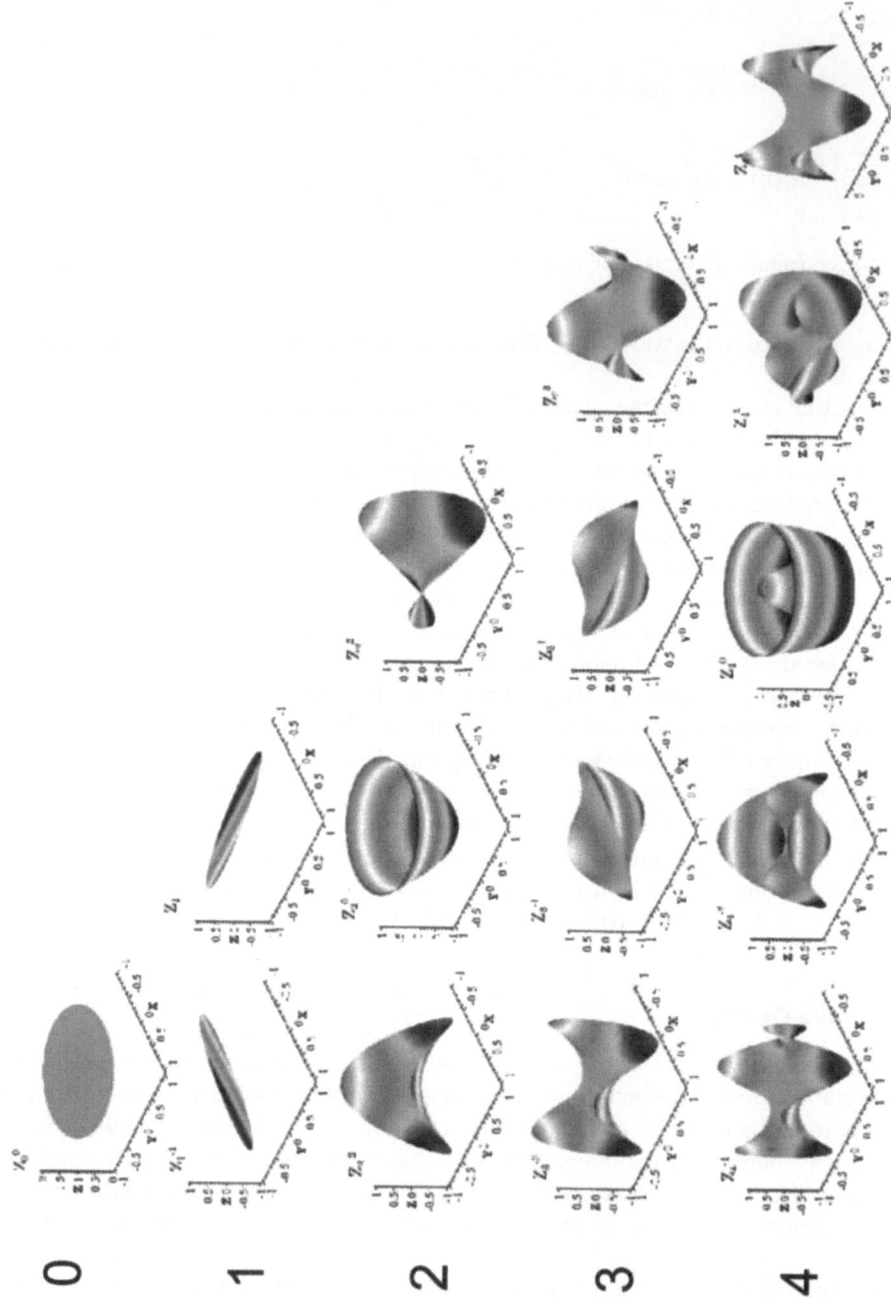

Figure 9.8 Graphic representations of Zernike polynomials.

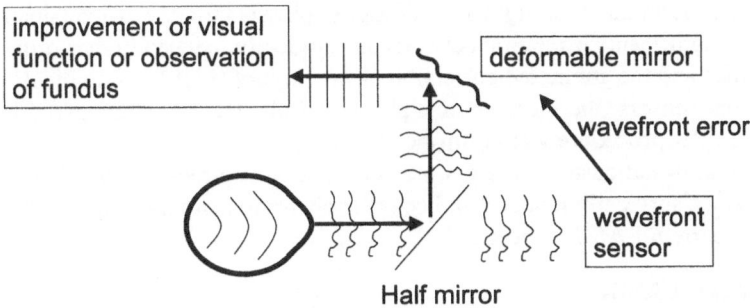

Figure 9.9 Principles of adaptive optics.

Babcock (8) arrived at the concept of adaptive optics in 1953, and this technology was used for military purposes for a long time. In 1991, much of the United States' military work in adaptive optics was declassified, and the astronomical community applied this technology to their field (9). In 1997, Liang and Williams corrected the monochromatic aberrations of normal human eyes with adaptive optics and showed that this improved the contrast sensitivity of the eye, and the imaging of cone cells in the living human retina. With adaptive optics, images of the cone mosaic (short-, medium-, and long-wavelength-sensitive cones) in living human eyes were observed (10).

If we use an excimer laser in place of the deformable mirror, we have the potential of correcting irregular astigmatism and obtaining supernormal vision by eliminating the inherent optical aberrations of normal human eyes. Although this might not be classified as adaptive optics by the strictest definition, this concept has become one of the most discussed topics in refractive surgery.

C. WAVEFRONT-GUIDED ABLATION IN LASIK

1. Optical Quality in Current LASIK Procedures

The question arises whether the current LASIK procedures are satisfactory. For correcting refractive changes, current LASIK procedures have reasonably good predictability for mild to moderate myopia and low hyperopia. As a result, most patients are satisfied with the outcome. This is the one of the major reasons why LASIK has been accepted by the public in such a short period. However, we have also noticed that the optical quality of the eye following LASIK is not optimal, and LASIK patients sometimes complain about problems such as halo, glare, or difficulty with night driving. It is also very difficult to treat irregular astigmatism with conventional LASIK procedures. Thus we must realize that current techniques, while quite satisfactory, still have room to be improved.

The effect of corneal shape on the optical quality of the eye can be calculated as corneal wavefront aberrations using corneal topography. It is possible to estimate the surgically induced higher-order aberrations of the eye from the measurement of corneal wavefront aberrations, because wavefront aberrations of the lens should be stable despite the refractive corneal surgeries. The measurement of corneal aberrations showed that higher-order aberrations of the cornea increased following PRK (11,12,13) and LASIK

(12). This trend was more prominent for night vision (large pupil) than for day vision (small pupil). Also, there is a significant correlation between the surgically induced higher-order aberrations of the cornea and the attempted correction of the surgery (11,13). With the development of wavefront sensors, the increase of higher-order aberrations of the eye following a conventional PRK procedure was confirmed (14).

These results suggest that custom ablation methods that can correct irregular astigmatism or that can reduce surgically induced higher-order aberrations might reduce some of the problems of the current LASIK procedures.

2. Wavefront-Guided LASIK

When wavefront-guided refractive surgery is performed, the following requirements should be satisfied for the wavefront sensing and the photo ablation. For the measurement of wavefront aberrations, wavefront sensors and softwares that can calculate the aberration are essential. Since 1999, many prototype wavefront sensor instruments have been introduced (Table 1). Figures 9.10, 9.11, and 9.12 show examples of wavefront sensors and their outputs. Although all of these instruments are prototypes, they should soon be commercially available.

Based on the measured wavefront aberrations, not only spherical and cylindrical errors but also irregular astigmatism (higher-order wavefront aberrations) should be correctable with the excimer laser. For that purpose, very fine processing of the corneal shape is required including asymmetrical or local ablations. Therefore laser instruments should be equipped with a flying spot scanning system or an equivalent mechanism, and an active eye tracking system is essential for precise ablation (Table 2). In addition, an algorithm that

Table 1   Examples of Wavefront Sensors

Wavefront sensor	Company	Principle	Corneal topography	Excimer laser
CustomCornea wavefront system	Zeiss Humphrey	Hartmann–Shack		Alcon/Summit/ Autonomous
WaveScan	20/10 Perfect Vision	Hartmann–Shack		VISX
Zywave	Technolas	Hartmann–Shack	Slit scanning (Orbscan IIz)	Technolas
Dresden wavefront analyzer	Technomed	Tscherning		Wavelight, Schwind
Ray-tracking refractometer	Tracey	Ray tracing Aberrometry		
ARK-10000	Nidek	Optical path difference	Videokeratoscope	Nidek
Wavefront analyzer	Topcon	Hartmann–Shack	Videokeratoscope	
COAS	Wavefront Sciencies	Hartmann–Shack		Meditec

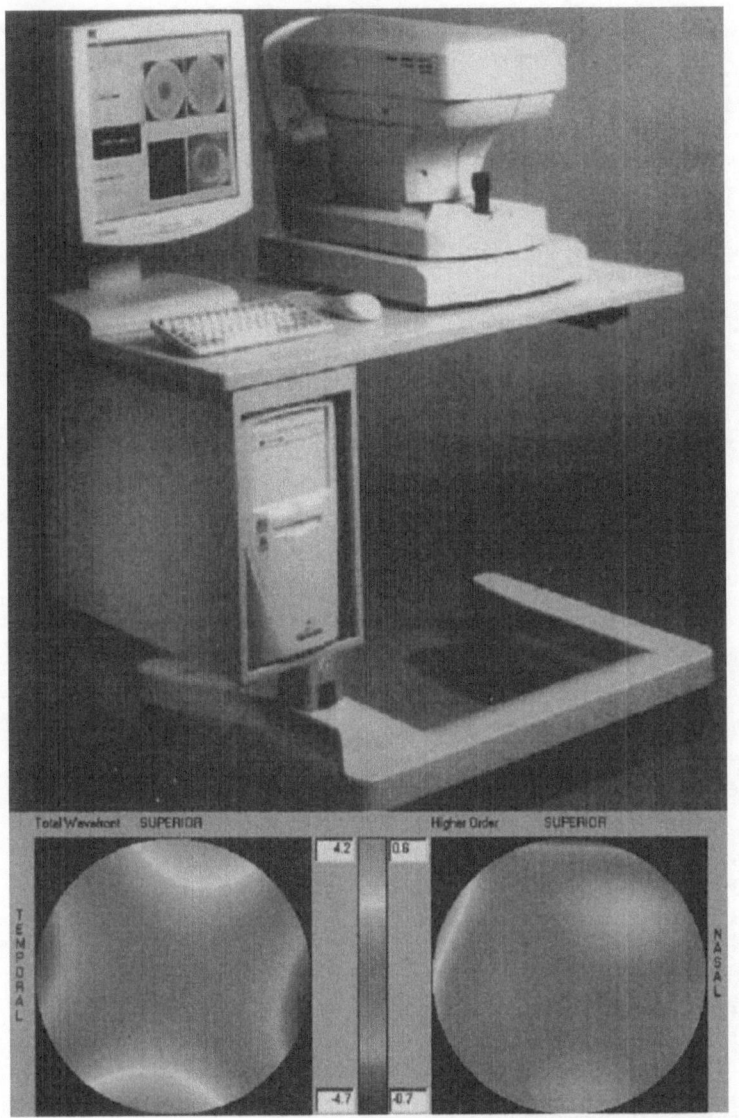

Figure 9.10 Alcon/Summit/Autonomous Custom cornea wavefront system. (Courtesy of Alcon/ Summit/Autonomous Inc.)

can perform aberration correction (15) should be provided. The speed of light in the air is faster than that in the corneal stroma. Therefore the corneal stroma where the wavefront is delayed should be ablated in order to correct aberrations. The areas that are displayed with cooler colors in the wavefront map should be cut to reduce the wavefront aberrations including sphere, cylinder, and higher-order aberrations.

On June 12, 1999, Seiler and his coworkers reported the first application of wavefront-guided LASIK. The early results in three eyes (16) were published by his group using the Wavelight Allegretto excimer laser. The results of this report were promising, as all

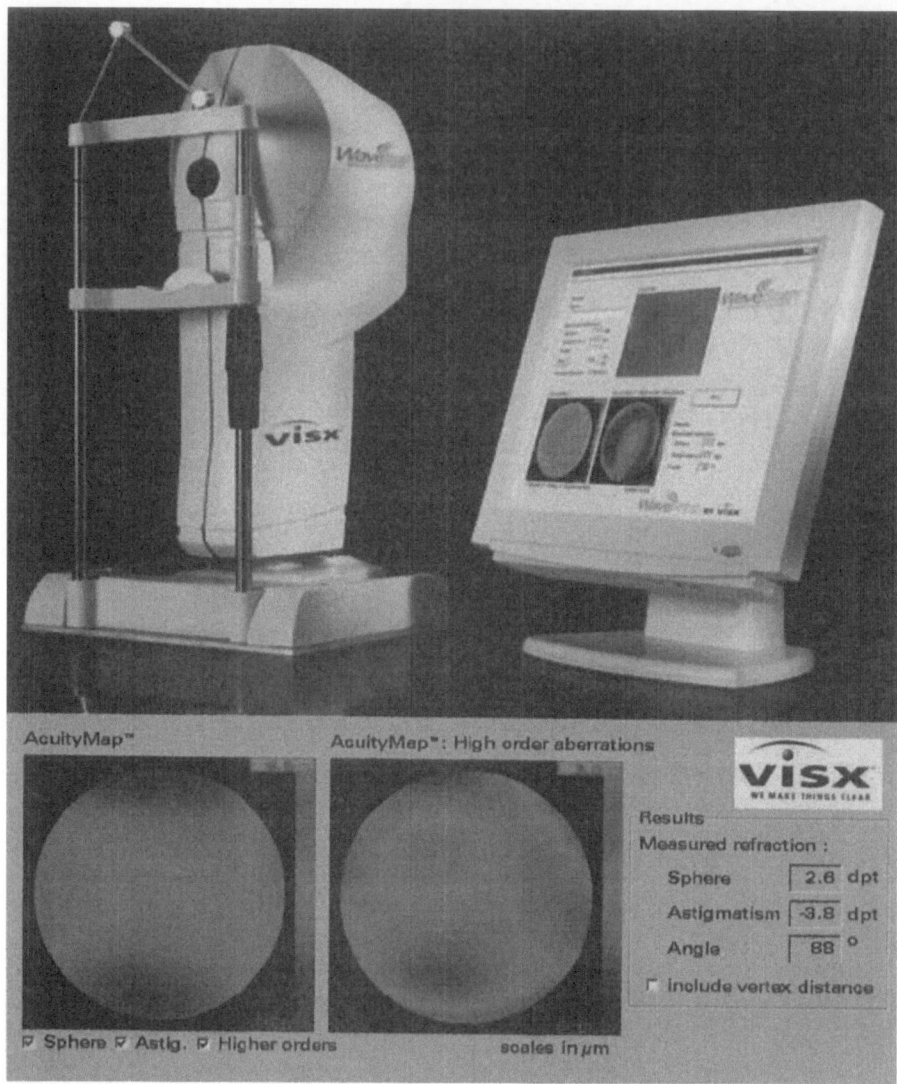

Figure 9.11   VISX WaveScan. (Courtesy of VISX.)

three eyes gained up to two lines of visual acuity, and the wavefront deviations were re-duced by 27% on the average. In the United States, McDonald started the first wavefront-guided LASIK with the Autonomous system on October 1999. She has been performing a comparative study by doing conventional LASIK in one eye and the wavefront-guided LASIK in the other eye for myopia and hyperopia. Although wavefront-guided LASIK pro-duced similar uncorrected visual acuity compared to conventional LASIK, a reduction of higher-order aberrations by wavefront-guided LASIK was found in some cases. Also, VISX and other laser companies have started clinical trials that evaluate the wavefront-guided ablations. The safety and the efficacy of this procedure should be reported soon.

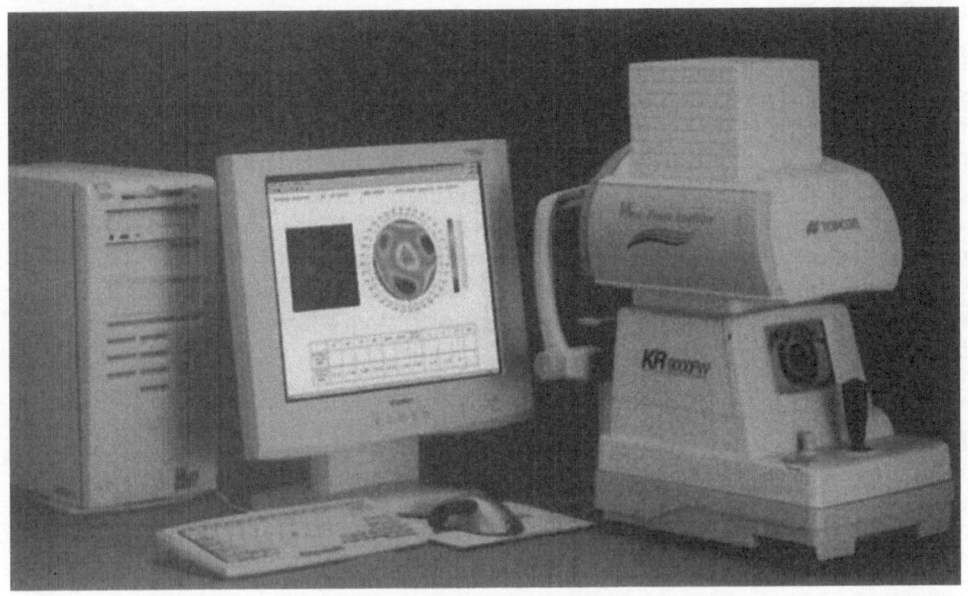

Figure 9.12 Topcon wavefront analyzer. (Courtesy of Topcon Inc.)

Table 2 Examples of Excimer Lasers

Laser	Company	Ablation	Eye tracking (sampling rate)
LadarVision 4000	Alcon/Summit/ Autonomous	Flying spot (0.8–0.9 mm)	Laser radar tracker (4000 Hz)
Star S3	VISX	Broad beam followed by scanning spot	Infrared tracker (60 Hz)
EC-5000CX	Nidek	Scanning slit followed by scanning spot	Infrared tracker (60 Hz)
MEL 70 G-Scan	Asclepion-Meditec	1.5 mm flying spot	Infrared tracker (50 Hz)
Technolas 217Z	B & L	Dual-diameter flying spot (2 and 1 mm)	Infrared tracker (120 Hz)
Allegretto	Wavelight	1 mm flying spot	Infrared tracker (250 Hz)
ESIRIS	Schwind	1 mm flying spot	Infrared tracker (300 Hz)
LaserScan LSX	Lasersight	Flying spot (0.8–1 mm)	Infrared tracker (60 Hz)

D. SUMMARY

It is reasonable for refractive surgeons to remove pathological irregular astigmatism or surgically induced aberrations that correlate with pupil diameter or attempt correction by refractive surgeries. On the other hand, we will need to know the clinical significance of supernormal vision, and also when we should correct for higher-order aberrations because aberrations of refractive surgery candidates do change with age (17,18).

Wavefront-guided refractive surgery has just begun. Many aspects must be improved to obtain better results than the conventional techniques, as many newly developed surgical procedures have problems for the first time. We need to know that conventional refractive surgeries induce higher-order aberrations, and custom ablation appears to be the only solution.

REFERENCES

1. J Liang, DR Williams, DT Miller. Supernormal vision and high-resolution retinal imaging through adaptive optics. J Opt Soc Am A 1997;14:2884–2892.
2. RK Tyson. Principles of Adaptive Optics. 2d ed. Boston: Academic Press, 1998.
3. MS Smirnov. Measurement of the wave aberration of the human eye. Biofizika 1961;6:687–703.
4. B Howland, HC Howland. Subjective measurement of high-order aberrations of the eye. Science 1976;193:580–582.
5. J Liang, B Grimms, S Goelz, JF Bille. Objective measurement of wave aberrations of the human eye with the use of a Hartmann–Shack wavefront sensor. J Opt Soc Am A 1994;11:1949–1957.
6. LN Thibos, X Hong. Clinical applications of the Shack–Hartmann aberrometer. Optom Vis Sci 1999;76:817–825.
7. J Liang, DR Williams. Aberrations and retinal image quality of the normal human eye. J Opt Soc Am A 1997;14:2873–2883.
8. HW Babcock. The possibility of compensating astronomical seeing. Publ Astron Soc Pac 1953;65:229–236.
9. RQ Fugate, DL Fried, GA Ameer, BR Boeke, SL Browne, PH Roberts, RE Ruane, LM Wopat. Measurement of atmospheric wavefront distortion using scattered light from a laser guide star. Nature 1991;353:144–146.
10. A Roodra, DR Williams. The arrangement of the three cone classes in the living human eyes. Nature 1999;397:520–522.
11. CE Martinez, RA Applegate, SD Klyce, MB McDonald, JP Medina, HC Howland. Effect of papillary dilation on corneal optical aberrations after photorefractive keratectomy. Arch Ophthalmol 1998;116:1053–1062.
12. T Oshika, SD Klyce, RA Applegate, HC Howland, MA El Danasoury. Comparison of corneal wavefront aberrations after photorefractive keratectomy and laser in situ keratomileusis. Am J Ophthalmol 1999;127:1–7.
13. KM Oliver, RP Hemenger, MC Corbett, DPS O'Brart, S Verma, J Marshall, A Tomlinson. Corneal optical aberrations induced by photorefractive keratectomy. J Refract Surg 1997;13:246–254.
14. T Seiler, M Kaemmerer, P Mierdel, HE Krinke. Ocular optical aberrations after photorefractive keratectomy for myopia and myopic astigmatism. Arch Ophthalmol 2000;118:17–21.
15. J Schwiegerling, RW Snyder. Custom photorefractive keratectomy ablations for the correction of spherical and cylindrical refractive error and higher-order aberration. J Opt Soc Am A 1998;15:2572–2579.

16. M Mrochen, M Kaemmerer, T Seiler. Wavefront-guided laser in situ keratomileusis: Early results in three eyes. J Refract Surg 2000,16:116–121.

17. T Oshika, SD Klyce, RA Applegate, HC Howland. Changes in corneal wavefront aberrations with aging. Invest Ophthalmol Vis Sci 1999;40:1351–1355.

18. A Guirao, C Gonzalez, M Redondo, E Geraghty, S Norrby, P Artal. Average optical performance of the human eye as a function of age in a normal population. Invest Ophthalmol Vis Sci 1999;40:203–213.

10

Preoperative Considerations
Diagnosis, Classification, and Avoidance of Keratoconus Complications

PAUL CHUNG-SHIEN LU

Chang Gung Memorial Hospital, Taipei, Taiwan, and Harvard Medical School, Boston, Massachusetts, U.S.A.

DIMITRI T. AZAR

Massachusetts Eye and Ear Infirmary, Schepens Eye Research Institute, and Harvard Medical School, Boston, Massachusetts, U.S.A.

A. INTRODUCTION

Keratoconus patients have problems with contact lenses and poor visual acuity with glasses, which contributes to the patients' natural tendency to consider refractive surgery. Keratoconus is a progressive, bilateral, and noninflammatory corneal disease associated with central and paracentral stromal thinning; it is characterized by anterior and posterior corneal protrusion, irregular astigmatism, stromal scarring, and decreased visual acuity, which may reduce the patient's ability to achieve 20/20 corrected visual acuity with spectacles (1). Keratoconus may be associated with systemic diseases (Down's syndrome, Leber's congenital amaurosis, connective tissue disease), trauma (2) (contact lens wear, eye rubbing), and positive family history (3–5). Stromal thinning, epithelial iron ring (Fleischer ring), Vogt's striae, and scarring (6) are often noted on slit lamp examination. Hydrops (Fig. 10.1) is generally associated with advanced keratoconus. Due to the pathologic conditions surgical trauma may exacerbate the disease. The corneas may be weakened by a lamellar cut and cause further corneal instability.

Controversy of diagnosis of keratoconus exists especially in contact lenses wearers (warpage or molding effects) and in other eye conditions simulating keratoconus, such as pellucid marginal degeneration, and keratoglobus.

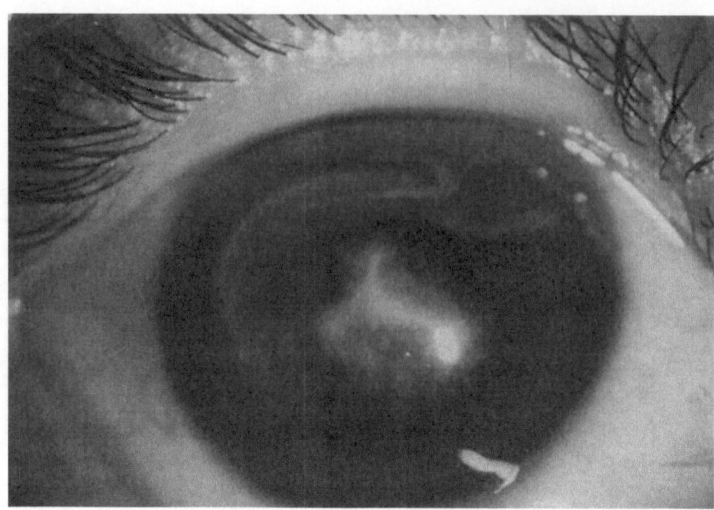

Figure 10.1 The advanced keratoconus with a hydrop in the central cornea. This patient does not pose a risk of being misdiagnosed. It is the more subtle changes on topography and examination that may be missed, if attention to this problem is not provided in the preoperative evaluation of LASIK surgery.

B. DIAGNOSIS

The diagnosis is based on clinical history, clinical examination, placido-based topography using modified Rabinowitz criteria, and scanning slit topography.

Videokeratographic signs (7,8) include increased K (anterior central corneal power) and I-S value (inferior versus superior difference in anterior central corneal power) (9).

The diagnosis of keratoconus is important for proper management with hard contact lenses (10,11) or penetrating keratoplasty (12) and to avoid unexpected adverse outcomes with refractive surgery (13–15). Rabinowitz and McDonnell classified keratoconus based on K, I-S value, and asymmetry of K between a patient's two eyes (16). Maeda, Klyce, and Smolek calculated the I-S value as corneal power difference between five inferior and five superior spots at 30° intervals 3 mm from the corneal vertex (17,18).

Maeda et al. developed a TMS-1 videokeratoscope guided by an automated system with eight indices (Simulated K1, Simulated K2, Surface Asymmetry Index, Differential Sector Index, Opposite Sector Index, Center/Surround Index, Irregular Astigmatism Index, Analyzed Area) which were used to diagnose keratoconus as differentiated from other causes of corneal irregularities (18). Patients were selected from the Louisiana State University Eye Center and had one of eight diagnoses: normal, keratoconus, keratoplasty, epikeratophakia, excimer laser photorefractive keratectomy, radial keratotomy, contact-lens-induced warpage (19,20), or other. Sensitivity and specificity were 98% and 99%, respectively (17).

The TMS-2 videokeratoscope used the modified Rabinowitz criteria to determine K and I-S value only. K of 47.2–48.7 D (diopters) was considered suspect for keratoconus, and K > 48.7 D was suggestive of keratoconus. Likewise, inferior–superior central anterior corneal power asymmetry between 1.4 and 1.9 D was considered suspect for keratoconus, and I-S value > 1.9 D was suggestive of keratoconus (21). Sensitivity and specificity of the modified Rabinowitz method were 96–100% and 85–89%, respectively (17,21).

M.E.E.I. KC Classification

Name_____

Patient ID #_____

			Score		
Kod-Kos	<1.9	0			
	>1.9	1			
Kod	<47.2	0			
	47.2-48.7	1			
	>48.7	2			
ISod	<1.4	0			
	1.4-1.9	1			
	>1.9	2			
≥2 Findings on hx (atopy, down), FH and exam (Fleisher, Vogt, Munson, nerves, scaring)	No	0			
	Yes	2			
Corneal Hydrops (by exam or hx) OD	No	0			
	Yes	2			
		Total Score			OD

			Score		
Kos-Kod	<1.9	0			
	>1.9	1			
Kos	<47.2	0			
	47.2-48.7	1			
	>48.7	2			
ISos	<1.4	0			
	1.4-1.9	1			
	>1.9	2			
≥2 Findings on hx (atopy, down), FH and exam (Fleisher, Vogt, Munson, nerves, scaring)	No	0			
	Yes	2			
Corneal Hydrops (by exam or hx) OS	No	0			
	Yes	2			
		Total Score			OS

SCORE	DIAGNOSIS
(Zero)	Normal
(1-3)	Suspect
(4-5)	Early KC
(6-9)	Advanced KC

Diagnosis_____ OD

Diagnosis_____ OS

Figure 10.2. The Azar-Lu MEEI keratoconus scoring system.

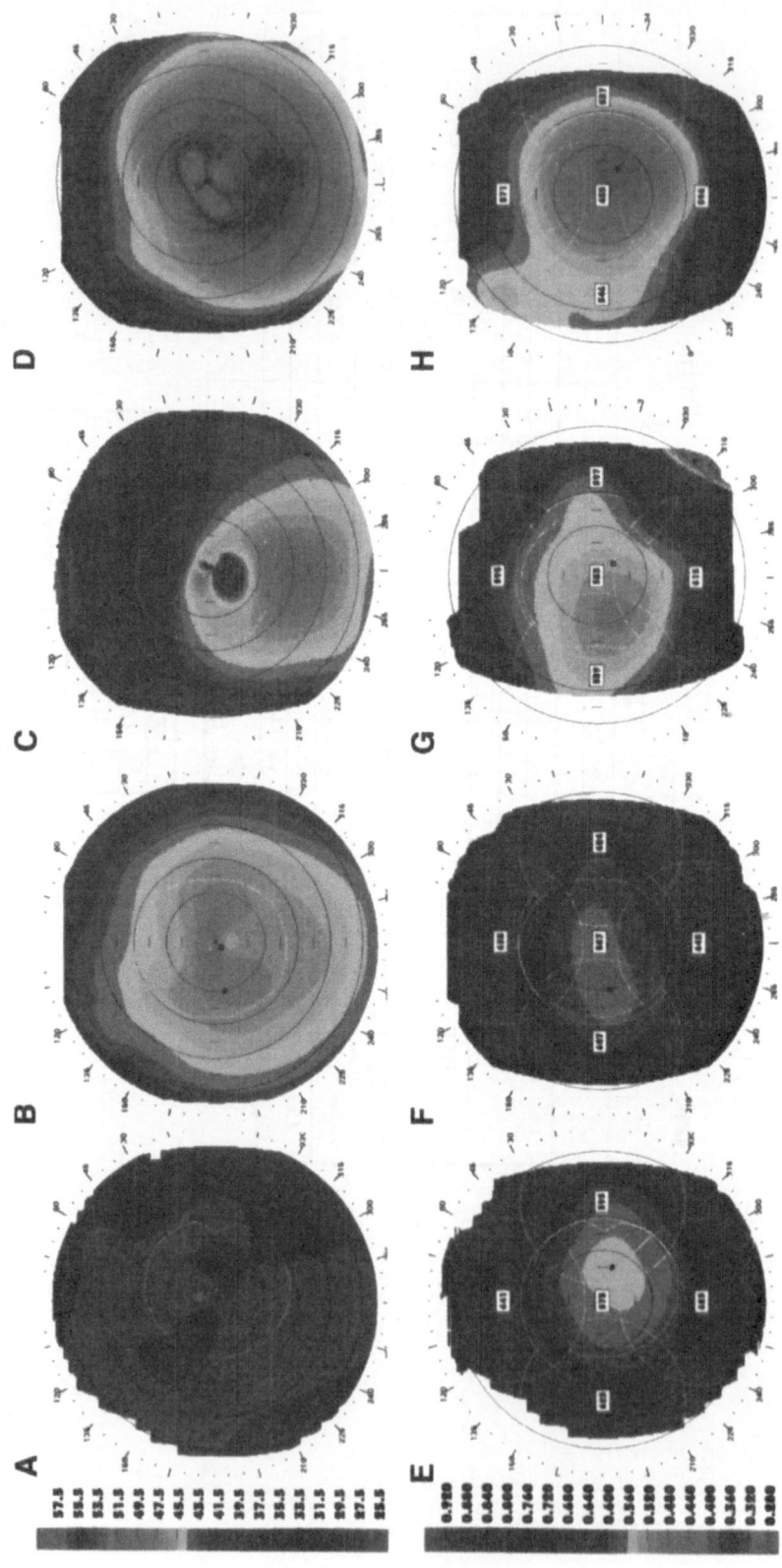

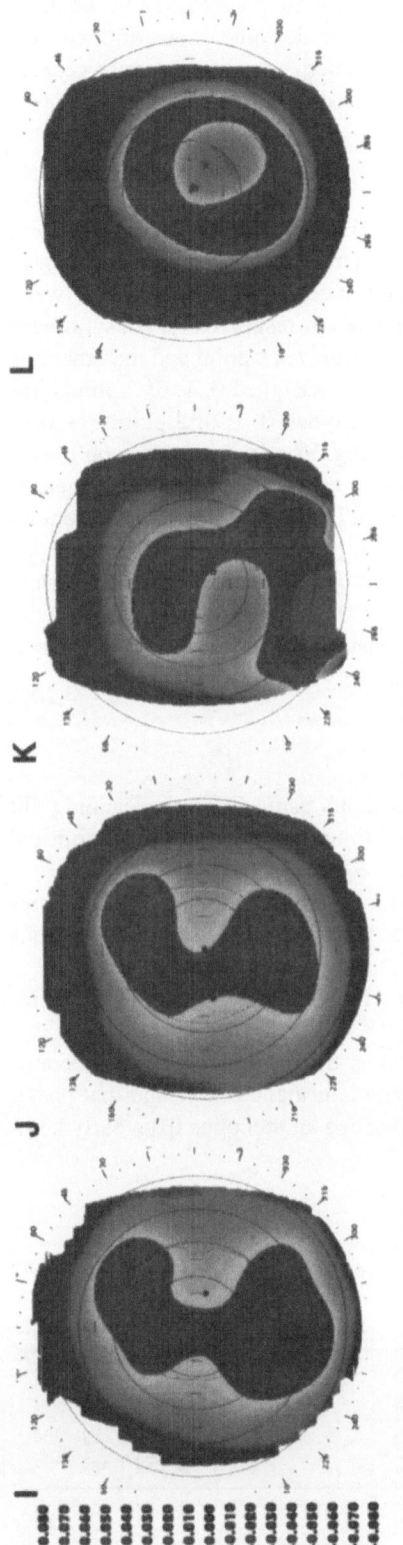

Figure 10.3 (Top lane) The central axial keratometry maps: normal controls (A), keratoconus suspects (B), early keratoconus (C), and advanced keratoconus (D). (Middle lane) The Pachymetry maps: normal controls (E), keratoconus suspects (F), early keratoconus (G), and advanced keratoconus (H). Note that corneal thinning is greatest in advanced keratoconus. (Bottom lane) The posterior best fit (B.F.) sphere maps: normal controls (I), keratoconus suspects (J), early keratoconus (K), and advanced keratoconus (L). Note increased posterior corneal curvature in advanced keratoconus. [Color in original.]

Controversy exists regarding the significance of ultrasonic pachymetry in the diagnosis of keratoconus (22,24). In preliminary investigations of the value of posterior corneal curvature in keratoconus, we have observed a potential benefit of using posterior corneal curvature data in differentiating advanced from early keratoconus (25).

C. CLASSIFICATION

The eyes were divided into four groups based on the MEEI keratoconus scoring system (Fig. 10.2), which is based on clinical history, clinical examination, scanning slit topography, and modified Rabinowitz criteria. Asymmetric anterior central corneal power between left and right eyes ≤ 1.9 D or >1.9 D is assigned 0 or 1 point, respectively. If asymmetry > 1.9 D is present, the eye with the higher corneal power receives 1 point and the other eye receives 0 points. K < 47.2 D, 47.2–48.7 D, or >48.7 D is assigned 0, 1, or 2 points, respectively. I-S value <1.4 D, 1.4–1.9 D, or >1.9 D is assigned 0, 1, or 2 points, respectively. If at least two findings on examination (Fleischer ring, Vogt's striae, Munson's sign, scarring) or history (atopy, Down's family history) are present, 2 points are assigned; if fewer than two findings are present, 0 points are assigned. If corneal hydrops is present on examination or elicited from history, 2 points are assigned; otherwise, 0 points are assigned. A total score of 0, 1–3, 4–5, or 6–9 points for an eye gives a diagnosis of normal control, keratoconus suspects, early keratoconus, or advanced keratoconus, respectively (Fig. 10.3). Orbscan corneal topography was used to measure pachymetry and the posterior best fit spheres.

D. DISCUSSION OF ORBSCAN FINDINGS

In one of our studies, we analyzed 180 eyes of 98 patients using Orbscan scanning slit corneal topography to determine central axial keratometry, I-S value, and optical pachymetry.

Table 1 presents the pachymetry and the posterior best-fit sphere data. Table 2 presents the comparisons of pachymetry and of posterior best-fit sphere among the various groups.

Statistical analyses were performed by one-way ANOVA with Tukey multiple comparisons at the .05 significance level.

From that study, we observed that pachymetry may differentiate early keratoconus and advanced keratoconus from keratoconus suspects and normal controls and that posterior corneal curvature is valuable in differentiating advanced keratoconus from early keratoconus, keratoconus suspects, and controls.

Table 1 Pachymetry and Posterior Best Fit Sphere Measurements

Eye groups	n	Pachymetry (μm); mean (SD)	Posterior best fit (mm); mean (SD)
Controls	83	551.59 (26.76)	6.55 (0.21)
Suspects	43	534.72 (36.03)	6.56 (0.32)
Early KC	22	497.40 (47.85)	6.35 (0.28)
Advanced KC	32	442.44 (57.52)	5.93 (0.58)

Suspects = keratoconus suspects, KC = keratoconus.

Table 2   Multiple Comparisons‡ of Pachymetry and Posterior Best Fit Sphere

			Pachymetry (μm) (n = 180); mean difference (95% CI)	P value	Posterior best fit sphere (mm) (n = 180); mean difference (95% CI)	P value
Advanced KC	vs.	Early KC	−54.97* (−86.67 to −23.27)	<.001	−0.42* (−0.66 to −0.18)	<.001
	vs.	Suspects	−92.28* (−119.01 to −65.56)	<.001	−0.64* (−0.84 to −0.43)	<.001
	vs.	Controls	−109.15* (−132.97 to −85.33)	<.001	−0.63* (−0.81 to −0.44)	<.001
Early KC	vs.	Suspects	−37.31* (−67.32 to −7.31)	.008	−0.22 (−0.44 to 0.01)	.071
	vs.	Controls	−54.18* (−81.63 to −26.73)	<.001	−0.20 (−0.41 to 0.01)	.056
Suspects	vs.	Controls	−16.87 (−38.38 to 4.63)	.182	−0.01 (−0.15 to 0.17)	.998

‡: Tukey Multiple Comparison, CI = confidence interval, KC = keratoconus, * = statistically significant. Suspects = KC suspects.

Ultrasonic pachymetry may provide corroborative evidence for the diagnosis of keratoconus, but Rabinowitz et al. have shown that this technique is less valuable than videokeratography-derived indices in distinguishing keratoconus from the normal condition (24). Other studies suggest that pachymetry data are important because corneal stromal thinning may be associated with disease progression (22,23). Bohm et al., using ultrasound pachymetry, showed that normal subjects had a central corneal thickness of 548 ± 30 μm, compared to 505 ± 42 μm in the corneal center and 424 ± 41 μm on the conus peak in keratoconus subjects (23). Stromal thinning occurs commonly in the inferotemporal quadrant; in one study, comparisons of pachymetry of keratoconus and normal eyes showed similarities in all except this quadrant (26).

These variations in corneal pachymetry findings in the normal population may contribute to its inability to differentiate keratoconus eyes from normal controls. Our study revealed significant differences in pachymetry in normal controls vs. early keratoconus and advanced keratoconus, keratoconus suspects vs. advanced keratoconus, and early keratoconus vs. advanced keratoconus, but not in normal controls vs. keratoconus suspects. This finding implies that pachymetry is a predictor of progression of keratoconus, especially in the much advanced stage.

Measurements of posterior best sphere (25,27) may be important, possibly because it may represent advanced disease progression. As the cornea thins and protrudes forward, the posterior corneal curvature may show more dramatic steepening than does the anterior corneal curvature. Posterior corneal curvature is a minor determinant of dioptric corneal power. Our study revealed significant difference in posterior best sphere in advanced keratoconus vs. controls, keratoconus suspects, and early keratoconus, suggesting that posterior corneal curvature changes to an extreme extent at the end stage of keratoconus progression.

Most previous keratoconus classifications used either topographical (28–32) quantitative indices or clinical findings only. The MEEI classification, using a scoring system, combines history, examination, topographical maps, and modified Rabinowitz criteria to establish stricter criteria for distinguishing normal controls, keratoconus suspects, and early and advanced keratoconus. Smolek and Klyce (21) modified the Rabinowitz criteria and identified the anterior central corneal power (K) between 47.2 and 48.7 D as suspect and K > 48.7 D as suggestive of keratoconus. The modified Rabinowitz criteria also identified the inferior–superior central anterior corneal power asymmetry (I-S value) between 1.4 and 1.9 D as suspect and I-S > 1.9 D as suggestive of keratoconus. Given these limits, we established three groups of central cornea power (K) (<47.2 D, 47.2–48.7 D, >48.7D) and inferior–superior corneal power asymmetry (I-S value) (<1.4 D, 1.4–1.9 D, >1.9 D) and assigned 0, 1, and 2 points, respectively. In other words, the higher the K and I-S value measurement, the more severe the disease and the higher the score assigned. Asymmetry of the central corneal power between one eye and the fellow eye greater than 1.9 D is assigned one point only because this asymmetry can be a normal variant. If asymmetry >1.9 D is present, the eye with the higher corneal power is assigned 1 point and the other is assigned 0 points. The presence of two or more findings by examination (Fleischer ring, Vogt's striae, Munson's sign, prominent nerves, scarring) and history (atopy, Down's, family history) is assigned two points, but the presence of one finding is assigned zero points. Corneal hydrops of examination or from history is assigned two points because it is easily diagnosed and is of definitive value since it is a sign of severe late stage keratoconus. Future studies incorporating optical pachymetry and posterior corneal curvature into current videokeratography-derived indices may improve the accuracy in distinguishing among keratoconus suspects and early and advanced keratoconus.

E.   KERATOCONUS AND LASIK/PRK

LASIK/PRK are effective and precise refractive surgery. Recently, however, there are many articles reporting disappointing results after performing LASIK or PRK on keratoconus suspects or early keratoconus patients (33–37). Seiler and Quurke reported a case of forme fruste keratoconus revealing a central steeping with rapid progression one month postoperatively (33). Speicher and Gottinger reported 4 eyes from 2 patients that got progressive corneal ectasia of up to 7 diopters within a few months after LASIK treatment (34). Buzard et al. used LASIK to treat mild to moderate keratoconus in 16 eyes of 9 patients and conclude that longer term results, even the initial visual results, appear promising, and they revealed regression of the refractive outcome in some cases. Moreover, despite improvement in the postoperative spherical equivalent and uncorrected visual acuity in most cases, the risk of loss of BCVA and the necessity of performing PKP in three cases lead us to consider LASIK as not a primary solution for keratoconus (35). Holland et al. also noted that 4 eyes in 2 patients with possible forme fruste keratoconus showed worsening irregular astigmatism after LASIK or PRK treatments (36). Schmitt-Bernard et al. reported a keratoconus suspect receiving two LASIK procedures and one PRK performed on his left eye, and three LASIK procedures on his right eye. After these surgeries, a dramatic corneal ectasia and grade III haze occurred in both eyes, with a clinical diagnosis of keratoconus. The best spectacle-corrected visual acuity was as low as 20/1200 bilaterally. Both eyes displayed dramatic corneal protrusion with corneal scarring (37).

F.   THE PATIENTS WITH ECTASIA AFTER LASIK/PRK

The cases revealing ectasia after LASIK or PRK treatments may be the undiagnosed keratoconus, forme fruste keratoconus (33,34,36,37), or may be due to corneal weakening and unstable after surgery. We cannot overemphasize the need for thorough preoperative evaluations of corneal conditions, such as slit lamp examination, corneal thickness measurement, and detailed analysis of videokeratographs. Thinning corneal disorders such as keratoconus, keratoconus suspects, or pellucid marginal degeneration should be considered as contraindications for excimer laser ablative refractive procedures (35–37).

G. INTRAOPERATIVE PACHYMETRY TO AVOID COMPLICATIONS

For cases without keratoconus, if the pachymetry is less than 500 μm or the refractive error more than -6 diopters, in order to preserve posterior corneal residual thickness, more than 250 μm (note the variable flap thickness); intraoperative pachymetry can be used to avoid serious complications after LASIK or PRK treatments. If the residual corneal thickness cannot meet that criterion undercorrection is recommended.

REFERENCES

1. YS Rabinowitz, AB Nesburn, PJ McDonnell. Videokeratography of the fellow eye in unilateral keratoconus. Ophthalmology 1993;100:181–186.
2. SE Wilson, DTC Lin, SD Klyce, JJ Reidy, MS Insler. Topographic changes in contact lens-induced corneal warpage. Ophthalmology 1990;97:734–744.
3. YS Rabinowitz, J Garbus, PJ McDonnell. Computer-assisted corneal topography in family members of patients with keratoconus. Arch Ophthalmol 1990;108:365–371.
4. J Parker, WW Ko, G Pavlopoulos, PJ Wolfe, YS Rabinowitz, ST Feldman. Videokeratography of keratoconus in monozygotic twins. J Refract Surg 1996;12:180–183.
5. V Gonzalez, PJ McDonnell. Computer-assisted corneal topography in parents of patients with keratoconus. Arch Ophthalmol 1992;110:1412–1414.
6. RH Kennedy, WM Bourne, JA Dyer. A 48-year clinical and epidemiologic study of keratoconus. Am J Ophthalmol 1986;101:267–273.
7. YS Rabinowitz. Videokeratographic indices to aid in screening for keratoconus. J Refract Surg 1995;11:371–379.
8. SE Wilson, DTC Lin, SD Klyce. Corneal topography of keratoconus. Cornea 1991;10:2–8.
9. YS Rabinowitz. Keratoconus. Surv Ophthalmol 1998;42:297–319.
10. YS Rabinowitz, JJ Garbus, C Garbus, PJ McDonnell. Contact lens selection for keratoconus using a computer-assisted video-photokeratoscope. CLAO J 1991;17:88–93.
11. MJ Mannis, K Zadnik. Contact lens fitting in keratoconus. CLAO J 1989;15:282–289.
12. MJ Crews, WT Driebe Jr, GA Stern. The clinical management of keratoconus: 6 year retrospective study. CLAO J 1994;20:194–197.
13. JH Lass, RG Lembach, SB Park, DL Hom, ME Fritz, GM Svilar, IF Nuamah, WJ Reinhart, EG Stocker, RH Keates. Clinical management of keratoconus: a multicenter analysis. Ophthalmology 1990;97:433–445.
14. AB Nesburn, S Bahri, J Salz, YS Rabinowitz, E Maguen, J Hofbauer, M Berlin, JI Macy. Keratoconus detected by videokeratography in candidates for photorefractive keratectomy. J Refract Surg 1995;11:194–201.
15. YS Rabinowitz, SD Klyce, J Krachmer, L Nordan, J Rowsey, J Sugar, S Wilson, P Binder, R Damiano, M McDonald, A Neumann, T Seiler, K Thompson, P Wyzinski, L O'Dell. Keratoconus, videokeratography, and refractive surgery. Refract Corneal Surg 1992;8:403–407.
16. YS Rabinowitz, PJ McDonnell. Computer-assisted corneal topography in keratoconus. Refract Corneal Surg 1989;5:400–408.
17. N Maeda, SD Klyce, MK Smolek. Comparison of methods for detecting keratoconus using videokeratography. Arch Ophthalmol 1995;113:870–874.
18. N Maeda, SD Klyce, MK Smolek, HW Thompson. Automated keratoconus screening with corneal topography analysis. Invest Ophthalmol Vis Sci 1994;35:2749–2757.
19. J Ruiz-Montenegro, CH Mafra, SE Wilson, JE Jumper, SD Klyce, EN Mendelson. Corneal topographic alterations in normal contact lens wearers. Ophthalmology 1993;100:128–134.
20. N Maeda, SD Klyce, H Hamano. Alteration of corneal asphericity in rigid gas permeable contact lens induced warpage. CLAO J 1994;20:27–31.
21. MK Smolek, SD Klyce. Current keratoconus detection methods compared with a neural network approach. Invest Ophthalmol Vis Sci 1997;38:2290–2299.

22. V Yaylali, SC Kaufman, HW Thompson. Corneal thickness measurements with the Orbscan Topography System and ultrasonic pachymetry. J Cataract Refract Surg 1997;23:1345–1350.
23. A Bohm, M Kohlhaas, RC Lerche, B Bischoff, G Richard. Messung des intraokularen druckes bei keratokonus: einfluss der veränderten biomechanik. (Measuring intraocular pressure in keratoconus: effect of the changed biomechanics.) Ophthalmologe 1997;94:771–774.
24. YS Rabinowitz, K Rasheed, H Yang, J Elashoff. Accuracy of ultrasonic pachymetry and videokeratography in detecting keratoconus. J Cataract Refract Surg 1998;24:196–201.
25. PC Lu, S Samapunphong, DT Azar. Posterior corneal curvature and keratoconus: quantitative and qualitative analysis. Asia-Pacific Journal of Ophthalmology 1999;11:28–31.
26. J Colin, Y Sale, F Malet, B Cochener. Inferior steepening is associated with thinning of the inferotemporal cornea. J Refract Surg 1996;12:697–699.
27. C Edmund. Posterior corneal curvature and its influence on corneal dioptric power. Acta Ophthalmol (Copenh) 1994;72:715–720.
28. TT McMahon, JB Robin, KM Scarpulla, JL Putz. The spectrum of topography found in keratoconus. CLAO J 1991;17:198–204.
29. JS Chan, RB Mandell, DS Burger, RE Fusaro. Accuracy of videokeratography for instantaneous radius in keratoconus. Optom Vis Sci 1995;72:793–799.
30. DA deCunha, EG Woodward. Measurement of corneal topography in keratoconus. Ophthalmic Physiol Opt 1993;13:377–382.
31. SE Wilson, SD Klyce. Advances in the analysis of corneal topography. Surv Ophthalmol 1991;35:269–277.
32. LJ Maguire, WM Bourne. Corneal topography of early keratoconus. Am J Ophthalmol 1989;108:107–112.
33. T Seiler, AW Quurke. Iatrogenic keratectasia after LASIK in a case of forme fruste keratoconus. J Cataract Refract Surg 1998;24:1007–1009.
34. L Speicher, W Gottinger. Progressive corneal ectasia after laser in situ keratomileusis. Klin Monatsbl Augenheilkd 1998;213:247–251.
35. KA Buzard, A Tuengler, JL Febbraro. Treatment of mild to moderate keratoconus with laser in situ keratomileusis. J Cataract Refract Surg 1999;25:1600–1609.
36. SP Holland, S Srivannaboon, DZ Reinstein. Avoiding serious corneal complications of laser assisted in situ keratomileusis and photorefractive keratectomy. Ophthalmology 2000;107:640–652.
37. CF Schmitt-Bernard, C Lesage, B Arnaud. Keratectasia induced by laser in situ keratomileusis in keratoconus. J Refract Surg 2000;16:368–70.

11

Corneal Stability and Biomechanics after LASIK

**ESEN KARAMURSEL AKPEK, RANA ALTAN-YAYCIOGLU,
and WALTER J. STARK**

*The Wilmer Eye Institute, Johns Hopkins University School of Medicine,
Baltimore, Maryland, U.S.A.*

A. BIOMECHANICAL PROPERTIES OF THE CORNEA

The elastic properties of any material are described by the relationship between the applied stress, or force per unit cross section, and the resultant strain, or relative deformation. The proportionality factor, Young's modulus (Y), is expressed in units of newtons per square meter (N/m^2). The smaller the value of Y, the more elastic is the material—that is, the less it deforms with stress.

For viscoelastic materials, unlike metals, Y is not constant (1). The cornea responds to stress as a typical viscoelastic material (2): for a given level of stress, the resultant strain changes with time. That is, an immediate elastic response (Y_i) is followed by the steady state response (Y_s). Y_i reflects the elastic properties of the collagen fibers, whereas Y_s reflects the elastic properties of the corneal matrix (3). In the steady state, Y_i is 100 times Y_s.

Ocular rigidity (E) is a volume elasticity coefficient that reflects the elastic response of ocular tunics: cornea, uvea, and sclera. E is related to Y_i by the equation

$$E = \frac{T \times Y_i}{\pi \times R^4 \times P_o} \tag{1}$$

where T is the uniform thickness, R is the radius, and P_o is the intraocular pressure. This equation suggests that a change in any of these parameters would affect ocular rigidity, possibly increasing the tendency toward deformity.

Under physiological conditions, the tensile strength of normal cornea is twice that of the keratoconic cornea (3,4), mainly due to a decrease in Y_i in keratoconus. This suggests

163

that, assuming the biomechanical parameters are constant throughout the cornea, a normal corneal thickness can be reduced twofold before its elasticity is reduced to that of a keratoconic cornea. That is, assuming a normal corneal thickness of about 540 μm, a total residual corneal thickness of more than 270 μm should be sufficient to provide the elasticity of a normal cornea. Unfortunately, this assumption is proven wrong by the long-term results of corneal refractive surgeries. Iatrogenic keratectasia, that is, progressive corneal thinning and weakening, remains an uncommon yet vision-threatening complication following refractive surgery.

B. LESSONS FROM INCISIONAL REFRACTIVE SURGERY

Refractive keratotomy was first described by European ophthalmologists in the late 1800s, developed in Japan after the Second World War, and evolved into its modern form in Russia in the 1970s (5–7). The first radial keratotomy in the United States was performed in 1978 (8). Before the LASIK era, radial keratotomy was the most widely used refractive surgical procedure to correct myopia. Approximately 250,000 radial keratotomy operations were performed annually in the United States (9).

Numerous articles described the initial short-term favorable outcomes of this procedure. In 1986, Deitz et al. (10) first reported a trend toward progressive hyperopic shift in postoperative refraction in a series of 150 patients who had undergone 225 metal-blade radial keratotomy procedures. Between 12 months to 4 years after surgery, 31% of the patients had hyperopic shifts of at least 1.00 D (mean shift, 0.51 D). Then in the Prospective Evaluation of Radial Keratotomy (PERK) series (11), in which patients received diamond-blade radial keratotomy, 43% of 693 eyes underwent a hyperopic change in refractive power of 1.00 D or more, 10 years after surgery. The mean rate of change was approximately 0.10 D per year. The investigators estimated that each year, an additional 5% of eyes would reach the level of 1.00 D hyperopic shift. The hyperopic shift showed no signs of slowing, confirming the long-term results of the metal-blade study that hyperopic shift could last as long as 12 years after the radial keratotomy procedure (12).

Most corneal surgeons initially thought the hyperopic shift was due to a continuation of the basic biomechanical change in the cornea that produces the initial central corneal flattening after surgery—perhaps an increase in the length of the incision. It took more than five years to recognize that the progressive hyperopic shift was in fact due to weakening of the paracentral cornea leading to iatrogenic keratectasia.

C. LESSONS FROM LAMELLAR CORNEAL SURGERY

Automated lamellar keratoplasty provided the most extensive experience with lamellar refractive surgery before the LASIK era. In this procedure, a 4.2 mm diameter lamellar disc is removed from the center of the visual axis, creating a uniform thinning of the entire corneal bed in that area. In LASIK, however, excimer ablation using the single-zone or multizone technique results in a gradient of thinning in the ablation zone. Maximum removal of tissue occurs only at the central 0.25 mm, depending on the first opening of the diaphragm, while the remaining posterior stromal tissue maintains substantially more thickness.

The type of lamellar surgery that penetrates most deeply into the cornea is hyperopic automated lamellar keratoplasty. This procedure uses a 5.6 to 6.6 mm diameter lamellar dissection extending to 53 to 74% of the corneal thickness to induce central ectasia. The

Ruiz nomogram for hyperopic automated lamellar keratoplasty suggested that a 300 μm cut in corneas ranging in thickness from 490 to 575 μm would produce a 1.0 D myopic shift due to the subsequent controlled corneal ectasia (13). Ruiz observed that microkeratome cuts of more than 60% of the central corneal thickness could produce uncontrolled ectasia (14). Similarly, Gris et al. (15) found that a microkeratome cut of more than 350 μm could produce corneal ectasia. Given the average central corneal thickness of approximately 540.5 ± 38.5 μm, automated lamellar keratoplasty can produce corneal ectasia with 180 to 275 μm of posterior stromal tissue. Lyle and Jin (16) reported a 26% incidence of iatrogenic keratoconus following hyperopic automated lamellar keratoplasty with a lamellar cut depth of 52 to 70% of corneal thickness. However, this series included corneas that had undergone prior radial keratotomy and were presumably weaker than naive corneas. Although a residual corneal stromal bed of less than 250 μm thickness is usual in hyperopic automated lamellar keratoplasty, when performed in primary cases this procedure rarely leads to keratectasia (17). Ghiselli et al. (18) looked for evidence of corneal ectasia in 38 eyes that had undergone hyperopic automated lamellar keratoplasty; mean residual corneal bed thickness was 195 μm (range, 126 to 230 μm). Multiple regression analysis showed no statistical evidence of corneal ectasia in the short term.

Barraquer (19), based on his extensive experience with myopic keratomileusis, in which corneal tissue is removed from the entire 7 to 8 mm diameter of the resected bed, suggested the need for a minimum of 300 μm total thickness of treated cornea, including a 100 μm sutured lamella. Slade has pointed out that a 15 year follow-up of his earlier myopic keratomileusis studies has not shown any loss of structural integrity or ectasia in eyes with a residual bed thickness of 200 μm (personal communication, October 1998).

D. CORNEAL BIOMECHANICS AFTER LASIK

Since Barraquer more than 50 years ago first introduced the myopic keratomileusis procedure with cryolathing of a freehand dissected corneal disc (20), substantial improvements have been made in lamellar corneal refractive surgery. LASIK combines the lifting of a corneal flap with a microkeratome and refractive photoablation of the stromal bed by means of a 193 nm argon fluoride excimer laser (21). Because of the accurate and consistent flap cut and the extreme precision of tissue removal, along with patients' more comfortable recuperation and rapid visual recovery, LASIK has become the most popular corneal refractive surgery.

This procedure, however, substantially weakens the mechanical strength of the cornea, the extent of weakening depending on the degree of refractive error. Depth of keratectomy is related to the diameter of the ablation zone and the attempted correction (22) (Fig. 11.1) by the equation

$$\text{Ablation depth} = \frac{(\text{Diameter of ablation})^2 \times \text{Attempted correction in diopters}}{3} \quad (2)$$

The state-of-the-art diameter for photorefractive keratectomy (PRK) is 6 mm, and from the early PRK reports we know that ablation zones less than 5 mm in diameter result in severe glare and halos (23,24). Therefore, according to Eq. (2), the excimer laser ablates about 12 μm per 1.00 D of myopic correction for a 6 mm ablation zone (Fig. 11.2). Similarly, for a 6.5 mm ablation zone the excimer laser ablates about 14 μm for the correction of 1.00 D myopia. One advantage of LASIK over older forms of lamellar corneal surgeries is that, as noted earlier, maximum removal of tissue occurs only at the central 0.25 mm, de-

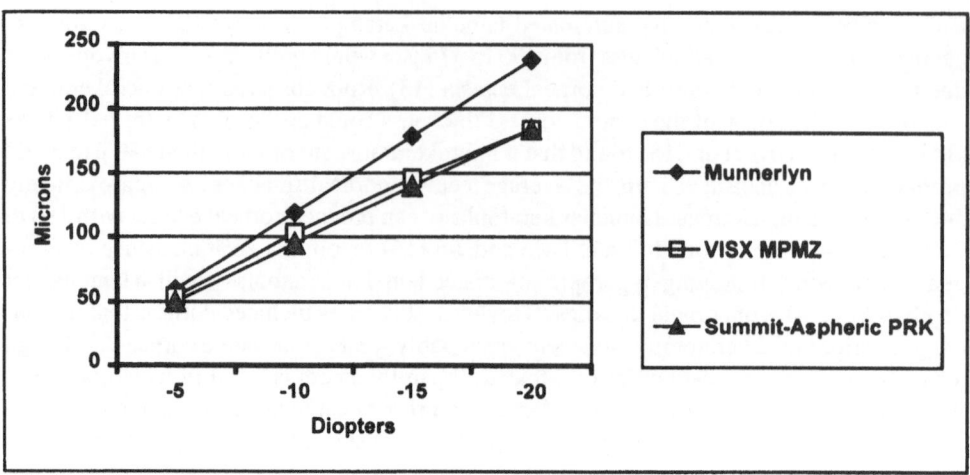

Figure 11.1 The schematic diagram of keratotomy depths for particular diopters of myopia according to Munnerlyn formula.

pending on the first opening of the diaphragm, and the remaining posterior stromal tissue maintains more of its normal thickness. A 200 μm LASIK-created bed therefore has more stress-bearing tissue than a 200 μm automated lamellar keratoplasty-created bed.

E. POSTERIOR CORNEAL CHANGES AFTER LASIK

Corneal shape is determined by the interplay among intraocular pressure, the elastic properties of the corneal tissue, and the amount and central/peripheral distribution of the corneal tissue mass (3). Thus the photosubtraction of corneal tissue with the lamellar cut during LASIK may affect corneal shape and lead to ectasia. Indeed, in a study of postoperative

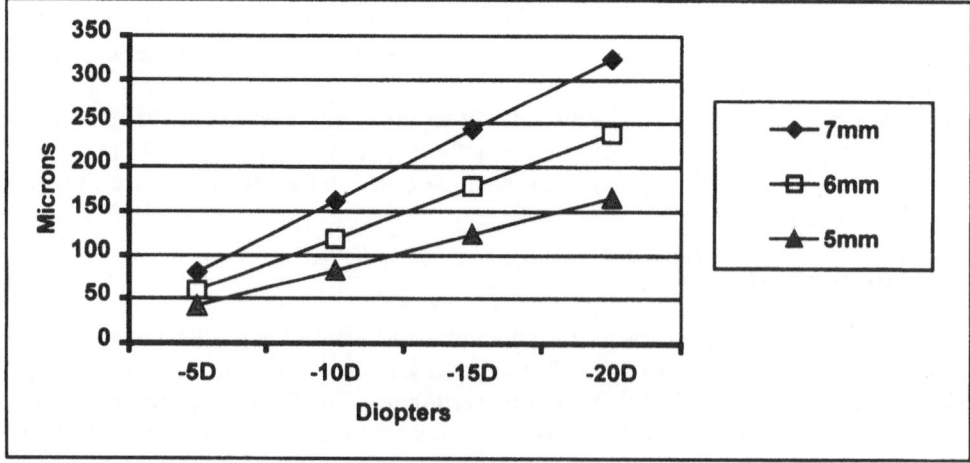

Figure 11.2 The difference of ablation depths in microns with different ablation diameters for attempted correction of particular diopters of myopia.

changes in the posterior corneal surface after LASIK, Wang et al. (25) reported that the thinner the residual corneal bed after ablation, the greater the postoperative ectasia. A residual corneal bed thickness of 250 μm was found to be a reasonable limit to prevent iatrogenic keratoconus. The authors also suggested that the post-LASIK regression might be due in part to induced central corneal ectasia. However, mainly because of the limitations of currently available corneal topography units (26), more investigations need to be performed before a final conclusion can be drawn.

F. IATROGENIC KERATECTASIA AFTER LASIK

One vision-threatening complication of LASIK is iatrogenic keratectasia (Fig. 11.3). Seiler et al. (27) first reported the occurrence of post-LASIK keratectasia in three eyes 1 to 8 months after surgery for 10.00 to 13.00 D of myopia. In all three cases the estimated residual corneal bed thickness was less than 250 μm. In a recent report, Joo and Kim (28) described two cases of postoperative corneal ectasia occurring 1.5 to 9 months after surgery (28). These surgeons used a manual microkeratome and an estimated flap thickness of 150 μm. The residual stromal bed thickness after the procedure was 232 to 257 μm. The authors recommended that half the original stromal bed thickness and more than 250 μm of residual stroma should be preserved after LASIK. They also reported corneal perforation *during* LASIK in two other patients (29). In both cases the residual bed thickness was less than 250 μm and there was a lag between the creation of the corneal flap and the laser application. The authors concluded that excessive dehydration of the cornea must be avoided and that the corneal shape should be carefully watched to prevent corneal perforation during LASIK.

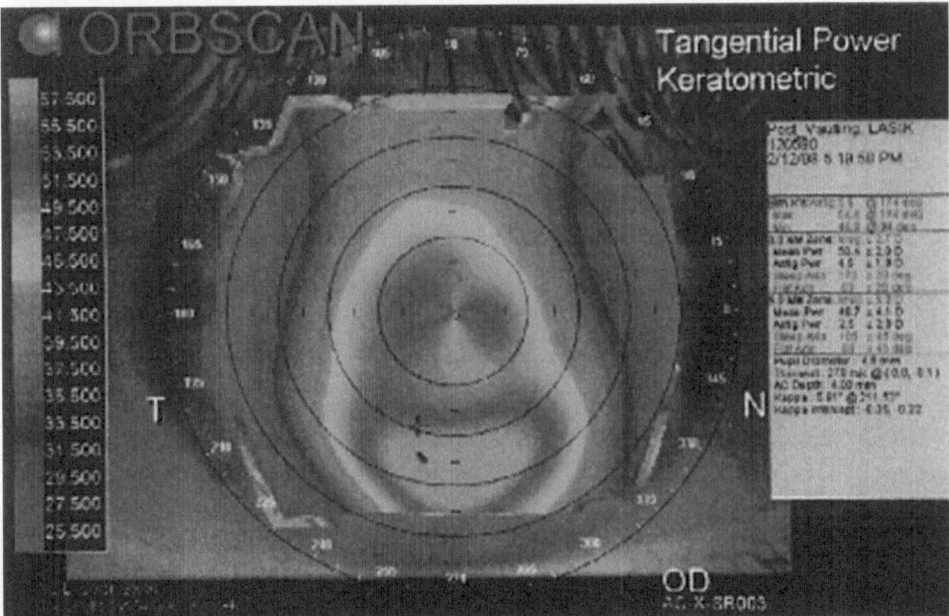

Figure 11.3 An Orbscan corneal tangential topography showing keratectasia after LASIK. (Courtesy of Donald Sanders, M.D., Ph.D.)

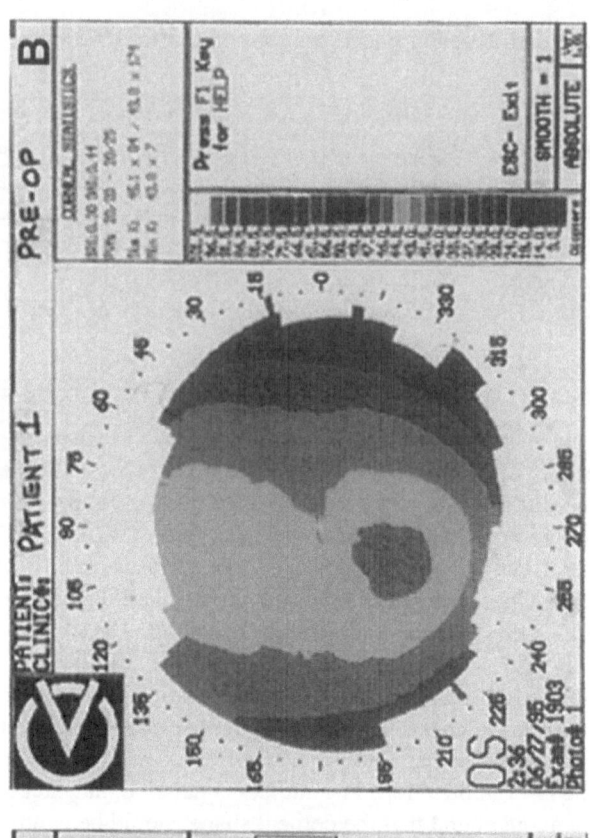

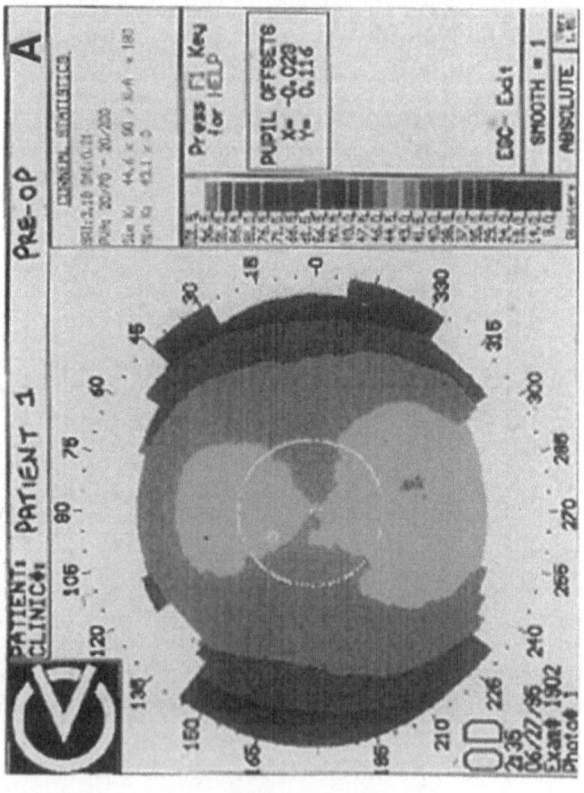

168

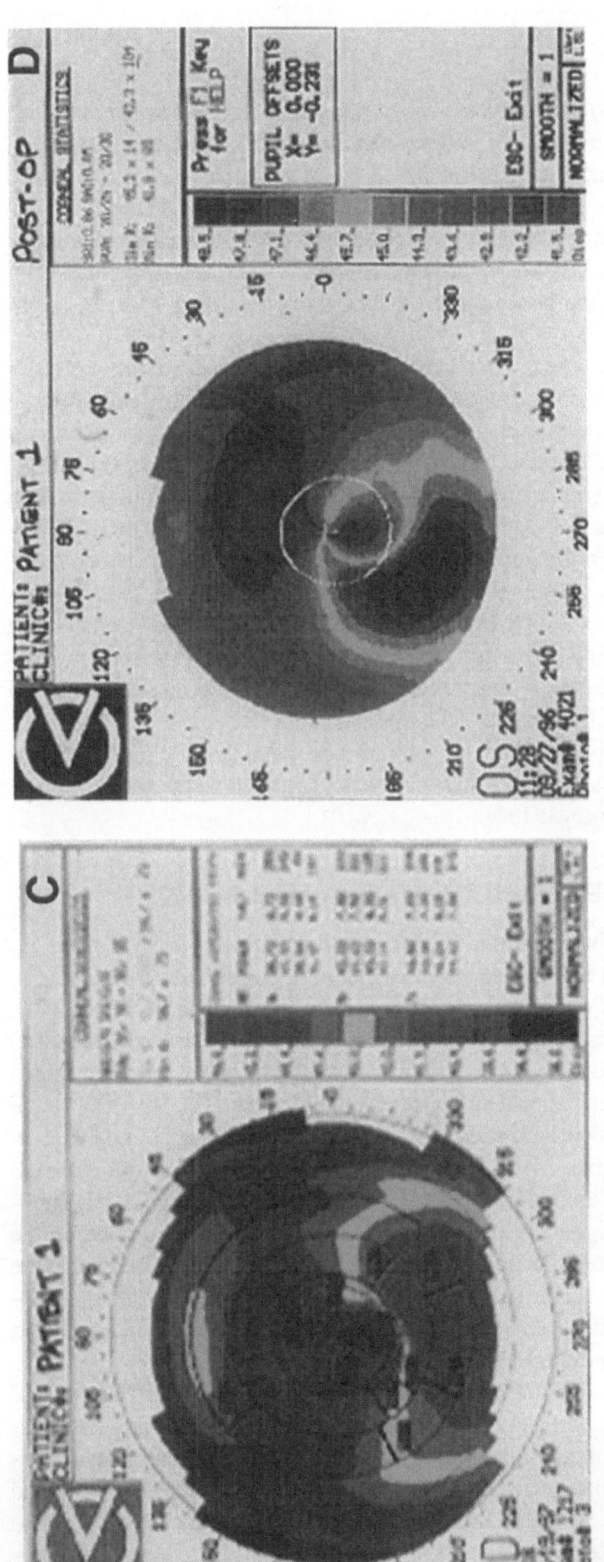

Figure 11.4 (A) Pre-LASIK topography in the right eye. (B) Pre-LASIK topography in the left eye. (C) Right eye: Frank inferior keratectasia 20 months postoperatively. (D) Left eye: topography showing marked inferonasal keratectasia 15 months postoperatively. (From Ref. 34.)

Geggel and Talley (30) described a patient who developed iatrogenic keratectasia after bilateral LASIK with enhancements. The authors documented a thinning of the total central corneal thickness; initial pachymetry was 449 μm and gradually decreased to 260 μm over a period of 9 months.

Several different authors have also reported progressive keratectasia induced by LASIK in keratoconic corneas (31,32). One interesting finding is the occurrence of keratectasia even in corneas with a residual stromal bed thickness of more than 250 μm in patients with keratoconus.

Preoperative corneal thickness measurement is of utmost importance in ruling out any corneal thinning disorders as well as in estimating the possible maximum amount of tissue ablation. Schmitt-Bernard et al. (33) reported on a patient with post-LASIK keratectasia resulting from a failure to perform preoperative pachymetry even though the topographic findings suggested keratoconus. They emphasized that corneal disorders with thinning such as keratoconus, suspected keratoconus, forme fruste keratoconus, or pellucid marginal degeneration are *absolute* contraindications for any corneal stromal ablative refractive procedures.

In a case series of 13 eyes, Amoils et al. (34) reported iatrogenic keratectasia following LASIK for myopia of −4.0 to −7.0 D. In one of the cases the calculated corneal bed thickness was 297 μm (right eye) and 300 μm (left eye). Preoperative topographic evaluation did not suggest keratoconus. However, the patient developed keratoconus with marked inferior steepening and thinning of the corneas 18 months postoperatively (Fig. 11.4A–D). The occurrence of LASIK-induced keratectasia even with a residual corneal bed thickness of more than 250 μm can perhaps be attributed to the considerable variation in biomechanical properties of individual corneas (35).

G.   IS THERE A SAFE CORNEAL BED THICKNESS AFTER LASIK?

As is apparent from the ocular rigidity equation, Eq. (1), corneal thickness is clearly one parameter of concern in LASIK. T in this equation represents total central corneal thickness. Given that the strength of a normal cornea is only twice that of the keratoconic cornea (4), as noted earlier, one might conclude that a normal 540 μm cornea could be reduced to 270 μm before its elasticity is reduced to that of a keratoconic cornea. This assumption is too optimistic, however, because the anterior corneal flap after LASIK does not contribute to the tensile strength of the cornea; the stress is supported only by the residual bed (27). Also, current ablation depth nomograms are based on results of PRK, in which Bowman's membrane and the anterior part of the stroma are ablated (36). In midstroma and deeper layers, however, per-pulse ablation rates are higher. Hence, owing to differences in water content, the actual ablation depth might be greater than calculated in LASIK (37). We also know that the deep posterior stroma has less biomechanical strength than the anterior layer (35). Thus ablating the same amount of tissue under a 160 μm flap might leave a weaker residual bed than ablating under a 130 μm flap, even though the final bed thickness is the same.

In order to extend the range of refractive correction by LASIK, thinner flaps would be an option. Ideally, a microkeratome should produce consistent corneal flap thickness within a 10% range of error, controlled by the thickness of the microkeratome plate. However, clinical studies have shown that actual flap thickness is usually thinner than intended and the range of error is wider (38,39). Thin, incomplete, or irregular flaps are difficult to deal with and may result in glare, decreased spectacle-corrected acuity, or loss of best-corrected visual acuity. Seiler et al. (27) estimated that an intended flap thickness of less than 110 μm would automatically create cutting errors in more than 5% of cases.

Corneal radius of curvature (R) is another parameter that affects corneal tensile strength. As the steepness of the cornea increases, tensile strength decreases by the fourth power of the increase in radius of curvature; Eq. (1). Therefore patients with high myopia are expected to have a significantly decreased corneal tensile strength. Maldonado et al. (40) have recently demonstrated that when performing LASIK in eyes with 12.0 D or more of myopia, a thicker than intended flap may occur due to unusual steepness of the cornea, leaving an unexpectedly thinner residual bed. Another, striking finding of the same study was a statistically significant mean difference (14.6 μm) between the predicted and the actual central ablation depth. This difference was weakly associated with the degree of preoperative ametropia and accordingly with the dose and duration of the laser treatment. The authors recommended adding a safety margin of 15 μm thickness to preoperative calculations for LASIK corrections.

Another factor to be considered is that the tensile strength (Y_i) of normal cornea varies by as much as ± 25% (35). Unfortunately, because currently available technology cannot measure patients' corneal elasticity preoperatively, the safe minimal residual bed thickness will have to be established by trial and error. At present it seems that a thickness of at least 250 μm is reasonable to minimize the risk of ectasia. However, a long-term follow-up of 5 years or more is required to establish reliable guidelines.

REFERENCES

1. YCB Fung. Stress-strain-history relations of soft tissue in simple elongation. In: YCB Fung, N Perrone, M Anliker, eds. Biomechanics, Its Foundation and Objectives. Englewood Cliffs, NJ: Prentice Hall, 1972, pp 181–208.
2. GW Nyquist. Rheology of the cornea: experimental techniques and results. Exp Eye Res 1968;7:183–188.
3. C Edmund. Corneal elasticity and ocular rigidity in normal and keratoconic eyes. Acta Ophthalmol 1988;66:134–140.
4. TT Andreassen, AH Simonsen, H Oxlund. Biomechanical properties of keratoconus and normal corneas. Exp Eye Res 1980;31:435–441.
5. BH Schimmelpfenning, GO Waring. Development of refractive keratotomy in the nineteenth century. In: GO Waring, ed. Refractive Keratotomy for Myopia and Astigmatism. St Louis, MO: Mosby—Year Book, 1992, pp 171–178.
6. K Akiyama, H Shibata, A Kanai. Development of radial keratotomy in Japan, 1939–1960. In: GO Waring, ed. Refractive Keratotomy for Myopia and Astigmatism. St Louis, MO: Mosby–Year Book, 1992, pp 179–220.
7. GO Waring. Development of refractive keratotomy in the Soviet Union, 1960–1990. In: GO Waring, ed. Refractive Keratotomy for Myopia and Astigmatism. St Louis, MO: Mosby–Year Book, 1992, pp 221–236.
8. GO Waring. Development of refractive keratotomy in the United States, 1978–1990. In: GO Waring, ed. Refractive Keratotomy for Myopia and Astigmatism. St Louis, MO: Mosby–Year Book, 1992, pp 237–258.
9. DV Leaming. Practice styles and preferences of ASCRS members: 1993 survey. J Cataract Refract Surg 1994;20:459–467.
10. MR Deitz, DR Sanders, MG Raanan. Progressive hyperopia in radial keratotomy: long term follow-up of diamond knife and metal blade series. Ophthalmology 1986;93:1284–1289.
11. GO Waring, M Lynn, PJ McDonnell, and the PERK Study Group. Results of the Prospective Evaluation of Radial Keratotomy study 10 years after the surgery. Arch Ophthalmol 1994;112: 1298–1308.

12. MR Deitz, DR Sanders, MG Raanan, M DeLuca. Long-term (5- to 12-year) follow-up of metal-blade radial keratotomy procedures. Arch Ophthalmol 1994;112:614–620.

13. GM Kezirian, CM Gremillion. Automated lamellar keratoplasty for the correction of hyperopia. J Cataract Refract Surg 1995;21:386–392.

14. American Academy of Ophthalmology. Automated lamellar keratoplasty. Ophthalmology 1996;103:852–861.

15. O Gris, JL Guell, A Muller. Keratomileusis update. J Cataract Refract Surg 1996;22:620–623.

16. WA Lyle, GJ Jin. Hyperopic automated lamellar keratoplasty: complications and visual results. Arch Ophthalmol 1998;116:425–428.

17. Y Burnstein, AL Robin. Pressure or progression? (letter). Arch Ophthalmol 1999, 117:417–419.

18. G Ghiselli, EE Manche, R Maloney. Factors influencing the outcome of hyperopic lamellar keratoplasty. J Cataract Refract Surg 1998;24:35–41.

19. JI Barraquer. Querato Mileusis y Queratofaquia. Bogota, Colombia: Instituto Barraquer de America, 1980, p 342.

20. JI Barraquer. Queratomileusis para la correccion de la miopia. Arch Soc Am Oftamol Optom 1964;5:27–48.

21. IG Pallikaris, DS Siganos. Excimer laser in situ keratomileusis and photorefractive keratectomy for correction of high myopia. J Refract Corneal Surg 1994;10:498–510.

22. CR Munnerlyn, SJ Koons, J Marshall. Photorefractive keratectomy: a technique for laser refractive surgery. J Cataract Refract Surg 1988;14:46–52.

23. DS O'Brart, DS Gartry, CP Lohmann, M Kerr Muir, J Marshall. Excimer laser photorefractive keratectomy for myopia: comparison of 4.0 and 5.0 millimeter ablation zones. J Refract Corneal Surg 1994;10:87–94.

24. T Seiler, J Wollensak. Results of a prospective evaluation of photorefractive keratectomy at 1 year after surgery. Ger J Ophthalmol 1993;2:135–142.

25. Z Wang, J Chen, B Yang. Posterior corneal surface topographic changes after laser in situ keratomileusis are related to residual corneal bed thickness. Ophthalmology 1999;106:406–410.

26. RK Maloney. Discussion of "Posterior corneal surface topographic changes after laser in situ keratomileusis are related to residual corneal bed thickness." Ophthalmology 1999;106:409–410.

27. T Seiler, K Koufala, G Richter. Iatrogenic keratectasia after laser in situ keratomileusis. J Refract Surg 1998;14:312–317.

28. C-K Joo, T-G Kim. Corneal ectasia detected after laser in situ keratomileusis for correction of less than −12 diopters of myopia. J Cataract Refract Surg 2000;26:292–295.

29. C-K Joo, T-G Kim. Corneal perforation during laser in situ keratomileusis. J Cataract Refract Surg 1999;25:1165–1167.

30. HS Geggel, AR Talley. Delayed onset keratectasia following laser in situ keratomileusis. J Cataract Refract Surg 1999;25:582–586.

31. FM Clair, B Schmitt, C Lesage, B Arnaud. Keratectasia induced by laser in situ keratomileusis in keratoconus. J Refract Surg 2000;16:368–370.

32. T Seiler, AW Quurke. Iatrogenic keratectasia after LASIK in a case of forme fruste keratoconus. J Cataract Refract Surg 1998;24:1007–1009.

33. CFM Schmitt-Bernard, C Lesage, B Arnaud. Keratectasia induced by laser in situ keratomileusis in keratoconus. J Refract Surg 2000;16:368–370.

34. SP Amoils, MB Deist, P Gous, PM Amoils. Iatrogenic keratectasia after laser in situ keratomileusis for less than −4.0 to −7.0 diopters of myopia. J Cataract Refract Surg 2000;26:967–977.

35. DA Hoetzel, P Altman, K Buzard, K Choe. Strip extensiometry for comparison of the mechanical response of bovine, rabbit and human corneas. J Biomech Eng 1992;114:202–215.

36. DD Koch. The riddle of iatrogenic keratectasia. J Cataract Refract Surg 1999;25:453–454.

37. R Turss, J Friend, M Reim, CH Dohlman. Glucose concentration and hydration of the corneal stroma. Ophthalmic Res 1971;2:253–260.
38. W-M Yi, C-K Joo. Corneal flap thickness in laser in situ keratomileusis using an SCMD manual microkeratome. J Cataract Refract Surg 1999;25:1087–1092.
39. A Behrens, B Seitz, A Langenbucher, MM Kus, C Rummelt, M Kuchle. Evaluation of corneal flap dimensions and cut quality using the automated corneal shaper microkeratome. J Refract Surg 2000;16:83–89.
40. MJ Maldonado, L Ruiz-Oblitas, JM Munuera, D Aliseda, A Garcia-Layana, J Moreno-Montanes. Optical coherence tomography evaluation of the corneal cap and stromal bed features after laser in situ keratomileusis for high myopia and astigmatism. Ophthalmology 2000;107:81–87; discussion 88.

12

LASIK Techniques

DIMITRI T. AZAR and KATHRYN COLBY

*Massachusetts Eye and Ear Infirmary, Schepens Eye Research Institute,
and Harvard Medical School, Boston, Massachusetts, U.S.A.*

DOUGLAS D. KOCH

Cullen Eye Institute, Baylor College of Medicine, Houston, Texas, U.S.A.

For most surgeons, the first few LASIK cases involve a concentrated learning effort focused primarily on the function of the microkeratone. As they gain more experience with LASIK, they begin to realize that the microkeratome step is only one of several important steps necessary for the achievement of successful LASIK outcomes (Fig. 12.1). We have divided the section on LASIK intraoperative techniques into three stages. Stage I is the preparation and suction ring stage. Stage II includes microkeratome advancement and flap lifting. Stage III involves laser ablation and flap realignment. Each case, however, is unique and may challenge the surgeon to individualize the treatment while still maintaining the overall surgical plan.

A. LASIK STAGE I. PREPARATION AND SUCTION RING

Post-LASIK infections are rare but potentially vision threatening. With the increasing number of LASIK procedures performed, a 1/2000 infection rate may translate to 800 to 1000 cases of flap infection annually in the U.S. Surgeons may be tempted to abandon the use of a sterile or aseptic technique during LASIK, because of the low infection rate, increasing emphasis on efficiency. However, sterile LASIK technique requires only minor modifications of technique by the surgeon and minimal reeducation of the surgical assistants, which may help to ensure optimal LASIK outcomes. The laser and instrument manufacturers are increasingly providing means of ensuring sterility during LASIK, and the use of a sterile field, sterile equipment, and sterile gloves is becoming a standard of care in LASIK surgery

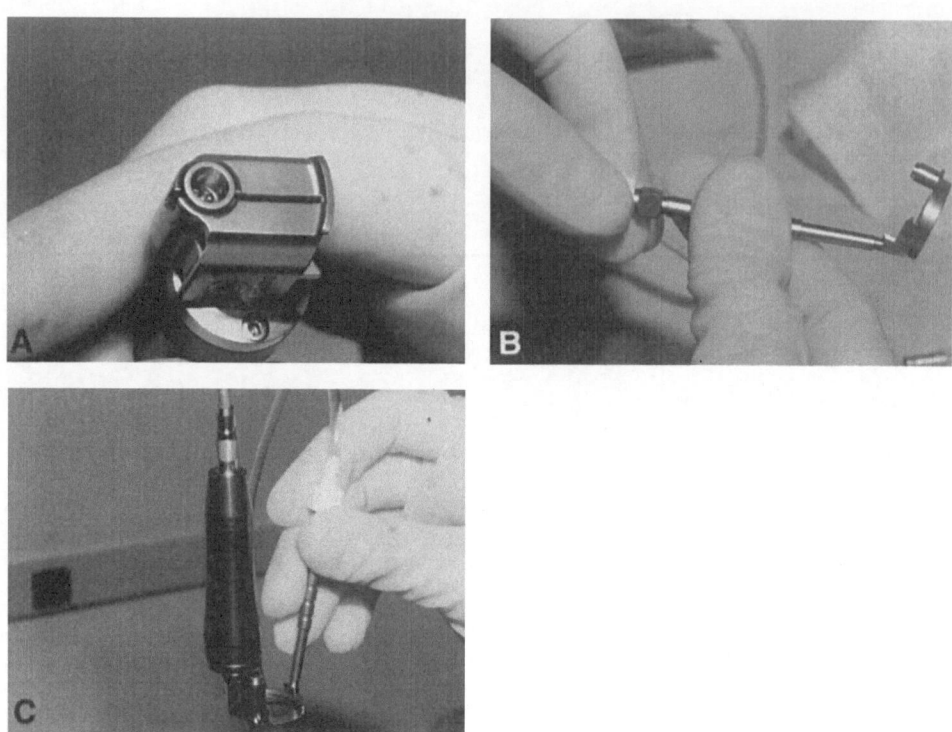

Figure 12.1 (A) Mickrokeratome head inspection. (B) Suction ring inspection. (C) Microkeratome testing.

(Fig. 12.2). The use of preoperative prophylactic antibiotics is a valuable adjunct, but not a replacement, for proper sterile technique.

1. Preoperative Topical Anesthetics/Pachymetry

Many surgeons give drops of topical anesthetic while the patients are in the pre-op area. However, we have observed that prior instillation of topical anesthetic does not add to the overall anesthetic effect and may predispose to epithelial defects. Accordingly, we prefer to delay the application of topical anesthetic until the patient is in the operating room. After the patient is positioned on the laser bed, a drop of topical anesthetic is applied. One of us (DTA) routinely obtains 2 or 3 measurements of central pachymetry in succession and records the lowest of these. The patient is instructed to keep the eyes gently closed after anesthetic has been applied.

2. Skin and Eyelash Scrubbing

Either in the preoperative holding area or in the operating room, betadine is applied over the skin surface in preparation for LASIK (Fig. 2A). We do not recommend application of betadine in the fornices in LASIK surgery, since it may weaken epithelial integrity and may also cause subsequent pain and irritation, which may lead to ocular movement. To avoid this problem, we recommend limiting the betadine scrubs to the eyelid surface and recommend the use of preoperative broad-spectrum antibiotics beginning one-half hour before surgery. Irrigation of the ocular surface may be necessary after eyelash scrubbing if the patient did not follow the preoperative instructions to clean the lids and remove makeup. However, this irrigation should not be done routinely because it can flush meibomian secretions into the tear film and therefore predispose to their becoming trapped in the interface after flap creation.

3. Sterile Drape

The betadine may be dabbed with sterile gauze and allowed to air dry for approximately 1 minute. A sterile drape is then applied over the lids to ensure an aseptic field (Fig. 12.2B). Several kinds of drapes are available for this purpose. When choosing a drape, the surgeon should consider the ability of the drape to cover the eyelashes, ease of application without break of sterile technique, ease of subsequent speculum insertion, and ease of removal at the end of the procedure. If the drape is applied on iodine-soaked skin, the drape may slip and the lashes may not be completely covered.

The lashes should be isolated not only for sterility but also to prevent them from jamming the microkeratome (Fig. 12.2B). Several alternatives to the surgical drape exist, including the use of 3M Tegaderm adhesive or a closed-blade speculum. One of us (DDK) uses the 3M Tegaderm adhesive to isolate the lashes and a blank drape to cover the forehead and temporal region. A similar drape is applied over the control panel of the laser microscope, ensuring that the surgeon's gloved hands do not touch unsterile surfaces.

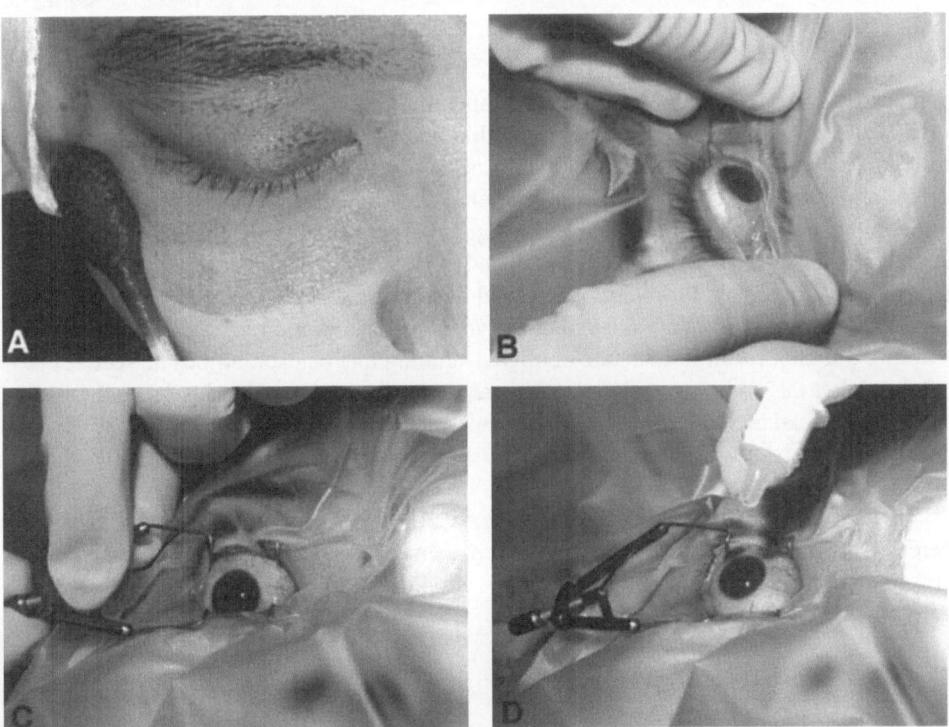

Figure 12.2 (A) Skin and eyelash scrubbing. (B) Sterile drape placement. (C) Wire speculum application. (D) Proparacaine instilled in inferior fornix.

4. Speculum

After the drape is placed, a lid speculum is introduced and opened slowly to avoid excessive eyelid pain (Fig. 12.2C). The aim of this step is to allow maximal exposure for the suction ring and ensure a clear path for the microkeratome. The choice of eyelid speculum often depends on the anatomical configuration of the patient's eyelids and orbits. For larger palpebral fissures, a long speculum blade may be appropriate. For narrower fissures a smaller speculum blade may be useful. A hexagonal eyelid opening after speculum application is ideal, for it allows for maximal surface area. A square opening is less good but may be better than a rectangular one. A solid blade speculum with rounded blades may be useful in such patients by providing a more rounded lid opening capable of accepting the suction ring and the microkeratome. It may be difficult to predict the ideal speculum design and size for an individual patient with narrow palpebral fissures. Switching from one design to another with suction ring placement rehearsals may be necessary to optimize this step if the initial suction application is unsuccessful.

5. Proparacaine in Fornix

If insertion or widening of the lid speculum causes eye pain or discomfort, the speculum should be narrowed, the patient instructed to look sideways or upwards, and topical anesthetic applied in the fornix (Fig. 12.2D). The patient is asked to look in the opposite direction and another drop of anesthetic is applied, avoiding corneal application. After a short waiting period, the speculum is widened, and the patient is reassured that the surgeon is aware of possible discomfort and that this step may be the most painful part of the surgery.

6. Corneal Preplaced Marks

Preplaced corneal marks help to ensure proper flap alignment at the completion of the surgery and are particularly useful in the unlikely event of a flap complication, such as a free cap. In this situation, asymmetric application of the marks assists in preventing inadvertent replacement of the cap with the epithelial surface facing down. Several markers are available, including existing radial keratotomy markers and specialized LASIK markers. Excessive ink on the marks should be avoided (Fig. 12.3A). The marks should be applied lightly to avoid epithelial toxicity or physical damage, and razor-sharp markers should be avoided. One option is to use rose bengal dye, since it is not toxic to the epithelium and therefore does not result in punctate epithelial staining that can sometimes be seen for several days after the use of gential violet. To prepare this, rose bengal strips are moistened in a pool of artificial tears (the authors' preference is Computer Tears, which seem to give the most consistent results). The strip is then brushed over the surface of the marker, which is allowed to air dry.

If epithelial loosening occurs during LASIK, the epithelial marks can shift and are therefore no longer a reliable guide for flap replacement. As a result, the surgeon should determine flap position by the gutter symmetry, which is in all cases the best measure of flap realignment.

7. Laser/Microkeratome Readiness

Suction time should be as short as possible to minimize optic nerve head and retinal ischemia during LASIK. Therefore it is critical that the surgeon confirm microkeratome readiness prior to suction ring application (Fig. 12.1A). Choice of suction ring and

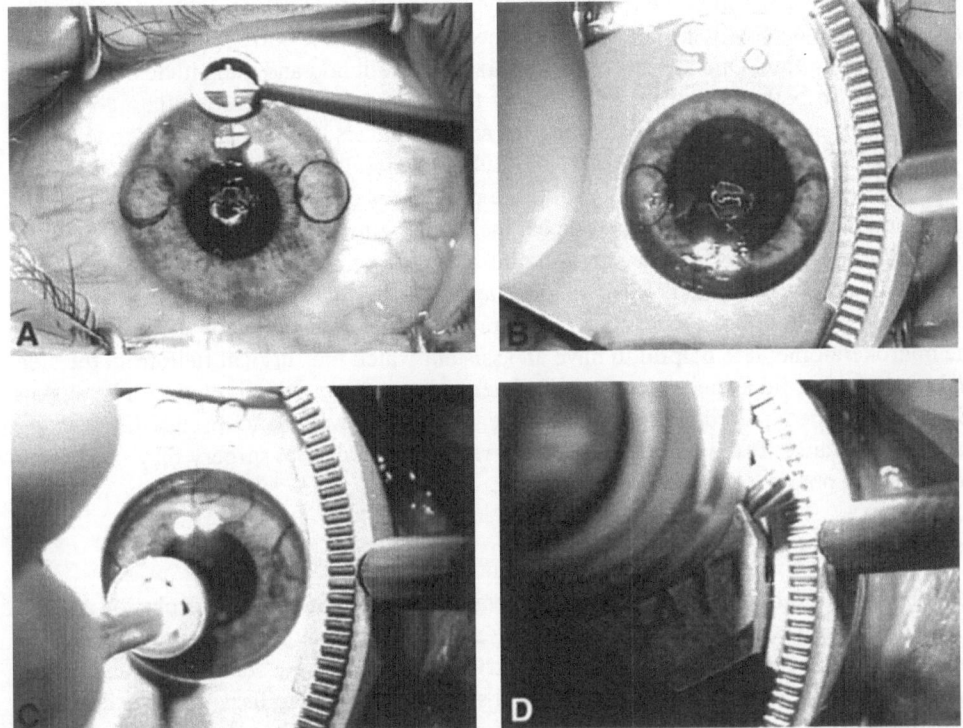

Figure 12.3 (A) Corneal preplaced marks. (B) Suction ring application. (C) Intraocular pressure check with pneumatonometer. (D) Microkeratome advance and reverse.

microkeratome settings should be individualized for each patient, taking into account ablation size, surgical eye (OD vs. OS), keratometry, refractive error, and pachymetry. Readiness of the microkeratome and integrity of the microkeratome blade should be checked before suction is applied. Laser readiness, including refractive error to be treated, should be confirmed as well. Laser recalibration should be performed prior to opening the eyelids for speculum application because, if performed at this stage, recalibration may be time consuming and may result in epithelial desiccation and stromal drying and thinning.

8. Suction Ring Application

In patients with adequate exposure, suction ring placement is relatively straightforward: close to the limbus, with approximately 0.5 mm decentration towards the flap hinge. In deep orbits, placement of the suction ring is facilitated by gentle pressure on the speculum to proptose the globe (Fig. 12.3B).

One of the most demanding steps for perfecting the LASIK surgical technique is ensuring suction ring centration. The suction ring should be intentionally decentered towards the hinge by approximately 0.5 mm to ensure flap centration relative to the pupil center. For certain microkeratomes, the suction ring may drift as suction builds up, more commonly in microkeratomes that have a relatively slow buildup of suction; the direction of the drift is toward the vacuum port (e.g., nasally with the Hansatome). This may not be always obvious. The surgeon should have a relatively low threshold to release suction, to inspect, and to fix any decentration. One or two diametrically opposite corrections may be necessary for recentration. One approach to minimize the likelihood and magnitude of drift is to push firmly on both sides of the suction ring for 2 to 5 seconds before initiating suction. This seats the suction ring in the conjunctiva and minimizes its tendency to migrate.

Small lid fissures, lid squeezing, and Bell's phenomenon may limit adequate placement and centration of the suction ring. If the problem is excessive lid squeezing, the surgeon should reassure the patient and repeat the instructions. A lid block may be necessary. For small orbits, options include (1) switching to a different lid speculum, particularly one that opens more widely and is less bulky; (2) applying the suction ring without a lid speculum, which warrants extra precaution to insure that lashes or lid skin are not in the path of the microkeratome; it is helpful to have an assistant watch the surgical field from the side and retract either lid as necessary, and (3) lateral canthotomy, which requires a local skin block and can be repaired with a single suture. It may be advisable to discuss this with the patient in advance. If the patient has already received a sedative, surgery may need to be postponed to obtain proper informed consent.

9. IOP Check

Most microkeratomes provide an auditory or visual indicator of adequate occlusion and the sound of the pump changes. As suction increases, the surgeon should ensure that scleral engagement is achieved as opposed to conjunctival occlusion of the suction ring and development of pseudosuction. Indicators of good suction include pupillary dilation, dimming of patient vision, and sympathetic forward movement of the globe upon the lifting of the suction ring. The IOP can be measured qualitatively with digital pressure on the globe or quantitatively with a fixed tonometer (e.g., Barraquer tonometer) or a device that measures the pressure such as a pneumotonometer (Fig. 12.3C). IOP measurement with a tonometer is advisable especially for beginning surgeons until they are comfortable relying upon the other signs of adequate suction. During the cutting of the flap, the suction ring can again be gently lifted to enhance unobstructed passage of the microkeratome.

B. LASIK STAGE II.   MICROKERATOME ADVANCEMENT AND FLAP LIFTING

1.   Preoperative Familiarity with Equipment

As discussed in Chap. 4, several microkeratomes may be used for LASIK, but none is ideal. As certain features are incorporated, additional limitations may be introduced. Furthermore, the LASIK microkeratome changes may require a different surgical technique and approach. The surgeon may thus have constantly to ensure preoperative familiarity with equipment prior to engaging the microkeratome head. Fortunately, most newer microkeratomes do not require a prolonged learning curve and result in far fewer complications, given surgeon familiarity and experience with the equipment.

2.   Patient Concerns

The surgeon may engender good cooperation by anticipating and paying attention to patient concerns. Preoperatively and at the beginning of surgery, we reassure the patient that the feelings of pressure and pain in the eye are not unexpected and that the vision may fade and disappear after suction application. The patient is told to expect a "cold sensation" during the following step of wetting the cornea.

3. Microkeratome Lubrication and Inspection

Several solutions may be used to wet the corneal surface. Proparacaine is recommended by several microkeratome manufacturers because it contains glycerin, which lubricates the ocular surface and therefore may minimize initial resistance and subsequent friction during the passage of the microkeratome head. This lubrication is an essential step that is often overlooked by the surgeon, who may be eager to pass the microkeratome, and one that requires attention on the part of the surgical assistant. The surgeon is handed the previously inspected microkeratome head for engagement on the suction ring. The surgeon and the assistant should ensure that there are no potential impediments such as eyelids, drape, or speculum in the path of the microkeratome head.

4. Advance/Reverse Microkeratome

Several microkeratomes are available; they are described in detail in Chapter 4. For horizontal microkeratomes, the head is engaged, and once a clear path is ensured, the foot pedal is used to advance the microkeratome in a temporal-to-nasal direction. Once the microkeratome cut is completed, the surgeon reverses the microkeratome.

For vertical microkeratomes, the head is dropped on the pivot prior to engagement of the microkeratome (Fig. 12.3D). It is sometimes helpful to rotate the eye slightly superiorly to minimize the risk of engaging the lower lid. The head is activated by depressing the foot pedal and rotates to create a superiorly based hinge. For manual vertical microkeratomes, the surgeon's index finger may provide assistance to ensure a constant speed of operation. The auditory signal indicating completion of the flap allows the surgeon to reverse the direction of the microkeratome head prior to disengagement. If the microkeratome stops prematurely, an attempt at continued forward advancement is acceptable after clearing any possible obstructions, as long as the microkeratome is not reversed. If the jam requires reversal, the microkeratome should be removed without attempting to go forward.

In most microkeratomes, the blade oscillates on the backward pass. Some surgeons elect to release suction prior to the automated backward pass. However, this can predispose to flap injury: if the patient moves the eye in any direction other than nasal for a horizontal microkeratome or superiorly for a vertical microkeratome, the flap can be lacerated by the oscillating blade. An alternative approach is to stop both suction and blade oscillation and simply slide the microkeratome off the eye after the forward pass. This shortens suction time and reduces friction between the flap and microkeratome during the reversal step; this may reduce the incidence and/or magnitude of epithelial injury. This approach is routinely used by one of us (DDK) when using the Hansatome.

In patients with deep-set orbits and prominent brows, a chin-up position may be helpful. In cases of prominent lower cheek and overhanging skin over the lower blade of the speculum, the assistant may have to retract the skin to ensure unobstructed passage of the microkeratome. It is important to release suction as soon as the reverse pass is completed in order to reduce the duration of the elevated IOP and minimize potential retinal and optic nerve injury.

5. Forniceal Drying

Drying of the fornices after removal of the microkeratome and suction ring is important to minimize the movement of meibomian and other tear debris into the flap interface. This can be done by using dry Murocel sponges, initiating vacuum with an aspirating speculum, or reapplying the suction ring lightly into the upper and lower fornices. Drying the ocular surface may also provide better visualization of the gutter around the flap and may reveal any epithelial irregularities.

6. Chayet Ring Application

Prior to lifting the flap, the application of a conventional or a modified Chayet ring (Fig. 12.4A) serves two purposes: (1) providing an elevated step for the everted flap to rest on, which will minimize tear fluid migration from the fornix to the undersurface of the flap, and (2) providing a relative barrier to the centripetal migration of debris onto the bed upon irrigation in preparation for and during flap repositioning.

7. Proper Centration of the Laser

The dehydration rate of the cornea increases after the flap is elevated. This is believed to alter corneal ablation rate, which may decrease the predictability of the procedure. It is therefore important to ensure proper centration of the laser prior to flap lifting. This will not

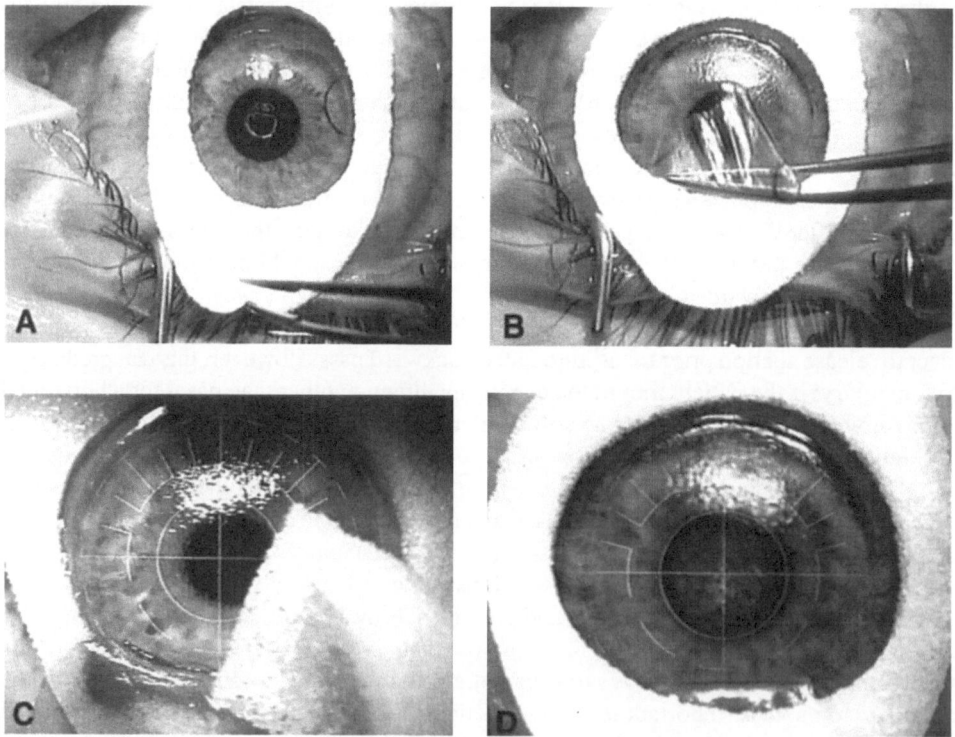

Figure 12.4 (A) Chayet ring application. (B) Lifting the flap. (C) Wiping off blood from ruptured limbal vessels. (D) Pupil centration and laser ablation.

only minimize the interval between lifting and ablation but also provide the patient with an opportunity to visualize the blinking target while the flap is in place. The patient should be instructed that the target may fade and change color as the flap is lifted.

8. Lifting the Flap

Several instruments may aid in lifting the flap, including an irrigating cannula, a modified hook, or a modified curved tying forceps (Fig. 12.4B). The advantage of the forceps is that as the flap is lifted the surgeon can separate the tips of the forceps by releasing the grasp on the forceps, thus preventing folding of the flap. The flap is then positioned on the Chayet ring. Gentle sweeps with a dry forceps on the undersurface of the flap may be necessary to prevent flap wrinkling while it dries on the ring. The flap can also be folded in half in the "taco" fold. This shields the undersurface of the flap from the laser in instances in which the ablation might slightly overlie the hinge.

A dry Murocel sponge may be necessary to wipe any fluid or blood pooling straddling the flap edge, especially at the hinge (Fig. 12.4C). This process may have to be repeated prior to laser ablation, but the time from flap turning to ablation should be minimized to avoid excessive stromal dehydration.

9. Ablation Depth and Pachymetry

The calculated ablation depth is reconfirmed prior to laser ablation. In patients in whom the calculated residual bed thickness approaches 250 μm, pachymetry is obtained intraoperatively. Because the flap thickness chosen for a particular procedure provided by the microkeratome manufacturer may vary dramatically from actual flap thickness, it may be risky to use the microkeratome thickness setting for calculating residual bed thickness. Optical pachymetry avoids touching the cornea and may underestimate ultrasound pachymetry by 15 to 20 μm. The use of an ultrasound pachymeter requires precalibration to measure pachymetry readings below 200 μm. Furthermore, the alcohol used to sterilize the tip of the pachymeter must be air dried prior to touching the cornea to avoid altering corneal ablation rates. This may be confirmed by sweeping the pachymeter tip in the surgeon's sterile glove prior to touching the stromal bed.

10. Residual Bed Calculations

Once the pachymetry is measured, residual bed calculations are performed and the laser parameters may be reconfirmed or altered to suit these calculations. If the flap is thinner than expected, the treatment diameter may be increased in patients with larger pupils. If the residual bed is smaller than expected, the surgeon should consider undercorrection to leave an adequate untreated bed and reduce the risk of subsequent ectasia. In cases of astigmatism ≥1 D, prior to finalizing the modified laser setting, if needed, the surgeon should confirm alignment of the cylinder marks to avoid axis shift.

C. LASIK STAGE III. LASER TREATMENT AND FLAP REALIGNMENT

1. Dim Oblique Illumination

Direct illumination is helpful in the first two stages of LASIK, but laser treatment may sometimes be achieved with greater patient cooperation if only dim oblique illumination is utilized. This allows physiologic dilation of the pupil, decreased light sensitivity, and greater ability to fixate on the blinking target. Alternatively, a ring light illuminator on its lowest setting may assist the patient in locating the fixation light and in some patients seems to increase the sharpness of the fixation target, perhaps because of the reduced pupil size.

The patient is instructed to maintain fixation on the target while the eye is monitored for any movement (Fig. 12.4D). If the laser system has no tracker, the surgeon may consider using a suction ring on low suction to assist a patient who cannot maintain fixation, but this is rarely required. Verbal contact with the patient is initiated at this step and continued throughout the laser treatment.

2.   Side View to Confirm Alignment

Additional confirmation of appropriate centration by an assistant or the surgeon may be necessary. This is facilitated by viewing the eye from the side to confirm alignment. Not infrequently, the patient may fixate on a target other than the fixation target. When this is suspected, the patient can be asked to describe the target (in order to correct fixation). The surgeon may have to dim all other microscope and room lights to ensure patient cooperation. Problems with proper fixation can usually be prevented by having the patient fixate on the target just before lifting the flap, which enables the patient to recognize the blurrier image of the fixation light as viewed through the exposed stromal bed.

3.   Pupil Centration

The laser treatment is centered on the pupil. Laser manufacturers provide several methods of centration. Decentration relative to the flap or the geometric center of the cornea should be disregarded. Once the pupil and the target are aligned, target fixation is confirmed by the patient, and the patient's head is held in place (Fig. 12.4D). Alternatively the laser joystick is used to track the eye. In lasers with active trackers, it may still be important to minimize eye and head movement to reduce postoperative aberrations.

4.   Head Holding

Head holding is preferred even in lasers with a tracker. It helps not only with tracking and correcting involuntary eye movement but also with regard to patient reassurance. A disadvantage is the possibility of change of plane of focus. Accordingly, the surgeon should estimate the customary amount of induced defocus and take it into consideration when centering the laser prior to holding the patient's head. Most often the surgeon's hand brings the head away from the microscope; thus defocus can be prevented by prior focusing on the iris plane.

5.   Updates During Surgery

As the laser procedure proceeds, the surgeon should keep updating the patient regarding the progress of laser ablation and reassuring the patient that he or she is fixating adequately. This coaching may help increase the patient's ability to maintain fixation and avoid giving up fixation prior to termination of the laser ablation.

Instead of asking a patient who has lost fixation to refixate during surgery, the surgeon should stop the laser and recenter prior to continuing the treatment. In hyperopic patients, these tasks have to be performed while protecting the flap, but priority should be given to fixation and centration rather than flap protection.

6. Flap Repositioning and Interface Irrigation with BSS

After congratulating the patient at the end of the treatment, one of the authors (DTA) routinely uses a long BSS cannula to wet the stromal bed (Fig. 12.5A). Such a cannula may offer the advantages of high squirting pressure and low volume of irrigation. It is advisable to have a dedicated syringe and cannula for this purpose and avoid introducing any other instruments into the interface, particularly the instrument previously used to lift the flap, which may theoretically reduce the chance of introducing epithelial cells in the interface. During this step, the surgeon may consider explaining to the patient that there will be blurring and apparent movement of the fixation target.

7. Flap Refloating

The flap is repositioned using one of several devices, such as a spatula or the same forceps initially used to lift the flap (Fig. 12.5B) to refloat it onto the stromal bed. The techniques of flap refloating vary among surgeons, but the speed of replacing the flap should be commensurate with the speed of the free fall of the flap, which may depend on patient age and flap thickness. Fast replacement may stretch the flap; slow replacement may predispose to incongruent edges and flap folding.

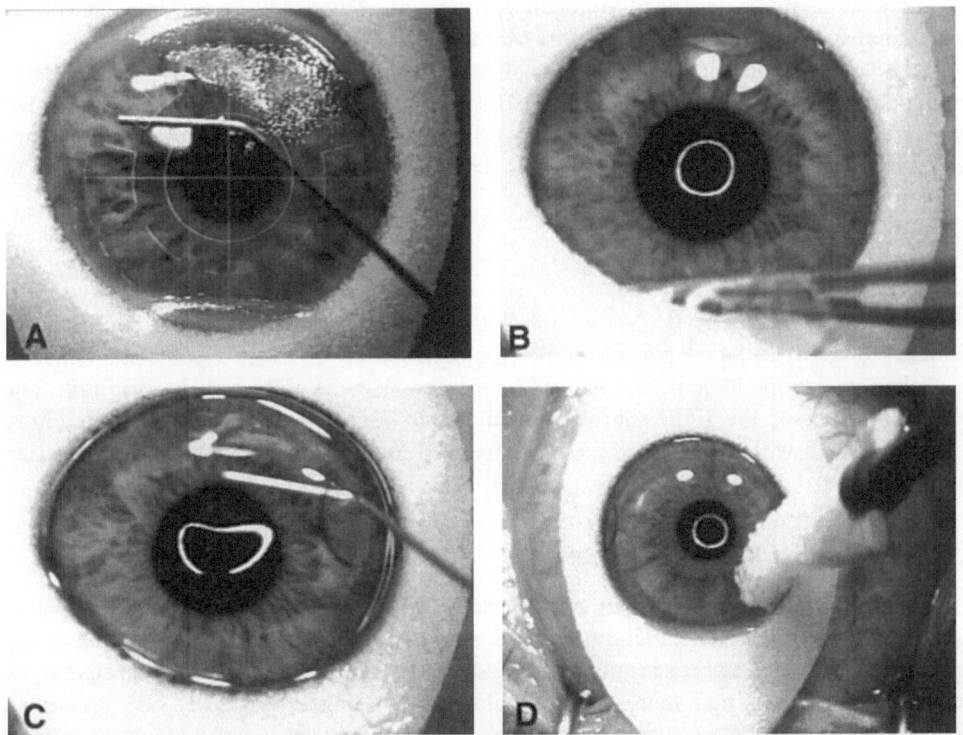

Figure 12.5   (A) Interface irrigation. (B) Flap repositioning. (C) Flap refloating. (D) Murocel drying of gutter.

8.   Interface Reirrigation

Some surgeons reirrigate the interface only if the initial flap replacement resulted in inadequate reapposition of the flap. Others, including the authors, routinely reirrigate the interface to loosen adherent debris and to assure technique consistency and presumed increased accuracy of outcomes (Fig. 12.5C). The fluid should be injected vigorously to flush debris from the interface without fluid pooling. If injecting from both sides of the flap, the direction of the injection should be centrifugal. If injecting from only one side, the injection should begin with the cannula tip just under the flap edge, moving the cannula centrally to flush material out of the opposite side of the flap. Irrigation should be continued while the cannula is being removed. Excess fluid irrigation should be avoided to minimize edema and may need to be aspirated with suction or with a Murocel sponge.

9.   Murocel Drying of Gutter and Flap Realignment

The endpoint is flap repositioning in a symmetrical gutter, realignment of the preplaced corneal marks, and absence of air, fibers, and debris in the interface Most surgeons use a noncellulose, nonfragmenting sponge (Murocel) to dry the gutter around the flap and to sweep the epithelial surface of the flap (Fig. 12.5D). Our approach is to apply a dry Murocel sponge just outside the flap margin adjacent to the inner margin of the Chayet ring. This allows centrifugal movement of fluid from the interface with minimal osmotic exchange of fluid from the tear film in the fornices and around the ring. This is followed by a gentle sweep with the moist expanded Murocel, starting at the hinge, and by multiple centrifugal pararadial sweeps with a (blotted) moist Murocel.

Even in the absence of basement epithelial membrane dystrophy, epithelial defects and loose epithelium may occur after flap dissection, especially if excessive proparacaine was used or if LASIK flaps were created with a rotating microkeratome. After repositioning of the flap stroma, loose epithelium is realigned. A moist Murocel is very helpful to achieve this goal without inducing striae.

10.   Direct Illumination

At this point one of us (DTA) switches the light source to the direct illumination mode, preferably using the placido single-ring light source. To avoid a Bell's phenomenon or other ocular movement, the patient is warned that the light will be brighter. The corneal reflex of the light source is valuable to identify striae and flap stretching (Fig. 12.6A). It will be helpful in deciding the need for and degree of sweeping of the flap once dried.

11.   Pararadial/Radial Sweeping

For one of us (DTA), the endpoint of corneal sweeping should be observation of a round placido reflex in the case of ring illumination as in the VISX laser. The direction of the pararadial and radial sweeps is guided by the shape of the light reflex and should start at the center aiming at making it more or less circular and avoiding folds (Fig. 12.6B). The reflex obtained after wetting the surface often appears more circular and more regular than reality (Fig. 12.6C). Furthermore, the wet corneal surface may prevent detection of flap folds or stretch marks.

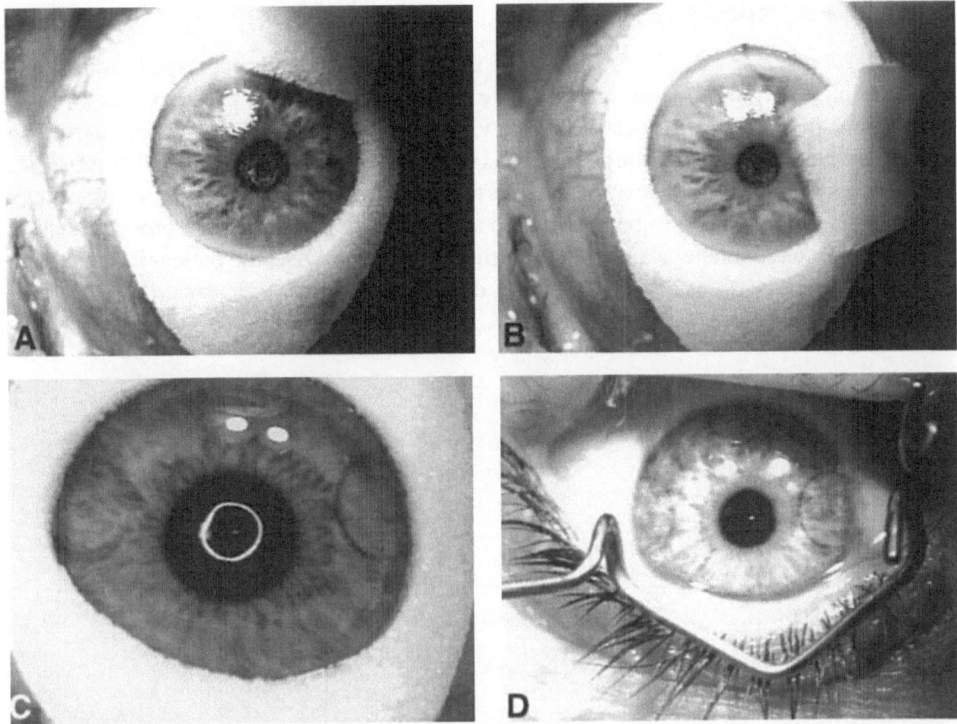

Figure 12.6 (A) Radial sweep. (B) Pararadial sweep. (C) Direct illumination and waiting period for adequate flap apposition. (D) Speculum removal.

12. Waiting Period for Adequate Flap Apposition

Once the sweeping with the moist sponge is complete, a 2 to 5 minute period of waiting ensues. The ocular surface should not be allowed to dry completely during the waiting period. Topical antibiotics, steroids, and nonsteroidal anti-inflammatory eyedrops are applied during the waiting period. After unintentional eye movement, observation of a circular light reflex should reassure the surgeon regarding the adequacy of flap apposition. Most surgeons use the waiting time to review postoperative precautions of avoiding eye rubbing and lid squeezing.

Alternatively, if the hinge is superior, one of us (DDK) does not wait once the flap is aligned. Antibiotic drops, preservative-free nonsteroidal drops, and preservative-free artificial tears are administered at 15 second intervals prior to removing the lid speculum.

13. Speculum Removal

At the conclusion of surgery, the lid speculum and drape are removed. This should be done with care to avoid flap dehiscence and folds (Fig. 12.6D). The speculum may be rotated superiorly prior to removal to minimize displacement or injury of the flap. Reinspection of the flap after removal of the speculum is valuable to ensure an adequate flap position.

14. Recheck Period and Discharge

Following surgery, the eye is inspected at the slit lamp to insure correct flap alignment and absence of clinically significant interface debris. The patient is then asked to wait 20 to 40 minutes with the eyelids gently closed. Following the waiting period, the surgeon can again examine the patient using slit lamp biomicroscopy to ensure flap and epithelial mark alignment, gutter symmetry, and clarity of the interface. In addition, flap folds and wrinkles may be seen. The flap may need to be re-elevated and irrigated and the patient brought back to the operating room to manage any abnormalities noted. Otherwise, the patient is discharged after receiving instructions and is followed 1 day after surgery.

13

Microkeratomes and Laser Settings

WILLIAM J. LAHNERS

University of South Florida, Tampa, and Center for Sight, Sarasota, Florida, U.S.A.

DAVID R. HARDTEN

*University of Minnesota and Minnesota Eye Consultants,
Minneapolis, Minnesota, U.S.A.*

A. INTRODUCTION

Advances in microkeratome design and laser technology have propelled LASIK to the forefront of refractive surgery. The newest generation of microkeratomes has reduced the risk and increased the accuracy of creating the lamellar flap—the step that historically has been the most challenging. Laser technology has produced improved treatment accuracy and predictability, and software updates allow the avoidance of certain pitfalls such as central islands and the treatment of refractive errors that were previously untreatable. The two most important instruments in LASIK are the microkeratome and the laser, and as such careful attention must be given to their calibration and settings. This chapter has been written to provide general guidelines for the use of these two instruments. The analysis of features and specifications of instruments made by individual manufacturers changes continuously and is beyond the scope of this chapter. In addition to the recommendations presented here, the surgeon is urged to become familiar with the nuances and eccentricities of the particular unit used.

B. MICROKERATOME SETTINGS

1. Suction Ring Size

One of the first decisions that must be made concerns the choice of suction ring size. Because the suction ring diameter determines how much of the cornea will protrude into the microkeratome, it is the primary determinant of flap diameter. In general, if a larger diam-

eter suction ring is chosen then a larger diameter flap will result. The preoperative keratometry values play a significant role in the diameter of the flap (1,2). As the cornea becomes steeper, more of the cornea will pass through the ring, producing a larger diameter
flap. Conversely, a flat cornea will not protrude into a given suction ring as much, and
would produce a flap of reduced diameter.

In a patient with a very steep cornea, use of a large diameter suction ring, such as a
9.5 mm ring, could produce a flap that exceeds the clear cornea diameter, potentially in-
juring the limbus and causing unnecessary bleeding. In patients with a history of long-term
soft contact lens wear and peripheral corneal neovascularization, it is possible to cause
bleeding by cutting into these vessels. Steep corneas are also more likely to produce button-hole complications during the microkeratome pass. This is most likely due to buckling
of the cornea against the microkeratome footplate. A larger diameter ring size may increase
the potential for this phenomenon. For this reason we recommend using a smaller diameter ring size for significantly steep corneas. Using the Hansatome we have had success using 46 D as a cutoff point: we use the 8.5 mm ring for corneas equal to or steeper than 46
D, when performing myopic or small optical zone corrections, and use the 9.5 mm ring for
corneas flatter than 46 D provided there is adequate corneal diameter. For hyperopic, or
large optical zone ablations, we use a K reading of 49 D as the cutoff point, using the 8.5
mm ring for 49 D and higher Ks and the 9.5 mm ring for lower Ks.

Patients with flatter corneas present less tissue through a given ring size, and produce
smaller diameter flaps. Corneas that are very flat are at higher risk for producing a free cap
during the creation of the flap. This occurs when relatively less of the corneal dome protrudes above the level of the ring, and subsequently a flap is produced which is so small that
it is completely excised. For these reasons, when performing myopic ablations, we recommend a larger ring size, a 9.5 mm or 10.0 mm ring, for corneas with Ks below 46 D. A small
flap, even if it is not a free cap, can be a problem for other reasons as well. Patients with
flatter corneas are more commonly presenting for hyperopic correction, which requires a
larger ablation zone. When attempting large ablations for hyperopia or mixed astigmatism,
we utilize the 9.5 mm suction ring in patients with K readings below 49 D.

The above guidelines will typically allow creation of a flap that is significantly
larger than the diameter needed for the ablation zone. This is beneficial for several reasons. Having a larger flap gives the surgeon a larger area for ablation, especially with
newer, larger transition zones. A larger stromal bed makes decentration of the microkeratome cut less likely to interfere with the ablation area. The flap hinge is moved farther
away with larger flaps, reducing the likelihood of accidental treatment of the back of the
flap, and reducing the effects of fluid collection at the flap edge. Moving the flap further
away from the ablation also prevents the surgeon from having to protect the flap or having to dry the fluid collecting at the flap edge. These extra maneuvers may slow the case,
increasing the variability of the treatment effect. Having a larger flap is also probably advantageous when performing LASIK following radial keratotomy, astigmatic keratotomy,
and penetrating keratoplasty. This allows a greater flap size to reduce the potential separation of the RK, AK, or penetrating keratoplasty incisions. In the event of an overcorrection leading to consecutive hyperopia, it is convenient to have a larger flap to perform
the hyperopic treatment (usually requiring a larger ablation zone) rather than having to
cut a new, larger flap. It has not been demonstrated in a controlled study that larger flaps
are any more, or less, likely to be dislocated by late trauma, but larger flaps clearly have
a larger area of adherence (a 9.5 mm flap has 84% more surface area than a 7.0 mm flap)

which may stabilize the flap. Larger flaps have edges closer to the limbus, in closer proximity to the limbal stem cells, which may speed the healing of the epithelial wound (3). Larger flaps will become increasingly important as we move to larger ablation zones and even larger transition zones.

Disadvantages of larger flaps include more fluid beneath the flap, which may require greater time at surgery to allow adherence of the flap. They may also require more stretching at the time of surgery to remove the extra fluid under the flap to reduce the incidence of striae. The cornea also is deformed to a greater extent, which can increase the incidence of epithelial defects. Placing the edge of the flap closer to the stem cells also may increase epithelial ingrowth rate, although if it were to occur it would be further from the visual axis.

There are instances when a smaller diameter ring, and thus flap diameter, is advantageous. If the flap is placed too close to the limbus, problems with bleeding can occur owing to transection of the limbal vessels. This is more of a problem with larger flaps. Long-term soft contact lens wearers can have a significant peripheral neovascular ingrowth, and in these patients a smaller ring size may be more prudent to avoid the nuisance of bleeding that can occur if the flap extends into these vessels.

2. Flap Thickness

Most microkeratomes designed for LASIK on the market today offer multiple footplate depths to produce a range of flap thicknesses. When deciding which one to choose, several factors must be considered. The two most important patient factors to be considered are the corneal thickness and the preoperative refractive error. There are also advantages and disadvantages of thicker and thinner flaps. Another important factor to consider when choosing the head plate depth is that the actual flap depth produced by the same microkeratome with the same head can vary substantially (4–7). Preoperative pachymetry can be one of the biggest determinants of flap thickness (2,5,7). Thinner corneas tend to produce thinner flaps, and thicker corneas yield thicker flaps. As the blade on the microkeratome gets duller, the flaps cut will be thinner and more likely to be irregular (5,6,8). Increasing translational speed (forward progress during the cut) results in thinner flaps, and this can cause problems with flap depth consistency in manually advanced microkeratomes (9). Intraocular pressure can affect flap thickness as well, with lower pressures resulting in thinner flaps. In microkeratomes with replaceable depth plates, the plate can be inserted incorrectly, resulting in a deeper than intended cut with possible entry into the anterior chamber (Figure 13.1). Newer microkeratomes with a fixed depth plate are less likely to cause this complication.

One of the most important factors to consider when choosing flap depth is the limitation imposed by the patient's central corneal thickness and level of ametropia. It is not known exactly how much residual posterior stromal thickness (RPST) is required to prevent consecutive ectasia following LASIK. It has become common at most institutions that 250 microns represents a minimum for RPST (10). This is clearly a controversial area, and few data are available to provide a definite answer. An RPST of 250 microns is probably more than necessary in most cases, but there probably will be rare cases where ectasia can occur even with a RPST of greater than 250 microns (11). From the patient's minimal central thickness we must subtract this 250 microns and the flap thickness to determine how much ablation can be performed. The ablation depth can be calculated using the Munner-

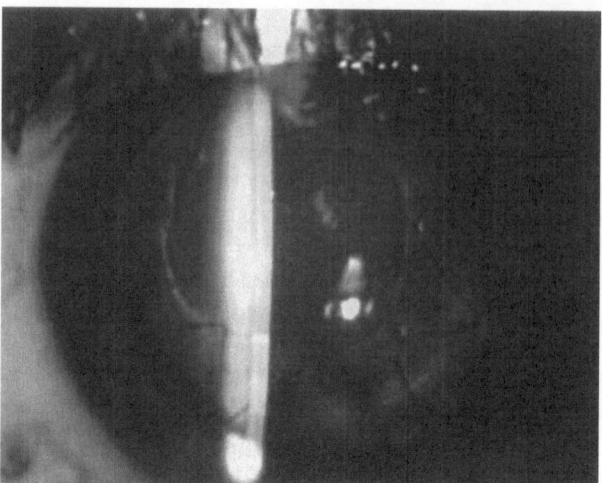

Figure 13.1 Inadvertent corneal penetration from failure to assemble microkeratome footplate. An eight bite 10-0 nylon suture was used to repair the wound.

lyn formula (depth of ablation = diopters of correction × (ablation diameter)^2/3) (12). In some cases of high refractive errors, thin central corneal thickness, or both, it may be necessary to choose a thinner flap to allow for more ablation. It should also be noted that thinner corneas tend to yield thinner flaps, and this may be advantageous in cases where residual stromal thickness is an issue (5). In any case in which the computation is close, the safest maneuver is to measure the residual thickness with ultrasonic pachymetry after the flap is reflected back. This will eliminate the unknown factor of flap thickness and alert the surgeon to a flap that may be thicker than expected.

While the ideal flap thickness has not been determined in any controlled studies, we believe that in most cases a flap thickness of around 180 microns is the best choice. This thicker flap has numerous advantages: it is easier to manipulate during surgery, has a lower incidence of folds and striae and a lower incidence of irregular astigmatism, and it is more likely to resist injury during manipulation and future enhancements if needed. In addition, a problem during the microkeratome cut resulting in a thinner flap is less potentially devastating if a thicker flap was initially targeted. The chief disadvantage of a thicker flap is that less residual stroma remains for ablation; this could become an issue in cases with high refractive errors, thinner corneas, or both.

The decision to use a lower footplate setting, and thus a thinner flap, is probably only advantageous in a setting where there is a risk of exceeding the minimum safe residual stromal bed thickness of 250 microns. In these cases, the disadvantages of the thinner flap (higher risk of folds, higher risk of irregular astigmatism, more difficulty handling thinner flaps, more difficulty lifting flap for enhancements, and a smaller margin of error when cutting the flap) must be weighed against the disadvantages of decreasing the treatment zone diameter to preserve tissue, or using an alternative technology such as a phakic intraocular lens. This decision should be made on a case-by-case basis, and patient factors that must be considered include patient's pupillometry and special visual needs (driving at night, etc.). In our experience it is probably better to preserve residual bed thickness by using a thinner flap than decreasing treatment zone size, because smaller treatment zones are more likely to result in optical distortions. In cases where using a thinner flap does not allow at least a

6 mm optical zone with 250 microns of residual stromal bed thickness, it is best to utilize another technology such as a phakic IOL implantation.

3. Vacuum Setting

Achieving and maintaining adequate vacuum during the microkeratome pass is critical to producing an accurate flap. The suction system should always be checked prior to every procedure. Suction should be sufficient to raise the intraocular pressure to at least 65 mmHg for most microkeratomes. When using the Hansatome, the vacuum level required to achieve this intraocular pressure is approximately 20 to 27 inches of Hg, depending on altitude. This will vary for different microkeratomes. Lower pressures can produce thinner cuts and irregular flaps. Pressures that are much higher than necessary increase the risk of chemosis, subconjuntival hemorrhages, and optic nerve injury. The intraocular pressure should be checked after the suction is activated to make certain that it is high enough to proceed with the microkeratome pass. If proper suction is not achieved, the cut should not be performed; if suction is lost during the cut, forward progress should be stopped immediately or transection of the flap can occur. Newer microkeratomes have safety features that stop blade oscillation and forward progress if there is loss of suction. Some microkeratomes have user adjustable vacuum settings designed for calibration at altitudes that differ from sea level.

4. Blade Selection

Blade assembly and inspection are critical to the success of the procedure. The surgeon should inspect the blade assembly, even if it is performed by trained personnel, in every case. An examination under the microscope should be done looking for a smooth finish, good edge quality with no pitting, and no residue or metal shavings. Any blade irregularities can seriously affect flap quality and final visual outcome (Fig. 13.2). Blade quality can

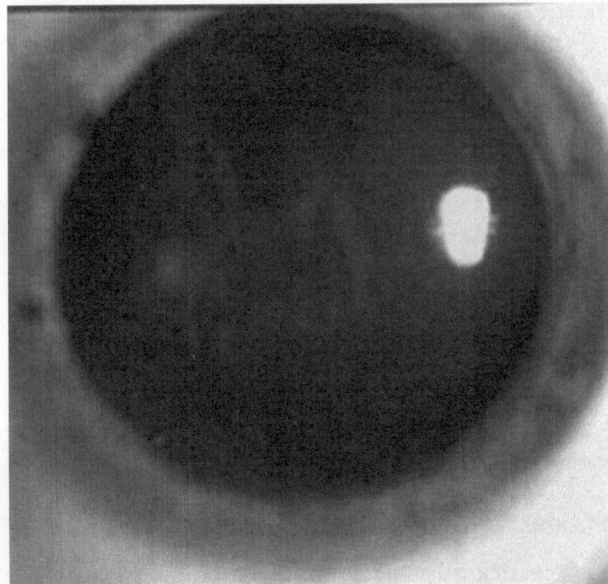

Figure 13.2   Intraoperative photograph of an irregular flap secondary to poor blade quality.

vary from unit to unit, and poor quality blades should uniformly be rejected and replaced. Blades should never be reused unless expressly designed for such use by the manufacturer. It has been shown that dull blades produce thinner flaps and increase the risk of irregular flaps (5,6). Many centers allow for the same blade to be used on both eyes of the same patient, but not more than this. Even in this usage it has been demonstrated that the second flap cut is somewhat thinner than the first (6).

C. GUIDELINES FOR LASER SETTINGS

It is a popular misconception that lasers are computer-controlled devices that are incapable of producing a less than perfect outcome. In reality these devices, while capable of great accuracy, must be carefully maintained and calibrated to achieve proper performance. When setting up the excimer laser the following parameters merit special attention: laser room environment, fluence testing, and beam homogeneity.

The laser room environment is an important variable that must be controlled. The room should be kept cool for optimal laser performance. This varies from laser to laser, but a temperature of 18 to 24 degrees Celsius should be maintained. The ambient humidity should be kept low (40 to 50% relative humidity) and as steady as possible. Humidity can significantly affect the ablation rate of corneal tissue, with overcorrections more likely in very dry conditions and undercorrections more likely in more humid conditions (13). The room should be kept free from particulate debris, which can adversely affect ablation regularity if it is deposited on the optical system of the laser. This can be achieved with an active filtration system using a HEPA (high efficiency particulate air) filter. These systems are capable of removing particles as small as 0.1 micron, including bacteria. The system should be in operation continuously, as shutdown periods will allow particulate matter to coat the optics of the laser system.

Laser fluence is a measure of the energy density and is described as the amount of energy applied per unit area with each pulse. This is measured in millijoules per centimeter squared (mJ/cm^2). The minimum fluence necessary for proper photoablation of the cornea is approximately 50 to 60 mJ/cm^2. The fluence of the laser should be checked before every ablation, which is usually automatically performed in most lasers. If the fluence is low, this is an indication that the gas concentrations should be raised to prevent undercorrections, which may occur due to inadequate tissue ablation. Gas levels that are too high can cause higher fluence and overcorrections.

Beam homogeneity is a measure of the consistency of the distribution of energy applied over the ablation area. Homogeneity is an important parameter in broad beam lasers, and if it is poor, it can lead to an irregular ablation and potential loss of best spectacle corrected visual acuity. It is of much less significance in small scanning spot/slit lasers, as any inhomogeneity present would be spread out evenly over the ablation area. Manual verification of beam homogeneity is essential in broad beam delivery systems. This is usually accomplished by test ablations into appropriate substrate materials as provided by the individual laser manufacturer. Visual evidence of poor homogeneity is reason to cancel the procedure until the problem can be remedied.

1. Adjustments to Standard Laser Nomograms

It should come as no surprise to any experienced surgeon that the laser is very much like any other surgical instrument in that an adjustment must be included in the treatment plan to allow for different surgical variables. While the primary determinant of the tissue ablation pattern and final visual outcome is the treatment design that is included in the laser software, this does not lessen the importance of developing personal nomograms. Today's surgeon has the advantage of using ablation software that has evolved through several generations and provides for advanced features such as wider optical zones, multiple treatment zones, transition zones, and software to reduce surface irregularities such as central islands. However, each laser is used in different settings, and surgeons have individual variations in technique and operating environment. To allow for these differences, individual nomograms should be developed to improve the accuracy and predictability of treatments. Increasing the standardization of the technique will improve the standard deviation of the achieved effect, and adjusting the nomogram by the average achieved effect will move the mean towards the desired result, which is typically emmetropia.

There are many factors that can contribute to the final visual and refractive outcome after LASIK. These include patient age, gender, preoperative keratometry, preoperative pachymetry, degree of planned correction, laser type, software version, room temperature, room humidity, facility altitude, accuracy in laser calibration, depth of keratectomy, degree of corneal hydration used by the surgeon, time that the flap is raised and the total procedure duration, whether or not forced air (or vacuum) is used across the stromal bed during ablation, postoperative inflammation (e.g., diffuse lamellar keratitis), and postoperative medications. It is the job of the surgeon to control as many of these factors as possible (e.g., temperature, humidity, technique, time of surgery, postoperative medications), as this is the first step in achieving precise outcomes. For the factors that are not controllable, it is important to examine how they affect refractive outcomes using statistical methods so that the accuracy of the ablation can be improved, decreasing the rate of over- and undercorrections.

Differences in technique can make a large difference in the final ablation. Even small variables should be sought out and eliminated if possible. For example, lifting the flap with nontoothed forceps instead of an irrigating cannula removes the risk of accidental introduction of fluid into the interface. Even a small amount of fluid can hydrate the stroma, resulting in decreased tissue ablation and undercorrection. The dryer the stromal tissue is, the more tissue is ablated per pulse of the laser (13). Increasing the amount of time that the flap is raised increases the evaporation and decreases the hydration of the bed. This can result in significantly increased ablation and thus overcorrection. The time to perform the entire technique from start to finish, and especially the time while the flap is lifted, should be consistent from case to case. If the surgeon chooses to wipe the bed, then the same technique should be performed in every case, including the dampness/dryness of the sponge and the number of wipes during the ablation. When choosing an initial nomogram one should choose one from a surgeon who ideally has experience on the same laser, at the same facility, and who uses a similar technique. This will give the beginning surgeon a starting point.

Patient age is a very important consideration when designing nomograms. The same laser will typically have more effect in an older patient. Older patients also have less accommodative amplitude, which will make them less tolerant of hyperopia. We are less aggressive when treating myopia in patients over 40 for these reasons. Some surgeons will include an adjustment for mild residual myopia in older patients where the nondominant eye treatment is reduced by 5 to 10%. Younger patients show a greater tendency towards regression and can tolerate small overcorrections owing to their increased accommodative amplitudes. For these reasons it is appropriate to be somewhat more aggressive in younger patients.

The development of a personal nomogram begins with the collection of data including the patient's age, refractive error, gender, pachymetry, keratometry, and postoperative manifest refractions, including data with the longest follow-up time possible; typically 6 months to 1 year is ideal. While in most cases the patient's refractive error will stabilize at 3 months, higher refractive errors may take longer, sometimes 6 to 12 months. It is important to collect and include this data, if it is available. The data is then analyzed using multiple regression analyses, and the resulting information is used to create a personal nomogram. There are also commercial programs on the market that will assist in nomogram development (Table 1).

Other factors should also be considered. As was mentioned above, it may be desirable to attempt slight hyperopia to achieve fewer myopic undercorrections in younger patients, and mild myopia on overage in older patients to reduce undesirable hyperopia. It must be remembered that treatments for overcorrection of myopia can be technically more difficult than the initial surgery, especially if a small flap was originally used, and the retreatment requires the cutting of a new flap. Because of the relative difficulty and poorer predictability in hyperopic treatments, some surgeons structure their nomograms so that the rate of enhancement for an overcorrection is less than the rate of enhancement for an undercorrection.

The nomograms should also be altered to allow for differences in corneal response following PRK, LASIK, radial keratotomy, or penetrating keratoplasty. Concerning retreatments, several trends can be observed. Patients who have shown large amounts of regression may be more likely to underrespond to retreatments as well. For this reason, some surgeons are more aggressive when treating an initial undercorrection. We tend to use the same nomogram for retreatment of initial undercorrections, unless it is clear why the patient originally underresponded, attempting to avoid problems with overtreatment. When treating overcorrections after previous LASIK, most surgeons reduce the correction, because these eyes have a tendency to overrespond to the second treatment.

The frequency of updating nomograms is a matter of personal choice. Some surgeons use a more rapid cycle when recalculating their nomograms and change nomograms every few months. This can allow for a more rapid adjustment to a new technique, new instruments, or other factors. Other surgeons prefer to make fewer adjustments on their nomograms, opting to refine their nomogram only when larger patient numbers and more follow-up data indicate that a change is necessary. Beginning refractive surgeons should begin data collection and analysis in a timely manner but should avoid the tendency to start changing the nomogram until an adequate amount of data has been collected at a stable time point postoperatively.

Table 1 Commercially Available Outcomes and Data Analysis Software

Software name	Designed by	Contact information
The Refractive Surgery Consultant	Guy M. Kezirian, MD and Jack T. Holladay, MD	480-348-9299; www.RefractiveConsultant.com
LASIK/PRK Outcomes Analysis	Perry S. Binder, MD	858-756-4462; email: LASIKSupport@aol.com

Table 2 Myopic LASIK. (David R. Hardten, M.D.; VISX Star S3 Smoothscan, Minneapolis, MN)

Age (yrs)	0–0.9 D (%)	1–1.9 D (%)	2–3.9 D (%)	4–5.9 D (%)	6–7.9 D (%)	8–11.9 D (%)
20–29	58	28	11	4	−1	0
30–39	45	22	8	1	−2	−5
40–49	32	14	3	−1	−4	−6
50–59	19	7	0	−2	−5	−7
60+	9	1	0	−3	−6	−8

Achieved effect = 1.11 PRK setting − 0.012 Age + 0.93, based on 1 month results with 5% additional regression to 1 year. Use the above adjustment to spherical equivalent (patient's spherical equivalent is the horizontal axis and age is the vertical); enter full cylinder without correction.

As an example we have included our nomograms from two surgeons (David R. Hardten, MD and Richard L. Lindstrom, MD) using the Visx Star S3 Smoothscan in Minneapolis, MN (Tables 2–4). The altitude of our facility is approximately 1000 feet above sea level, our temperature between 68 and 74 degrees F, and our humidity 20 to 40%. To use the nomogram we convert to spherical equivalent and then use the percentage adjustment indicated to change the sphere of the patient's refractive error. We enter cylinder directly as we have not found that this parameter requires independent adjustment. The differences between the nomograms illustrate effects of variation in technique between two surgeons using the exact same laser and operating setting.

Based on our experience we have found that the factors that influence our results most are age and preoperative refractive error. This does not mean that other factors do not contribute to the accuracy of the treatment. Using multiple regression analyses the surgeon can determine the contribution of different variables and calculate adjustment factors for each. While setting up nomograms can be a laborious task for the busy clinician, it is an important step that should not be overlooked, as it can contribute greatly to more accurate surgical outcomes and more satisfied patients.

Table 3 Myopic LASIK. (Richard L. Lindstrom, MD; VISX Star S3 Smoothscan, Minneapolis, MN)

Age (yrs)	0–0.9 D (%)	1–1.9 D (%)	2–3.9 D (%)	4–5.9 D (%)	6–7.9 D (%)	8–11.9 D (%)
20–29	68	32	10	0	−5	−9
30–39	45	22	3	−4	−7	−10
40–49	32	10	−3	−8	−10	−11
50–59	19	−3	−9	−12	−13	−14
60–69	−14	−15	−16	−16	−17	−17

Achieved effect = 1.26 PRK setting − 0.023 Age + 1.53, based on 1 month results with 5% additional regression to 1 year. Use the above adjustment to spherical equivalent (patient's spherical equivalent is the horizontal axis and age is the vertical); enter full cylinder without correction.

Table 4   Hyperopic LASIK. (David R. Hardten, MD; VISX Star S3 Smoothscan, Minneapolis, MN)

Age (yrs)	0–1.9 D (%)	2–3.9 D (%)	4–6 D (%)	After RK (%)	After LASIK (%)
20–29	0	10	20	−4	−14
30–39	10	18	25	−2	−10
40–49	17	23	28	−1	−1
50–59	30	30	30	0	4
60	35	32	31	2	8

Columns to far right are for consecutive hyperopia. Use the above adjustment to spherical equivalent (patient's spherical equivalent is the horizontal axis and age is the vertical); enter full cylinder without correction.

D. CONCLUSION

LASIK continues to evolve into a very safe and effective technique. The proper selection of microkeratome settings and the development of personal laser nomograms are important elements of a successful LASIK procedure. It is only by diligent attention to details and the continuous analysis of variables that we can continue to advance the state of the art, while providing the greatest accuracy and best possible vision for our patients.

REFERENCES

1. C Argento, MJ Cosentino, G Valenzuela. Influence of keratometry on the flap size. ASCRS Symposium on Cataract, IOL, and Refractive Surgery, San Diego, 1998, p 119.
2. YI Choi, SJ Park, BJ Song. Corneal flap dimensions in laser in situ keratomileusis using the Innovatome automatic microkeratome. Korean J Ophthalmol 2000;14(1):7–11.
3. HS Dua, JV Forrester. The corneoscleral limbus in human corneal epithelial wound healing. Am J Ophthalmol 1990;110(6):646–656.
4. PS Binder, M Moore, RW Lambert, DM Seagrist. Comparison of two microkeratome systems. J Refract Surg 1997;13(2):142–153.
5. E Donnenfeld, R Wertheimer, A Wallerstein, H Perry, L Landrio, E Rahn. Predictors of corneal flap thickness in LASIK surgery. ASCRS Symposium on Cataract, IOL and Refractive Surgery, San Diego, 1998, p 63.
6. FR Villareal, PR Valdes, EB Garza. Reproducibility of corneal flap thickness with Hansatome microkeratome: comparison between first and fellow eye using the 180-micron head. ASCRS Symposium on Cataract, IOL and Refractive Surgery, Boston, 2000, p 14.
7. WM Yi, CK Joo. Corneal flap thickness in laser in situ keratomileusis using an SCMD manual microkeratome. J Cataract Refract Surg 1999;25(8):1087–1092.
8. A Behrens, B Seitz, A Langenbucher, MM Kus, C Rummelt, M Kuchle. Evaluation of corneal flap dimensions and cut quality using the Automated Corneal Shaper microkeratome. J Refract Surg 2000;16(1):83–89.
9. R Suarez, R Yee. Are manual microkeratomes reliable? ASCRS Symposium on Cataract, IOL and Refractive Surgery, Boston, 2000, p 33.
10. T Seiler, K Koufala, G Richter. Iatrogenic keratectasia after laser in situ keratomileusis. J Refract Surg 1998;14:312–317.
11. SP Amoils, MB Deist, P Gous, PM Amoils. Iatrogenic keratectasia after laser in situ keratomileusis for less than −4.0 to −7.0 diopters of myopia. J Cataract Refract Surg 2000;26(7):967–977.
12. CR Munnerlyn, SJ Koons, J Marshall. Photorefractive keratectomy: a technique for laser refractive surgery. J Refract Surg 1988;14:46–52.

14

Centration of LASIK Procedures

MARSHA C. CHEUNG

*Massachusetts Eye and Ear Infirmary and Harvard Medical School,
Boston, Massachusetts, U.S.A.*

CHUN CHEN CHEN and DIMITRI T. AZAR

*Massachusetts Eye and Ear Infirmary, Schepens Eye Research Institute,
and Harvard Medical School, Boston, Massachusetts, U.S.A.*

A. EFFECT OF IMPROPER CENTRATION

Many corneal procedures such as LASIK and photorefractive keratectomy demand proper centration on the cornea. The optical zone is the part of the cornea that refracts light rays to form the image on the fovea. Many corneal surgical procedures can cause scarring in the peripheral cornea, leaving behind a central optical zone. If this optical zone is too small or improperly centered, visual function can be adversely affected by glare or irregular astigmatism. Glare and blurred images are especially noted at night when the pupil is dilated, thereby demanding the largest scar-free optical zone. Numerous other complications such as monocular diplopia, unpredictable visual acuity outcomes, and poor contrast sensitivity can also be attributed to improper centration of the optical zone (2). Since the majority of refractive surgeries such as LASIK (1) operate on eyes that can be corrected to 20/20 visual acuity and (2) are elective procedures, all these complications affecting visual outcome are significant. By careful attention to proper centration of corneal procedures, many of the optical problems following the refractive surgical procedures including LASIK may be decreased.

The question then arises as to what method should be used to determine the optical zone and how this zone should be centered. Many axes of the eye can be described such as the optical axis, visual axis, pupillary axis, line of sight, line of fixation, etc. Over the years, confusion and conflicting definitions over these various axes have been sources of much controversy surrounding the question of what is the proper centration technique. In this chapter, we review the relevant definitions, examine the evolution of the current centration methods, and describe the most current clinical approach to centering corneal refractive surgery.

B. INITIAL CENTRATION TECHNIQUES: USING THE OPTICAL AXIS AND THE VISUAL AXIS

Every optical system has an optical axis defined by the line passing through the center of curvature of each component of the system (3). However, the human eye does not represent a perfectly aligned optical system, so the eye cannot be assigned an optical axis. As shown in Fig. 14.1, the incoming ray of light hits a primary nodal point and then continues toward the fovea from a second nodal point with the identical angle to the optical axis (4). The Gullstrand model of the eye deals with the nonideal nature of the human eye by considering it a centered system with a pair of nodal points. The visual axis is an interrupted line that connects the point of fixation with the fovea, passing through multiple nodal points (3). Figure 14.2 shows how the eye would be if it were a perfectly centered optical system.

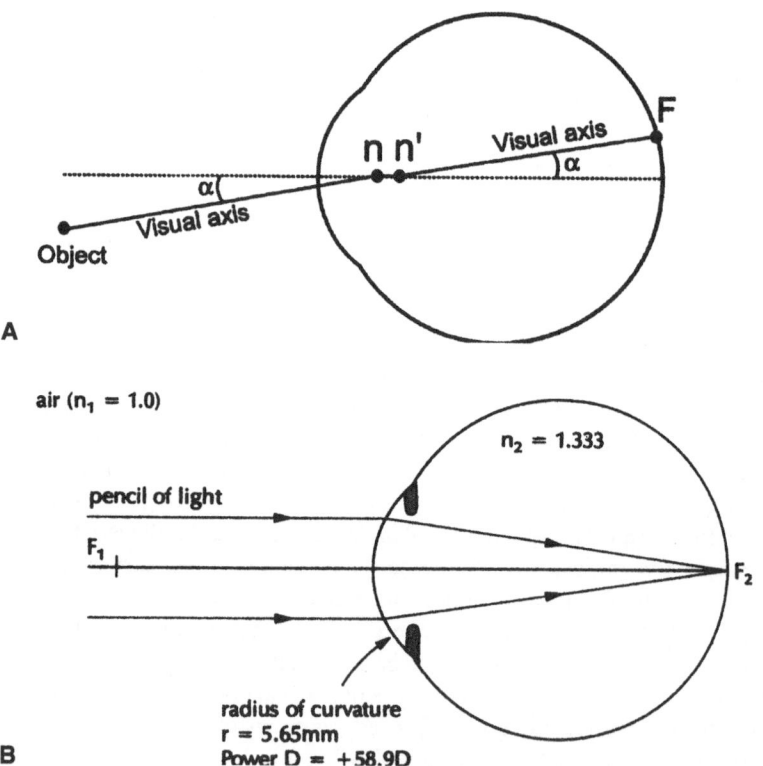

Figure 14.1 (A) The simplified schematic eye: in this simplified model of the eye as an optical system, the visual axis connects the object to the fovea via two nodal points. This model relates the object and image sizes and distances but does not take into account the real path of light as it passes through the human eye. (From Ref. 1.) (B) Pencils of parallel light rays in an emmetropic eye will be bent by the cornea and lens to focus on the retina. (From Ref. 59.)

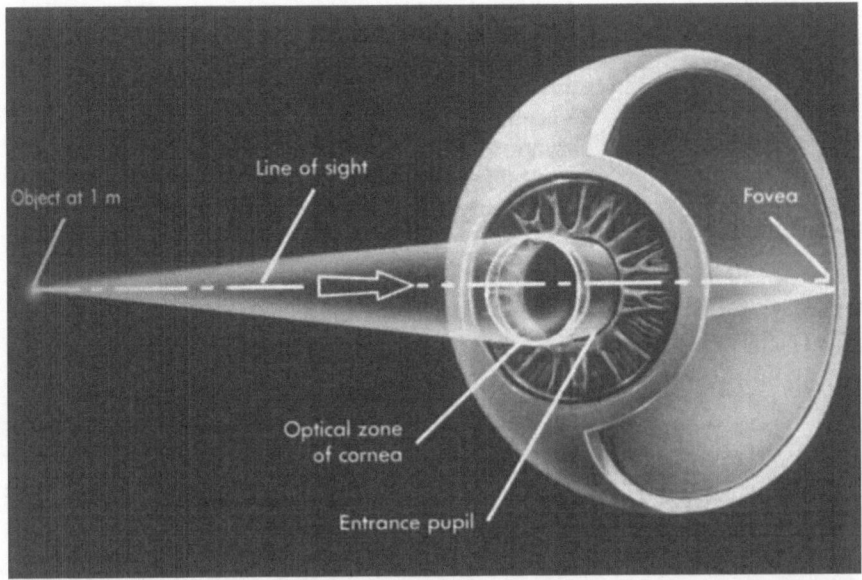

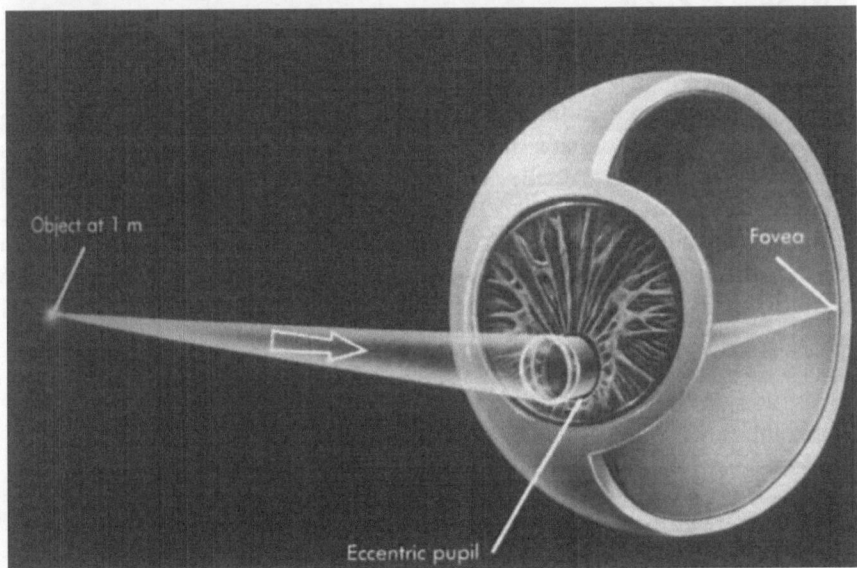

Figure 14.2   If the human eye were a perfectly centered system, then all optical elements including the corneal intercept of the visual axis, the corneal light reflex, the corneal center of curvature, and the foveal image would all be perfectly aligned. (From Ref. 7.)

The visual axis may be useful in terms of allowing optical calculations for the eye such as the refraction and magnification of objects and their images. However, given that these models are based on a false assumption of the human eye being a centered system, these models are insufficient in making optical calculations for patients with especially decentered systems.

The initial proposed centering techniques in the 1980s were based on this erroneous assumption that the eye is centered according to this visual axis. Despite the theoretical usefulness of the early models, they cannot be used for the human eye. There are numerous elements that may contribute to a patient's eye being a decentered system—for example, an eccentric pupil or a large angle between the visual and optical axes. While the visual axis may be useful for theoretical circumstances and mathematical calculations relating objects and image sizes and distances, it is not of much value when evaluating the path of actual rays as they pass through the human eye.

C. CURRENT CENTRATION TECHNIQUES: CENTERING BASED ON THE ENTRANCE PUPIL

In the mid-1980s, Walsh and Guyton and then Uozato and Guyton transformed the initial thinking on centering techniques (5,6). They emphasized that the former method of using the visual axis of the eye was poorly defined and inaccurate; they reported that these methods should not be used for centering corneal surgical procedures. Instead, these authors brought to light the notion of centering based on the entrance pupil.

D. THE ENTRANCE PUPIL

As shown in Fig. 14.3, the pupil can be thought of as it exists in three different planes: the entrance pupil, the real pupil, and the exit pupil. When we look at the human eye, we see a virtual image of the pupil and the iris that is based on the refractive properties of the cornea and aqueous. The entrance pupil is that virtual image of the pupil. Clinically, measurements have been taken showing that the entrance pupil is approximately 0.30 mm anterior to and 14% larger than the human pupil (8). It is located about 5 mm behind the front surface of the cornea (6). As the patient fixates on an object, a collection of light rays will fall onto the eye surface, but only those that specifically are within the boundaries of the entrance pupil will go into the eye. Similarly, the exit pupil of the eye is the image of the real pupil formed by refraction through the crystalline lens.

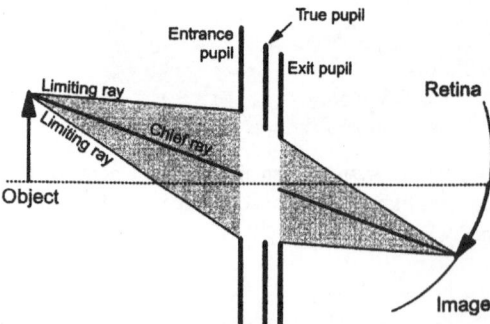

Figure 14.3 The pupil can be thought of as it exists in three different planes: the entrance pupil, the real pupil, and the exit pupil. The entrance pupil is a virtual image of the pupil based on the refractive properties of the cornea and aqueous, located approximately 0.30 mm anterior to the real pupil and approximately 14% larger. The exit pupil is the virtual image of the real pupil formed by the refraction through the crystalline lens. (From Ref. 1.)

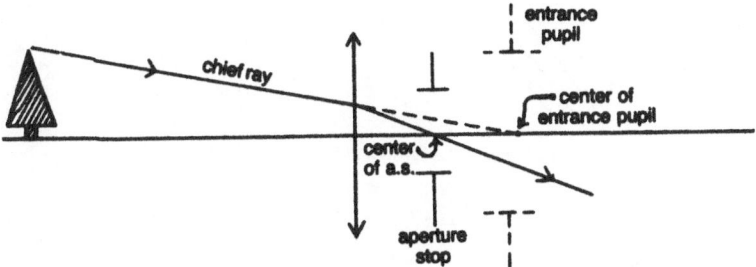

Figure 14.4   The line of sight is defined as the line connecting the fixation point to the center of the entrance pupil. In geometrical optic terms, this is equivalent to the chief ray. (From Ref. 58.)

E.   THE OPTICAL ZONE

There is a critical portion of the cornea used to see the fixation point—this portion of the cornea overlies the entrance pupil and is termed the *optical zone* as described by Maloney which is shown in Fig. 14.3 (9). The optical zone is centered on the "line of sight" which matches the chief ray in geometrical optical terminology, but only in a perfectly aligned optical system (10). This line of sight or chief ray joins the object to the center of the entrance pupil to the foveal image as shown in Fig. 14.4. Since the entrance pupil is circular, the bundle of rays passing through it is circular as well. These rays strike the corneal surface in a circular fashion—the optical zone—which is centered on the intersection of the line of sight with the cornea.

These definitions are of critical importance to the corneal surgeon. Uozato and Guyton first emphasized that the intersection of this line of sight, or the chief ray, is located at the desired center of the optical zone for corneal surgical procedures such as LASIK or PRK (6). They also pointed out how irregular and unpredictable refraction and glare may result from any corneal scarring or irregularities overlying the entrance pupil. On the other hand, irregularities or scarring that are peripheral to the optical zone of the cornea affect only the light rays that do not reach the fovea; in other words, scarring peripheral to the corneal surface over the entrance pupil will not affect the foveal image. However, light from peripheral locations in the patient's visual field does pass through the eccentric portions of the cornea to reach the entrance pupil; thus peripheral corneal irregularities or scarring can affect the patient's peripheral image quality (6).

Figure 14.5 displays how the light rays pass through the optical zone to reach the fovea. It also shows the path of peripheral rays to reach the parafovea. A corneal scar within the optical zone can scatter the light, leading to a blurred foveal image as shown in Fig. 14.6. Figure 14.7 shows how in LASIK, even a properly centered ablation zone can have peripheral rays outside of the optical zone leading to unwanted visual side effects such as glare.

F.   THE PUPILLARY AXIS AND THE ANGLE LAMBDA

The pupillary axis has been described as the line perpendicular to the cornea that passes through the center of the entrance pupil and is shown relative to the line of sight in Fig. 14.8 (1,6). It also passes through the center of curvature of the corneal surface. Therefore clinically it can be located as the surgeon centers the corneal light reflex in the center of the patient's pupil; in doing so, it is important that the surgeon take great caution to sight monocularly from directly behind the light source. While the pupillary axis and the line of sight

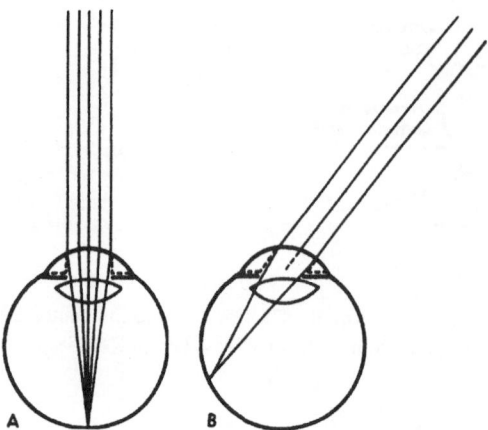

Figure 14.5 (A) Light rays pass through the optical zone, or the area of the cornea overlying the entrance pupil to reach the fovea. (B) Peripheral rays can pass through eccentric portions of the cornea to reach the entrance pupil to reach the parafovea. Thus peripheral irregularities in the cornea affect the quality of the peripheral image. (From Ref. 3.)

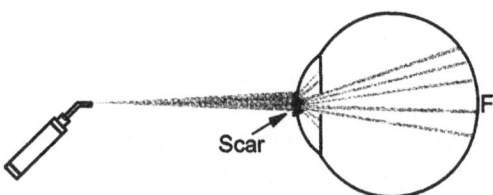

Figure 14.6 Light striking irregularities or scarring on the corneal surface is scattered, blurring the foveal image. (From Ref. 1.)

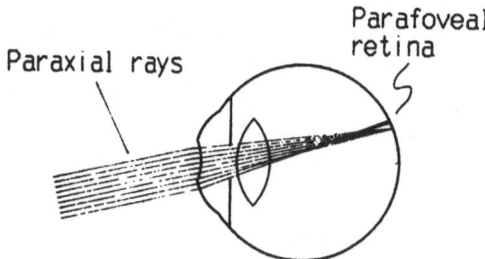

Figure 14.7 The LASIK ablated zone is shown in this figure. Even if the ablated zone is properly centered for foveal vision, peripheral rays from an object may miss the ablated zone leading to foveal blur or glare. (From Ref. 9.)

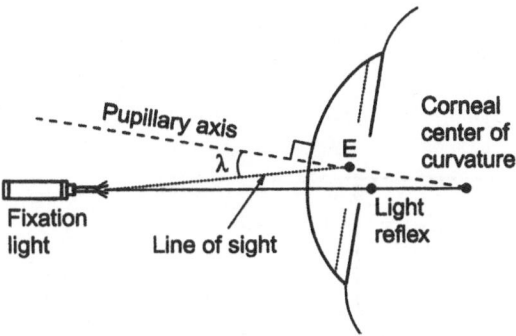

Figure 14.8 Both the pupillary axis and the line of sight pass through the center of the entrance pupil. The angle between these two axes is the angle lambda. (From Ref. 1.)

both pass through the center of the entrance pupil, it is important to distinguish between the two. The angle between them is the angle lambda and has been clinically measured to be around 3 to 6 degrees as shown in Fig. 14.8 (11). Another angle that is frequently described, but is impossible to measure in the eye, is the angle kappa, which is the angle between the pupillary axis and the theoretical visual axis (11).

As shown in Fig. 14.9 (Uozato and Guyton), if the surgeon sights monocularly directly behind the fixation light, the patient's corneal light reflex will appear to be decentered nasally in the pupil; the projection of the corneal light reflex onto the corneal surface will correspondingly be located nasal to the point where the line of sight and the cornea intersect. In other words, the corneal light reflex will be located nasal to the optimal centration point for corneal surgical procedures. If the corneal light reflex is used to guide centration, there will be error in marking the center. The center of the entrance pupil should be used to guide centration; this will ensure that the point where the line of sight and the cornea intersect—the optimal point for proper centration—will be appropriately identified.

G. CONTROVERSY OVER CENTRATION TECHNIQUES: CENTERING BASED ON THE CORNEAL LIGHT REFLEX

The corneal light reflex has been described alternatively as the basis of centration techniques. When a light source is reflected by the anterior surface of the cornea, a virtual image is created behind the cornea. This virtual image of the light source is the corneal light reflex, also know as the first Purkinje–Sanson image. The exact position of this image changes depending on the location of the point source of light and the direction of gaze of the eye. When the light source is located at infinity, the corneal light reflex will be located halfway back to the center of curvature, exactly at the focal point of the anterior corneal surface; for example, when the corneal radius of curvature is 7.80 mm, the corneal light reflex is located 3.90 mm behind the cornea surface (6). Using Gulstrand's model of the eye, the position of the corneal light reflex is calculated to be about 0.85 mm behind the plane of the entrance pupil (6). As the light source is moved closer to the eye in clinical practice, the corneal light reflex moves closer to the cornea. Also, as the surgeon behind the light source observes, the corneal light reflex can be seen to move from side to side as the patient's direction of gaze shifts.

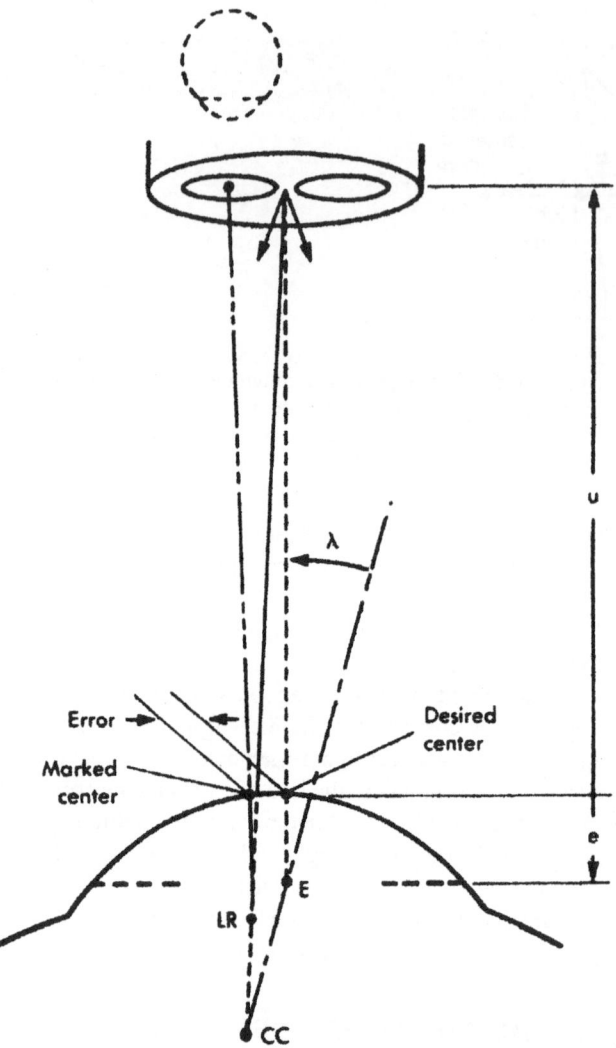

Figure 14.9 The point where the line of sight and the cornea intersect is the optimal centration point for corneal surgical procedures. If the surgeon sights monocularly directly behind the fixation light, the center of curvature and corneal light reflex appear nasally decentered in the pupil. If the corneal light reflex is used to guide centration, there will be error in marking the center. The center of the entrance pupil should be used to guide centration; this will ensure that the point where the line of sight and cornea intersect is appropriately marked. (From Ref. 6.)

In 1993, Pande and Hillman disputed the existing theories that the center of the entrance pupil should be the optimal point of centration (18). These authors used a modified autokeratometer to photograph the cornea in 50 subjects to mark the following four geometric points: (1) the geometric corneal center, (2) the entrance pupil center, (3) the corneal light reflex, and (4) the visual axis. Their results showed the relative positions of the entrance pupil, the corneal light reflex, and the geometric corneal center from the corneal intercept of the visual axis. Based on these measurements, Pande and Hillman concluded: (1)

that the ideal physiologic centration point is the corneal intercept of the visual axis and (2) given the practical difficulty of marking this point, the coaxially sighted corneal light reflex was the closest to the corneal intercept of the visual axis (18). In other words, these authors reported that the corneal light reflex should be used for centration of corneal surgical procedures in place of the entrance pupil.

Numerous authors have since disputed the findings of Pande and Hillman. First, it has been pointed out by Mandell that their method, which was based on their definitions of the visual axis, did not actually even use the true visual axis (19). In their discussion, Pande and Hillman correctly defined the visual axis as a line joining the fovea to the point of fixation. However, in their actual methods, they marked the point on the cornea joining the keratometer target to the corneal center of curvature—this is by definition the line that passes through the corneal light reflex (19). Uozato and Guyton discounted this technique themselves and reported that the corneal light reflex should not be used due to error arising from the angle lambda (6). Guyton also disputed Pande and Hillman's methods noting that the authors ignored the path of light rays as they travel through the eye, thus treating the human eye as if it were a perfectly aligned optical system from the autokeratometer straight to the fovea (20). Furthermore, he pointed out that their work was based on a theoretical assumption that the visual axis is the best centration point while failing to substantiate this assumption.

H. THE PREVAILING METHOD FOR CENTRATION: USING THE ENTRANCE PUPIL

Ellis and Hunter reviewed the papers of numerous authors who agreed with Uozato and Guyton's recommendation that refractive surgical procedures should be centered on the entrance pupil of the eye (1). Maloney reported that corneal refractive procedures should be centered on the pupil while the patient is fixating coaxially with the surgeon (9). He noted that small or decentered optical zones could decrease the quality of visual outcomes by negatively affecting visual acuity, reducing contrast sensitivity scores, and creating glare.

Mandell discussed the alignment error in videokeratoscopy between the optic axis of the instrument and the central reference axis of the eye (12). He reported that the videokeratoscope ought to be aligned with the patient's line of sight, which again is defined by the line connecting the fixation point with the center of the entrance pupil. Mandell emphasized that the line of sight is the most relevant axis leading from the fixation point through the eye's optics to the fovea; he pointed out how redirecting the videokeratoscope so that is it aligned with the line of sight could be accomplished by centering the system using the patient's entrance pupil as viewed through the instrument (12).

Klyce and Smolek likewise used topographical analysis to evaluate the center of the excimer laser ablations relative to the center of the pupil (15). In the past, the success of keratorefractive surgery was evaluated primarily be refraction comparing the attempted change to the induced change. Additional measurements are necessary to evaluate the induced changes in the corneal curvature. Therefore Klyce and Smolek's work was significant in reporting the use of corneal surface topography to determine the success of keratorefractive surgeries.

Similarly, Cavanaugh et al. evaluated PRK centration in 49 patients using the Eye-Sys topography system to measure the location of the treatment zone relative to the pupillary center and the corneal vertex (13). Performing their treatments using the technique of centration based on the entrance pupil, these authors showed that centration of PRK relative to the pupillary center (0.40 mm) was more accurate than to the corneal vertex (0.44 mm) (13). Their study also used topographical methods to measure centration of corneal procedures accurately from the pupil. They strongly supported the notion that corneal surgical procedures should be centered on the line of sight that passes through the center of the entrance pupil as both the patient and the surgeon are fixating coaxially.

Roberts and Koester, in their studies on the effect of the optical zone diameter on glare production, also agreed that the optical zone should be centered on the line of sight as it passes through the entrance pupil (16). They noted that if the optical zone were centered on the corneal light reflex instead, the optical zone would be off center with respect to the pupil, and that an optical zone of a particular diameter would lessen the glare-free field in all directions as shown in their study.

Ellis and Hunter reviewed the findings of the aforementioned authors regarding the proper use of the entrance pupil for centration techniques in refractive corneal procedures (1). As further evidence, Ellis and Hunter raise four interesting scenarios including (1) a reduced schematic eye with a coaxial cornea, pupil, lens, fovea, and fixation point, (2) an eye with an eccentric pupil, (3) an eye with aligned optical elements, but with variations in corneal curvature and clarity, and (4) a model eye with centered optical elements and a centered pupil, but with an eccentric fovea. The authors' discussions on each of these four scenarios leads to the same conclusion, that the visual axis is of no use in evaluating the rays of light as they are acted upon within the eye. Therefore they emphasize that even if the human eye were in perfect alignment, there would be no actual use in determining the intercept of the visual axis on the cornea. In their review on the subject, they are in agreement with all of the authors who support the prevailing method: the center of the entrance pupil is the best and most accurate centration point for corneal refractive surgical procedures (1,6,9,12,13,15,16).

I. THE IMPORTANCE OF ACCURATE CENTRATION

Improper centration can lead to undesired side effects. For example, one key concern in photorefractive surgery is the side effect of glare. This can be induced by beams of light entering the pupil through the cornea beyond the edge of ablation. As the pupil size increases with dilation, more of these rays will enter the eye to reach the retina. This leads to degradation of the image both in the fovea and in the area surrounding the fovea. This glare can be produced when light is incident on an irregular interface that reflects, scatters, or refracts light toward the fovea or parafovea. Thus the optical zone should ideally be free of scarring or irregularities. Even a seemingly insignificant error in centration can cause the edge of the ablation treatment zone to overlap into the critical optical zone.

In his review on the optical zone location in photorefractive keratectomy, Maloney calculated that, if a 4 mm optical zone is decentered by 0.5 mm, 16% of the light rays that fall on the retina will have missed the optical zone (9). With even further subtle decentration distances, that percentage increases so that with a decentration of 1, 2, and 4 mm, 31%, 61%, and 100% of the light rays reaching the retina will have missed the optical zone (9).

The light rays that are refracted within the optical zone are the only ones that will reach the fovea, so the corneal power of this region bears a special significance. Decentration translates to unpredictable corneal curvatures within the optical zone affecting refractive outcomes. For example, in the myopic eye, decentration of the myopic optical zone causes the unablated zone of a higher refractive power over the entrance pupil. The light rays that pass through the cornea peripheral to the ablated zone will be refracted more strongly than those taking the path through the zone that has been ablated. In this case, one might expect that the patient would experience monocular diplopia with a second blurred image. Similarly, in a patient with hyperopia, decentration of the optical zone could also lead to blurriness and undesired refractive outcomes.

How big should the optical zone be? Roberts and Koester report that the optical zone must be larger than the entrance pupil in order to avoid the side effect of glare (16). Based on their studies using an optical analysis computer program to define the edge of the optical zone, these authors further reported that the minimum optical zone diameter increases with increasing pupil size, anterior chamber field depth, and the desired glare-free visual field angle (16). In order to create a good parafoveal image, the ablated zone should be larger than the entrance pupil. If the optical zone and the entrance pupil are exactly equivalent, a portion of the light rays that focus on the parafoveal retina will miss the optical zone. Areas of the retina that receive the light rays that miss the optical zone may have decreased image clarity or poor contrast sensitivity. On the other hand, with a greater diameter of the ablated zone, a larger portion of the parafoveal retina obtains a good image.

J. RECOMMENDED CENTRATION TECHNIQUE

The technique used by the surgeon for corneal refractive procedures is of critical importance. Based on the aforementioned understanding of ocular optics and the clinical data, we recommend the following technique for centration.

First, the patient's nonoperative eye should be occluded. The patient should then be asked to use the operative eye to fixate on a lighted target that is coaxial with the surgeon's eye. It has been noted by Fay and coauthors that miosis can displace the entrance pupil in a superonasal direction as the pupil constricts (35). If the principal ray of the miotic pupil is used as a guide, this can be misleading, as it may lead to a decentered ablation zone when the pupil assumes its normal diameter in ambient light. For this reason, it is important that the pupil be in its most natural state, not under the influence of any medications that affect pupillary constriction.

What degree of illumination should be used during the centration of the entrance pupil? Klyce and Smolek described a technique whereby the center of the entrance pupil is determined at three different levels of illumination provided by the fixation light (15). The ablation is then centered according to the average of the three measurements. Ellis and Hunter suggest that if these three marks do not coincide, the mark should be placed at a pupil diameter of 3 to 4 mm (1).

The patient's nonoperative eye should be occluded. As the patient fixates on the target and the surgeon sights monocularly through the microscope tube containing the fixation spot, the surgeon should then center the procedure on the spot on the cornea overlying the center of the entrance pupil. The corneal light reflex should be ignored. By using this method, many of the problems related to improper centration—glare, poor contrast sensitivity, monocular diplopia, ghost images, unpredictable refractive outcomes—can be minimized, thereby achieving the desired visual outcomes.

K. CORNEAL TOPOGRAPHY: AXIAL AND TANGENTIAL TOPOGRAPHY

In the field of photorefractive surgery, corneal topography has emerged as an invaluable tool for refractive surgeons. Clinically, topographic analysis allows description of the topographic surface of the normal human cornea as well as numerous irregularities such as irregular astigmatism, keratoconus, and contact-lens-induced changes (21–23). Postoperative complaints may include glare, reduced night vision, monocular diplopia, and halos (27). A patient with postoperative complaints following refractive surgery can have topographic testing to detect for decentration, corneal irregularities, islands, and optical zone characteristics. In addition, topographic techniques allow the comparison of preoperative corneal contour with postoperative results, which can be used to show whether the intended postoperative change in refractive power was accomplished (13,24,25). Furthermore, topographical analysis has gained an important role in determining the location of the treatment zone and whether the ablation zone was properly centered (13,14,17,25,26).

Two methods of topographically analyzing the corneal surface have been described, axial and tangential (31,44,45). In both cases, a Placido disk, a series of concentric rings, is reflected off of the front surface of the cornea, and the resultant image is analyzed by a computer program designed to reconstruct the corneal contour (28). Numerous studies on PRK have used axial topography to analyze the corneal changes postoperatively (13,15,17,24, 29,30). The axial power at a given point in the cornea represents the average of instantaneous powers to that specific point (31). Axial analysis has been shown to underestimate refractive power in the periphery of the ablated cornea and to overestimate the power of the normal cornea (32). Tangential topography provides the instantaneous radius of curvature information; this is especially useful in identifying focal characteristics of the corneal curvature. In this way, tangential or instantaneous topography is more precise than methods of axial measurement.

L. SOME DEFINITIONS: DECENTRATION, SHIFT, AND DRIFT

1. Decentration and Measuring Axial Decentration

As discussed in depth in the earlier segments of this chapter, proper centration is important in photorefractive surgical procedures. Decentered treatments have been associated with poor visual acuity and undesired visual effects such as halos and glare (30). Using topographical techniques, a number of different types of decentration have been described. The term *decentration* has been commonly used to refer to a treatment in which the resulting flattest part of the cornea does not lie over the pupillary center (14). In other words, the zone of maximum ablation postoperatively, as determined by topographical methods, does not coincide precisely with the center of the entrance pupil, regardless of the actual intraoperative events leading to this situation.

Lin et al. described the method for measuring centration using axial topographic maps (17). Azar and Yeh used this technique to measure what they referred to as axial decentration (33). One can determine the distance between the center of ablation and its displacement from the pupillary center using the pupillary center as the origin. The maximum edges of the ablation in the x-axis and y-axis are marked, and the center of ablation is estimated to be the intersecting site of the four positions. The axial decentration, or the distance from the center of the ablation to the pupillary center, based on the axial maps, can therefore be quantified in this way.

Distinguishing another set of terms from the term decentration, Azar and Yeh first defined the difference between treatment displacement and intraoperative drift using the method of topographical analysis of myopic patients after PRK (33).

2. Treatment Displacement and Measuring Tangential Displacement

Azar and Yeh described shift or treatment displacement as a misalignment between the location of the intended treatment and the actual resulting treatment (33). Treatment displacement occurs if there is an error in the initial aiming of the laser or in patient fixation resulting in the final treatment zone being different from the intended treatment zone. Treatment displacement, or shift, is therefore a consequence of misalignment from the beginning of treatment. In their study, they defined treatment displacement as the distance from the ablation center to the center of the pupil.

These authors devised a mathematical way to calculate the treatment displacement. Using the properties of a geometric circle, it is possible to determine the center of the ablation using the pupillary center as a reference of origin. The locations of the ablation edges are identified using the map, and the temporal (T), nasal (N), superior (S), and inferior (I) intercepts are recorded. The distance from the origin, the pupillary center, to each of these four positions is measured. When only three points are identifiable, one can use the formula $X_1 \times X_2 = Y_1 \times Y_2$. The center of ablation can be determined using this data and then marked on the map. The distance from the center of the ablation to the pupillary center, using tangential topography, or the tangential displacement (r), is calculated using the formula (33,38) $r = [(T - N)^2 + (S - I)^2]^{1/2}$

In addition, one can compare it to the intended treatment radius; the radius (R) of the treatment zone of each map can also be estimated using the formula $R = \frac{1}{4} \{[(T - N)^2 + (S + I)^2]^{1/2} + [(T + N)^2 + (S - I)^2]^{1/2}\}$

3. Drift and Measuring the Drift Index

Drift, as described by Azar and Yeh, is gradual movement during treatment that can occur either passively or through correctional means (33). Passive drift occurs either as the result of unintentional eye movement or movement of the laser. Correctional drift occurs during intentional movement when either the patient or the surgeon attempts to correct a situation of misalignment. They defined drift as the zone of greatest flattening relative to the ablation center. When drift occurs, the result is an irregular ablation area with the flatter treatment zone shifted peripherally, leaving the central area of the ablation zone with a higher corneal surface power difference. Since the area of greatest flattening is moved away from the center of the ablation zone, this creates an uneven and unpredictable corneal surface overlying the pupillary axis. Since laser drift, such as with the subtle involuntary movements of the eyeball, can occur irrespective of the initial centration, displacement and drift should be considered independent. A treatment that is perfectly centered initially can be affected by drift when movement, by either the patient or the surgeon, occurs during the course of the treatment. Conversely, an ablation may be displaced or decentered and yet be characterized by minimal drift, thus maintaining uniformity of the corneal surface.

The work by Azar and Yeh was significant in defining a quantitative method to analyze drift. In their study, they established the drift index by establishing three important variables, P, H, and L. P represents the rate of change of curvature within the central 4 mm^2, which may correspond to the degree of drift across the central pupillary axis. The greater the change in power (in diopters), the greater the drift index will be across the central cornea. H corresponds to the drift distance, the measured distance between the inner transition of the flattest to the second flattest zone to the center of ablation. The greater H is, the farther the drift of the laser ablation. L is measured by the arc length in radians of the area of greatest ablation. In other words, L is approximately proportional to the area of greatest flattening, so the greater L value means the lesser drift from the pupillary axis. Therefore L is noted to be inversely proportional to the amount of drift during the laser ablation treatment. Given these three variables, there can be a relationship between them and the drift index, as

$$\text{Drift index} \quad \frac{PH}{L}$$

M. DECENTRATION AND CLINICAL OUTCOMES

Various studies have disagreed as to the relative importance of decentration on clinical outcome in terms of best corrected visual acuity (BCVA) and undesired visual side effects. Factors that may have contributed to this disagreement include different measuring techniques, differing degrees of decentration, and various levels of intended correction. This controversy may have come into being due to the initial use of axial topography in the early studies, which theoretically cannot offer the same degree of precision as tangential mapping of the edge of the ablation zone.

Several authors have reported no correlation between centration and best corrected visual acuity (15,17,34). Klyce and Smolek evaluated decentration from the center of the pupil and found that the amount of decentration did not correlate with best corrected visual acuity (15). Lin et al. did studies using corneal topography to calculate the SRI, a measure of irregular astigmatism, and found that it did not correlate with decentration (17).

On the other hand, a handful of other authors reported a decrease in visual acuity associated with decentration (13,24,35–37). Cavanaugh et al. performed a retrospective study of PRK and concluded that decentration of greater than 1 mm may be associated with decreased best corrected visual acuities; however, they measured decentration from the corneal vertex, not the entrance pupil (13). Cantera et al. also performed studies evaluating PRK centration using videokeratography (36). These authors reported a correlation between the amount of decentration and best corrected visual acuity, with postoperative astigmatism greatest in the group with the highest decentration. Cantera and coauthors also noted that the greater the diopteric correction attempted, the greater the ablation decentration.

Amano and coauthors and Uozato and Guyton have suggested that for photorefractive keratectomy, only decentrations of 0.5 mm or more are expected to influence postoperative visual function (6,26). However, Mulhern and coauthors suggest that decentrations of 1.0 mm or slightly more may be tolerated, with only slight or no subjective visual disturbance (50). According to these results, decentration less that 0.5 are optimal, those between 0.5 and 1.0 mm are acceptable, and those greater than 1.0 mm are considered severe and to be avoided if possible.

N. DRIFT EFFECT AS A BETTER PREDICTOR OF VISUAL ACUITY OUTCOMES

Azar and Yeh addressed the question of the difference between using axial and tangential topography, and their results suggested that axial topography may be insufficient to analyze clinically important intraoperative events (33). In their study, axial decentration did not correlate with visual acuity outcomes. The patients with the worst mean best corrected visual acuity had the lowest axial decentration, and those with the highest axial decentration had the best mean best corrected visual acuity. They noted that tangential topography is useful in distinguishing between treatment displacement (shift) and drift effect, which seemed better to predict visual acuity outcomes. Figure 14.10 shows a comparison between axial and tangential topography of the same eye.

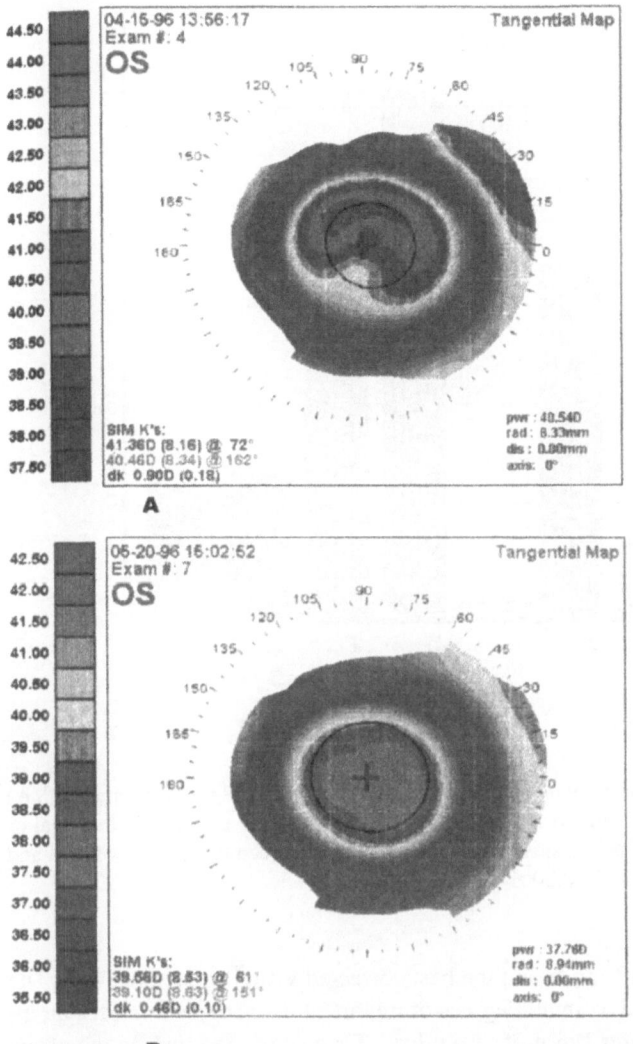

Figure 14.10 Corresponding axial (A) topography (B) of the same eye one month after an attempted myopic correction of −4.25 diopters. The tangential topographic (B) analysis shows a well-demarcated ablation edge with the center of the ablation minimally displaced inferotemporally. The black circle shows the pupillary margin and the black cross shows the center of the entrance pupil. (From Ref. 33.)

They noted that analysis of the zone of the greatest flattening relative to the ablation center may provide useful information on whether there was eye movement during the PRK treatment. These authors reported no significant correlation between the laser treatment displacement and the best corrected visual acuity as shown in Fig. 14.11.

In their study, treatment drift was better correlated with best corrected visual acuity than with axial or tangential treatment displacement, also shown in Fig. 14.11. Therefore, it may be very useful to make the distinction between laser treatment displacement and drift in corneal surgery decentration analysis. They did report a statistically signifi-

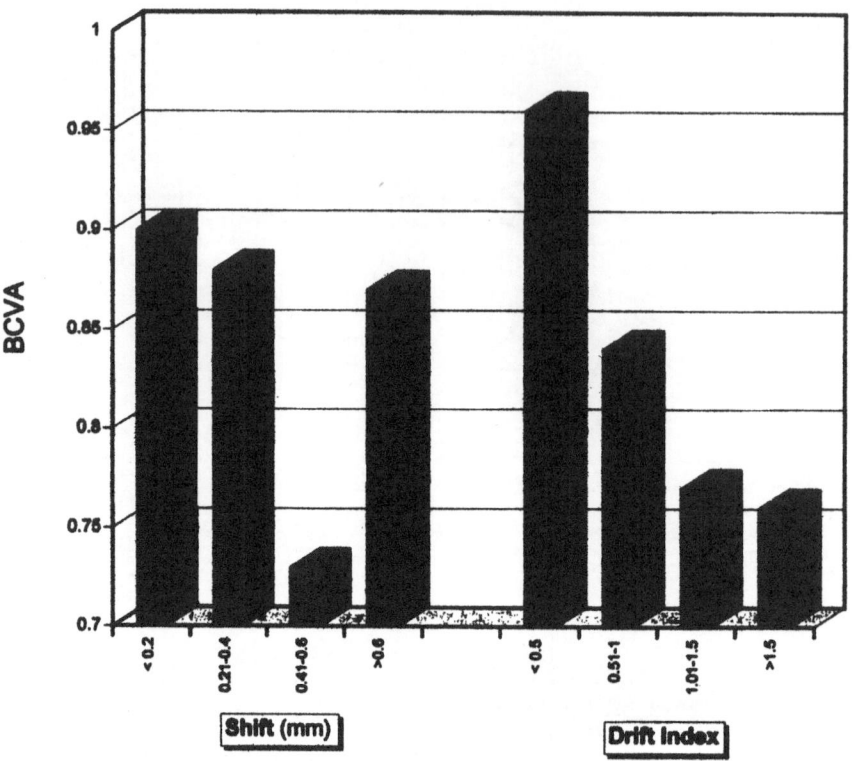

Figure 14.11   The bar graph shows the relationship between best corrected visual acuity (BCVA) and shift and drift index. No significant correlation was found between the BCVA and the axial or tangential decentration/shift. There is a positive inverse correlation between the amount of drift and best corrected visual acuity ($r-0.58$, $P<0.0001$). (From Ref. 33.)

cant correlation between the drift index and the best corrected visual acuity (BCVA). The authors suggested that compared to small degrees of treatment displacement (shift), an intraoperative drift may be a greater cause of visual loss. They suggested that, in the group of patients with no treatment displacement (nearly perfect centration of treatment), the nonuniformity overlying the pupillary axis that results secondary to drift may be responsible for loss of best corrected visual acuity. Figure 14.12 compares laser drift in two patients with similar degrees of treatment displacement using tangential topography.

They separated patients into categories based on the degree of displacement and drift, separating patients into four groups: low drift, low shift; low drift, high shift; high shift, low drift; and high shift, high drift, as shown in Fig. 14.13. Their results showed that the patients with low displacement and low drift had the best mean best corrected logMAR visual acuity. They found that the high shift, high drift group of patients, who had low decentration via axial topographical techniques, had the worst logMAR best corrected visual acuity. Interestingly, the group with high displacement and low drift had a better visual outcome than the patients with low displacement and high drift. Their results demonstrate that drift may be of greater importance as a determinant of visual acuity after corneal surgical procedures than treatment displacement. This is consistent with the concept of using a tracker during LASIK surgery which minimizes drift and improves visual outcomes.

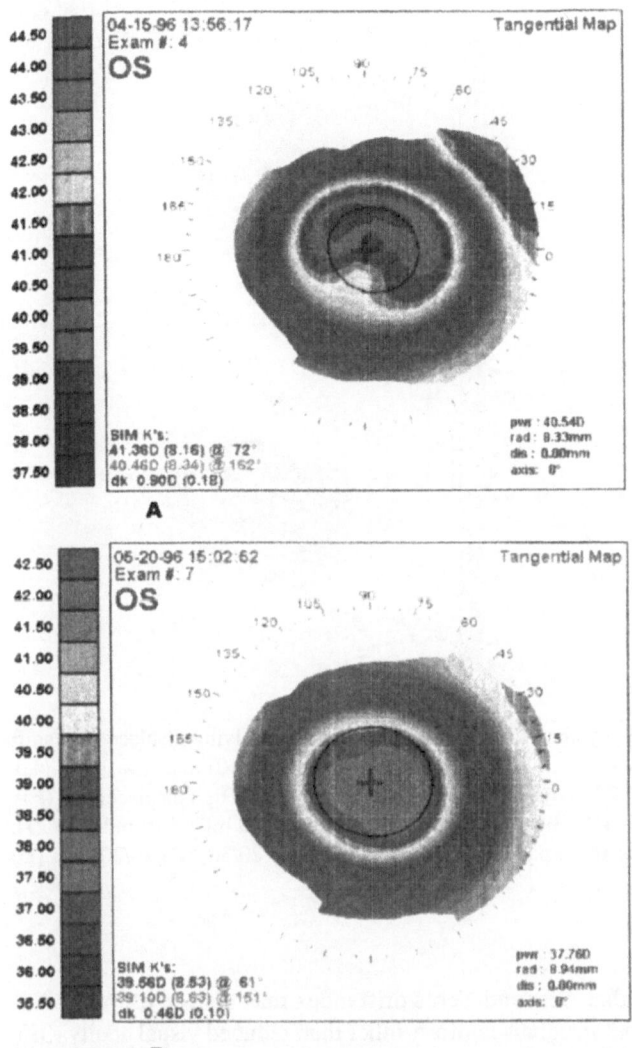

Figure 14.12 This figure compares laser drift in two patients with similar degrees of treatment displacement (decentration) using tangential topography. The pupillary contour (black circle) and the pupillary center (black cross) are displayed. Both maps show a similar degree of displacement with a shift in the inferotemporal temporal direction ($r = 0.31$ in both maps). (A) The left map shows that the area of greatest ablation (blue) was shifted upward, resulting in a nonuniform central ablation power. The drift index in this patient was calculated to be 0.98. The best corrected visual acuity 1 month after PRK was 20/40. (B) Compared with the panel on the left, the figure on the right shows how the central power is more homogenous, without gross drift effect (drift index = 0.03). The visual acuity was 20/20 postoperatively. (From Ref. 33.) [Color in original]

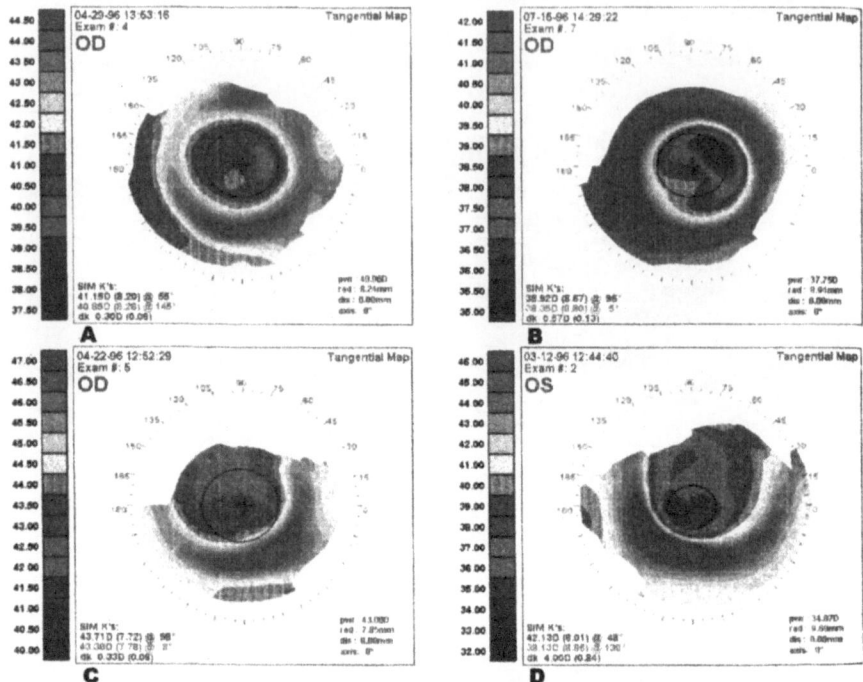

Figure 14.13 Tangential topography shows four possible scenarios involving displacement/shift and drift from the study by Azar and Yeh. (A) Low displacement ($r = 0.10$) and low drift index (0.23). (B) Low displacement ($r = 0.20$ mm) and high drift index (1.30). (C) High displacement ($r = 0.67$ mm) and low drift index (0.00). (D) High displacement (0.95 mm) and high drift index (3.27). The postoperative visual acuities for these patients were (A) 20/15, (B) 20/30, (C) 20/20, and (D) 20/40. (From Ref. 33.)

Sakarya et al. commented that Azar and Yeh's drift index may also be useful in illuminating why some patients report visual discomforts other than reduced visual acuity (39). They mentioned that the drift index may provide additional evidence about the causes of visual discomfort in patients who have satisfactory tangential topography.

O. THE ACCURACY OF CORNEAL TOPOGRAPHY IN PREDICTING PATIENT COMPLAINTS

Kampmeier et al. provide useful information about the correlation between corneal topography and patient satisfaction (40). They evaluated the sensitivity, specificity, and accuracy of postoperative corneal topography used by surgeons to predict the potential complaints of patients after PRK. They evaluated relative scale differences of 0.5 diopters (D) vs. 1.0 D. In addition, they studied whether the surgeon experience level in evaluating topographical images was a factor in cases of topographic analysis following PRK. These authors' results were that the topographies of the patients with complaints (sensitivity) compared to those without (specificity) were correctly distinguished in 53.2% overall, and in 44% and 63.5%, respectively. Experienced examiners were not significantly more accurate, and images of the 1.0 D scales were significantly more correct than those of 0.5 D scales. They stated, therefore, that subjective analysis of postoperative corneal topography by itself is not sufficient to predict potential patient complaints after PRK, and that the topographical findings should be interpreted within the context of the whole clinical picture.

P. FUTURE DIRECTIONS

As Uozato and Guyton emphasized, consistent centration of the corneal surgical procedures relative to the entrance pupil is critical for the success of refractive outcomes.

While various studies have disagreed as to the relative importance of decentration on clinical outcome in terms of best corrected visual acuity (BCVA) and undesired visual side effects, new topographical techniques and methods of assessing decentration are shedding light on this picture.

The method of using tangential topographic maps postoperatively to assess the laser ablation profile is useful to evaluate the correlation between the intraoperative events and the final visual outcome. Furthermore, these methods are useful in assessing the edges of photorefractive keratectomy ablation and to distinguish treatment displacement from intraoperative drift.

Even a small amount of eye movement during the laser ablation treatment changes the uniformity of the intended ablation. A well centered ablation is still subject to drift during the laser treatment. It has been shown as described in this section that laser drift may be a more important determinant of postoperative visual acuity after photorefractive keratectomy than treatment displacement. Furthermore, the issue has been raised whether laser drift may affect outcomes in terms of visual quality beyond simply visual acuity.

The question then arises, When initial decentration occurs, are the conventional methods of recentering treatment, either by patient refixation or by the surgeon's correctional efforts of recentration, the best approach? Or can this result increase the drift, thereby increasing the risk of irregular astigmatism and reduced visual acuity? Further study of these questions and further development of the current techniques being used to evaluate these questions will, we hope, shed additional light on this topic of decentration. Until then, it seems that a slightly decentered treatment without a drift (using a tracker) may be the preferred approach.

Q. THE IMPORTANCE OF PATIENT FIXATION DURING REFRACTIVE SURGERY

During laser in situ keratomileusis (LASIK) or photorefractive keratectomy (PRK), eye movement can lead intraoperative drift as described in an earlier section. If the eye is not perfectly aligned with the excimer laser throughout the treatment, the regions of corneal tissue that are removed with each pulse will also not be perfectly aligned. This can result in an undesired ablation pattern in which the laser ablation regions are not properly lined up with the visual axis.

There are numerous causes of unintentional eye movement. For example, haziness of the desiccated corneal surface can hinder the patient's attempt to maintain a steady fixed stare on the lighted target (47). Secondly, as described by Amano et al., there can be a tendency of the eye for downward decentration, which may be a result of the reflex upward movement of the eye, demonstrated by Bell's phenomenon, resulting from the topical anesthesia (26). Or, the eye may be characterized by subtle movements that correlate with heart pulsations (48). And of course, the patient may voluntarily move the eye.

R. PATIENT SELF-FIXATION

Two different techniques have been utilized to keep the globe immobile during photorefractive surgical procedures. In one method, the patient fixes on a target in order to maintain eye position. In other words, there is no mechanical restraint of the eye. The patient should fixate on a light or target that is coaxial with the surgeon's sighting eye. One way to do this is to place a fixation spot exactly in the center of one of the viewing cylinders of the microscope.

Many surgeons currently use the method of patient unassisted fixation, but this method has numerous shortcomings (47). There is the assumption of patient cooperation. Also, patients may be distracted or disturbed by the sounds of the laser pulsations. Patients may be prepared preoperatively with patient education such as videos and by trial ablations on methylcellulose to allow them to hear what the laser treatment will sound like prior to the actual procedure. However, even the most cooperative and prepared patients are not free from the physiological difficulties inherent in patient self-fixation. It is difficult for the patient to remain steadily fixed on the target when the ablated surface of the cornea becomes dry during the laser treatment. Also, the saccadic eye movements of the patient cannot be eliminated. Furthermore, Bell's phenomenon can cause some patients to have upward eye movement with attempted lid closure, which may result in wetting of the superior part of the cornea within the ablation zone. Sher et al. explained how this event can lead to uneven ablations, because of the laser's altered ablation rate on the hydrated cornea compared to the dehydrated cornea (47). Furthermore, as the techniques to correct astigmatism and higher myopia develop and the total laser time increases, patient self-fixation becomes increasingly challenging.

Schwartz-Goldstein and Hersh discussed a number of ways in which the surgeon can encourage patient fixation during the photoablation treatment (29). For example, proper and comfortable positioning of the patient in the patient surgical chair should be ensured prior to starting the procedure. The patient should be encouraged throughout the whole surgical procedure to keep looking at the lighted target to maintain proper fixation. Gentle support of the patient's head may also help to maintain maximum centration.

S. SURGEON ASSISTED FIXATION OF THE GLOBE

Alternatively, the globe can be immobilized by the surgeon using mechanical devices with a suction ring around the limbus. This technique uses a suction ring or a Thorton ring that is held by the surgeon to maintain corneal centration during the laser treatment (17,46). These handheld instruments used to stabilize the eye also have a number of drawbacks (47). They can cause pain, augment patient anxiety, and lead to subconjunctival hemorrhage. They can affect intraocular pressure and have been noted to contribute to torsion of the globe. Since these forceps or suction ring instruments are handheld devices, they may be applied to the eye at various angles with uneven forces, possibly leading to distortion of the corneal surface.

T. STUDIES ADDRESSING PATIENT FIXATION VS. MECHANICAL
IMMOBILIZATION

Terrell et al. studied the question of which method results in better centration of the ablation zone over the entrance pupil, unassisted patient fixation during photorefractive keratectomy (unassisted by the surgeon) or mechanical immobilization by the surgeon using a cornealschleral limbus mounted ring (42). Using a retrospective study, they showed a significant difference in the accuracy of centration of the ablated zone between the two groups, depending upon the method used for globe fixation. The group of unassisted patient fixation showed more accurate centration of the ablation zone than did surgeon fixation. Based on their results, they recommended unassisted patient fixation, even for very experienced surgeons, to stabilize the globe.

In contrast, Lin et al. reported a decentration of 0.36 ± 0.25 mm by fixation with the surgeon's control—better than the results of fixation by the patient in Terrell's study (17). Their last 20 eyes had an even lower decentration of 0.20 mm. Terrell's group raised the notion that the difference in the results of the two research groups may be explained by a difference in the experience of the surgeons (42).

Work by Mulhern et al. also contradicted the results of Terrell's group (50). These authors studied ablation decentration with LASIK and PRK. Their procedures were performed using the aid of a suction ring on an Aesculap Meditec device. They noted improved centration with the use of this device in centration in LASIK patients. This may be explained by the differences between LASIK and PRK. The conclusions of Terrell et al. may have limited application in the context of LASIK vs. PRK.

U. EYE TRACKING SYSTEMS: EARLY DEVELOPMENTS

Eye tracking devices are important developments to address the issue of eye fixation during refractive surgery. The newer excimer lasers are equipped with active eye tracking systems that are designed to keep the laser beam correctly aimed on the cornea. With these systems, the excimer laser beam follows the eye's movements to help prevent decentration.

Gobbi et al. developed an eye tracking system that is based on the pupillary margin (51). They used an eye tracker characterized by its design as a device to be added on to a commercial laser system. They reported that the device did not interfere with the laser pathway or the operator's observation. Using this device, they reported that they were able to track the pupil with an accuracy of better than 0.1 mm in a 6×6 mm^2 tracking field with a response time of less than 100 ms. Using this device, they noted that eye motions in the horizontal direction tended to be greater than those in the vertical direction. They proposed that such a system might be an effective way to compensate for patient eye movements during photorefractive procedures.

Schwiegerling and Snyder reported the development of a new video tracking technique that can follow a specific point though the course of surgery (52). By marking the coordinates of the pupil center from the onset, the pupillary center can be followed throughout the surgery. In addition, the system that they described follows a landmark feature, such as a scleral rim, blood vessels, or ink marks. The pupillary center and landmark are tracked through the course of the procedure relative to the laser axis of the VISX Star S2 System. Their results showed the mean centration of the 5 eyes in the study to be approximately 0.25 mm of the laser axis with a standard deviation of 0.10 mm. They suggested that this new video tracking technique may be useful in assessing quantitatively intraoperative motion and centration.

A recent study by Tsai and Lin evaluated the ablation centration following active eye tracker assisted photorefractive keratectomy and laser in situ keratomileusis (53). They reported that centration was better in the patient's second eye, which they attributed to the effect of learning, suggesting that patient-related factors are significant. They mentioned that patients were more cooperative during the second eye surgery because they were familiar with the sound and smell and knew when to focus on the lighted target. Furthermore, their study showed more decentration in eyes with high myopia. The authors attributed this to the notion that patients with higher myopia have a more difficult time fixating on the light of the excimer laser. In contrast, in their evaluation of surgeon-related factors, they found no significant difference between the surgeon's first 50 LASIK procedures and their last 50 procedures. The authors concluded that the use of an eye tracker in which the laser beam follows the patient's eye movements is helpful to prevent decentration. However, their work showed that an eye tracking system alone is not sufficient to ensure proper centration and that patient fixation and cooperation are also important.

Recent work by Coorpender et al. evaluated the topographic characteristics of photorefractive keratectomy for low myopia using a small beam (0.9 mm) excimer laser with tracking capabilities (54). Theoretically, when depending on patient self fixation, the longer time required for a scanning laser could increase the risk of decentration due to eye movements. The tracking system used by these authors was used in part to overcome this increased risk. They reported comparable results with similar studies using wide-beam lasers and differential power maps measuring centration (26,29,50). They noted that the similarity in the degree of decentration compared to the others suggests that the tracking system may have effectively eliminated any additional increased risk of decentration caused by the small beam scanning laser.

V. FDA APPROVED EYE TRACKERS

The LADAR, or laser radar device, was the first and only FDA approved active eye tracker in commercial distribution in the United States. Recent data by Alcon-Summit Autonomous shed additional light on the topic of eye movement and high speed eye tracking systems. A study of eye movements during ablation on 554 eyes created average displacements from the starting location of 0.04 to 1.16 mm, with a mean of 0.35 mm ± 0.19 mm (56). LADAR is an active eye tracking system that actively transmits an infrared signal to the eye and analyzes the re-emitted wavefront to track the target, thus compensating for eye motion during surgery. It was reported that 150 mm/s of eye movement can be tracked to a precision of ± 30 microns. Furthermore, the tracker was able to compensate for eye movement leading to refractive outcomes that were independent of the degree of eye motion. Specifically, those patients who had large eye movements during surgery had no significant difference in visual acuity from those with lesser eye movements during surgery. In addition, the study on tracking effectiveness included computer simulations of what would have happened had the treatment been conducted without the tracking system; the results indicated that significant height errors between the actual treatment shape and the desired shape of ± 20 microns would have resulted, suggesting that the clinical outcomes of 20/20 UCVA can be attributed to the tracking system, which is now available on most laser platforms.

Looking ahead, further refinement is most likely to occur in terms of the technological advances of laser delivery systems and their eye tracking mechanisms. It is clear that improvements in the tracking systems such that they can effectively eliminate or reduce alignment errors will improve the accuracy and efficacy of corneal surgical procedures such as PRK and LASIK. While it has been suggested that active eye tracking leads to overall good centration and may reduce decentration, larger controlled studies will be needed to address the role of active eye tracking in significantly reducing decentration and assuring proper centration in corneal surgical procedures.

W. DIRECTIONAL DISPLACEMENT: COMPARATIVE DATA FROM NUMEROUS DECENTRATION STUDIES

Several authors have analyzed the meridian displacement associated with decentration, as shown in Table 1. Cavanaugh et al. have reported a mean superior deviation (13). In contrast, an inferior displacement has been reported by Mulhern et al. (50) and Amano et al. (26). Terrell et al. noted a mean superior deviation in the patient fixation group and a mean inferior displacement in those patients whose eyes were stabilized using a suction ring (42). Schwartz-Goldstein and Hersh reported an inferonasal displacement in both eyes (29). Table 1 shows how the meridional decentration has varied significantly among the results of the different groups. This may be because the meridional direction of mean decentration has no real significance. Alternatively, differences in surgical technique and the methods of analysis may produce significant variations.

X. FLAP CENTRATION

We have discussed the topic of centration/decentration of the treatment zone in LASIK and PRK. With the LASIK procedure, the creation of a flap with a microkeratome creates an additional issue to be addressed, namely, that of centration/decentration of the flap itself. Numerous studies have addressed many of the complications involved in the creation of a corneal flap in LASIK including flap wrinkles, corneal flap melting, corneal haze, epithelial ingrowth, endothelial cell loss, glare, and halos. However, the topic of flap decentration or flap displacement and its effect on refractive outcomes has not received as much attention.

Table 1 Optical Zone Decentration and Retinal Image Quality

Amount of decentration of the optical zone (mm)	Percentage of light rays falling on the retina that will miss the optical zone
0	0
0.5	16
1	31
2	61
3	86
4	100

Source: From Maloney, 1990.

Table 2 Mean Decentration Shown in Recent Studies

Study	Procedure	Total mean decentration	Meridional displacement
Cavanaugh et al. (13)	PRK	0.40 mm	OD Superotemporal OS Inferonasal Overall—
Lin (24)	PRK	0.34 mm	—
Amano et al. (26)	PRK	0.51 mm	Inferior
Schwartz-Goldstein and Hersh (29)	PRK	0.46 mm	OD Inferonasal OS Inferonasal Overall Inferotemporal?
Terrell et al. (42)	PRK	0.41 (patient fixation) 0.63 (suction ring)	Superior Inferior
Pallikaris and Siganos (55)	PRK LASIK	0.81 (suction ring) 0.96 (suction ring)	— —
Mulhern et al. (50)	PRK LASIK	0.48 0.90	Inferior "To the left"
Tsai and Lin (53)	PRK	0.33	OD nasal/left OS—
	LASIK	0.35	OD nasa/left OS—

Normally, the surgeon performing LASIK will center the microkeratome on the corneal surface to create a centered flap. The proper position of the flap naturally depends upon the proper position of the treatment zone. As discussed in great detail earlier in this chapter, the center of the entrance pupil should be used for centering corneal surgical procedures. Light rays from a point on which a patient fixates will fall upon the entire surface of the eye—but only the rays bounded by the entrance pupil will actually enter the eye. The only portion of the cornea that is used to see the fixation point is that portion centered on the line of sight. It is the intersection of the line of sight with the cornea that marks the proper center for the optical zone of corneal surgery such as LASIK or PRK.

In the patient with a properly centered pupil, the center of the entrance pupil will be aligned with the center of the cornea. When performing LASIK on such a patient, the surgeon should accordingly center the microkeratome on the cornea to create a properly centered flap in alignment with the center of the entrance pupil. This technique will lead to a properly centered ablation zone, thereby minimizing the numerous side effects such as glare, halos, monocular diplopia, astigmatism, and unpredictable refractive outcomes that have been associated with improper centration of the ablation zone.

Y. FLAP DECENTRATION

Displacement of the corneal flap refers to the distance between the center of the corneal flap and the center of the pupil. Final decentration of the flap created in LASIK is influenced by two factors. First, the initial displacement of the positioning of the microkeratome can lead to a decentered flap. Second, there may be drift during suction that can contribute to un-predictable location of the microkeratome, thus altering the flap position during the proce-dure. In other words, there can be intentional flap displacement as desired by the corneal surgeon or there may be unintentional flap displacement resulting from mechanical mat-ters. These two factors will be discussed in turn.

Z. INTENTIONAL FLAP DISPLACEMENT

1. An Eccentric Pupil

Figure 14.14 distinguishes between a normal pupil and an eccentric pupil and shows how even in the case of pupil eccentricity the image will remain focused on the fovea. In the case of the eccentric pupil, the corneal light reflex is in the same position as in a normal eye. However, with an eccentric pupil, the patient's optical zone and the line of sight are dis-placed from the corneal light reflex. How does the eye with an eccentric pupil still create an image on the fovea?

  If the pupil in an optical system is decentered, the image will indeed still be focused on the fovea. The light rays from the object must still pass through the entrance pupil to reach the fovea. This bundle of rays must therefore still pass through and be refracted by the optical zone of the cornea. If the patient is asked to fixate on a lighted target while the surgeon observes monocularly from directly behind the target, the patient's optical zone of the cornea should be marked concentric with the pupil. Thus the patient's optical zone is decentered as well, although the patient's corneal light reflex is in the same position as in the case of a centered pupil.

  As seen in Fig. 14, in the case of an eccentric pupil, the visual axis and the line of sight are no longer in alignment. How can the appropriate image as perceived by the pho-toreceptors be formed? It has been shown that in a living eye, the photoreceptors can actu-ally reorient their axis toward the center of an eccentric pupil instead of the visual axis.

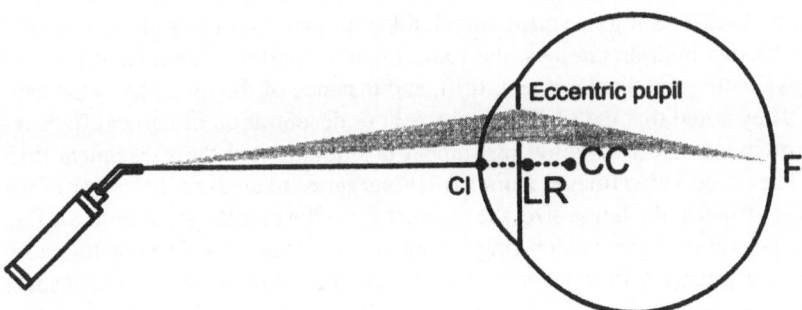

Figure 14.14 In the case of an eccentric pupil, the image is still focused on the fovea as in the nor-mal pupil. However, the corneal intercept of the visual axis is not involved in the refraction of light rays to the fovea. This is a good example of how the "visual axis" is useful theoretically, but practi-cally it has very limited applications to the human eye because it fails to take into account the actual path of light rays as they pass through the eye. (From Ref. 1.)

Therefore the image will remain on the fovea even if the pupil is decentered within the optical system.

2. Indication for Flap Decentration

Normally, the corneal surgeon performing LASIK creates a corneal flap centered on the eye. However, as described above, the patient with an eccentric pupil presents a unique situation. If the flap were centered on the cornea as usual with the ablation zone centered within the exposed corneal tissue following lifting of the flap, the ablation zone would be centered on the corneal light reflex, but not on the center of the entrance pupil. If the center of the treatment zone is not centered within the area under the lifted flap, then a number of complications may arise, including the incomplete delivery of laser energy to the intended zone of corneal stromal tissue or the unintentional laser ablation of the flap hinge itself. Ablation of the flap hinge could lead to areas of double treatment, unpredictable refractive outcomes, and irregular astigmatism. Any corneal irregularity or scarring overlying the entrance pupil can lead to glare and unpredictable refraction.

Therefore intentional decentration of the flap should be performed in the case of a patient with an eccentric pupil. Decentering the flap in such a patient, the corneal surgeon should center the flap according to the location of the desired treatment zone—so the flap should be centered on the entrance pupil. In other words, in all patients, regardless of the pupil location, the most important issue is that the treatment must be centered on the optical zone, the center of which should be the center of the entrance pupil.

AA. UNINTENTIONAL FLAP DISPLACEMENT

Alternatively, the flap may be unintentionally decentered or displaced due to initial ring mal-positioning or to the drift of the suction ring of the microkeratome. In this sense, drift here refers to the movement of the eye with respect to the suction ring during vacuum. One would expect that by minimizing the amount of intraoperative drift it would be possible to attain maximum control of the flap placement, thereby minimizing the final amount of displacement.

A recent study by Ufret-Vincenty et al. aimed to compare the displacement of corneal flaps created during LASIK using two different microkeratomes (57). The authors analyzed the flaps created by two microkeratomes, the Hansatome 8.5 and the Automated Corneal Shaper (ACS), evaluating the displacement, drift, and distance of the hinge from the center of the pupil. They noted that the final displacement or decentration of corneal flaps results from the combined effect of initial instrument positioning and the subsequent drift during suction. They used video images from LASIK surgeries to analyze the center of the pupil to flap hinge distance, the hinge size, the distance from the pupillary center to the flap margins, and the positions of the suction ring before and after vacuum. The coauthors reported that there was greater drift induced by the Hansatome, which seemed to contribute to the horizontal final decentration of the corneal flaps. Furthermore, this drift during suction was reported for the Hansatome microkeratome to be of a size and direction such that the pupillary center to hinge distances fell below the radius of the laser treatment. The authors concluded that identifying the drift and pupillary to hinge distances unique to each microkeratome is useful in terms of correcting for final unintentional flap decentration. It is unknown whether the drift and pupillary center to hinge distance can be correlated to visual refractive outcomes in LASIK.

REFERENCES

1. EJ Ellis, DG Hunter. Centering refractive corneal surgical procedures. In: DT Azar, ed. Refractive Surgery. Stamford, CT: Appleton & Lange, 1997, pp 125–134.
2. PS Binder. Optical problems following refractive surgery. Ophthalmology 1986;93:739–745.
3. WB Lancaster. Terminology in ocular motility and allied subjects. Am J Ophthalmol 1943;26: 122.
4. KS Ogle. Optics, 2nd ed. Springfield, IL: Charles C Thomas, 1968, p 149.
5. PM Walsh, DL Guyton. Comparison of the two methods of marking the visual axis on the cornea during radial keratotomy (Letter). Am J Ophthalmol 1984;97:660–661.
6. H Uozato, DL Guyton. Centering corneal surgical procedures. Am J Ophthalmol 1987;103: 264–275.
7. H Uozato, DL Guyton, GO Waring III. Centering corneal surgical procedures. In: GO Waring III, ed. Refractive Keratotomy for Myopia and Astigmatism. St Louis: Mosby–Year Book, 1992, pp 491–505.
8. AG Bennett, JL Francis. The eye as an optical system. In: H Davson, ed. The Eye. New York: Academic Press, 1962;4:101.
9. RK Maloney. Corneal topography and optical zone location in photorefractive keratectomy. Refract Corneal Surg 1990;6:363–371.
10. GA Fry. Geometrical Optics. Philadelphia: Chilton, 1969, p 110.
11. WB Lancaster. Terminology in ocular motility and allied subjects. Am J Ophthalmol 1993;100: 1230–1237.
12. RB Mandell. The enigma of corneal contour. CLAO J 1992;18:267–273.
13. TB Cavanaugh, DS Durrie, SM Riedel, JD Hunkeler, MP Lesher. Centration of excimer laser photorefractive keratectomy relative to the pupil. J Cataract Refract Surg 1993;19(suppl):144–148.
14. TB Cavanaugh, DS Durrie, SM Riedel, J Hunkeler, MP Lesher. Topographical analysis of the centration of excimer laser photorefractive keratectomy. J Cataract Refract Surg 1993;19 (suppl):136–143.
15. SD Klyce, MK Smolek. Corneal topography of excimer laser photorefractive keratectomy. J Cataract Refract Surg 1993;19(suppl):122–130.
16. CW Roberts, CJ Koester. Optical zone diameters for photorefractive corneal surgery. Invest Ophthalmol Vis Sci 1993;34:2275–2281.
17. DTC Lin, HF Sutton, M Berman. Corneal topography following excimer photorefractive keratectomy for myopia. J Cataract Refract Surg 1993;19(suppl):149–154.
18. M Pande, JS Hillman. Optical zone centration in keratorefractive surgery. Ophthalmology 1993;100:1230–1237.
19. RB Mandell. Optical zone centration for keratorefractive surgery (Letter). Ophthalmology 1994;101:216–217.
20. DL Guyton. More on optical zone centration (Letter). Ophthalmology 1994;101:793–794.
21. SE Wilson, DT Lin, SD Klyce. Corneal topography of keratoconus. Cornea 1991;10:2–8.
22. SA Dingeldein, SD Klyce. The topography of normal corneas. Arch Ophthalmol 1989;107: 512–518.
23. SE Wilson, DT Lin, SD Klyce, JJ Reidy, MS Insler. Topographic changes in contact lens induced corneal warpage. Ophthalmology 1990;97:734–744.
24. DTC Lin. Corneal topographic analysis after excimer photorefractive keratectomy. Ophthalmology 1994;101:1432–1439.
25. SE Wilson, SD Klyce, MB McDonald, JC Liu, HE Kaufman. Changes in corneal topography after excimer laser photorefractive keratectomy for myopia. Ophthalmology 1991;98:1338–1347.
26. S Amano, S Tanaka, K Shimizu. Topographical evaluation of centration of excimer laser myopic photorefractive keratectomy. J Cataract Refract Surgery 1994;20:616–619.

27. JJ Salz, E Maguen, AB Nesburn, C Warren, JI Macy, JD Hofbauer, T Papaioannou, M Berlin. A two-year experience with excimer laser photorefractive keratectomy for myopia. Ophthalmology 1993;100:873–882.

28. SD Klyce. Computer assisted corneal topography: high-resolution graphic presentation and analysis of keratoscopy. Invest Ophthalmol Vis Sci 1984;25:1426–1435.

29. BH Schwartz-Goldstein, PS Hersh, the Summit Photorefractive Keratectomy Topography Study Group. Corneal topography of PHASE III excimer laser photorefractive keratectomy. Ophthalmology 1995;102:951–962.

30. JF Doane, TB Cavanaugh, DS Durrie, KM Hassanein. Relation of visual symptoms to topographic ablation zone decentration after excimer laser photorefractive keratectomy. Ophthalmology 1995;102:42–47.

31. SA Klein, RB Mandell. Axial and instantaneous power conversion in corneal topography. Invest Ophthalmol Vis Sci 1995;36:2155–2159.

32. J Wang, DA Rice, SD Klyce. A new reconstruction algorithm for improvement of corneal topographical analysis. Refract Corneal Surg 1989;5:379–387.

33. DT Azar, PC Yeh. Corneal topographic evaluation of decentration in photorefractive keratectomy: treatment displacement vs intraoperative drift. Am J Ophthalmol 1997;124:312–320.

34. SD Klyce, MB McDonald. Computerized corneal topography of surface ablations with the Tomey (TMS-1). In: JJ Salz, PJ McDonnell, MB McDonald, eds. Corneal Laser Surgery. St. Louis: Mosby, 1995, pp 100–101.

35. AM Fay, SL Trokel, JA Myers. Pupil diameter and the principal ray. J Cataract Refract Surg 1992;18:348–351.

36. E Cantera, I Cantera, L Olivieri. Corneal topographic analysis of photorefractive keratectomy in 175 myopic eyes. Refract Corneal Surg 1993;9(suppl):19–22.

37. LJ Maguire, RW Zabel, P Parker, RL Lindstrom. Topography and raytracing analysis of patients with excellent visual acuity 3 months after excimer laser photorefractive keratectomy for myopia. Refract Corneal Surg 1991;7:122–128.

38. S Xunlun. Corneal topographic evaluation of decentration in photorefractive keratectomy: treatment displacement vs. intraoperative drift. Am J Ophthalmol 1999;128(2):259.

39. Y Sakarya, V Ozatep, SS Ermip. Drift index to explain patient complaints after PRK. J Cataract Refract Surg 2000;26:161.

40. J Kampmeier, DJ Tanzer, H Er, SC Schallhorn, L LaBree, PJ McDonnell. Significance of corneal topography in predicting patient complaints after photorefractive keratectomy. J Cataract Refract Surg 1999;25:492–499.

41. LJ Maguire, S Bechara. Epithelial distortions of the ablation zone margin after excimer laser photorefractive keratectomy for myopia. Am J Ophthalmol 1994;117:809–810.

42. J Terrell, SJ Bechara, A Nesburn, GO Waring III, J Macy, RK Maloney. The effect of globe fixation on ablation zone centration in photorefractive keratectomy. Am J Ophthalmol 1995;119:612–619.

43. T Seiler, W Reckmann, RK Maloney. Effective spherical aberration of the cornea as a quantitative descriptor in corneal topography. J Cataract Refract Surg 1993;19(suppl):155–165.

44. C Roberts. Characterization of the inherent error in a spherically biased corneal topography system in mapping radially aspheric surface. J Cataract Refract Surg 1994;10:103–116.

45. C Roberts. The accuracy of "power" maps to display curvature data in corneal topography systems. Invest Ophthalmol Vis Sci 1994;35:3525–3532.

46. MB McDonald, JM Frantz, SD Klyce, RW Beuerman, R Varnell, CR Munnerlyn, TN Clapham, B Salmeron, HE Kaufman. Central photorefractive keratectomy for myopia: the blind eye study. Arch Ophthalmol 1990;108:799–808.

47. NA Sher, T Burba, A Bergin. The eye fixation speculum: a new instrument to immobilize the eye during refractive surgery. In: JM Jeffery, ed. Excimer Laser Refractive Surgery. Thorofare, NJ: SLACK, 1996, pp 108–109.

48. HD Hoskins, M Kass. Becker-Shaffer's Diagnosis and Therapy of the Glaucomas. 7th ed. St. Louis, MO: CV Mosby, 1989, p 71.

49. PS Hersh, BH Schwartz-Goldstein. Corneal topography of phase III excimer laser photorefractive keratectomy. Ophthalmology 1995;102:963–978.

50. MG Mulhern, A Foley-Nolan, M O'Keefe, PI Condon. Topographical analysis of ablation centration after excimer laser photorefractive keratectomy and laser in situ keratomileusis for high myopia. J Cataract Refract Surg 1997;23:488–494.

51. PG Gobbi, F Carones, R Brancato, M Carena, A Fortini, F Scagliotti, A Morico, E Venturi. Automatic eye tracker for excimer laser photorefractive keratectomy. J Refract Surg 1995;11 (suppl):S337–S342.

52. J Schwiegerling, RW Snyder. Eye movement during laser in situ keratomileusis. J Cataract Refract Surg 2000;26:345–351.

53. YY Tsai, JM Lin. Ablation centration after active eye-tracker-assisted photorefractive keratectomy and laser in situ keratomileusis. J Cataract Refract Surg 2000;26(1):28–34.

54. SJ Coorpender, SD Klyce, MB McDonald, MW Doubrava, CK Kim, AL Tan, S Srivannaboon. Corneal topography of small-beam tracking excimer laser photorefractive keratectomy. J Cataract Refract Surg 1999;25:675–683.

55. IG Pallikaris, DS Siganos. Excimer laser in situ keratomileusis and photorefractive keratectomy for correction of high myopia. J Refract Corneal Surg 1994;10:498–510.

56. B Haffey, A Sacharoff. Data presented at CREST 2000. The importance of high speed high quality eye tracking in laser refractive surgery.

57. R Ufret-Vincenty, RJ Chen, DT Azar. Flap displacement in LASIK: comparison of the Hansatome and ACS Microkeratomes, Am J Ophthalmology. In Press.

58. MP Keating, ed. Geometric, Physical, and Visual Optics. Stoneham: Butterworth, 1998, p 272.

59. DT Azar, L Strauss. Principles of applied clinical optics. In: Albert and Jacobiec, eds. Principles and Practice of Ophthalmology. Philadelphia: W.B. Saunders, 2000, p 5337.

15

Surgical Caveats for Managing Difficult Intraoperative Situations

SAMIR G. FARAH

Massachusetts Eye and Ear Infirmary, Boston, Massachusetts, U.S.A.

DIMITRI T. AZAR

Massachusetts Eye and Ear Infirmary, Schepens Eye Research Institute, and Harvard Medical School, Boston, Massachusetts, U.S.A

The majority of LASIK complications occur intraoperatively. Preoperative complications are related to inadequate preparation for surgery (Table 1). Postoperative complications are almost always related to events that occurred during surgery. Many complications unique to LASIK are microkeratome related. With improvement in microkeratome technology, the incidence of LASIK complications has been substantially reduced and may decrease further as instrumentation becomes more sophisticated (1). In a study by Stulting et al. (2), the incidence of intraoperative complications decreased from 2.1% during the first 3 months to 0.7% during the last 9 months of the study, proving that the complication rates can be reduced as the surgical team gains experience. Most intra- and postoperative complications are common to myopic and hyperopic LASIK. Several complications may be prevented if slit lamp examination is performed in the immediate postoperative period.

A. DIFFICULT MICROKERATOME-RELATED SITUATIONS

Difficult situations are primarily encountered during the steep learning curve of microkeratome use. Experience with the Hansatome, Moria, and automated sliding microkeratomes suggests that their use will minimize the occurrence of difficulties during surgery and substantially reduce the incidence of serious LASIK complications.

Table 1   Preoperative Difficulties

Etiology

Anesthesia: (1) Patient unable to cooperate or fixate, (2) risks associated with the anesthesia itself. *Para/peribulbar:* (1) Retrobulbar hemorrhage, (2) globe perforation, (3) mydriasis, (4) conjunctival chemosis, (5) subconjunctival hemorrhage. *Topical anesthesia:* (1) Epithelial toxicity, edema, fragility, (2) epithelial defects and sloughing, (3) drape. *Epithelial trauma:* (1) Inadequate lid/lash covering and retraction, (2) speculum. *Fluids/secretion in the fornix:* (1) Malfunction of the vacuum pump, (2) contamination of the field.

Corneal marking

Pen (gentian violet): (1) Epithelial toxicity, (2) contamination of the interface with dye debris, (3) epithelial irregularity during the cut.

Metallic marker: (1) Epithelial defects, (2) inadequate marking.

Management

(1) Topical anesthesia preferred, (2) reduced dose topical anesthesia, (3) retrobulbar anesthesia must be performed correctly, (4) use the adhesive drape positioned carefully with a moist cornea, (5) carefully control/speculum positioning, (6) irrigate the fornices prior to applying the suction ring, then dry the fornices, (7) and check integrity and smoothness of the marker/use only a small amount of gentian violet sufficient but not excessive impressions. In the event of problems (conjunctival chemosis, etc.), delay for a few hours or postpone the operation.

1.   Incomplete or Irregular Cut (Tables 2 and 3)

These may be created by poor gear advancement (1) or the nonuniform cutting speed of the microkeratome. It is also caused by inadequate suction or loss of suction during passage of the microkeratome head (3). Several papers (4–8) reported incomplete or irregular flaps with rates reaching up to 4%. Steep non-rigid corneas predispose to these complications.

Table 2   Incomplete Flap

Etiology

(1) Incorrect setting of the stop device, (2) power failure, (3) power loss or motor breakdown/malfunction, (4) accidental blocking or stopping of the foot pedal, (5) microkeratome blockage due to obstacles along the pass: from the speculum—the drap—cell debris—salt granules from dehydrated saline solutions—eyelashes—eyelid margins—incorrect assembly of the microkeratome—poor cleaning of the microkeratome, (6) partial or total detachment of the suction ring/loss of suction.

Results

(1) Unable to proceed with the ablation; (2) the ablation may be performed but with greater difficulty and decreased ablation size.

Avoidance and Intraoperative Management

(1) Total surgeon- and assistant-comfort with the type of microkeratome used, (2) adequate globe exposure using lateral canthotomy if necessary, (3) perfect assembly—clean and check the microkeratome and suction ring prior to every procedure, (4) make sure the microkeratome is advancing and returning smoothly in the track prior to each procedure, (5) avoid excess fluid prior to using the microkeratome, (6) avoid salt-containing solution prior to the cut, (7) pay attention to all clues that may suggest loss of suction, (8) if the laser ablation is performed, protect the hinge with a sponge or metal protector, and (9) if the ablation is not possible, reposition the flap and postpone the laser ablation.

Table 3 Irregular Cut

Etiology
(1) Irregular speed of microkeratome pass (plow-up), (2) uneven blade edge, (3) microkeratome slips because of accidental movement by the surgeon, (4) block during the cut phase from speculum—eyelashes—drape—redundant conjunctiva, (5) loss of suction.

Result
(1) Irregular cut surface in terms of smoothness and regularity of the stromal surface.

Avoidance and Intraoperative Management
(1) Test the microkeratome pass prior to each procedure, (2) check the blade edge and replace it before each procedure, (3) wet the track, (4) make sure there are no obstacles in microkeratome advancement, (5) check that the correct depth plate has been inserted, (6) check that the orifice of the suction ring is open and free, (7) check that the conjunctiva is smooth and flat, (8) avoid excessive topical anesthesia that may cause detachment of the epithelium, (9) assume a relaxed, comfortable operating position, (10) make sure all cords, tubes, etc. are unrestricted and will not bend, (11) check the values of voltage and current (voltmeter and ammeter), (12) smoothen the cut stromal surface using the excimer laser (PTK), (13) abort the ablation, reposition the flap, and repeat the operation 3 to 6 months later, or perform a homoplastic operation at least 6 months later.

Occasionally the microkeratome head will stop before clearing the 6 mm diameter zone needed for unhindered application of the laser. Application of the laser treatment with such a flap will result in nasal flattening and irregular astigmatism, even if the hinge of the flap is protected from the laser beam.

2. Free Cap (Table 4)

This may be due to inadvertent omission of the stopper or to the use of a thin suction ring on a steep cornea (Moria microkeratomes). Several studies (7–13) reported the occurrence of a free cap ranging from 0.7 to 10%. In case a free cap is not visible on the surface of the

Table 4 Free Cap

Etiology
(1) Corneal anatomy: large flat cornea (generally less than 41 D but also depends on the type of microkeratome), (2) inadequate suction, (3) incorrect applanation of desired resection, (4) a ring that does not allow sufficient exposure of the globe, (5) low intraoperative IOP, (6) removal of the suction ring with the flap adhered to it, (7) incorrect positioning or setting of the stopper, (8) defective stop device.

Results
(1) Free cap, (2) more difficult to reposition, (3) easier to dislocate, (4) easier to completely loose, (5) the ablation can be performed.

Avoidance and Intraoperative Management
(1) Always mark correctly, (2) check the microkeratome prior to every operation, (3) check correct positioning and setting of the stop device, (4) advise patients with flat corneas of the increased risk, (5) ensure that the mark is retained or remark prior to removing it from the microkeratome head, (6) place the free cap in an antidesiccation chamber, (7) replace the cap, right side up, on the stromal bed, (8) correctly align the flap, (9) ensure adhesion between the flap and stroma (wait 3 to 8 minutes before removing the speculum), (10) place sutures if necessary, and (11) use a bandage contact lens if the epithelium has been altered.

Table 5   Thin or Perforated Buttonhole Flap

Etiology

(1) Inadequate suction, (2) corneal anatomy, (3) very flat corneas, (4) very steep corneas, (5) irregular surface curvature, (6) severe astigmatism, (7) torsion induced by the weight of the microkeratome, (8) poor blade quality.

Results

(1) Impossible to perform the ablation, (2) risk of epithelial growth, (3) risk of irregular astigmatism.

Avoidance and Intraoperative Management

(1) Do not begin the pass with less than perfect suction (IOP management), (2) caution patients with high or low keratometry readings of the increased risk, (3) check that the plate is inserted correctly, (4) consider using a thicker plate on steeper corneas, (5) check the microkeratome each time before using, (6) use a new blade for each patient, (7) gently support the handle of the microkeratome during the run, (8) carefully replace the thin or perforated flap, (9) carefully examine the flap and check adhesion, (10) continue the operation if it is possible to lift the flap, despite it being difficult, (11) recut the flap 2 to 3 months later with a thicker plate, (12) use contact lenses, and (3) totally remove the flap in severe cases.

cornea, the microkeratome head should be carefully inspected and if need be disassembled, since the cap is probably inside the instrument.

3. Perforated Lenticule or Button Hole (Table 5)

If the suction is broken during passage of the microkeratome, the blade will surface; an irregular cap with a cut through the central cornea may result.

If the intraocular pressure is too low during passage of the head, a thin or donut-shaped flap or cap is likely to be created; it will likely be small in diameter.

Nonuniform cutting speed (14) in case of a manually advanced microkeratome may also predispose to this complication. The rate may reach up to 4% (5,7,15).

4. Intraocular Penetration (6) (Table 6)

All LASIK surgeons should possess a good understanding of the mechanics, assembly, and calibration of the microkeratome being used.

This complication is almost always due to human error in placing the plate, controlling the depth of the cut, into instruments such as the Automated Corneal Shaper. The result is penetration of the cornea under high intraocular pressure and serious damage to the iris, lens, and other structures in the eye.

Table 6   Globe Perforation

Etiology

Simple perforation: (1) Cornea is thinner than usual in just one spot, (2) old corneal ulcer scar, (3) old corneal wound, (4) keratoconus, (5) previous refractive surgery. *Perforation with damage to the iris and crystalline lens with no vitreous loss*: (1) Incomplete insertion or absence of the plate. *Perforation that may also jeopardize the posterior segment, vitreous loss, expulsive hemorrhage*: (1) Incomplete insertion or absence of the plate.

Avoidance and Intraoperative Management

(1) Precise assembly of the microkeratome, (2) check the microkeratome prior to use, (3) obligatory preoperative examinations: slit lamp—corneal topography—pachymetry, (4) treatment varies from case to case on the basis of severity of the situation.

Table 7 Inadequate Globe Exposure

Etiology
(1) Orbit anatomy: sunken eyes, small eyes, (2) prominent brows, (3) narrow palpebral fissures, (4) tight eyelids, (5) squeezing, (6) previous surgery of the orbit or eyelids, (7) previous trauma of the orbit or eyelids, (8) poor drape application and retraction, (9) poor choice of speculum.
Results
(1) Difficult to position the suction ring, (2) difficult to achieve suction, (3) incomplete microkeratome pass, (4) interference from the speculum, (5) interference with the drape, (6) interference with eyelashes.
Avoidance and Intraoperative Management
(1) Accurate positioning of the drape to maximize exposure, (2) use an appropriate speculum, (3) have alternate speculums available, (4) position the patient's head with the chin up or down as needed to obtain better exposure, (5) have the assistant exert downward pressure on the speculum during the microkeratome pass, (6) lateral canthotomy if necessary, (7) retrobulbar injection if necessary, (8) perform the operation without the speculum.

5. Poor Coupling to the Eye (Table 7)

Microkeratome placement is more difficult in sunken globes and in eyes with narrow palpebral fissures and small corneas (5). The use of the newer generation microkeratomes with the down–up flap has overcome this obstacle. By turning the head of the patient slightly to the opposite side or by exerting a gentle pull and tilt on the eye through the suction ring handle, these cases can be operated easily. Other authors advise using a manual dissection (16) of the corneal flap or another refractive procedures.

6. Corneal Epithelial Defects (17,18) (Table 8)

This complication is usually caused by the microkeratome head passage over a dry corneal surface. It also happens in case of reoperation on a previously operated eye with PRK or when dissecting the interface while re-elevating the flap for a retreatment. In the case of a

Table 8 Epithelial Complications

Etiology
(1) Drying the flap surface, especially on the conjunctiva, (2) manipulation of the flap, (3) microkeratome pass, (4) excessive topical anesthesia preoperatively, (5) gentian violet markings, (6) a suction ring that has perilimbal support, (7) suction transmitted through the suction ring, (8) phototoxicity, (9) microtrauma from the forceps or instruments during the operation, (10) eye movement as the speculum is being removed, (11) blinking as the speculum is being removed, (12) damage is increased in superficial corneal dystrophies.
Results
(1) Discomfort for the patient, (2) epithelial ingrowth, (3) longer functional recovery, (4) loss of the gentian violet mark.
Avoidance and Intraoperative Management
(1) Avoid operating, or cautiously operate on patients with superficial corneal dystrophies, (2) avoid excessive flap drying, (3) reduce manipulation of the flap, (4) reduce preoperative anesthesia, (5) take care in applying and removing the speculum, (6) in the event of displacement, reposition the epithelium, (7) remove the epithelium if it cannot be replaced, (8) apply a bandage contact lens, and (9) use antibiotic cover.

microkeratome-related epithelial defects, inadequate irrigation and wetting of the cornea and microkeratome head may be the cause. This complication should not be overlooked while under the laser. Slit lamp examination in the immediate postoperative is necessary.

7. Wound Dehiscence

This complication may occur when a flap is being cut on a cornea-grafted eye. The high intraocular pressure exerted during the application of the suction ring is the cause. Several surgeons find LASIK a good treatment for the myopic and astigmatic refractive errors after a penetrating keratoplasty (PK). Yet the time of surgery is still debatable. The consensus is to delay the LASIK procedure as much as possible after a PK. The presence of a good wound scar and the documentation of refractive and topographic stability for at least 3 months after removal of all keratoplasty sutures are good signs to do the surgery (19). Surgeons should always warn their patients about this potential complication.

8. Pizza Slicing

This complication may occur when a flap is cut in an eye that had radial keratotomy (RK) with the incisions extending beyond the 8 to 9 mm central area. The inadequate healing of the RK incisions causes a part of the flap to separate in a triangular shape. An epithelial plug in the incision almost always precipitates this complication. Always check the RK incisions under the microscope before cutting the flap.

9. Corneal Bleeding (18) (Table 9)

This usually occurs when the microkeratome blade hits limbal vessels in case of a decentered flap or corneal pannus in contact lens wearers. Attention should be made to have a clear stromal bed before laser application. Gentle pressure on the oozing vessels or on their limbal feeders with a murocel is usually sufficient, followed by good irrigation of the stromal bed. Phenylephrine should be avoided for fear of irregular pupillary dilation and loss of centration landmarks, with subsequent decentration of the treatment.

Table 9   Intraoperative Corneal Bleeding

Etiology
(1) Corneal neovascularization, (2) very large flaps: very steep corneas—Very small corneas.
Results
(1) Ablation delayed until bleeding is stopped, (2) blood must be removed, (3) reduced visibility to the surgeon, (4) overhydration of the stroma, (5) blockage of the incident laser ray (asymmetric ablation), (6) erroneous flap ablation.
Avoidance and Intraoperative Management
Primary: (1) decentration of the suction ring and flap, (2) preoperative argon laser photoablation, (3) use a smaller diameter ring to have a smaller cut. *Secondary*: (1) Use a Chayet or Gimbel–Chayet sponge, (2) use suction pressure briefly, (3) use manual pressure on the ring, (4) use 2.5% phenylephrine on a merocel, (5) use pressurized air flow, (6) interrupt the ablation, (7) remove blood from the stromal bed, (8) eliminate any blood in the interface by irrigation under the repositioned flap, (9) leave the flap in position and wait for clotting; the operation can then be continued, (10) apply a dry sponge to the bleeding, exert slight pressure and continue with ablation.

Table 10 Decentered Cut

Etiology
(1) Surgeon error in centering the optical axis, (2) error in paracentral marking, (3) incorrect centration of the suction ring on the corneal surface, (4) globe torque when suction is engaged, (5) poor patient cooperation during surgery.
Results
(1) Inadequate exposure of the central stroma for a well centered complete ablation.
Avoidance and Intraoperative Management
(1) Check centration of the optic axis, (2) a nonmydriatic pupil to center the optical axis, (3) accurate marking, (4) center the suction ring correctly and stabilize the cornea as suction is engaged, (5) patient education and reassurance, (6) postpone the procedure instead of reattempting to reapply the suction ring, (7) perform the ablation if adequate bed is available, (8) replace the flap and repeat the operation after 3 or 4 months.

10. Others

Other difficulties include decentered cut, (Table 10), irregular thickness flaps (Table 11), and inadequate suction (Table 12).

B. PHOTOABLATION RELATED DIFFICULTIES

1. Decentration (Table 13)

Significant decentration is defined as ablation center displacement from the pupil center by 0.5 mm or more. Decentration may be precipitated by a decentered laser beam prior to ablation (shift) or to eye drift during ablation (drift); see Chapter 14.

Centration is worse in LASIK than in PRK (20,21), the magnitude of displacement being almost twice as high. Decentration in LASIK may be precipitated by the higher amount of correction attempted; the duration of the treatment is longer, so there is much more time for patient drift to occur. The poor unaided vision of the high myopes combined with the progressive decrease in visibility of the fixation target during ablation exacerbates the existing fixation difficulties (20).

Decentration can cause irregular postoperative astigmatism, glare, ghosting, halo effect, loss of best corrected visual acuity (BCVA), decreased contrast sensitivity, and monocular diplopia. Decentration may be more critical in hyperopic treatments than in myopic treatments.

Table 11 Flap With Irregular Thickness

Etiology
(1) Interference with the suction ring, (2) scleroconjunctival cysts and irregularities, (3) pterygium, (4) dents, damage, or debris on the suction ring tracks, (5) inadequate suction during the cut, (6) poor blade quality, (7) lateral displacement of the microkeratome during the cut.
Results
(1) Not a serious problem if excimer laser ablation is planned (as opposed to ALK).
Prevention
(1) Check and clean the suction ring tracks, (2) check the microkeratome, (3) change and inspect the blade after each procedure, and (4) examine the blade edge under high magnification.

Table 12 Inadequate Suction

Etiology

(1) Suction pump malfunction, (2) small diameter cornea with redundant conjunctiva, (3) conjunctival chemosis, (4) relaxed conjunctiva, (5) squeezing of lids, (6) excessive elasticity in severely
myopic eyes because of an excess in orbit fat, (7) iatrogenic reasons: the suction pedal is accidentally depressed, (8) intraoperative manipulations of the suction ring, drape, or speculum, (9) previous vitreoretinal surgery.

Results

(1) Thin or superficial flap, (2) buttonhole or interrupted flap, (3) irregular flap.

Avoidance and Intraoperative Management

(1) Preoperative patient sedation, (2) good globe exposure, (3) keep the suction ring firmly against
the globe until suction has been activated correctly, (4) practice using the pedals, (5) avoid manipulating the suction ring, drape, and speculum once good suction is achieved, (6) always measure
IOP, (7) always remeasure IOP if there has been manipulation, (8) treat any induced chemosis, (9)
conjunctival incision, (10) conjunctival squeezing (milk the chemosis into the fornix), (11) conjunctival peritomy, (12) wait 30 to 45 minutes, (13) postpone the operation.

The reported rates of decentration ranged from none to 16% (4,6,9,10,13,20,22–24).
Decentration was reported in several studies (4,20,22,25). Condon et al. (20) had eight eyes
(16%) with significant decentration.

Bas and Onnis (4) found three cases of decentration (<1.0 mm) in 97 eyes, while
Fiander and Tayfour (10) found five cases in 124 eyes. Pallikaris and Siganos (23) reported
that centration in their PRK and LASIK groups were comparable. They reported a mean deviation of 0.96 mm of the ablation center from the center of the pupil, which did not affect
the final visual outcome. In their second study (6), the mean deviation of the ablation center from the center of the pupil was 0.89 mm (0.11 to 1.84 mm); this was determined by
subtraction topography between the 1 month postoperative and preoperative topographies.
In Pérez-Santonja et al.'s series (9), 6.5% of eyes had a decentration of more than 0.75 mm.

2.   Central Islands (Table 14)

Central islands are diagnosed on corneal topography as central steep areas within the treatment zone and are defined by their width (≥2 mm) and diopteric height (≥3 keratometric
diopters). Central islands may be related to the size of the ablation zone. They may be

Table 13 Decentered Ablation

Etiology

(1) Poor fixation by the patient, (2) poor centration of the laser beam by the surgeon, (3) poor eye
stabilization if a ring is used, (4) eye tracker malfunction.

Results

(1) Irregular astigmatism, (2) mixed astigmatism, (3) problems with nighttime vision, (4) halos,
(5) ghost images, (6) glare, (7) reduced BCVA, (8) diploma.

Avoidance and Intraoperative Management

(1) Calm, accurate instruction on patient fixation, (2) use of a fixation ring if necessary, (3) proceed
with the ablation if possible, (4) reposition the flap and postpone the operation, (5) enhancement
in the event of undercorrection.

Table 14 Central Islands

Etiology
(1) Central vortex plume, (2) deterioration of laser optics, (3) differential hydration and lower central acoustic shock wave.
Results
(1) Blurred vision, (2) ghost images, (3) monocular diplopia.
Avoidance and Intraoperative Management
(1) Anticentral island pretreatment software, (2) plume suction, (3) scanning slit beam and flying spot lasers, (4) observe versus laser ablation.

caused by the presence of fluid on the stromal bed, the difference in ablation rate between the central and peripheral stroma due to the centripetal intrastromal water movement, the insufficient or inadequate removal of debris within the center of a large ablation zone, or the deterioration of the laser mirror system. The reported rate may be as high as 20% (7) depending on the timing of the postoperative topography. Central islands can cause irregular postoperative astigmatism, glare, ghosting and halo effect, loss of BCVA, and monocular diplopia.

When faced with the diagnosis of a central island, always rule out iatrogenic keratectasia of the posterior corneal surface, especially in high myopia correction.

C. WRINKLES (TABLE 15)

Two types of flap wrinkles are described. Those that occur intraoperatively are due to malpositioning of a thin flap (undetectable intraoperative misalignment of the corneal flap on the stromal bed). These wrinkles may not be detected with the operating laser microscope. Surgeons should inspect the flap at the slit lamp immediately after surgery to insure that flap wrinkles are not present.

The second type occurs in the early postoperative period and might be caused by eye rubbing or by eyelid pressure during blinking. This type is almost always accompanied by slight sliding or dislodgment of the flap. After instillation of fluorescein dye in the eye, an uneven pattern of pooling in the tear film may be detected. This fluorescein test may be useful in detecting minimal striae in the corneal flap (26) (Please refer to Figures 17.3 and 17.4).

Table 15 Flap Wrinkles

Etiology
(1) Incorrect positioning of the flap during ablation, (2) excessive desiccation of the flap, (3) rough manipulation of the flap.
Results
(1) Wrinkling of the flap will cause irregular astigmatism and visual aberrations.
Avoidance and Intraoperative Management
(1) During the ablation, gently place the flap in a cupped position on a damp sponge, (2) use a moistened merocel sponge to smoothen from the hinge and then from the center to the edges, (3) do not allow fluid to remain under the flap, (4) using a spatula or sponge, smoothen the flap with centrifugal motion, (5) gently replace the flap to its original position, (6) epithelial wrinkling often disappears spontaneously within a few days; if it has not disappeared within 5 to 6 days, raise the flap and reposition correctly.

Table 16   Debris in the Interface

Etiology

(1) Regurgitation of fluid in the fornix, (2) debris from sponge, drape, gauze, (3) debris from the microkeratome blade, (4) debris from the cannula, syringe, bottles, (5) powder/talc from surgical gloves, (6) dust particles in the operating room, (7) debris from blepharitis that was not treated preoperatively, (8) blood or epithelial cell residues.

Result

(1) May affect best corrected visual acuity and induce glare and inflammation.

Avoidance and Intraoperative Management

(1) Irrigate and dry the fornices preoperatively to remove any mucous/lipid debris, (2) avoid excess fluid in the surgical field, (3) carefully check the microkeratome prior to each operation, (4) carefully clean and dry all cannulas, (5) use disposable syringes, (6) use powder-free gloves, (7) use HEPA air filters, (8) treat blepharitis prior to surgery, (9) reduce movement of personnel in the operating room, (10) carefully examine the interface and flap prior to removing the drapes and speculum, (11) irrigate the edges to remove any peripheral debris, (12) raise the flap and reposition it following irrigation to remove significant debris seen at the slit lamp flap check.

D.   INTERFACE DEBRIS (5,15,20,22,27–29) (TABLE 16)

These may arise from conjunctival or skin epithelial cells swept onto the interface by excessive irrigation or excessive tearing. The debris can also be caused by the meibomian secretions, by the powder of the gloves or from the swabs used to clean the interface, by metal fragments from the microkeratome blade, by mucus from the ocular surface, or by blood from cut pannus. The use of the Chayet ring, the suction lid spectrum, and the merocel have tremendously decreased this complication. The debris may not be detected by the operating laser microscope. Surgeons should inspect the interface at the slit lamp immediately after surgery to insure that interface debris is not present.

E.   VASOVAGAL OR OCULOCARDIAC REFLEX

The sudden high intraocular pressure (IOP) exerted by the suction ring in LASIK can cause bradycardia (30,31). A study of 20 patients who underwent LASIK (30) reported that 20% had a heart rate drop of more than 10% at the time of suction. 20% had a heart rate increase more than 10% at the time of positioning under the laser, and 60% had no heart rate change during the procedure.

Table 17   Pain

Etiology

(1) Pressure from the speculum, (2) pressure from the suction ring, (3) poor apposition of the flap edge and bed, (4) epithelial defects, (5) dislocation of the flap, (6) loss of the flap.

Avoidance and Intraoperative Management

(1) Give accurate information to the patient, (2) avoid any movements that may cause alteration to the flap or the epithelium, (3) carefully reposition the flap, (4) check that the flap and epithelium are in place and intact, (5) reassure the patient, (6) use analgesics/sedation when appropriate, (7) use NSAID, (8) use bandage contact lenses when there is epithelial damage, (9) artificial tears/ointment lubrication.

Table 18 Flap Dislocation During Surgery

Etiology

(1) Sudden eye movement when an instrument is near the limbus, (2) eye movement during the striae test, (3) blinking or squeezing when the speculum and drapes are removed.

Results

(1) Dislocation or wrinkling of the flap.

Avoidance and Intraoperative Management

(1) Have the patient fixate at the light when the striae test is being done and warn the patient about pressure, (2) ask the patient to not blink and stare straight ahead when the drape and speculum are removed, and have the assistant retract the lids during these maneuvers, (3) immediately refloat and reposition the flap.

Table 19 Flap Edema

Etiology

(1) Prolonged manipulation of the flap, (2) excessive irrigation.

Results

(1) Retraction of the flap edge, (2) adhesion to the stromal bed is more difficult.

Avoidance and Intraoperative Management

(1) Minimally manipulate the flap, (2) minimally irrigate under the flap, (3) try gently to distend the flap with an almost dry sponge or blunt spatula, (4) suture if necessary.

Table 20 Flap Shrinkage

Etiology

(1) Excessive dryness of the flap (due to delays during surgery).

Results

(1) The flap must be stretched, (2) sutures may be required.

Avoidance and Intraoperative Management

(1) Avoid delay during surgery, (2) decrease time between flap reflection and ablation, (3) decrease time between ablation and flap repositioning, (4) gently stretch and distend the flap, (5) lift and rehydrate the flap a second time, (6) suture if necessary.

Table 21 Flap Stretching and Displacement of the Epithelium

Etiology

(1) Prolonged manipulation, (2) excessively aggressive smoothening and positioning.

Results

(1) Difficulty in positioning the flap and/or epithelium, (2) striae that affect vision.

Avoidance and Intraoperative Management

(1) Minimize manipulation of the flap, (2) delicately strike with a damp sponge when smoothing or positioning the flap, (3) gently reposition the epithelium, (4) eliminate redundant epithelium, (5) use a bandage contact lens if necessary (there is a risk of flap dislocation when the contact lens is removed).

Table 22 Irreversible Damage or Complete Destruction of the Flap

Etiology

(1) Faulty blade, (2) cut performed on an excessively dry cornea, (3) significant ablation of the flap undersurface, (4) lack of flap and/or hinge protection during the ablation.

Prevention

(1) Prior to performing the lamellar cut, ensure that the corneal surfaces are not excessively dry, (2) protect the flap and hinge during the ablation.

Treatment

(1) Homoplastic tissue may be needed, (2) proceed with the refractive ablation and apply a contact lens (PRK), (3) perform a PTK and then refractive ablation, (4) perform a second very thin lamellar cut, followed by PTK, and then refractive ablation, (5) abort the operation, use a bandage contact lens, allow re-epithelization, and then perform a transepithelial PTK.

LASIK surgeons should be aware of the possibility of the oculocardiac reflex in their patients. Patients should be asked during the preoperative evaluation about cardiac or cerebrovascular disease.

F. OTHERS

Other difficulties are pain (Table 17), flap dislocation during surgery (Table 18), flap edema (Table 19), flap shrinkage (Table 20), flap stretching (Table 21), and destruction of the flap (Table 22).

REFERENCES

1. V Filatov, JS Vidaurri-Leal, JH Talamo. Selected complications of radial keratotomy, photorefractive keratectomy, and laser in situ keratomileusis. Int Ophthalmol Clin 1997;37(1):123–148.
2. RD Stulting, JD Carr, KP Thompson, GO Waring III, WM Wiley, JG Walker. Complications of laser in situ keratomileusis for the correction of myopia. Ophthalmology 1999;106:13–20.
3. L Buratto, M Ferrari. Indications, techniques, results, limits and complications of laser in situ keratomileusis. Curr Opin Ophthalmol 1997;8(4):59–66.
4. AM Bas, R Onnis. Excimer laser in situ keratomileusis for myopia. J Refract Surg 1995; 11(suppl):S229–S233.
5. HV Gimbel, S Basti, GB Kaye, M Ferensowicz. Experience during the learning curve of laser in situ keratomileusis. J Cataract Refract Surg 1996;22:542–550.
6. IG Pallikaris, DS Siganos. Laser in situ keratomileusis to treat myopia: early experience. J Cataract Refract Surg 1997;23:39–49.
7. MC Knorz, A Liermann, V Seiberth, H Steiner, B Wiesinger. Laser in situ keratomileusis to correct myopia of −6.00 to −29.00 diopters. J Refract Surg 1996;12:575–584.
8. A Marinho, MC Pinto, R Pinto, F Vaz, MC Neves. LASIK For high myopia: one year experience. Ophthalmic Surg Lasers 1996;27(suppl):S517–S520.
9. JJ Pérez-Santonja, J Bellot, P Claramonte, MM Ismail, JL Alio. Laser in situ keratomileusis to correct high myopia. J Cataract Refract Surg 1997;23:372–385.
10. DC Fiander, F Tayfour. Excimer laser in situ keratomileusis in 124 myopic eyes. J Refract Surg 1995;11(suppl):S234–S238.
11. JL Guell, A Muller. Laser in situ keratomileusis (LASIK) for myopia from −7 to −18 diopters. J Refract Surg 1996;12:222–228.

12. T Salah, GO Waring III, A El-Maghraby, K Moadel, SB Grimm. Excimer laser in situ keratomileusis under a corneal flap for myopia of 2 to 20 diopters. Am J Ophthalmol 1996;121: 143–155.

13. CJ Argento, MJ Cosentino. Laser in situ keratomileusis for hyperopia. J Cataract Refract Surg 1998;24:1050–1058.

14. YH Kim, JS Choi, HJ Chun, CK Joo. Effect of resection velocity and suction ring on corneal flap formation in laser in situ keratomileusis. J Cataract Refract Surg 1999;25(11):1448–55.

15. SF Brint, DM Ostrick, C Fisher, SG Slade, RK Maloney, R Epstein, RD Stulting, KP Thompson. Six-months results of the Multicenter Phase I Study of Excimer Laser Myopic Keratomileusis. J Cataract Refract Surg 1994;20:610–615.

16. M Gomes. Laser in situ keratomileusis for myopia using manual dissection. J Refract Surg 1995;11(suppl):S239–S243.

17. R Zaldivar, JM Davidorf, S Oscherow. Laser in situ keratomileusis for myopia from −5.5 to −11.5 diopters with astigmatism. J Refract Surg 1998;14:19–25.

18. J Davidorf, R Zaldivar, S Oscherow. Results and complications of laser in situ keratomileusis by experienced surgeons. J Refract Surg 1998;14:114–122.

19. AS Forseto, CM Francesconi, RAM Nose, W Nose. Laser in situ keratomileusis to correct refractive errors after keratoplasty. J Cataract Refract Surg 1999;25:479–485.

20. PI Condon, M Mulhern, T Fulcher, A Foley-Nolan, M O'Keffe. Laser intrastromal keratomileusis for high myopia and myopic astigmatism. Br J Ophthalmol 1997;81:199–206.

21. MG Mulhern, A Foley-Nolan, M O'Keefe, PI Condon. Topographical analysis of ablation centration after excimer laser photorefractive keratectomy and laser in situ keratomileusis for high myopia. J Cataract Refract Surg 1997;23:488–494.

22. L Buratto, M Ferrari, C Genisi. Keratomileusis for myopia with the excimer laser (Buratto technique): short term results. Refract Corneal Surg 1993:9(suppl):S130–S133.

23. IG Pallikaris, DS Siganos. Excimer laser in situ keratomileusis and photorefractive keratectomy for correction of high myopia. J Refract Corneal Surg 1994;10:498–510.

24. MC Knorz, B Wiesinger, A Lierman, V Seiberth, H Liesenhoff. Laser in situ keratomileusis for moderate and high myopia and myopic astigmatism. Ophthalmology 1998;105:932–940.

25. FB Kremer, M Dufek. Excimer laser in situ keratomileusis. J Refract Surg 1995;11(suppl): S244–S247.

26. YS Rabinowitz, K Rasheed. Fluorescein test for the detection of striae in the corneal flap after laser in situ keratomileusis. Am J Ophthalmol 1999;127(6):717–718.

27. I Kremer, M Blumenthal. Myopic keratomileusis in situ combined with VISX 20/20 photorefractive keratectomy. J Cataract Refract Surg 1995;21:508–511.

28. LW Hirst, KW Vandeleur. Laser in situ keratomileusis interface deposits. J Refract Surg 1998;14:653–654.

29. HM Stein. Powder-free gloves for ophthalmic surgery. J Cataract Refract Surg 1997;23:714–717.

30. M Paciuc, G Mendieta, R Naranjo. Oculocardiac reflex during laser in situ keratomileusis. J Cataract Refract Surg 1998;24:1317–1319.

31. M Paciuc, G Mendieta, R Naranjo, E Angel, E Reyes. Oculocardiac reflex in sedated patients having laser in situ keratomileusis. J Cataract Refract Surg 1999;25(10):1341–1343.

Bilateral Simultaneous LASIK
Advantages, Disadvantages, and Surgical Caveats

**DAVID R. HARDTEN, ELIZABETH A. DAVIS,
and RICHARD L. LINDSTROM**

University of Minnesota and Minnesota Eye Consultants, Minneapolis, Minnesota, U.S.A.

WILLIAM J. LAHNERS

University of South Florida, Tampa, and Center for Sight, Sarasota, Florida, U.S.A.

A. INTRODUCTION

Refractive surgery has rapidly evolved over the last decade, with LASIK emerging as the procedure of choice for most degrees of myopia and hyperopia. One reason for this rapid acceptance is that patient satisfaction is very high, with excellent visual results. The safety has also proven to be quite high, especially in the hands of experienced surgeons. It is also extremely convenient for patients in that the visual recovery is very rapid, typically allowing a return to work within 24 hours. This has lead to the predominance of LASIK patients choosing to have both eyes operated on at the same surgical setting. In this situation one eye has surgery and the second eye follows a few minutes later. This should probably be termed bilateral sequential same-day surgery, but in keeping with common terminology we will refer to this as bilateral simultaneous surgery. In addition, we will refer to staged surgery where the eyes are operated on in separate sessions, whether they be separated by days or months, as bilateral sequential surgery. There is still, though, quite a bit of controversy concerning whether LASIK should be done in both eyes on the same day, or whether the second eye should be delayed until the first has healed.

B. ADVANTAGES OF BILATERAL SIMULTANEOUS LASIK

When should the second eye of a patient with bilateral ametropia be operated on with LASIK? Many surgeons have taken different viewpoints on this issue, yet most would agree that it is not wise to operate on the second eye until you are confident that the first eye will experience a satisfactory recovery. But how much of a delay is in the patient's best interest? Here we must apply the benefit/risk ratio. In early laser photorefractive keratectomy and LASIK studies in the United States, we waited 12 months between eyes. We occasionally noticed a late complication, such as regression, haze, epithelial erosion, epithelial ingrowth, or keratitis. The safest means never to have a bilateral complication is never to operate on the second eye. Yet we found patients wanted their second eye done, in spite of the possibility that a late complication may not have yet manifested in their first eye.

After almost 10 years of careful study and analysis, the delay between eyes has decreased from 12 months to 6 months, 3 months, 1 month, 1 week, 1 day, and now to 5 minutes in the majority of our patients. The benefit/risk ratio favors surgery 5 minutes apart for most patients because the benefits increase while the risks remain the same. To date, no study demonstrates an increased risk to bilateral same-day LASIK surgery performed a few minutes apart compared to performing the second-eye surgery a day to a year later. The patient convenience and functional benefits are clear, significant, and highly appreciated.

Because LASIK is nonpenetrating eye surgery, it avoids many of the potentially devastating complications of intraocular procedures. The classic teaching that bilateral intraocular surgery is rarely indicated is a good one, although no such teaching should be universally applied. There is no such classical ethic for extraocular procedures. How many ophthalmologists have performed strabismus surgery sequentially on both eyes at the same sitting (accepting the risk of endophthalmitis, retinal detachment, globe perforation, etc.)? How many ophthalmologists have performed bilateral oculoplastic procedures on both eyes at the same sitting (accepting the risk of bilateral blindness from intraorbital hemorrhage, preseptal cellulitis, exposure keratitis, and the like)?

From the patient's perspective, one of the most obvious advantages of bilateral simultaneous LASIK is the savings in time. Refractive surgery patients tend to be very active, and frequently have very demanding occupational and personal schedules. Having both eyes treated in the same session translates to less time away from work: one less day of surgery and fewer postoperative visits. In addition, both eyes recover in one day to functional vision, reducing the total recovery time from two (separate) days to one. Simultaneous bilateral surgery saves time and represents potentially less missed work for the person who must accompany the patient as well.

While convenience issues are important, there are functional issues that favor bilateral surgery. Many refractive surgery patients are requesting refractive surgery because they are no longer able to wear their contacts. This can be due to a variety of reasons including intolerance, hypoxic complications, giant papillary conjunctivitis, and others. Monocular treatment of a patient with more than a few diopters of ametropia will induce potentially intolerable anisometropia if spectacles must be worn postoperatively in only one eye. Even in patients who are not contact lens intolerant, this anisometropia can be a problem during the days before treatment of the second eye when contact lens wear must be stopped to reduce lens-induced warpage.

By treating both eyes in the same session we decrease the amount of time that patients spend in their cars traveling to and from the office. This savings in travel time has a potential, if difficult to measure, reduction in the risk of travel related injury. Every year in the United States over 40,000 people are killed in automobile crashes and 5 to 6 million are injured (United States Department Of Transportation, National Highway Transportation Safety Association, 1997 report). Obviously these risks are relatively small, but they are real and should not be omitted from consideration.

One of the reasons cited for performing sequential surgery has been the fear of excessive malpractice awards for cases of bilateral visual loss. However, it is not in the patient's best interest to withhold the benefits of bilateral LASIK, oculoplastics, or strabismus surgery, primarily because of the perceived medicolegal risk. This type of defensive medicine increases the patient's cost, probably reduces the patient's benefit, and has no meaningful impact on the patient's ultimate risk.

The experience of the surgeon is important in this discussion as well. Inexperienced LASIK surgeons are more likely to have complications, especially during creation of the flap. Novice LASIK surgeons should not perform bilateral same-day surgery until they are confident of a successful outcome in the first eye. Obviously, even experienced surgeons should postpone treatment of the second eye if there are any questions about the success of the first. If problems occur during creation of the flap, in most cases laser ablation should not be performed, and the flap should be reapproximated. In many cases, successful LASIK can safely be performed 3 to 6 months later by recutting a new flap (1–3).

C. DISADVANTAGES OF BILATERAL SIMULTANEOUS LASIK

One disadvantage of having both eyes done at the same sitting is that patients cannot be certain that they are satisfied with the quality of their vision, in terms of glare, halos, and night driving, before proceeding with the second eye. Several authors have reported LASIK or PRK patients who have chosen not to proceed with surgery on their second eye because of subjective visual complaints, preferring their contact lens in the unoperated eye (JJ Salz, MB McDonald, DD Koch, ON Serdarevic, RL Abbott. Bilateral LASIK should be performed on sequential days. Eye World, August 1998, pp 16–18). These subjective visual complaints, frequently involving night vision, can be difficult to predict preoperatively. The option to treat one eye only is eliminated if surgery is performed on both eyes on the same day.

There are several risks that may not be apparent at the completion of the operation, including infections, displaced or lost flaps, interface haze and inflammation, epithelial ingrowth, flap melt, irregular astigmatism, and retinal complications. Some of these may not be apparent for 3 to 4 weeks postoperatively. Because these complications can present weeks after surgery, performing simultaneous surgery risks bilateral occurrence. With sequential surgery one can identify these late complications and treat them before proceeding to the second eye, or in some cases, withhold surgery on the second eye altogether. This can allow the patient to retain functional vision in at least one eye, should an unusual complication occur.

Another disadvantage of bilateral surgery is that the risks of complications in both eyes of one patient may not be truly independent. The risk of epithelial defect, for example, is approximately 1–4%, but once we recognize a defect in one eye we know that the other eye is more likely to experience this complication. The occurrence of an epithelial defect in the first eye, depending on its severity, can be a reason to postpone the second eye. In this type of complication the problem can be recognized immediately. This is different in cases of infectious keratitis where again the risks are probably not independent (same lid flora, degree of blepharitis, hygiene, etc.), but the complication cannot be recognized immediately. This higher likelihood of certain complications occurring in the second eye of patients in whom they occur in the first eye may apply to other problems as well (e.g., epithelial ingrowth, macular hemorrhage, retinal detachment).

We have had two cases of presumed infectious keratitis (culture negative) in more than 25,000 lamellar refractive procedures. These responded quickly to topical antibiotics, with no loss of visual acuity. Both of these infections did not become apparent for 3 weeks following the procedure, suggesting that unless we waited one month between eyes, we still could have been dealing with a complication in both eyes at the same time. We have had intermittent cases of diffuse lamellar keratitis in the first postoperative week with most responding to frequent topical steroids or interface irrigation. With appropriate current management techniques of DLK, the risk of loss of best corrected vision from DLK is extremely low.

The principal risk of performing bilateral simultaneous LASIK is, therefore, only related to adverse events occurring in the first 2 to 4 weeks (or whatever interval is chosen for sequential surgery) after the surgery that cannot be anticipated by the surgeon at the time of surgery. This excludes intraoperative complications, which would prevent surgery on the second eye (or could only happen to the second eye if surgery was uneventful on the first), and later complications, which would occur after the intereye waiting period.

D. COMPARATIVE STUDIES

A prospective randomized study by Waring et al. looked at the results of simultaneous and sequential bilateral LASIK for the correction of myopia (1). They looked at 357 patients who desired surgical correction of myopia ranging from -2 to -22.50 diopters. The patients were randomized to simultaneous or sequential bilateral LASIK. They had 378 eyes that were enrolled in the simultaneous group and 331 eyes in the sequential group. With a mean follow-up of 10 months, they found no significant difference in the complication rate between the two groups ($P = 0.55$). They also found no significant difference in the loss of two or more lines of best spectacle-corrected visual acuity ($P = 0.87$). The number of patients were similar that had correction within ± 0.50 diopters between both of these groups. They did see a slightly higher, yet unexplained, frequency of epithelial ingrowth in a simultaneous group (2.9%) than in the sequential group (0.6%). While it might seem as though this could be from transfer of epithelial cells, it was not found to be more common in the second eye of the simultaneous cases. In summary, this study demonstrated no benefit in safety or efficacy in sequential versus same-day bilateral surgery, although its statistical power was limited due to sample size.

We also performed a randomized prospective clinical trial at our institution (PP Rath, DR Hardten, RL Lindstrom, B Witte. Bilateral sequential versus unilateral sequential laser in situ keratomileusis (LASIK) for the treatment of myopia. Submitted for publication). We randomized 508 patients into two groups: bilateral simultaneous surgery (5 minutes apart) and bilateral sequential surgery (1 month apart). The mean preoperative spherical equivalent was -5.96 ± 2.76 D, with a range of -1.00 to -15.63 D. There were 272 eyes in the bilateral group and 236 eyes in the sequential group, with both groups having 1 year follow-up. In the bilateral group, at last follow-up, 92% had UCVA of 20/40 or better, and 50% had UCVA of 20/20 or better. In the unilateral group 90% had UCVA of 20/40 or better, and 50% had UCVA of 20/20 or better. These results did not achieve a statistically sig-

Table 1 Results of Two Prospective Randomized Studies Comparing Bilateral Simultaneous Versus Sequential LASIK

	Waring et al.[1]			Rath et al.[2]	
	Simultaneous [% (no. of eyes)]	Sequential [% (no. of eyes)]	Statistical Significance [P (power %)]	Simultaneous [% (no. of eyes)]	Sequential [% (no. of eyes)]
UCVA >20/40	88.9 (305/343)	91.8 (281/306)	0.26 (10)	92 (250/272)	90 (212/236)
UCVA >20/20	44.6 (153/343)	36.6 (112/306)	0.05 (30)	50 (136/272)	50 (118/236)
Predictability ± 1.0 D	84.5 (306/362)	82.6 (266/322)	0.57 (10)	88 (236/272)	86 (201/236)
Predictability ± 0.5 D	58.6 (212/362)	53.1 (171/322)	0.17 (10)	68 (182/272)	67 (155/236)
Loss of 2 lines of BCVA	4.0 (15/378)	3.9 (13/331)	0.9 (10)	1.5 (4/272)	0.4 (1/236)
Intraoperative complications*	1.4 (8/560)	2.1 (10/475)	0.55 (10)	0.3 (1/272)	1.2 (3/236)
Postoperative complications+	3.4 (19/560)	1.1 (5/475)	0.02 (30)	3.3 (9/272)	3.3 (8/236)
Infectious complications	0 (0/560)	0 (0/475)		0 (0/272)	0 (0/236)

[1] (From Ref. 47).
[2] (From Ref. 48).
* Intraoperative complications included incomplete flap, button-hole flap, free flap.
+ Postoperative complications included slipped flap, dislocated flap, epithelial ingrowth, sterile keratitis, significant folds.

nificant difference ($P = 0.73$). At one year follow-up 1.4% lost 2 or more lines in the bilateral group and 1.2% lost 2 or more lines in the unilateral group. The rate of enhancement in both groups was similar: 15.1% in the bilateral group and 17.4% in the unilateral group. The complication rate between the two groups was similar (refer to Table 1). In summary, there was no significant difference between the two groups in postoperative UCVA, BCVA, complication rate, enhancement rate, or loss of BCVA. As in the study by Waring et al., the statistical power of this study was limited by sample size.

Other authors have compared simultaneous to sequential LASIK retrospectively and found simultaneous surgery to be as safe and efficacious as sequential surgery (5,6).

E. PATIENT COUNSELING AND INFORMED CONSENT

No patient should be coerced or encouraged to undergo unilateral or bilateral same-day LASIK without an appropriate informed consent outlining the risks and benefits of surgery compared to the options of no correction, glasses, and contact lenses. A discussion of whether one or both eyes are to be done at the same setting is one of the most important aspects to be covered during this informed consent discussion. There are several points that need to be adequately covered to improve patient understanding, as well as to reduce medicolegal liability from an uninformed patient.

1. There is some risk of a problem occurring in both eyes, both intraoperatively and postoperatively. Even if the surgical procedure goes as planned as far as the surgeon can tell, several problems can still occur.

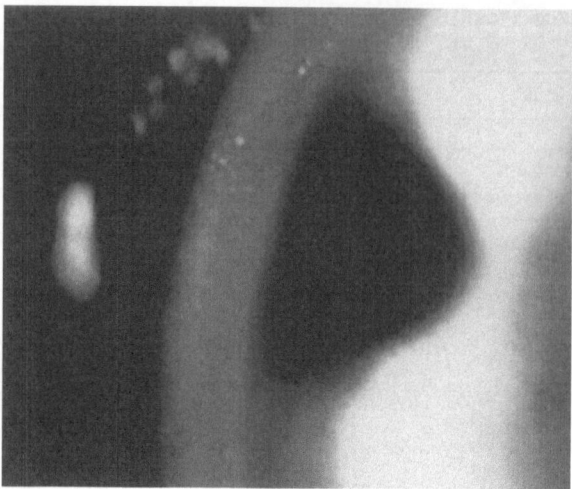

Figure 16.1   Striae in flap producing loss of best corrected visual acuity.

2.   Postoperatively, the flap may move out of the appropriate position, or it may be malpositioned at the end of the procedure but not be apparent to the surgeon (Fig. 16.1). This may not be recognized for up to 1 month after the surgical procedure, because edema may mask the typical signs of striae. Also, late trauma could cause dislocation of the flap. The latest traumatic flap dislocation that we are aware of occurred 3 years after the LASIK procedure. This usually requires surgical repositioning of the flap and may result in irregular astigmatism, permanent striae, or any other typical surgical risks (1,2).

3.   It is not uncommon after the procedure for patients to complain of dry eye symptoms or have more problems with their ocular surface related to blepharitis. These problems are usually worst the first month following the procedure and typically resolve within 3 to 4 months. Many investigators believe that this dryness is secondary to the neurotrophic state of the cornea caused by severing of the nerves during the LASIK procedure. It is not uncommon, though, for patients not to be fully aware of the implications of this problem until the next winter following the procedure. Postoperatively, they no longer have contact lenses or glasses to protect them the drying effects of the car heater or dryer air that comes from the furnace.

4.   Infectious keratitis can occur following any surgical procedure, and LASIK is no exception (Fig. 16.2). There have been case reports of bilateral infectious complications from other refractive procedures (7–9). There have been several reported cases of infectious keratitis after LASIK (10–23), and some of these have been bilateral, with reported loss of vision (24,25). This may not become obvious for several weeks following the surgical procedure, or may be associated with late traumatic dislocation of the flap. Typically, rapid institution of appropriate topical antibacterial, antifungal, or antituberculous medications will prevent permanent scarring. Some infections require surgical irrigation of the interface.

5.   In up to 1–9% of eyes, epithelial ingrowth may occur, occasionally requiring surgical removal (Fig. 16.3) (1,4,10). Epithelial ingrowth occurs more frequently in patients that have an epithelial defect at the time of the surgery (26) but can occur without an obvious break in the epithelium. Typically it is noted at the one-month examination, but in some

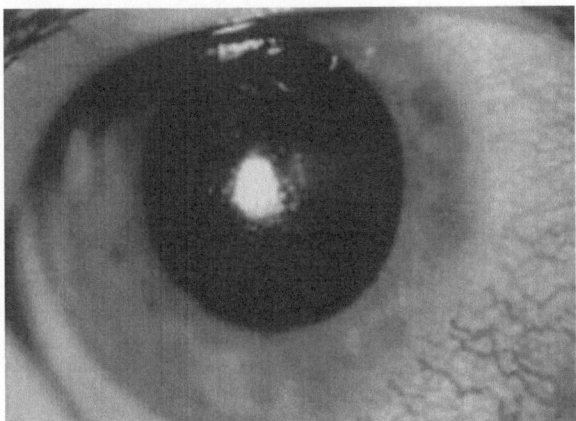

Figure 16.2   Infectious keratitis following LASIK.

cases interface debris and epithelial ingrowth can be difficult to distinguish for several months. Ingrowth encroaching on the visual axis or associated with melting of the flap mandates surgical removal. Recurrences occur in up to 24% of cases, due to the difficulty in complete removal (26). Complications from epithelial ingrowth include melting of the flap with permanent irregular astigmatism or scarring with loss of best corrected visual acuity (Fig. 16.4).

     6.   The ablation may be irregular due to asymmetric hydration of the stromal bed, decentration, laser calibration or alignment errors, or variations in the response of the corneal tissue to the laser. Typically these may be detected early postoperatively, but they may not become obvious for several months, when edema of the flap resolves and the epithelium returns to normal.

     7.   The healing response of the patient's cornea to the treatment may be irregular or asymmetric. This is usually noted in the first few months after the procedure but may take several months to become apparent.

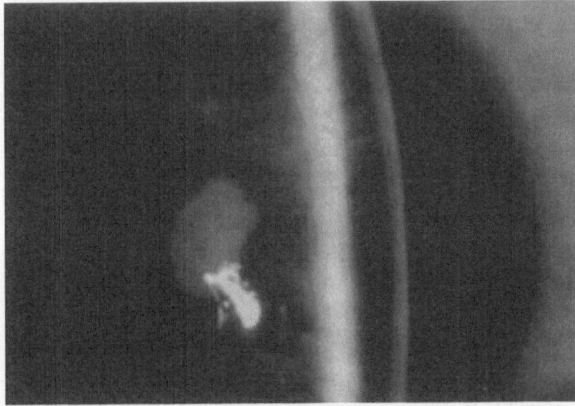

Figure 16.3   Epithelial ingrowth.

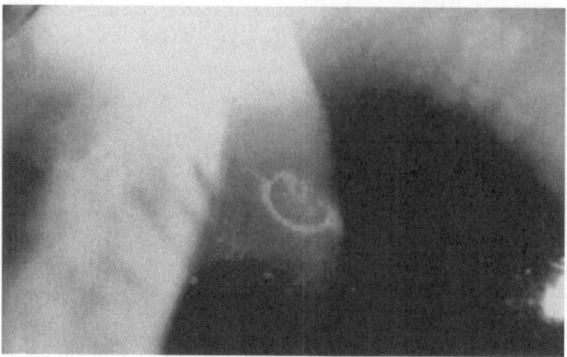

Figure 16.4 Epithelial ingrowth resulting in melting of the flap edge.

8.   The determination of the final refractive effect may take several months in some patients. Therefore it may not be apparent whether there are small degrees of residual myopia, hyperopia, or astigmatism for up to 18 months after the surgical procedure. Typically about 1 month per diopter of myopia treated and 3 months per diopter of hyperopia treated are required to determine the final refraction. This may be due to stromal wound remodeling or epithelial hyperplasia. Individual patients may respond in a different manner, due to unknown factors. It is not clear whether the response of one eye can predict the response in the other eye, as there are reports to support and oppose this hypothesis (4–6,27–30).

9.   Glare and halos may be noted by the patient postoperatively and are typically worse in the first few months postoperatively. These most likely are multifactorial in etiology, coming from small irregularities in the ablation zone, diffraction and scatter from the edge of the optical zone, increased oblate shape of the cornea, and an increase in nocturnal spherical aberration due to enlarging scotopic pupil size. Some glare or visual aberrations noted by the patient are also due to small residual amounts of myopia, hyperopia, or astigmatism. These can continue to improve up to 2 years after the surgical procedure, although in many cases small compromises in visual performance may persist (3,31–33).

10.   Diffuse lamellar keratitis following LASIK has been a dilemma for refractive surgeons (Fig. 16.5). For unknown reasons, occasional patients will develop more than the usual amount of inflammation postoperatively. The white cells may settle in the interface, and if a significant number remains a loss of stromal tissue with irregular astigmatism and corneal scarring can result. Several etiologies have been suggested, but we have not been able to eradicate the problem. This is most often bilateral (in cases of bilateral surgery), yet is typically worse in one eye than in the other. It almost always manifests in the first few days after surgery. Intervention with high-dose topical steroids or interface irrigation for severe cases can prevent loss of best corrected visual acuity.

11.   Increased intraocular pressure can result from the topical steroids used postoperatively. This may not become evident for several weeks after the procedure. Discontinuation of the steroids usually results in normalization of pressure. There have been cases reported of loss of best corrected vision from suspected steroid induced glaucoma (34,35).

12.   Retinal complications such as retinal detachment, posterior vitreous detachment, and macular hemorrhage can occur (1,36–44). In one report, bilateral macular hemorrhages occurred during bilateral simultaneous LASIK, resulting in profound visual loss

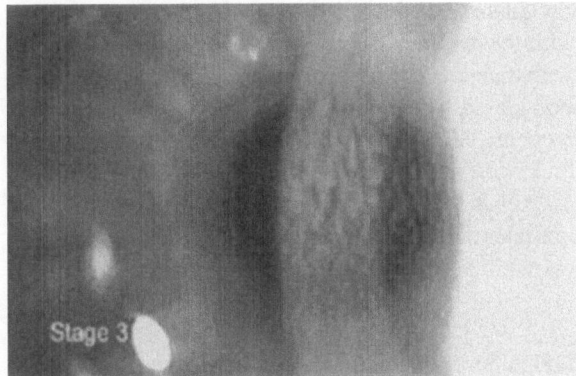

Figure 16.5 Diffuse lamellar keratitis, Stage 3.

in both eyes (41). High myopes are at higher risk of retinal detachment, which can occur several months after the procedure.

    13. After counseling about the risks and benefits of the procedure, as well as a discussion of unilateral versus bilateral surgery, about 90% of our patients choose same-day surgery, and about 10% of our patients choose to have their eyes operated on separately, usually 1 month apart. The time frame of most complications makes the risk/benefit ratio of waiting 1 to 3 days minimally different from operating on the same day.

F. SURGICAL CONSIDERATIONS FOR BILATERAL SURGERY

It is important for a surgeon to have enough experience to feel comfortable that he or she will be able to complete the surgical procedure successfully in the first eye before choosing bilateral surgery for the patients. It is also vital that the surgeon be able to recognize intraoperative occurrences that may lead to a slower visual recovery or the possibility of an increased risk for visual loss. The surgeon should be familiar with the use of the microkeratome as well as the laser to make certain that the procedure is as successful as possible.

    It is important to tape the nonoperative eye shut when working on the first eye. This will prevent fixation by the patient with the wrong eye and will reduce hydration changes in the corneal stroma that may occur if the second eye is allowed to dry while the first eye is being operated on. If the second eye dries too much or irregularly, overcorrection and irregular astigmatism can result. Additionally, if the eye dries too much, it can lead to localized areas of thinning, which can lead to buttonhole formation when the flap is cut. Some surgeons use the same blade for both eyes, while others change the microkeratome blade for the second eye. It is important to rinse the blade to remove debris or epithelium that can be deposited on the blade during the surgical procedure. Typically the second use of the blade will result in a thinner flap, owing to dulling of the edge (45,46). Surgeons that advocate the use of the same blade point out that the blade is known to have performed well in the first eye.

    Postoperative care in the patient that has had bilateral surgery is usually easier, because they can take care of both eyes at once. It is important for them to rest their eyes on the first postoperative day. This will reduce keratopathy that can occur from the topical anesthetics and the microkeratome cut.

It is important to let patients know that one of the unique aspects of their postoperative recovery is that they are dealing with the healing issues in both eyes at the same time. For most patients this is easier to deal with than the asymmetric situation present when each eye is treated separately. They may need glasses early postoperatively to assist them with the early hyperopia or myopia that may occur. There is also some chance that their best corrected vision may not be adequate to function early after the surgery for any of the reasons stated earlier. This is more common in higher levels of both myopia and hyperopia, and these patients may want to consider a unilateral approach.

G. CONCLUSIONS

Bilateral simultaneous same-day LASIK is becoming increasingly accepted and does not appear to pose a significantly higher risk to the patient. The patient should understand though that there is a possibility of complications in both eyes at the same time, resulting in bilateral loss of vision, such as an infection or diffuse lamellar keratitis occurring postoperatively. The risk of this occurring appears to be extremely low and has been below the threshold of measurement in all comparison studies thus far. The benefits of reduced anisometropia, quicker visual recovery, and convenience outweigh these in most patients. We anticipate increasing application of bilateral same-day LASIK among refractive surgeons.

REFERENCES

1. GO Waring III, JD Carr, RD Stulting, KP Thompson, W Wiley. Prospective randomized comparison of simultaneous and sequential bilateral laser in situ keratomileusis for the correction of myopia. Ophthalmology 1999;106(4):732–738.
2. HV Gimbel, JA van Westenbrugge, EE Penno, M Ferensowicz, GA Feinerman, R Chen. Simultaneous bilateral laser in situ keratomileusis: safety and efficacy. Ophthalmology 1999;106(8):1461–1467; discussion 1467–1468.
3. R Zaldivar, S Oscherow, G Ricur, V Piezzi. Bilateral simultaneous laser in situ keratomileusis. J Refract Surg 1999;15(2 suppl):S202–S208.
4. VM Tham, RK Maloney. Microkeratome complications of laser in situ keratomileusis. Ophthalmology 2000;107(5):920–924.
5. RD Stulting, JD Carr, KP Thompson, GO Waring III, WM Wiley, JG Walker. Complications of laser in situ keratomileusis for the correction of myopia. Ophthalmology 1999;106(1):13–20.
6. RA Beldavs, S al-Ghamdi, LA Wilson, GO Waring. Bilateral microbial keratitis after radial keratotomy [letter]. Arch Ophthalmol 1993;111(4):440.
7. RJ Duffey. Bilateral serratia marcescens keratitis after simultaneous bilateral radial keratotomy. Am J Ophthalmol 1995;119(2):233–236.
8. K Szerenyi, JM McDonnell, RE Smith, JA Irvine, PJ McDonnell. Keratitis as a complication of bilateral, simultaneous radial keratotomy. Am J Ophthalmol 1994;117(4):462–467.
9. RL Lindstrom, DR Hardten, DM Houtman, B Witte, N Preschel, YR Chu, TW Samuelson, EJ Linebarger. Six-month results of hyperopic and astigmatic LASIK in eyes with primary and secondary hyperopia. Trans Am Ophthalmol Soc 1999;97:241–255.
10. EK Kim, DH Lee, K Lee, SJ Lim, IS Yoon, YG Lee. Nocardia keratitis after traumatic detachment of a laser in situ keratomileusis flap. J Refract Surg 2000;16(4):467–469.
11. MS Sridhar, P Garg, AK Bansal, U Gopinathan. Aspergillus flavus keratitis after laser in situ keratomileusis. Am J Ophthalmol 2000;129(6):802–804.
12. KO Karp, PS Hersh, RJ Epstein. Delayed keratitis after laser in situ keratomileusis. J Cataract Refract Surg 2000;26(6):925–928.

13. MS Sridhar, P Garg, AK Bansal, S Sharma. Fungal keratitis after laser in situ keratomileusis. J Cataract Refract Surg 2000;26(4):613–615.

14. H Gelender, HL Carter, B Bowman, WE Beebe, GR Walters. Mycobacterium keratitis after laser in situ keratomileusis. J Refract Surg 2000;16(2):191–195.

15. MS Chung, MH Goldstein, WT Driebe, Jr., B Schwartz. Fungal keratitis after laser in situ keratomileusis: a case report. Cornea 2000;19(2):236–237.

16. T Dada, N Sharma, VK Dada, RB Vajpayee. Pneumococcal keratitis after laser in situ keratomileusis. J Cataract Refract Surg 2000;26(3):460–461.

17. MS Chung, MH Goldstein, WT Driebe, Jr., BH Schwartz. Mycobacterium chelonae keratitis after laser in situ keratomileusis successfully treated with medical therapy and flap removal. Am J Ophthalmol 2000;129(3):382–384.

18. PA Quiros, RS Chuck, RE Smith, JA Irvine, JP McDonnell, LC Chao, PJ McDonnell. Infectious ulcerative keratitis after laser in situ keratomileusis. Arch Ophthalmol 1999;117(10): 1423–1427.

19. M al-Reefy. Bacterial keratitis following laser in situ keratomileusis for hyperopia. J Refract Surg 1999;15(2 suppl):216–217.

20. JJ Perez-Santonja, HF Sakla, JL Abad, A Zorraquino, J Esteban, JL Alio. Nocardial keratitis after laser in situ keratomileusis. J Refract Surg 1997;13(3):314–317.

21. V Reviglio, ML Rodriguez, GS Picotti, M Paradello, JD Luna, CP Juarez. Mycobacterium chelonae keratitis following laser in situ keratomileusis. J Refract Surg 1998;14(3):357–360.

22. HM Kim, JS Song, HS Han, HR Jung. Streptococcal keratitis after myopic laser in situ keratomileusis. Korean J Ophthalmol 1998;12(2):108–111.

23. JA Hovanesian, EG Faktorovich, JD Hoffbauer, SS Shah, RK Maloney. Bilateral bacterial keratitis after laser in situ keratomileusis in a patient with human immunodeficiency virus infection. Arch Ophthalmol 1999;117(7):968–970.

24. H Watanabe, S Sato, N Maeda, Y Inoue, Y Shimomura, Y Tano. Bilateral corneal infection as a complication of laser in situ keratomileusis [letter]. Arch Ophthalmol 1997;115(12):1593–1594.

25. MY Wang, RK Maloney. Epithelial ingrowth after laser in situ keratomileusis. Am J Ophthalmol 2000;129(6):746–751.

26. H Bahcecioglu, A Ozdamar, R Aktunc, T Aktunc, M Karacorlu, C Ercikan. Simultaneous and sequential photorefractive keratectomy. J Refract Surg 1995;11(3 suppl):S261–S262.

27. PK Chiang, PS Hersh. Comparing predictability between eyes after bilateral laser in situ keratomileusis: a theoretical analysis of simultaneous versus sequential procedures. Ophthalmology 1999;106(9):1684–1691.

28. WH Coles. Simultaneous versus bilateral sequential LASIK [letter]. Ophthalmology 2000;107(5):818–820.

29. GO Waring III, JD Carr, RD Stulting, KP Thompson. Prospective, randomized comparison of simultaneous and sequential bilateral LASIK for the correction of myopia. Trans Am Ophthalmol Soc 1997;95:271–284.

30. CS Ahn, TE Clinch, M Moshirfar, JR Weis, CB Hutchinson. Initial results of photorefractive keratectomy and laser in situ keratomileusis performed by a single surgeon. J Cataract Refract Surg 1999;25(8):1048–1055.

31. MA el Danasoury. Prospective bilateral study of night glare after laser in situ keratomileusis with single zone and transition zone ablation. J Refract Surg 1998;14(5):512–516.

32. PS Hersh, RF Steinert, SF Brint. Photorefractive keratectomy versus laser in situ keratomileusis: comparison of optical side effects. Summit PRK-LASIK Study Group. Ophthalmology 2000;107(5):925–933.

33. JT Holladay, DR Dudeja, J Chang. Functional vision and corneal changes after laser in situ keratomileusis determined by contrast sensitivity, glare testing, and corneal topography. J Cataract Refract Surg 1999;25(5)663–669.

34. J Najman-Vainer, RJ Smith, RK Maloney. Interface fluid after LASIK: misleading tonometry can lead to end-stage glaucoma [letter]. J Cataract Refract Surg 2000;26(4):471–472.

35. WA Lyle, GJ Jin. Interface fluid associated with diffuse lamellar keratitis and epithelial ingrowth after laser in situ keratomileusis. J Cataract Refract Surg 1999;25(7):1009–1012.

36. C Aras, A Ozdamar, M Karacorlu, B Sener, H Bahcecioglu. Retinal detachment following laser in situ keratomileusis. Ophthalmic Surg Lasers 2000;31(2):121–125.

37. JF Arevalo, E Ramirez, E Suarez, G Antzoulatos, F Torres, R Cortez, J Morales-Stopello, G Ramirez. Rhegmatogenous retinal detachment after laser-assisted in situ keratomileusis (LASIK) for the correction of myopia. Retina 2000;20(4)338–341.

38. DG Charteris. Retinal detachment associated with excimer laser. Curr Opin Ophthalmol 1999;10(3):173–176.

39. J Fernando Arevalo, O Azar-Arevalo. Retinal detachment in myopic eyes after laser in situ keratomileusis [letter]. Am J Ophthalmol 2000;129(6):825–826.

40. HS Han, JS Song, HM Kim. Long-term results of laser in situ keratomileusis for high myopia. Korean J Ophthalmol 2000;14(1):1–6.

41. JD Luna, VE Reviglio, CP Juarez. Bilateral macular hemorrhage after laser in situ keratomileusis. Graefes Arch Clin Exp Ophthalmol 1999;237(7):611–613.

42. DO Mazur, R Hollifield, W Gee. Retinal detachment in myopic eyes after laser in situ keratomileusis [letter]. Am J Ophthalmol 2000;129(6):823–824; discussion 824–825.

43. A Ozdamar, C Aras, B Sener, M Oncel, M Karacorlu. Bilateral retinal detachment associated with giant retinal tear after laser-assisted in situ keratomileusis. Retina 1998;18(2):176–177.

44. JM Ruiz-Moreno, JJ Perez-Santonja, JL Alio. Retinal detachment in myopic eyes after laser in situ keratomileusis. Am J Ophthalmol 1999;128(5):588–594.

45. E Donnefeld, R Wertheimer, A Wallerstein, H Perry, L Landrio, E Rahn. Predictors of corneal flap thickness in LASIK surgery. ASCRS Symposium on Cataract, IOL and Refractive Surgery, San Diego, 1998, p 63.

46. FR Villarreal, PR Valdes, EB Garza. Reproducibility of corneal flap thickness with Hansatome microkeratome: comparison between first and fellow eye using the 180 micron head. ASCRS Symposium on Cataract, IOL and Refractive Surgery, Boston, 2000, p 14.

47. GO Waring III, JD Carr, RD Stulting, KP Thompson, W Wiley. Prospective randomized comparison of simultaneous and sequential bilateral laser in situ keratomileusis for the correction of myopia. Ophthalmology 1999;106(4):732–738.

48. PP Rath, DR Hardten, RL Lindstrom, B Witte. Bilateral sequential versus unilateral sequential laser in situ keratomileusis (LASIK) for the treatment of myopia. Submitted for publication.

17

Postoperative Management Protocols for Uncomplicated LASIK Procedures

MELANIE A. R. GRAHAM

Greater Baltimore Medical Center, Baltimore, Maryland, U.S.A.

DIMITRI T. AZAR

Massachusetts Eye and Ear Infirmary, Schepens Eye Research Institute, and Harvard Medical School, Boston, Massachusetts U.S.A.

Laser in situ keratomileusis (LASIK) is a rapidly advancing technique with evolving pre-operative, intraoperative, and postoperative strategies. Despite the efforts to evaluate surgical techniques critically, to compare instruments, and to minimize the incidence and optimize the management of post-operative complications, differences in protocols create confounding variables that prohibit an accurate compilation and analysis of data collected from multiple sites. Standardization allows for the manipulation and study of individual approaches. Standardized protocols also can improve the quality and efficiency of patient care by preparing patients and staff for an expected clinical course and therapeutic regimen. Lastly, standardized protocols foster the detection of situations of biologic variability that lead to suboptimal surgical outcomes.

A simplified and standardized postoperative protocol for uncomplicated LASIK procedures will be proposed and discussed in this chapter. A review of the LASIK literature reveals differences in postoperative medication profiles, in the use of bandage contact lenses, in preferences for bilateral sequential versus simultaneous LASIK, and in the scheduling of short- and long-term follow-up visits. Many of the proposed regimens in this chapter are simply preferences, and we hope that standardized protocols and future randomized controlled studies will enable the eventual optimization of all aspects of LASIK.

Acknowledgment: Dr. Kimberly Sippel helped with the figures and legends.

A. POSTOPERATIVE MEDICATIONS

In general, patients are prescribed antibiotic and steroid drops after uncomplicated LASIK. The choice of steroid and antibiotic and the frequency of application, however, are variable. The practice of tapering antibiotics is concerning. Tapering produces subtherapeutic antibiotic levels that can promote the emergence of drug-resistant bacteria. Given that the corneal epithelial barrier should be restored within a few days after uncomplicated LASIK, we prescribe a one-week course of antibiotics, without tapering. Antibiotic spectrum, cost and availability, and preferences for combination drops influence the choice of antibiotic for postoperative bacterial prophylaxis. Different antibiotics, however, are prepared with different preservatives that can variably affect the ocular surface. Hence antibiotic use ideally would be matched in studies comparing LASIK outcomes.

Although anecdotal, there may be a reduction in the incidence of diffuse lamellar keratitis with the use of higher potency steroid drops. Higher potency steroids, however, have a greater potential for inducing an elevation in intraocular pressure, typically noted after a two-week period of application. As with antibiotics, different steroid drops are prepared with formulations that have different ocular surface penetration and effect, and a uniform steroid regimen would reduce the number of confounding variables in studies of LASIK outcomes. We recommend the use of a high-potency topical steroid, tapered over a period of 7 to 10 days.

Additional therapeutic strategies that may be included in the armamentarium of LASIK surgeons include nonsteroidal anti-inflammatory agents (NSAIDS), artificial tears, and punctal occlusion. Vantesone and colleagues have reported an equivalent efficacy of NSAIDS and steroids in their postoperative LASIK patients and have recommended the consideration of NSAIDS after LASIK as steroid-sparing agents (1). Artificial tears have been reported to accelerate the recovery of the ocular surface in the LASIK postoperative period (2). In our practices, NSAIDS are rarely prescribed in the postoperative LASIK patient, artificial tears are recommended on an as needed basis, and punctal occlusion is performed on those patients with pre- or post-operative symptoms or signs of dry eye syndrome.

B. BANDAGE CONTACT LENSES

Bandage contact lenses are frequently used in the setting of such LASIK postoperative complications as large epithelial defects, poor flap adherence, flap displacement, and free caps, but the routine application of bandage contact lenses after uncomplicated LASIK is controversial. Certainly bandage contact lenses promote corneal epithelial healing and can improve patient comfort. Bandage contact lenses may also reduce flap movement secondary to eyelid excursions, thus theoretically reducing the development of flap wrinkles, flap displacement, and flap loss (3). Bandage contact lenses, however, pose an increased risk of bacterial keratitis. In a study by Detorakis and colleagues, 18.3% of 60 patients with bandage contact lenses after uncomplicated LASIK were found to have bacterial colonization of the lenses (4). The combination of colonized contact lenses and a surgically disrupted corneal epithelial barrier creates an environment suitable for corneal infection. Bandage contact lenses also introduce a potential for flap slippage at the time of removal, a potential for "tight lens syndrome", and an increased time and expense for the surgical procedure.

In our practices, bandage contact lenses are not used routinely after uncomplicated primary LASIK procedures. A randomized, controlled study evaluating the importance of bandage contact lenses after uncomplicated LASIK would require a very large patient population, but it might provide insight into the role, if any, of bandage contact lenses in reducing epithelial ingrowth and flap complications.

C. SCHEDULING THE SECOND EYE AFTER UNILATERAL LASIK

Simultaneous LASIK and sequential LASIK each have distinct advantages and disadvantages that need to be discussed at length with patients for proper informed consent. Simultaneous LASIK is convenient for both patient and surgeon, and studies have reported similar outcomes in simultaneous and sequential LASIK (5–7). Also, strabismus surgery and oculoplastic surgery commonly involve bilateral simultaneous ophthalmic procedures. Sequential LASIK, however, avoids the rare but possible incidence of a bilateral catastrophic complication such as bacterial keratitis (3), flap complication (8), central retinal vein occlusion, and submacular hemorrhage (9). Also, Waring and colleagues have demonstrated a slightly reduced risk of epithelial ingrowth in sequential LASIK (5), and Chiang and Hersh have reported improved outcomes in patients undergoing sequential LASIK. Chiang reported that by using information from the postoperative course of an individual's first eye, the targeted correction of the second eye was better achieved (10). This was described as a correlation in refractive predictability between the two eyes of an individual, and an improved targeted correction was noted in the fellow eye even after observing the first eye for only one week.

Based on this information, we counsel patients to schedule surgeries at least one week apart. Information is gathered in the first postoperative week on the operated eye, including post-operative manifest refraction and topography (Figures 17.1 and 17.2). Biological variability, which may predispose to under- or overcorrection, as well as to diffuse lamellar keratitis, is noted, and this information is used to guide the treatment of the fellow eye. Eyes with unexpected overcorrections are conservatively treated, and fellow eyes of patients with diffuse lamellar keratitis (DLK) are prophylactically treated with pre- and post-operative high dose topical steroids. Complications, which generally are noted within the first few days, are managed before treating the fellow eye.

Occasionally a patient insists on bilateral simultaneous surgery despite our recommendations. In order to minimize complications such as flap dislocation or a dislocated flap, the first eye is scheduled early and the second late in the day, allowing for settling and examination of the flap prior to the treatment of the second eye. This separation of treatments also ensures the use of sterilized blades and equipment for each eye, thus reducing the risk of bilateral contamination.

D. ROUTINE POSTOPERATIVE VISITS

Postoperative visit protocols for uncomplicated LASIK procedures vary among different centers, leading to difficulty in compiling and comparing outcome data from multiple centers. Most LASIK surgeons routinely see their patients 24 hours after surgery, but many do not schedule or report 1 week, 1 month, and/or 3 month visit examinations (11,12). Examination of the patient on the first post-operative day is essential for the evaluation of flap placement (Figures 17.3 and 17.4). The risk of striae formation is greatest during the first 24 post-operative hours, and prompt surgical treatment may provide optimal visual outcome (13). Flap positioning should be re-examined at the one-week visit, at which time topography and manifest refraction can also be obtained to guide treatment of the fellow eye.

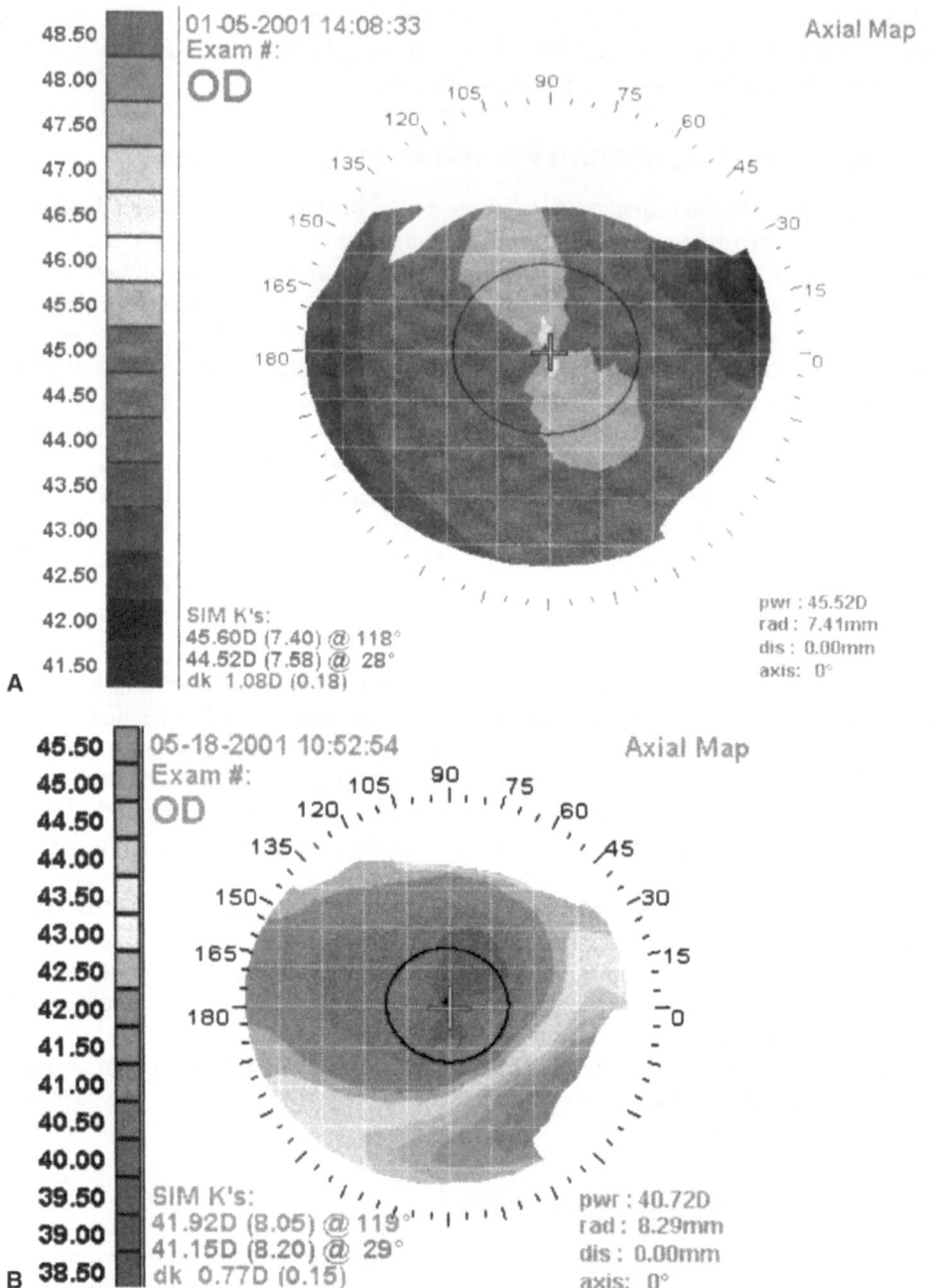

Figure 17.1 Preoperative (A) and postoperative (B) Eye Sys™ corneal topographic maps demonstrating a myopic ablation profile. After myopic LASIK treatment utilizing the VISX Star S2 laser, with treatment parameters of −4.40 − 1.00 × 003°, postoperative uncorrected visual acuity of 20/20 was achieved. Corneal topography demonstrates flattening of the central corneal curvature with reduction of power from 45.52 to 40.72 diopters.

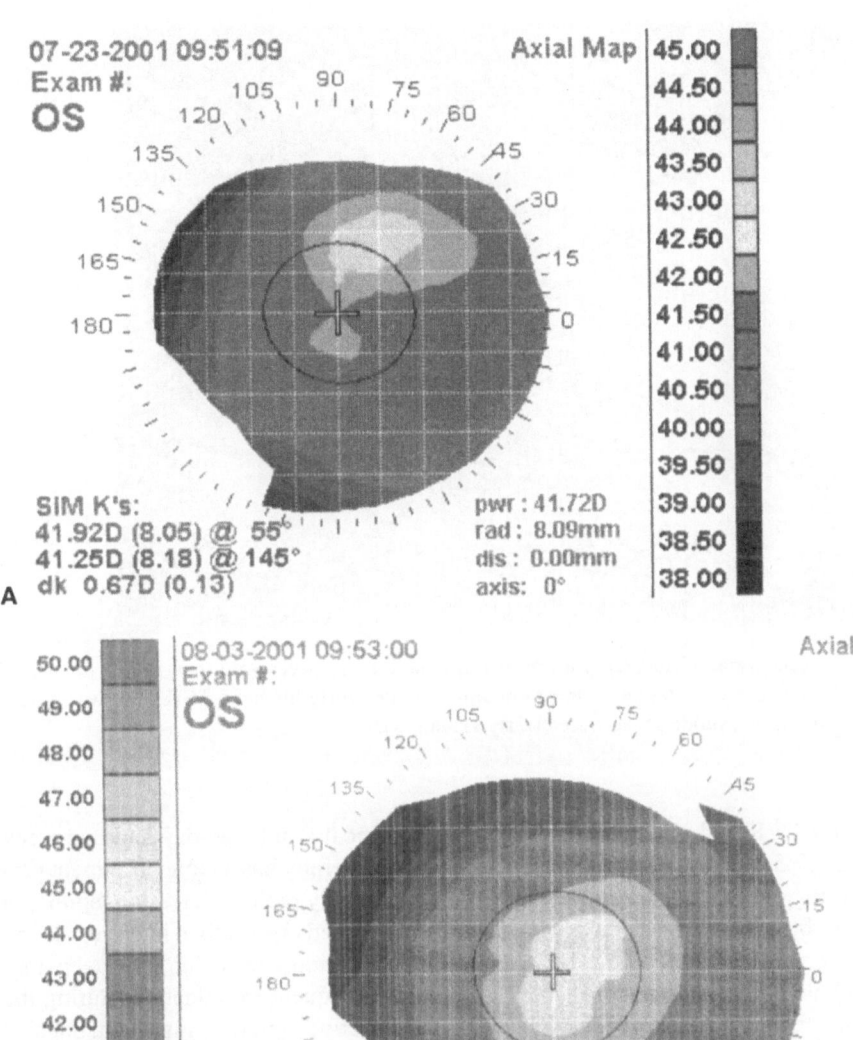

Figure 17.2 Preoperative (A) and postoperative (B) Eye Sys™ corneal topographic maps demonstrating a hyperopic ablation profile. After hyperopic LASIK treatment utilizing the VISX Star S2 laser, with treatment parameters of +3.00 + 0.50 × 090°, post-operative uncorrected visual acuity of 20/25⁻² at distance and J1 at near was achieved. Corneal topography demonstrates steepening of the central corneal curvature with an increase in power from 41.7 to 45.4 diopters.

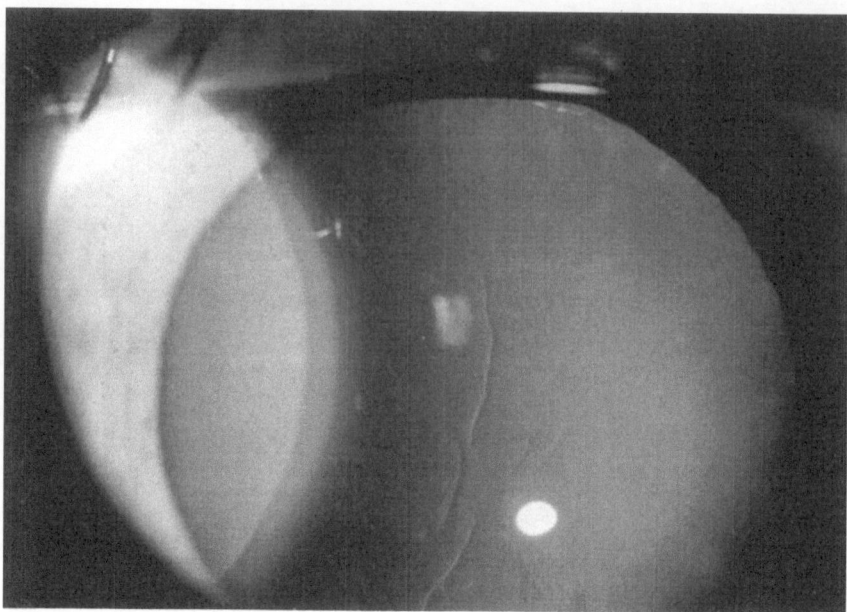

Figure 17.3 Flap striae visualized with retro-illumination. A 39-year-old man with a history of myopic LASIK presented with glare. On examination, a superiorly hinged LASIK flap was noted. With retro-illumination, subtle striae were clearly visualized.

Evaluation for DLK and epithelial ingrowth is also critical at the one-day and one-week visit (Figures 17.5 and 17.6). In contrast to DLK which generally has a more prominent presentation during the first postoperative week and a potentially rapid progression, epithelial ingrowth can be subtle. Epithelial ingrowth is distinguished from other interface debris such as meibomian gland secretions by gutter-staining and ridge formation, gradual extension an epithelial peninsula, and possible flap melting. Frequent examinations during the first postoperative months are not only important for detecting epithelial ingrowth, but also for evaluating patterns of corneal wound healing and for studying the efficacy of evolving LASIK techniques (14).

Currently, we recommend scheduling post-operative visits for the uncomplicated LASIK patient at 1 day, 1 week, 1 month, 3 months, 6 months, and 1 year. Slit lamp examination and manifest refraction are performed at each consultation. Applanation tonometry is deferred on the first postoperative day to prevent flap trauma. Topography is routinely performed at the 1, 3, 6, and 12 month visits, and earlier if there is a suspicion of irregular astigmatism, such as from a decentered ablation or central island, accounting for symptomatic ocular aberrations. Topography is also usually obtained at 1 week if the patient's eyes are scheduled for LASIK 1 week apart. For patients not enrolled in studies, we do not routinely perform tests measuring contrast sensitivity.

E.   LONG TERM FOLLOW-UP

Frequently studies report data with no information beyond a sixth month time-point (11,15). After the first year, we recommend yearly examinations for patients without postoperative complications. Serial corneal topography and refraction may be useful for future studies. Long-term follow-up will enable a more critical analysis of techniques such as wave-front-guided corneal ablations, in particular the effects of age-related changes in lenticular aberrations on post-operative visual acuity. Lastly, long-term care should include the maintenance of excellent records to allow for the calculation of intraocular lens power at the time of cataract surgery (16).

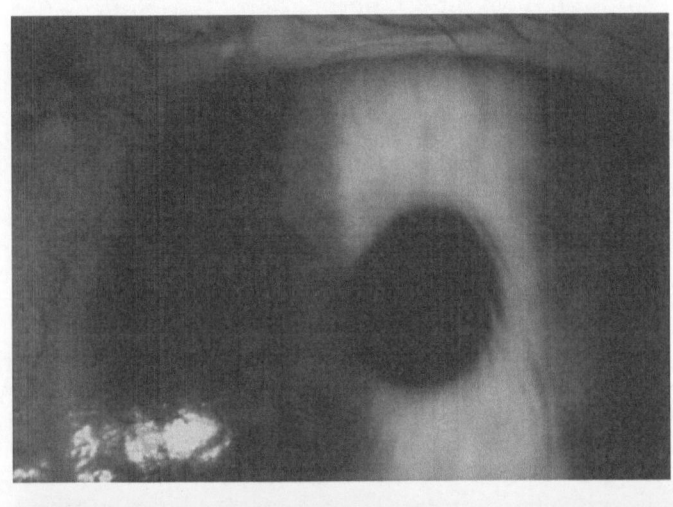

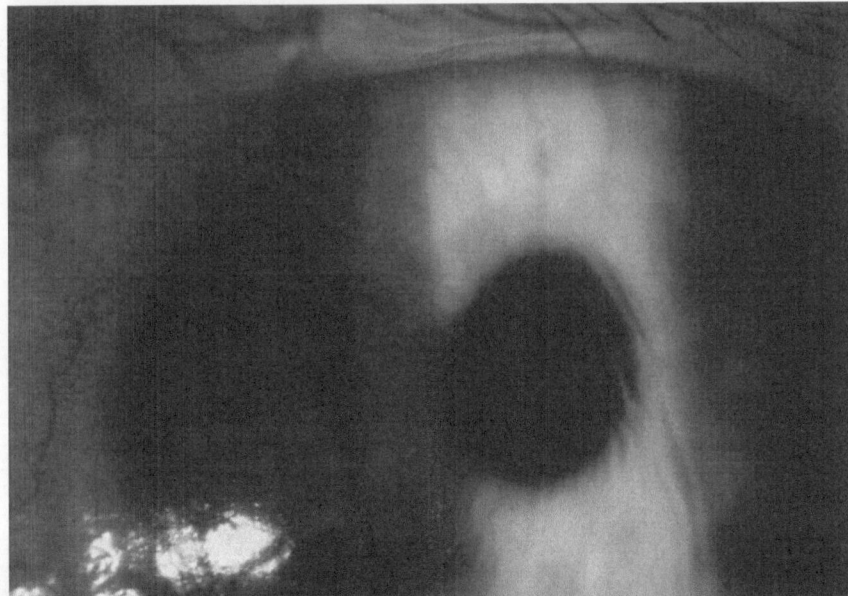

Figure 17.4 Flap striae visualized with fluorescein staining. A 57-year-old man underwent hyperopic LASIK with a superiorly hinged LASIK flap. He presented on the third postoperative day with pain. Examination revealed marked striae formation and staining with fluorescein dye enhanced visualization. [Color in original.]

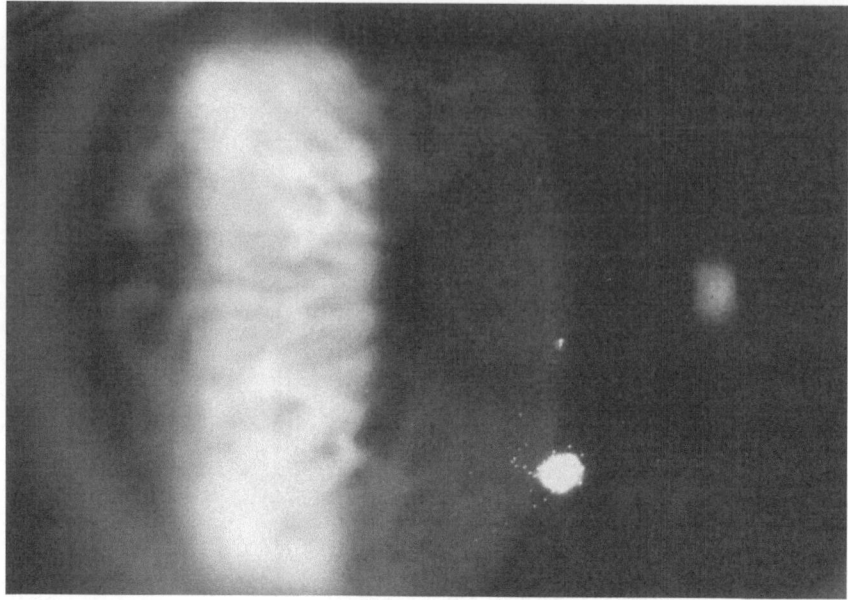

Figure 17.5   Diffuse lamellar keratitis. A 36-year-old man underwent myopic LASIK. Postoperative examination revealed a diffuse fine granular cellular infiltrate in the flap interface indicative of diffuse lamellar keratitis, prompting immediate therapeutic intervention.

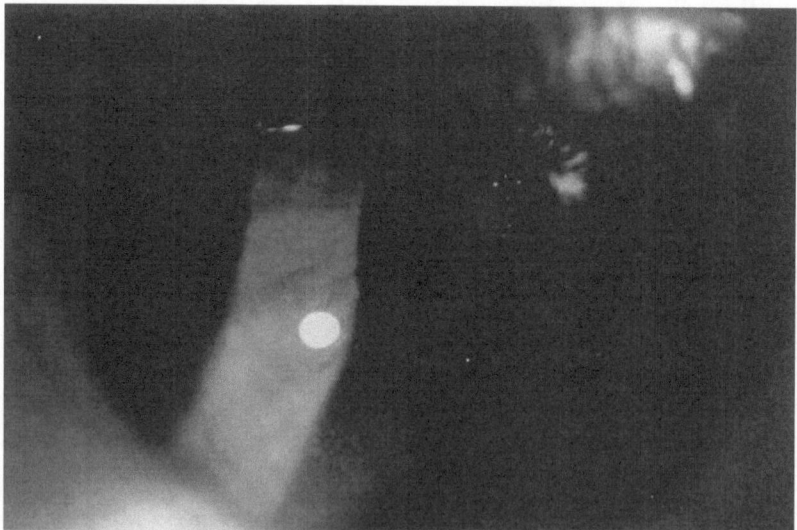

Figure 17.6   Epithelial ingrowth. A 65-year-old woman underwent hyperopic LASIK with a superiorly hinged flap two months prior to presentation. She was referred for evaluation of interface debris. Slit lamp examination revealed interface peninsulae and pearls, representing the linear extensions and nests of cells found in epithelial ingrowth.

F. CONCLUSION

As the strategies to perfect LASIK outcomes evolve, so must protocols for the uncomplicated LASIK procedure change and approach standardization. Limiting the number of confounding variables will allow the pooling of data from a number of centers. Large computerized databases will expedite the discovery of effective techniques. Simplification and standardization of protocols may also improve patient care and office productivity. We have proposed a reasonable postoperative medical regimen without the use of a bandage contact lens and with the surgical scheduling of an individual's eyes at least one week apart. We also have suggested guidelines for postoperative examination schedules. We hope that widespread use of a reasonable standardized postoperative protocol that fosters the collection and study of data from multiple centers will eventually enable the revelation of the optimal protocol for postoperative LASIK care.

REFERENCES

1. DL Vantesone, JD Luna, JC Muino, CP Juarez. Effects of topical diclofenac and prednisolone eyedrops in laser in situ keratomileusis patients. J Cataract Refract Surg 1999; 25:836–841.
2. LM Lenton, JM Albietz. Effect of carmellose-based artificial tears on the ocular surface in eyes after laser in situ keratomileusis. J Refract Surg 1999; 15:S227–S231.
3. SE Wilson. LASIK: management of common complications. Laser in situ keratomileusis. Cornea 1998; 17:459–467.
4. ET Detorakis, DS Siganos, VM Houlakis, et al. Microbiological examination of bandage soft contact lenses used in laser refractive surgery. J Refract Surg 1998; 14:631–635.
5. GO Waring III, JD Carr, RD Stulting, KP Thompson, W Wiley. Prospective randomized comparison of simultaneous and sequential bilateral laser in situ keratomileusis for the correction of myopia. Ophthalmology 1999; 106:732–738.
6. HV Gimbel, JA van Westenbrugge, EE Penno, M Ferensowicz, GA Feinerman, R Chen. Simultaneous bilateral laser in situ keratomileusis: safety and efficacy [see comments]. Ophthalmology 1999; 106:1461–1467; discussion 1467–1468.
7. GO Waring III, JD Carr, RD Stulting, KP Thompson. Prospective, randomized comparison of simultaneous and sequential bilateral LASIK for the correction of myopia. Trans Am Ophthalmol Soc 1997; 95:271–284.
8. SP Holland, S Srivannaboon, DZ Reinstein. Avoiding serious corneal complications of laser assisted in situ keratomileusis and photorefractive keratectomy. Ophthalmology 2000; 107:640–652.
9. JD Luna, VE Reviglio, CP Juarez. Bilateral macular hemorrhage after laser in situ keratomileusis. Graefes Arch Clin Exp Ophthalmol 1999; 237:611–613.
10. PK Chiang, PS Hersh. Comparing predictability between eyes after bilateral laser in situ keratomileusis: a theoretical analysis of simultaneous versus sequential procedures. Ophthalmology 1999; 106:1684–1691.
11. SG Farah, DT Azar, C Gurdal, J Wong. Laser in situ keratomileusis: literature review of a developing technique. J Cataract Refract Surg 1998; 24:989–1006.
12. C Barraquer, AM Gutierrez. Results of laser in situ keratomileusis in hyperopic compound astigmatism. J Cataract Refract Surg 1999; 25:1198–1204.
13. LE Probst, J Machat. Removal of flap striae following laser in situ keratomilieusis. Journal of Cataract and Refractive Surgery 1998; 24:153–155.
14. MC Knorz, B Jendritza. Topographically-guided laser in situ keratomileusis to treat corneal irregularities. Ophthalmology 2000; 107:1138–1143.
15. JC Casebeer, GM Kezirian. Outcomes of spherocylinder treatments in the comprehensive refractive surgery LASIK study. Semin Ophthalmol 1998; 13:71–78.
16. B Seitz, A Langenbucher. Intraocular lens calculations status after corneal refractive surgery. Curr Opin Ophthalmol 2000; 11:35–46.

18

Visual Outcomes After Primary LASIK

SAMIR G. FARAH

Massachusetts Eye and Ear Infirmary, Boston, Massachusetts, U.S.A.

DIMITRI T. AZAR

Massachusetts Eye and Ear Infirmary, Schepens Eye Research Institute, and Harvard Medical School, Boston, Massachusetts U.S.A.

For this chapter, we have compiled a list of articles on LASIK. We identified pertinent articles published in peer-reviewed journals through a multistaged, systematic approach. In the first stage, a computerized search of Medline databases from 1990 to 2000 was performed to identify all articles about the efficacy and safety of LASIK. The terms laser in situ keratomileusis, keratomileusis, and LASIK were used for a broad and sensitive search.

In the second stage, all abstracts were carefully scanned to identify articles, written in English, that described the results of a clinical series. Copies of the entire articles were obtained. Articles published before 1997 were grouped together because they reflected the early experience with LASIK surgery. Articles reported after January 1997 were divided into those describing series with a spherical equivalent (SE) ≤ -4 diopters (D), those describing series with a SE between -4 and -13 D, those describing series with SE ≥ -13 D, those describing series with SE $\leq +8$ D, and those reporting on astigmatism treatment. Bibliographies of these articles were searched for additional articles. All identified journals were manually searched up to and including the January 2000 issues using the same search guidelines.

In the third stage, articles were reviewed and analyzed according to preoperative and postoperative spherical equivalent, follow-up (F/U), uncorrected visual outcome (UCVA), predictability, and safety. Results in each category were used to calculate the weighted mean of that category.

A. EARLY STUDIES OF LASIK IN MODERATE AND HIGH MYOPIA

Several reports regarding LASIK in moderate and high myopia were published before January 1997 and are considered in the analysis. The total number of eyes reported in these papers was 1028.

a. Follow-Up

The follow-up ranged from 10 days to 24 months but was most often performed at 6 (1–8) or 12 months (9–13). In one study (14) it was ambiguous, and in others (15–18) only a mean follow-up was presented.

b. Preoperative Refraction

The preoperative refraction was generally in the range of moderate to high myopia. The lowest was 6.0 D and the highest (18), 37.0 D, with a mean of 12.59 D. Only Salah et al. (17) operated on a group with low myopia (2.0 to 6.0 D) in the series on which they reported clinical results. Arenas and Maglione (16) operated on four contact lens intolerant patients after PKP because of high residual myopia (mean 11.2 D) causing anisometropia.

1. Refractive Outcome and Predictability

a. Postoperative Refraction

An undercorrection was seen in most of the reviewed series. The postoperative result ranged from an overcorrection (1) of +6.63 to an undercorrection (3) of −9.5 D, with a mean of −1.1 D. Bas and Onnis (19) aimed at emmetropia in cases of low myopia and at overcorrection by 2.0 D in cases of high myopia because the myopia progresses over time and the cornea tends to bend its anterior surface slightly after surgery (stromal scar, molecular memory in collagen fibers, and intraocular pressure on the cornea). In the post-PKP study (16), the mean post-LASIK refraction was −2.37 D at a mean follow-up of 7 months. The scattergram in the series by Knorz et al. (3) showed that most eyes were somewhat undercorrected, with 22% beyond ±3.0 D. Analysis of these cases showed that the cause of this undercorrection was not related to the ablation algorithm. Pérez-Santonja et al. (5) had a mean postoperative refraction of +0.18 D ± 1.6 (SD) at 6 months. They found that the mean postoperative spherical equivalent was significantly higher with the 5.0/5.5/6.0 mm ablation profile (+0.47 ± 1.5D) than that with the 4.0/4.5/5.0 mm profile (−0.93 ± 2.1 D). In another study (18), six eyes between −20.0 and −40.0 D were undercorrected due to the limitation that 30% of the preoperative corneal thickness must be left undisturbed beneath the ablated area to avoid subsequent corneal ectasia.

b. Percentage Within ±1.0 D

The percentage of LASIK patients within ±1.0 D of emmetropia was 46.5% (19) and 70.0% (14) at 3 months postoperatively; 47.0% (2,3), 74.2% (4), 60.0% (5), and 85.0% (moderate myopia group), and −41.0% (high myopia group) (6), 67.65% (7), 72.0% (17), and 47.8% (8) at 6 months; and 57.0% (9), 66.6% (10), and 85.7% (13) at 1 year, with an overall mean of 67.0%.

The studies indicate that the predictability of LASIK decreases when the preoperative myopia is high. In one study (17), the group with low myopia (2.0 to 6.0 D) had the highest predictability; 92.5% at a mean follow-up of 5.2 months; whereas the groups with moderate (6.0 to 12.0 D) and high (12.0 to 20.0 D) myopia had predictabilities of 65.0%

and 43.0%, respectively (17). Guell and Muller (6) found that 85.0% of eyes with moderate myopia and only 41.0% of eyes with high myopia were within ± 1.0 D. In their study, Pérez-Santonja et al. (5) reported 72.4% with 8.0 to 12.0 D of myopia were within ±1.0 D at 6 months; this predictability was lower in the two groups with higher myopia.

2. Visual Outcome

In several studies, patients with reduced levels of preoperative corrected and uncorrected vision because of progressive myopic chorioretinal degeneration, anisometropic amblyopia, or both were included. To ensure that upcoming studies reflect the exact postoperative outcome, patients with a low preoperative best corrected visual acuity (BCVA) should be studied separately from those with a BCVA of 20/40 or better. Studies should specify the preoperative uncorrected visual acuity (UCVA), permitting comparisons between preoperative and postoperative acuities.

a. Postoperative UCVA of 20/40 or Better

The mean UCVA improved from 20/1000 preoperatively to 20/45 postoperatively at 6 months in one study (5). A UCVA of 20/40 or better was achieved by 49.9% (19) and 81.0% (14) at 3 months; by 66.0% (1,8), 81.0% (4), 71.4% (moderate myopia group), and 45.0% (high myopia group) (6), 71.0% (17), 29.2% (3), and 46.4% (5) at 6 months, and by 10.0% (9) and 75.0% (13) at 1 year, with an overall mean of 49.2%.

Salah et al. (17) reported a UCVA of 20/40 or better in 92.8% of patients in the low myopia group (2.0 to 6.0 D), 62.3% in the moderate myopia group (6.0 to 12.0 D), and 36.8% in the high myopia group (12.0 to 20.0 D) at 5.2 months after LASIK. In Guell and Muller's series (6), the postoperative UCVA in the moderate and high myopia groups was 71.4% and 45.0%, respectively. In the post-PKP study (16), no patient had a UCVA better than 20/40, but all four eyes improved to 20/150 or 20/100.

b. Postoperative UCVA of 20/20 or Better

A UCVA of 20/20 or better was achieved by 44.0% (15) and 50.0% (14) of patients at 2 to 3 months postoperatively; by 34.0% (1), 0% (6), 36.0% (17), and 7.8% (3) at 6 months; and by 0% (9) and 17.5% (13) at 1 year. The overall mean was 22.0%.

3. Astigmatism

Several studies do not mention correcting the astigmatic error (5,6,9,14,20). In the papers, the mean preoperative and postoperative astigmatism were 0.85 and 0.95 D, respectively.

Two studies (12,18) reported the attempted correction of the astigmatic error. In one, (18), the cylindrical component was reduced from a mean of −2.1 D (−0.5 to −6.0) to a mean of −0.5 (0 to −3.25). Two other studies (6,13) reported that after LASIK, the percentage of patients experiencing an increase in astigmatism was lower than the percentage experiencing a decrease (6.0% and 27.5% increase; 17.2% and 42.3% decrease). In the post-PKP study (16), there was an increase in mean astigmatism after LASIK.

4. Loss of BCVA

A reduction in BCVA is consistently seen in some eyes having LASIK. It can be due to interface abnormalities (7,18,21), central islands (3,18), or induced irregular astigmatism (3,7). In one study (18), it was attributed to the learning curve associated with this technique, particularly while the flap was being fashioned. The percentage of eyes that lost two or more lines was 8.0 (22), 21.3 (1), 13.4 (19), 20.0 (12), 0 (4,6), 10.0 (15), 8.82 (7), 3.6 (17), 5.5 (2), 12.0 (3), and 1.4 (5), with a mean of 8.0.

B. OUTCOMES OF LASIK IN LOW MYOPIA (−0.75 TO −4 D)

Reports about LASIK for low myopia have emerged in the recent 4 years. The concern during the first few years of LASIK practice was the treatment of moderate to high myopia; the range of myopia where PRK has increased the risk of scaring and complications. In recent years and after that LASIK proved to be a reliable and predictable procedure for moderate to high myopia, reports (23,24,25–27) on the treatment of low myopia with LASIK started to emerge in the literature showing similar results to those of the higher ranges of myopia (28).

The total number of eyes reported in these papers was 1125. The F/U ranged between 1 and 12 months with a mean of 4.5 months.

Preoperative Refraction

Articles reporting on series with a preoperative SE less than −4 D were included. The preoperative mean SE was −3.64 ± 1.28 D (mean ± st. dev.).

1. Refractive Outcome and Predictability

a. Postoperative Refraction

Postoperatively, a minimal undercorrection was noticed in most of the reviewed series. The postoperative refraction ranged from an overcorrection (29) of +2 D to an undercorrection (30) of −2.25 with a mean spherical equivalent of −0.2 ± 0.46 D.

b. Percentage Within ±1.0 D

The percentage of LASIK patients within ± 1 D of emmetropia was 89 (23), 96.4 (29), 100 (24,27), 91 and 89 (26), 93 and 87 (30), with a mean of 92.3.

c. Percentage Within ±0.5 D

The percentage of LASIK patients within ±0.5% of emmetropia was 71 (23), 92.8 (29), 87.5 (24), 78, and 73 (26), and 94 (27), with a mean of 80.

2. Visual Outcome

a. Postoperative UCVA of 20/40 or Better

A UCVA of 20/40 or better was achieved in 91% (23,30,31), 100% (24,27,29), and 93% (25,26), with a mean of 93.5%.

b. Postoperative UCVA of 20/20 or Better

A UCVA of 20/20 or better was achieved in 83% (23), 52% (29), 79.2% (24), 39% and 46% (26), 81% (27), 43% (31), and 60% and 37% (30), with a mean of 55.1%.

3. Loss of BCVA

The loss of two lines or more was reported as 1% (23), 10.7% (29), and 0% (24,26,27,30, 31), with a mean of 0.39%.

C. OUTCOMES OF LASIK IN THE MODERATE (−4 TO −9 D) TO HIGH (−9 TO −13 D) MYOPIA RANGE

The results of Knorz et al. (32) indicate that LASIK provides stability of manifest refraction and adequate UCVA as well as a high degree of patient satisfaction without significant visual loss in patients with myopia up to −10 D. Results still may be acceptable in patients with myopia up to −15D, but the rate of visual loss is higher and patient satisfaction is lower. For myopia greater than 15 D, accuracy and patient satisfaction were sufficiently poor to advise against the use of LASIK. Furthermore, patients with astigmatism correction were less pleased with the results than were patients who received spherical corrections only (32). The total number of eyes was 1373 in the moderate myopia group and 289 in the high myopia group.

a. Follow-Up

The follow-up ranged from 1 month to 25 months but was most often performed at 6 (29,33–37) or 12 months (32,38,39). In two studies (31,40), it was ambiguous and in another two (41,42), a mean follow-up was presented.

b. Preoperative Refraction

The preoperative refraction was in the range of moderate to high myopia. We arbitrarily chose to include in this group articles reporting on preoperative spherical equivalents between −4 and −13 diopters. We chose −13 as the highest limit because when using the Munnerlyn formula, and keeping in mind that a residual stromal bed thickness of 250 μ should be left, only 13 diopters of myopia can be treated with LASIK in a normal thickness cornea (550 μ) with a 150 μ thick flap. We divided this group into the moderate myopia group (spherical equivalent between −4 and −9 D) and the high myopia group (spherical equivalent between −9 and −13 D).

The mean preoperative spherical equivalent in the combined group was −8.12 D. It was −7.25 D in the moderate myopia group, and −11.36 D in the high myopia group.

1. Refractive Outcome and Predictability

a. Postoperative Refraction

An undercorrection was seen in most of the reviewed series. The postoperative spherical equivalent ranged from an overcorrection (34) of +1.62 to an undercorrection (35) of −5 D, with a mean of −0.31 D. It was −0.17 D in the moderate myopia group and −0.84 D in the high myopia group.

Most of the nomograms used took into consideration the age of the patient and the difference in ablation between deep and superficial stroma.

b. Percentage Within ±1.0 D

The percentage of eyes after LASIK within ±1.0 D of emmetropia was 83% (41) and 73% and 54.1% (26) at 3 months postoperatively; 78% (33), 80% (34), 40.7% (35), 90.7% (36), 83% (37), 72% and 100% (42), and 72.7% and 61.5% (29) at 6 months; and 85% and 72.75% (32), 54% (38), and 96% and 91% (39) at 1 year, with an overall mean of 71.6% for the combined group. It was 75% for the moderate myopia group and 56.3% for the high myopia group.

c.   Percentage Within ±0.5 D

The percentage of LASIK patients within ±0.5 D of emmetropia was 56% (41) and 52.5% and 39% (26) at 3 months postoperatively; 67% (33), 26% (34), 27% (35), 72% (36), 67% (37), 20% and 43.75% (42), and 50% and 53.8% (29) at 6 months; and 50% and 57.6% (32), 23% (38), and 68% and 75% (39) at 1 year, with an overall mean of 52.92% for the combined group. It was 55.8% for the moderate myopia group and 38.8% for the high myopia group.

2.   Visual Outcome

a.   Postoperative UCVA of 20/40 or Better

A UCVA of 20/40 or better was achieved by 77% (41) and 86% and 68% (26) at 3 months postoperatively; 73% (33), 69% (34), 55.7% (35), 79% (36), 91% (37), 84% and 100% (42), and 75% and 53.8% (29) at 6 months; and 77.7% and 84% (32), 85% (38), and 88% and 94.7% (39), at 1 year, with an overall mean of 77.6% for the combined group. It was 81% for the moderate myopia group and 61.3% for the high myopia group.

b.   Postoperative UCVA of 20/20 or Better

A UCVA of 20/20 or better was achieved by 22% (41) at 3 months postoperatively; 20% (33), 26% (35), 35% (36), 56% (37), 16% and 68.75% (42), and 29.2% and 15.4% (29) at 6 months; and 36% (38), and 76% and 55.4% (39), at 1 year, with an overall mean of 29% for the combined group. It was 32.9% for the moderate myopia group and 16% for the high myopia group.

3.   Loss of BCVA

A reduction in BCVA is consistently seen in some eyes having LASIK. It can be due to interface abnormalities, central islands, or induced irregular astigmatism. Loss of BCVA is reported in 1.2% (41) and 0% (26) at 3 months postoperatively; 4% (33,34), 3.2% (35), 2.32% (36), 3% (37), and 10.7% and 15.4% (29) at 6 months; and 6.3% and 0% (32), 2% (38), and 0% (39) at 1 year, with an overall mean of 2.65% for the combined group. It was 2% for the moderate myopia group and 6% for the high myopia group.

D.   OUTCOMES OF LASIK IN THE EXTREMELY HIGH MYOPIA RANGE (BEYOND −13 D)

a.   Follow-Up

The follow-up ranged from 1 month to 25 months with a mean follow-up of 10.5 months. The total number of eyes was 114.

b.   Preoperative Refraction

The preoperative spherical equivalent refraction was in the range of extremely high myopia (>-13 D). Beyond −13 D the residual stromal bed thickness is less than 250 μ, which was found in several studies (44–48) to be associated with progressive keratectasia and loss of BCVA. The mean spherical equivalent in this group was −17.7 D.

1. Refractive Outcome and Predictability

a. Postoperative Refraction

An undercorrection was seen in most of the reviewed series. The mean postoperative SE was -1.13 D.

b. Percentage Within ±1.0 D

The percentage of LASIK patients within ±1.0 D of emmetropia was 83% (41) and 73% and 54.1% (26) at 3 months postoperatively; 78% (33), 80% (34), 40.7% (35), 90.7% (36), 83% (37), 72% and 100% (42), and 72.7% and 61.5% (33) at 6 months; and 85% and 72.75% (32), 54% (38), and 96% and 91% (39) at 1 year, with an overall mean of 36.44%.

c. Percentage Within ±0.5 D

The percentage of LASIK patients within ±0.5 D of emmetropia was 56% (41) and 52.5% and 39% (26) at 3 months postoperatively; 67% (33), 26% (34), 27% (35), 72% (36), 67% (37), 20% and 43.75% (42), and 50% and 53.8% (29) at 6 months; and 50% and 57.6% (32), 23% (38), and 68% and 75% (39) at 1 year, with an overall mean of 23.18%.

2. Visual Outcome

a. Postoperative UCVA of 20/40 or Better

A UCVA of 20/40 or better was achieved by 77% (41) and 86% and 68% (26) at 3 months postoperatively; 73% (33), 69% (34), 55.7% (35), 79% (36), 91% (37), 84% and 100% (42), and 75% and 53.8% (29) at 6 months; and 77.7% and 84% (32), 85% (38), and 88% and 94.7% (39) at 1 year, with an overall mean of 34.53%.

b. Postoperative UCVA of 20/20 or Better

A UCVA of 20/20 or better was achieved by 22% (41) at 3 months postoperatively; 20% (33), 26% (35), 35% (36), 56% (37), 16% and 68.75% (42), and 29.2% and 15.4% (29) at 6 months; and 36% (38), and 76% and 55.4% (39) at 1 year, with an overall mean of 4.85%.

3. Loss of BCVA

A reduction in BCVA is consistently seen in some eyes having LASIK. It can be due to interface abnormalities, central islands, or induced irregular astigmatism. Loss of BCVA is reported in 1.2% (41) and 0% (26) at 3 months postoperatively; 4% (33,34), 3.2% (35), 2.32% (36), 3% (37), and 10.7% and 15.4% (29) at 6 months; and 6.3% and 0% (32), 2% (38), and 0% (39) at 1 year, with an overall mean of 4.55%.

E. OUTCOMES OF LASIK IN LOW (+0.5 TO +4 D) AND MODERATE HYPEROPIA (+4 TO +8D)

a. Follow-Up

The follow-up ranged from 1 month to 24 months with a mean follow-up of 7.5 months. The total number of eyes reported was 638.

b.   Preoperative Refraction

The preoperative refraction was in the range of low to moderate hyperopia (+0.5 to +8.0 D), with a mean spherical equivalent of +3.79 D for the combined group. The range was between +0.5 to +4 D (mean +2.37 D) for the low hyperopia group and between +4 to +8.5 D (mean +5.52 D) for the moderate hyperopia group.

1.   Refractive Outcome and Predictability

a.   Postoperative Refraction

An undercorrection was seen in most of the reviewed series. The postoperative spherical equivalent ranged from an overcorrection (49) of −1.13 to an undercorrection (50) of +1.5 D, with a mean spherical equivalent of +0.69 D. It was +0.34 D in the low hyperopia group and +0.88 D in the moderate hyperopia group. Most of the nomograms overcorrected the intended correction taking into account the regression of effect after hyperopic ablations.

b.   Percentage Within ±1.0 D

The percentage of LASIK patients within ±1.0 D of emmetropia was 86% (49), 75.9% (51), 85% and 58% (50), 72.7% and 56.5%, (52) 100, 95.3, and 71.4% (53) and 67% (54), with a mean of 83.4% for the combined group. It was 93.3% for the low hyperopia group and 69.9% for the moderate hyperopia group.

c.   Percentage Within ±0.5 D

The percentage of LASIK patients within ±0.5 D of emmetropia was 39% (51), 36.5% and 30.8% (52), and 42% (54), with an overall mean of 37% for the combined group. It was 38% for the low hyperopia group and 36.5% for the moderate hyperopia group.

2.   Visual Outcome

a.   Postoperative UCVA of 20/40 or Better

A UCVA of 20/40 or better was achieved by 93% (49), 66.7% (51), 95% and 90% (50), 70.6% and 78% (52), 94%, 100%, and 87.8% (53), and 91% (54), with an overall mean of 89.5% for the combined group. It was 94.4% for the low hyperopia group and 83% for the moderate hyperopia group.

b.   Postoperative UCVA of 20/20 or Better

A UCVA of 20/20 or better was achieved by 21% (49), 14.8% (51), 6.7% and 0% (52), 70.3%, 75%, and 45.3% (53), and 41% (54), with an overall mean of 51.5% for the combined group. It was 63.6% for the low hyperopia group and 34.4% for the moderate hyperopia group.

3.   Loss of BCVA

A reduction in BCVA is consistently seen in some eyes having LASIK. It can be due to interface abnormalities, decentration, or induced irregular astigmatism. Loss of BCVA is reported in 0% (49), 6.8% (51), 5% and 4.3% (50), 0% (52–54), and 2% (53), with an overall mean of 1.37% for the combined group. It was 1.1% in the low hyperopia group and 1.72% for the moderate hyperopia group.

F. OUTCOMES OF LASER ASTIGMATIC TREATMENT

In the myopic astigmatism group the total eye number was 610, and the mean preoperative and postoperative astigmatisms were -1.76 and -0.51 D, respectively. In the hyperopic astigmatism group, the total eye number was 181, and the mean preoperative and postoperative astigmatism were $+2.75$ and $+0.29$ D, respectively.

Several methods are used to analyze the outcome of astigmatic treatment, such as the vector analysis method (29,36,55) (Holladay's, Naeser's, or Alpins'), the ratio of the postoperative to the preoperative cylinder (39), and the analysis of the visual and refractive outcomes (29,31,37,55–57), The nomograms used targeted the full amount of cylinder in the majority of the studies (31,36,39). In others (29,56,58), the targeted cylinder was more than the refractive cylinder. To correct hyperopic astigmatism, Argento et al. (56) added 70% to the cylindrical correction in cylinders less or equal to $+1$ D; from 60% to 70% for cylinders between 1 and 2 D; and 50% for cylinders greater than 2 D. Salchow et al. (29) added 10% to the myopic cylindrical correction.

Undercorrection of the cylinder was the rule in most of the series reported (29,31,36, 37,39,55–59). This may be due to the inadequate nomograms and laser algorithms used and/or to the regression of effect (37,56,59).

In Zaldivar et al. series (58), 57% achieved the target refractive cylinder of 0.5 D, 27% had an undercorrection, and 4% had an overcorrection of the cylinder. In El Danasoury et al. series (39), the mean percent of cylindrical correction was 73% (range between 41.7% and 100%). The mean magnitude of the vectoral change in astigmatism was 1.23 D (range between 0.25 and 2.93 D), and the mean axis of the vectoral change was 0.37 degrees (range between -3.72 and $+13.07$ degrees) (39). In Chayet et al. series (55), 76% of eyes were within 0.5 D and 95% were within 1 D of the intended cylinder correction. Five eyes (12%) showed a cylinder overcorrection, from which only one eye was overcorrected for more than 1 D (55). At 6 months, Argento et al. (56) reported a reduction in the mean refractive cylinder from $+3.37$ to $+0.58$ D in the simple hyperopic astigmatism group, from $+3.34$ to $+0.12$ D in the compound hyperopic group, and from $+3.45$ to -0.11 D in the mixed astigmatism group. UCVA were 20/20 in 66.7%, 60.4%, and 76.5% of the groups, respectively.

Several variables may decrease the astigmatic laser treatment outcome. Among others, decentration of the treatment, the discrepancy between topographic and refractive axes, the misalignment of the corneal and laser beam astigmatic axes, posterior corneal surface astigmatism, wound healing, inaccurate laser nomograms, and regression of effect.

CONCLUSIONS

The LASIK procedure was originally practiced for the moderate to high myopia cases, but it slowly invaded the low myopia range due to its quicker and more stable visual rehabilitation than PRK. With current techniques and third-generation machinery, LASIK has proven to be a good procedure for all ranges of myopia (29–31).

The studies indicate that the predictability of LASIK decreases when the preoperative refractive error increases.

REFERENCES

1. SF Brint, DM Ostrick, C Fisher, SG Slade, RK Maloney, R Epstein, RD Stulting, KP Thompson. Six-months results of the Multicenter Phase I Study of excimer laser myopic keratomileusis. J Cataract Refract Surg 1994;20:610–615.

2. H-M Kim, HR Jung. Laser assisted in situ keratomileusis for high myopia. Ophthalmic Surg Lasers 1996;27(suppl):S508–S511.

3. MC Knorz, A Liermann, V Seiberth, H Steiner, B Wiesinger. Laser in situ keratomileusis to correct myopia of −6.00 to −29.00 diopters. J Refract Surg 1996;12:575–584.

4. FB Kremer, M Dufek. Excimer laser in situ keratomileusis. J Refract Surg 1995;11(suppl): S244–S247.

5. JJ Pérez-Santonja, J Bellot, P Claramonte, MM Ismail, JL Alio. Laser in situ keratomileusis to correct high myopia. J Cataract Refract Surg 1997;23:372–385.

6. JL Guell, A Muller. Laser in situ keratomileusis (LASIK) for myopia from −7 to −18 diopters. J Refract Surg 1996;12:222–228.

7. A Marinho, MC Pinto, R Pinto, F Vaz, MC Neves. LASIK for high myopia: one year experience. Ophthalmic Surg Lasers 1996;27(suppl):S517–S520.

8. SG Slade, SF Brint, SA Updegraff. Excimer laser myopic keratomileusis: United States experience. In: JJ Salz, ed. Corneal Laser Surgery. St Louis, MO, Mosby, 1995;195–196.

9. L Buratto, M Ferrari, C Genisi. Myopic keratomileusis with the excimer laser: one year follow up. Refract Corneal Surg 1993;9:12–19.

10. IG Pallikaris, DS Siganos. Excimer laser in situ keratomileusis and photorefractive keratectomy for correction of high myopia. J Refract Corneal Surg 1994;10:498–510.

11. IG Pallikaris, DS Siganos. Laser in situ keratomileusis to treat myopia: early experience. J Cataract Refract Surg 1997;23:39–49.

12. I Kremer, M Blumenthal. Myopic keratomileusis in situ combined with VISX 20/20 photorefractive keratectomy. J Cataract Refract Surg 1995;21:508–511.

13. SA Helmy, A Salah, T Badawy, AN Sidky. Photorefractive keratectomy and laser in situ keratomileusis for myopia between 6.00 and 10.00 diopters. J Refract Surg 1996;12:417–421.

14. DC Fiander, F Tayfour. Excimer laser in situ keratomileusis in 124 myopic eyes. J Refract Surg 1995;11(suppl):S234–S238.

15. T Salah, GO Waring III, A El Maghraby. Excimer laser keratomileusis in the corneal bed under a hinged flap: results in Saudi Arabia at the El-Maghrabi Eye Hospital. In: JJ Salz, ed. Corneal Laser Surgery. St Louis, MO, Mosby, 1995;187–195.

16. E Arneas, A Maglione. Laser in situ keratomileusis for astigmatism and myopia after penetrating keratoplasty. J Refract Surg 1997;13:27–32.

17. T Salah, GO Waring III, A El-Maghraby, K Moadel, SB Grimm. Excimer laser in situ keratomileusis under a corneal flap for myopia of 2 to 20 diopters. Am J Ophthalmol 1996;121: 143–155.

18. PI Condon, M Mulhern, T Fulcher, A Foley-Nolan, M O'Keefe. Laser intrastromal keratomileusis for high myopia and myopic astigmatism. Br J Ophthalmol 1997;81:199–206.

19. AM Bas, R Onnis. Excimer laser in situ keratomileusis for myopia. J Refract Surg 1995;11(suppl):S229–S233.

20. HV Gimbel, S Basti, GB Kaye, M Ferensowicz. Experience during the learning curve of laser in situ keratomileusis. J Cataract Refract Surg 1996;22:542–550.

21. IG Pallikaris, ME Papatzanki, DS Siganos, MK Tsilimbaris. A corneal flap technique for laser in situ keratomileusis; human studies. Arch Ophthalmol 1991;109:1699–1702.

22. L Buratto, M Ferrari, C Genisi. Keratomileusis for myopia with the excimer laser (Buratto technique): short term results. Refract Corneal Surg 1993:9(suppl):S130–S133.

23. Z Wang, J Chen, B Yang. Comparison of laser in situ keratomileusis and photorefractive keratectomy to correct myopia from −1.25 to −6 diopters. J Refract Surg 1997;13:528–534.

24. MA El Danasoury, A El Maghraby, SD Klyce, K Mehrez. Comparison of photorefractive keratectomy with excimer laser in situ keratomileusis in correcting low myopia (from −2 to −5.5 diopters). Ophthalmology 1999;106:411–421.

25. WA Pirzada, H Kalaawry. Laser in situ keratomileusis for myopia of −1 to −3.5 diopters. J Refract Surg 1997;13(suppl):S425–S426.

26. JC Casebeer, GM Kezirian. Outcomes of spherocylinder treatments in the comprehensive refractive surgery LASIK study. Semin Ophthalmol 1998;13(2):71–78.

27. M Montes, A Chayet, L Gomez, R Magallanes, N Robledo. Laser in situ keratomileusis for myopia of −1.5 to −6 diopters. J Refract Surg 1999;15:106–110.

28. SG Farah, DT Azar, C Gurdal, J Wong. Laser in situ keratomileusis: literature review of a developing technique. J Cataract Refract Surg 1998;24:989–1006.

29. DJ Salchow, ME Zirm, C Stieldorf, A Parisi. Laser in situ keratomileusis for myopia and myopic astigmatism. J Cataract Refract Surg 1998;24:175–182.

30. RL Lindstrom, DR Hardten, YR Chu. Laser in situ keratomileusis for the treatment of low, moderate, and high myopia. Trans Am Ophthalmol Soc 1997;XCV:285–306.

31. JM Davidorf, R Zaldivar, S Oscherow. Results and complications of laser in situ keratomileusis by experienced surgeons. J Refract Surg 1998;14:114–122.

32. MC Knorz, B Wiesinger, A Lierman, V Seiberth, H Liesenhoff. Laser in situ keratomileusis for moderate and high myopia and myopic astigmatism. Ophthalmology 1998;105:932–940.

33. F Lavery. Laser in situ keratomileusis for myopia. J Refract Surg 1998;14:S177–S178.

34. A Ozdamar, B Sener, C Aras, R Aktunc. Laser in situ keratomileusis after photorefractive keratectomy for myopic regression. J Cataract Refract Surg 1998;24:1208–1211.

35. PS Hersh, SF Brint, RK Maloney, DS Durrie, M Gordon, MA Michelson, VM Thompson, RB Berkeley, OD Schein, RF Steinert. Photorefractive keratectomy versus laser in situ keratomileusis for moderate to high myopia. Ophthalmology 1998;105:1512–1523.

36. GE Fraenkel, SK Webber, GL Sutton, MA Lawless, CM Rogers. Toric laser in situ keratomileusis for myopic astigmatism using an ablatable mask. J Refract Surg 1999;15:111–117.

37. DD Dulaney, RW Barnet, SA Perkins, GM Kezirian. Laser in situ keratomileusis for myopia and astigmatism: 6 month results. J Cataract Refract Surg 1998;24:758–764.

38. RF Steinert, PS Hersh. Spherical and aspherical photorefractive keratectomy and laser in situ keratomileusis for moderate to high myopia: two prospective randomized clinical trials. Trans Am Ophthalmol Soc 1998;96:197–221.

39. MA el Danasoury, GO Waring III, A El Maghraby, K Mehrez. Excimer laser in situ keratomileusis to correct compound myopic astigmatism. J Refract Surg 1997;13:511–520.

40. A Maldonado-Bass, R Onnis. Results of laser in situ keratomileusis in different degrees of myopia. Ophthalmology 1998;105:606–611.

41. R Zaldivar, JM Davidorf, S Oscherow. Laser in situ keratomileusis for myopia from −5.5 to −11.5 diopters with astigmatism. J Refract Surg 1998;14:19–25.

42. PM Pesando, MP Ghiringhello, P Tagliavacche. Excimer laser in situ keratomileusis for myopia. J Refract Surg 1997;13:521–527.

43. RJF Tsai. Laser in situ keratomileusis for myopia of −2 to −25 diopters. J Refract Surg 1997;13:S427–S429.

44. T Seiler, K Koufala, G Richter. Iatrogenic keratectasia after laser in situ keratomileusis. J Refract Surg 1998;14:312–317.

45. T Seiler, AW Quurke. Iatrogenic keratectasia after LASIK in a case of forme fruste keratoconus. J Cataract Refract Surg 1998;24:1007–1009.

46. Z Wang, J Chen, B Yang. Posterior corneal surface topographic changes after laser in situ keratomileusis are related to residual corneal bed thickness. Ophthalmology 1999;106:406–410.

47. HS Geggel, AR Talley. Delayed onset keratectasia following laser in situ keratomileusis. J Cataract Refract Surg 1999;25:582–586.

48. FW Price Jr, DL Koller, MO Price. Central corneal pachymetry in patients undergoing laser in situ keratomileusis. Ophthalmology 1999;106(11):2216–2220.

49. KA Buzard, BR Fundingsland. Excimer laser assisted in situ keratomileusis for hyperopia. J Cataract Refract Surg 1999;25:197–204.

50. K Ditzen, H Huschka, S Pieger. Laser in situ keratomileusis for hyperopia. J Cataract Refract Surg 1998;24:42–47.

51. S Goker, H Er, C Kahvecioglu. Laser in situ keratomileusis to correct hyperopia from +4.25 to +8 diopters. J Refract Surg 1998;14:26–30.
52. MC Knorz, A Lierman, B Jendritza, P Hugger. LASIK for hyperopia and hyperopic astigmatism. Semin Ophthalmol 1998;13:83–87.
53. CJ Argento, MJ Cosentino. Laser in situ keratomileusis for hyperopia. J Cataract Refract Surg 1998;24:1050–1058.
54. W Portellinha, K Nakano, M Olivieira, R Simoceli. Laser in situ keratomileusis for hyperopia after thermal keratoplasty. J Refract Surg 1999;15:S218–S220.
55. AS Chayet, R Magallanes, M Montes, S Chavez, M Robledo. Laser in situ keratomileusis for simple myopic, mixed, and simple hyperopic astigmatism. J Refract Surg 1998;14:S175–S176.
56. CJ Argento, MJ Cosentino, A Biondini. Treatment of hyperopic astigmatism. J Cataract Refract Surg 1997;23:1480–1490.
57. CC Barraquer, AM Gutierrez. Results of laser in situ keratomileusis in hyperopic compound astigmatism. J Cataract Refract Surg 1999;25:1198–1204.
58. R Zaldivar, JM Davidorf, MC Shultz, S Oscherow. Laser in situ keratomileusis for low myopia and astigmatism with a scanning spot excimer laser. J Refract Surg 1997;13:614–619.
59. O Ibrahim. Laser in situ keratomileusis for hyperopia and hyperopic astigmatism. J Refract Surg 1998;14:S179–S182.

19

Quality of Vision After LASIK

PATRICK C. YEH and DIMITRI T. AZAR

*Massachusetts Eye and Ear Infirmary, Schepens Eye Research Institute,
and Harvard Medical School, Boston, Massachusetts U.S.A.*

A. PATIENT SATISFACTION

Because of its relative safety, predictability, and quick recovery (1–8), excimer laser refractive surgery, specifically laser in situ keratomileusis (LASIK), has become widely accepted worldwide as a safe and effective method to treat refractive error. This is evidenced by the increasing popularity of the procedure among successful contact lens wearers (9).

Snellen chart visual acuity has been the "gold standard" and the most commonly utilized performance-based outcome measure both in the ophthalmic literature and in daily ophthalmic practice. In order to understand patient dissatisfaction and frustration, one needs to realize that good UVCA or best corrected visual acuity (BCVA) alone may not be enough to achieve satisfactory functional visual outcomes. Optical side effects and ocular aberrations may be detrimental to the patients' quality of vision following LASIK, and to overall their satisfaction.

Patient satisfaction has been regarded as a measure of quality of medical care and compliance with treatment regimens (10–11). Satisfaction is not easy to evaluate. A patient may be satisfied with the overall outcome of a procedure but may be dissatisfied with individual components, thereby compromising the overall quality. This concept is in particular relevant to refractive surgery. Ophthalmic refractive surgeons treat patients with relatively healthy eyes and normal preoperative corrected visual acuity, requesting high levels of postoperative outcomes.

Although LASIK can correct lower order aberrations, i.e., spherocyclinders, with great precision and success, we have come to realize that higher order aberrations of the cornea may increase after surgery (12). The satisfaction level has been relatively high after LASIK in terms of uncorrected visual acuity (UCVA) and refractive predictability and stability (13–16). However, dry eyes, glare, ghost images, and night vision disturbance can reduce quality of vision and thus patient satisfaction following laser refractive surgery (17,18).

B. STUDIES OF PATIENT SATISFACTION

Several studies have examined patient satisfaction following photorefractive keratectomy (PRK) (19–31), but only a few studies examined patient satisfaction after LASIK (7–8,17,32–33). In the most recent study by Miller et al. (17) of a patient population ranged from −0.75 to −15.75 D sphere and 0 to +4.50 D cylinder, a high level of patient satisfaction was achieved following LASIK myopic and myopic astigmatic correction. A high level of overall patient satisfaction has also been reported in other studies. As high as 90–97.9% of patients following low to moderate myopic (<10.00 D) (7,32–33) and 78–85% of high myopic correction (>10.00 D) (7–8) with LASIK were satisfied with an improved quality of life according to other publications. These studies suggest a correlation between higher satisfaction and a lower spherical correction. As with the findings observed in PRK patients (21,24), Miller et al. (17) showed a correlation between satisfaction and amounts of preoperative astigmatism. A higher mean satisfaction score was achieved among the groups with less than +2.00 D of astigmatism, with a statistical significance between the 0 to +0.75 D and +2.00 to +2.75 D cylinder groups.

When comparing PRK to LASIK, patients tend to prefer the LASIK procedure even though both PRK and LASIK have been shown to be equal in terms of efficacy, predictability, stability, and final visual outcome in correcting myopia (34–36). In a prospective randomized study of spherical equivalent correction from −2.00 to −5.50 D, el Danasoury et al. compared satisfaction of patients treated with PRK on one eye and LASIK on the fellow eye. They showed that, one year after the procedure, 83% were very satisfied with the LASIK eye while only 63% were very satisfied with the PRK eye. In an another prospective, randomized study by el Maghraby et al., LASIK produced a higher percentage of eyes (26% more eyes at 2 years) with an uncorrected visual acuity of 20/20 or better. Similarly, at one year, almost twice as many patients were highly satisfied with the LASIK-treated eye as opposed to the PRK-treated eye (90% versus 52%), although this difference became much less significant at two years (81% versus 71%).

C. OPTICAL ABERRATIONS

A number of self-perceived optical disturbances such as glare and halo have been reported after laser refractive surgery (27,32). After corneal refractive surgery, higher order aberrations of the cornea typically increase (12). Increased higher order aberrations after corneal laser surgery is also correlated with a significant decrease in quality of vision, especially under scotopic conditions (12,41,44–45). Aspheric changes in the cornea also limit visual performance under decreased illumination as pupil size increases (43). Roberts et al. have also shown that there is a persistent increase in elevation, curvature, and pachymetry outside the ablation zone (44,45). Peripheral elevation increases were strongly correlated with central flattening in a series of eyes after LASIK, suggesting a structural change in the cornea secondary to a biomechanical response over the entire cornea, independent of the ablation profile on the cornea. A 10-fold to 20-fold increase in ocular wavefront aberrations has also been reported in other studies (12,46,47).

The development of wavefront technology may help to minimize optical aberration of the eye and improve its visual quality and performance, especially under scotopic conditions. Using wavefront-guided LASIK, Seiler et al. (47) demonstrated that ocular aberrations are correctable in addition to myopia and astigmatism. An improved quality of the retinal image does not necessarily result in improved vision. Perhaps evolution has optimized the human eye to reach an optical quality that matches or exceeds the mosaic of the retinal photoreceptors (49). In addition, corneal healing after LASIK, though considered minimal, may be responsible for some regression of the refractive effect and thereby may influence spherical aberration afterwards. Mrochen and coauthors (50) conclude that wavefront-guided LASIK is not very predictable in reducing higher order optical aberrations. According to their study, only 22.5% have a significant reduction in the higher order optical aberrations, and on average there is an increase in optical aberrations by a factor of 1.44 after 3 months. Variation also exists in the effective correction among the types of aberrations, with a fair correction of coma and an insufficient correction of spherical aberrations.

D. REDUCED CONTRAST SENSITIVITY AFTER LASIK

A decrease in contrast sensitivity can deteriorate the quality of vision and impair visual function independent of Snellen visual acuity. Greater impairment in contrast sensitivity is on the other hand associated with difficulties with day and evening driving, and causes a higher number of at-fault motor vehicle accidents (48–51). After LASIK, patients may complain of reduced contrast sensitivity (52). Nakamura and coauthors (53) reported that patients with myopia ranging from -6.0 to -14.0 D experienced persistent decrease in intermediate and low CVA, while patients with -2 to -5.75 D experienced transient decreases (53).

Some authors report initial decreased contrast sensitivity, which recovers quickly with no significant change from the preoperative value at 3 months following LASIK (43). Mutyala et al. (54) report a slight decrease in contrast sensitivity at the higher frequencies (12 and 18 cycles/degree), which improves by 1 month after surgery at 18 cycles/degree, but remained depressed at 12 cycles/degree for at least 3 months after LASIK, which was within the normal range. Based on the results, they concluded that LASIK has little effect on contrast sensitivity for patients with up to -13.75 D of myopia and $+5.25$ of astigmatism.

E. EFFECT OF LASIK ON UNCORRECTED DAYTIME VISION

Miller et al. (17) noted that 96% of eyes treated with LASIK were able to enjoy freedom from corrective lenses. McGhee et al. (33) reported that 81% to 100% of patients had functional improvement and satisfaction across the spectrum of visual tasks assessed using a questionnaire-based cross-sectional study; 85.1% perceived improvement in reading without correction in natural light. Most patients also noted significant improvement in their ability to drive in daylight (94.0%), watch television (95.7%), or watch movie at a cinema (95.0%). Other functional tasks with a marked improvement after LASIK include the ability to play sports (97.5%), to swim (100%), and to shop (91.3%) without refractive aids. Only two patients expressed disappointment with the postoperative UCVA. However, both patients had had more than 5.00 D or anisometropia before LASIK, and only one eye was treated to balance the refraction with that in the untreated eye.

F. EFFECT OF LASIK ON NIGHT VISION

Reduced clarity with night vision was noted in 29% in the study by Miller et al. (17). McGhee et al. (33) identified 11.8% of patients with increased difficulty with nighttime driving with 8.8% reported being "much worse." The authors note that none of these patients had a central ablation zone diameter of less than 5.0 mm and all of them had an ablation centration within 0.5 mm of the center of the pupil.

Similar problems with nighttime vision were also identified in eyes treated with PRK (20,22–23,26). In one study of patient satisfaction after bilateral PRK (25), over 60% noted reduced quality of vision in dim light relative to daylight, and as high as 50% reported night driving difficulties. Freitas et al. (29), using pre- and post-PRK questionnaires, identified a net subjective functional improvement in night driving. Brunette et al. (31) reported that 66.1% of patients perceived poorer night vision relative to daytime vision, 20.2% of patients thought that their night vision was poor or very poor, 68.3% of patients noted that night vision was either the same or better than before surgery, and 31.7% reported that it was worse or much worse.

These findings demonstrate that difficulties with nighttime vision and driving still pose a significant problem for a fair number of patients, thus reducing the overall quality of vision. It is a potential side effect of refractive surgery that should not be underestimated or understated to the patients seeking refractive surgery.

The visual disturbances associated with decreased night vision are not unique to patients who receive surgical refractive correction. Patients using spectacles or contact lenses also report similar visual problems with glare, halo, and reduced contrast sensitivity, especially at night. Nevertheless, given the unique demographics and psychological profile of most patients seeking refractive surgery, patient expectations are high; many patients want perfect UCVA to get rid of their spectacles or contact lenses but without unwanted visual aberrations. Future advances in laser technology, such as the active eye tracking system, variable spot scanning laser, and wavefront analysis, may minimize these aberrations. The journey to achieving an aberration-free refractive vision correction, or the so-called super vision, is long. Until then, it is important to realize that visual acuity alone is not an indicator of patient satisfaction and visual function. Careful patient selection, thorough evaluation, patient education, and informed consent about these potential side effects cannot be overemphasized.

REFERENCES

1. T Seiler, J Wollensak. Myopic photorefractive keratectomy with excimer laser; one-year follow-up. Ophthalmology 1991;98:1156–1163.
2. DS Gartry, MG Kerr Muir, J Marshall. Excimer laser photorefractive keratectomy: 18 month follow-up. Ophthalmology 1992;99:1209–1219.
3. T Seiler, A Holschbach, M Derse, B Jean, U Genth. Complications of myopic photorefractive keratectomy with the excimer laser. Ophthalmology 1994;101:153–160.
4. SL Trokel, R Srinnivasan, B Braren. Excimer laser surgery of the cornea. Am J Ophthalmol 1983;96:710–715.
5. D Epstein, P Fagerholm, H Hamberg-Nystrom, B Tentroth. Twenty-four-month follow-up of excimer laser photorefractive keratectomy for myopia; refractive and visual acuity results. Ophthalmology 1994;101:1558–1563.
6. S Dutt, RF Steinert, MB Raizman, CA Puliafito. One-year results of excimer laser photorefractive keratectomy for low to moderate myopia. Arch Ophthalmol 1994;112:1427–1436.

7. MC Knorz, B Wiesinger, A Liermann, V Seiberth, H Liesenhoff. Laser in situ keratomileusis for moderate and high myopia and myopic astigmatism. Ophthalmology 1998;105:932–940.

8. A Marinho, MC Pinto, R Pinto, F Vaz, MC Neves. LASIK for high myopia: one year experience. Ophthalmic Surg Lasers 1996;27(5 suppl):S517–S520.

9. MK Migneco, JS Pepose. Attitudes of successful contact lens wearers toward refractive surgery. J Refract Surg 1996;12:128–133.

10. KJ Roghmann, A Hengst, TR Zastowny. Satisfaction with medical care: its measurement and relation to utilization. Medical Care 1979;17:461–477.

11. J Kincey, P Bradshaw, P Ley. Patients' satisfaction and reported acceptance of advice in general practice. J Roy Coll Gen Pract 1975;25:558–566.

12. T Oshika, SD Klyce, RA Applegate, HC Howland, MA El Danasoury. Comparison of corneal wavefront aberrations after photorefractive keratectomy and laser in situ keratomileusis. Am J Ophthalmol 1999;127:1–7.

13. DD Dulaney, RW Barnet, SA Perkins, GM Kezirian. Laser in situ keratomileusis for myopia and astigmatism: 6 month results. J Cataract Refract Surg 1998;24:758–764.

14. FB Kremer, M Dufek. Excimer laser in situ keratomileusis. J Refract Surg 1995;11(suppl):S244–247.

15. AM Bas, R Onnis. Excimer laser in situ keratomileusis for myopia. J Refract Surg 1995;11(suppl):S229–233.

16. A Maldonado-Bas, R Onnis. Results of laser in situ keratomileusis in different degrees of myopia. Ophthalmology 1998;105:606–611.

17. AE Miller, JP McCulley, RW Bowman, HD Cavanagh, XH Wang. Patient satisfaction after LASIK for myopia. CLAO 2001;27(2):84–88.

18. M Lipner. LASIK-related dry eyes: putting the condition on the map. Eye World 1999(Aug);20–22.

19. BL Halliday. Refractive and patient satisfaction results following bilateral photorefractive keratectomy for myopia. Refract Corneal Surg 1993;9(suppl):S5–S11.

20. A Ben-Sira, A Loewenstein, I Lipshitz, D Levanon, M Lazar. Patient satisfaction after 5.0 mm photorefractive keratectomy for myopia. J Refract Surg 1997;13:129–134.

21. AA Rushood, HM Nassim, T Azeemuddin. Patient satisfaction after photorefractive keratectomy for low myopia using the visual analogue scale. J Refract Surg 1997;13(suppl):S438–S440.

22. AS Al-Kaff. Patient satisfaction after photorefractive keratectomy. J Refract Surg 1997;13(suppl):S459–S460.

23. OB Hadden, CP Ring, AT Morris, MJ Elder. Visual, refractive, and subjective outcomes after photorefractive keratectomy for myopia of 6 to 10 diopters using the Nidek laser. J Cataract Refract Surg 1999;25:936–942.

24. S Shah, S Perera, A Chatterjee. Satisfaction after photorefractive keratectomy. J Refract Surg 1998;13:S226–S227.

25. HV Gimble, JA Van Westenbrugge, WH Johnson, et al. Visual, refractive, and patient satisfaction results following bilateral photorefractive keratectomy for myopia. Refract Corneal Surg 1993;9(suppl):S5–S10.

26. G Kahle, T Seiler, J Wollensak. Report on psychosocial findings and satisfaction among patients 1 year after excimer laser photorefractive keratectomy Refract Corneal Surg 1992;8:286–289.

27. W Verdon, M Bullimore, RK Maloney. Visual performance after photorefractive keratectomy. Arch Ophthalmol 1996;144:1465–1472.

28. CM Fichte, AM Bell. Ongoing results of excimer laser photorefractive keratectomy for myopia: subjective patient impressions. J Cataract Refract Surg 1994;20(suppl):268–270.

29. C Freita, BM Oliveiro, E Marques, EB Leite. Effect of photorefractive keratectomy on visual functioning and quality of life. J Refract Surg 1995;11(suppl):S327–334.

30. H Hamberg-Nystrom, B Tengroth, P Fagerholm, D Epstein, EM van der Kwast. Patient satis-
    faction following photorefractive keratectomy for myopia. J Refract Surg 1995;11(suppl):
    S335–336.

31. I Brunette, J Gresset, JF Boivin, M Pop, P Thompson, GP Lafond, H Makni. Functional out-
    come and satisfaction after photorefractive keratectomy. Part 2: Survey of 690 patients. Oph-
    thalmology 2000;107(9):1790–1796.

32. DJ Salchow, ME Zirm, C Stieldorf, A Parisi. LASIK for correction of myopia and astigmatism.
    Ophthalmologe 1998;95(3):142–147.

33. CNJ McGhee, JP Craig, N Sachdev, K Weed, AD Brown. Functional, psychological, and sat-
    isfaction outcomes of laser in situ keratomileusis for high myopia. J Cataract Refract Surg
    2000;26:497–509.

34. MA el Danasoury, A el Maghraby, SD Klyce, K Mehrez. Comparison of photorefractive kera-
    tectomy with excimer laser in situ keratomileusis in correcting low myopia (from −2.00 to
    −5.50 diopters). Ophthalmology 1999;106(2):411–421.

35. A el Maghraby, T Salah, GO Waring III, SD Klyce, O Ibrahim. Randomized bilateral compar-
    ison of excimer laser in situ keratomileusis and photorefractive keratectomy for 2.50 to 8.00
    diopters of myopia. Ophthalmology 1999;106(3):447–457.

36. IG Pallikaris, DS Siganos. Excimer laser in situ keratomileusis and photorefractive keratectomy
    for correction of high myopia. J Refract Corneal Surg 1994;10:498–510.

37. CNJ McGhee, D Orr, B Kidd, C Stark, IG Bryce, CN Anastas. Psychological aspects of excimer
    laser surgery for myopia: reasons for seeking treatment and patient satisfaction. Br J Ophthal-
    mol 1996;80:874–879.

38. MK Powers, BE Meyerowitz, PN Arrowsmith, RG Marks. Psychosocial findings in radial ker-
    atotomy patients two years after surgery. Ophthalmology 1984;91:1193–1198.

39. AA Ghaith, J Daniel, RD Stulting, KP Thompson, M Lynn. Contrast sensitivity and glare dis-
    ability after radial keratotomy and photorefractive keratectomy. Arch Ophthalmol 1998;116:
    12–18.

40. CP Lohmann, F Fitzke, D O'Brart, MK Muir, G Timberlake, J Marshall. Corneal light scatter-
    ing and visual performance in myopic individuals with spectacles, contact lenses, or excimer
    laser photorefractive keratectomy. Am J Ophthalmol 1993;115:444–453.

41. KM Oliver, RP Hemenger, MC Corbett, DP O'Brart, S Verma, J Marshall, A Tomlinson.
    Corneal optical aberrations induced by photorefractive keratectomy. J Refract Surg 1997;13:
    246–254.

42. JW Blaker, PS Hersh. Theoretical and clinical effect of preoperative corneal curvature on ex-
    cimer laser photorefractive keratectomy. J Refract Corneal Surg 1994;10:571–574.

43. JT Holladay, DR Dudeja, J Chang. Functional vision and corneal changes after laser in situ ker-
    atomileusis determined by contrast sensitivity, glare testing, and corneal toppography. J
    Cataract Refract Surg 1999;25:663–669.

44. C Roberts, A Mahmoud, EE Herderick, G Chan. Characterization of corneal curvature changes
    inside and outside the ablation zone in LASIK. Invest Ophthalmol Vis Sci 2000;41(suppl):
    S679.

45. C Roberts. Future challenges to aberration-free ablative procedures. J Refract Surg 2000;
    16(suppl):S623–S629.

46. C Martinez, R Applegate, S Klyce, M McDonald, I Medina, CK Howland. Effects of pupillary
    dilation on corneal optical aberrations after photorefractive keratectomy. Arch Ophthalmol
    1998;116:1053–1062.

47. T Seiler, M Kaemmerer, P Mierdel, HE Krinke. Ocular optical aberrations after photorefractive
    keratectomy for myopia and myopic astigmatism. Arch Ophthalmol 2000;118:17–21.

48. JM Wood, R Troutbeck. Elderly drivers and simulated visual impairment. Optom Vis Sci
    1995;72:115–124.

49. GS Rubin, KB Roche, P Prasada-Rao, LP Fried. Visual impairment and disability in older
    adults. Clin Vis Sci 1994;71:750–756.

50. K Ball, C Owsley, ME Sloane, DL Roenker, JR Bruni. Visual attention problems as a predictor of vehicle crashes in older drivers. Invest Ophthalmol Vis Sci 1993;34:3110–3123.

51. C Owsley, K Ball, G McGwin Jr. Visual processing impairment and risk of motor vehicle crash among older adults. JAMA 1998;279:1083–1088.

52. JJ Perez-Santonja, HF Sakla, JL Alio. Contrast sensitivity after laser in situ keratomileusis. J Cataract Refract Surg 1998;24:183–189.

53. K Nakamura, H Bissen-Miyajima, I Toda, Y Hori, K Tsubota. Effect of laser in situ keratomileusis correction on contrast visual acuity. J Cataract Refract Surg 2001;27:358–361.

54. S Mutyala, MB McDonald, KA Scheinblum, MD Ostrick, SF Brint, H Thompson. Contrast sensitivity evaluation after laser in situ keratomileusis. Ophthalmology 2000;107(10):1864–1867.

LASIK for Hyperopia, Hyperopic Astigmatism, and Presbyopia

NEAL A. SHER

*University of Minnesota Medical School and Phillips Eye Institute,
Minneapolis, Minnesota, U.S.A.*

A. INTRODUCTION

Until recently, the surgical correction of hyperopia and presbyopia has lagged behind the surgery of myopia in terms of patient demand and investigative efforts. Early surgical attempts at hyperopic correction included hexagonal keratotomy (1), automated lamellar keratoplasty (2), epikeratophakia (3), and keratophakia (4). These procedures all had very limited success. They were either very difficult to perform or were unstable and unpredictable and caused irregular astigmatism.

When we reviewed this subject for a textbook in 1997 (5), the number of papers published on the surgery for hyperopia and presbyopia was a small fraction of those published on myopia. Although the amount of research effort and published material is now much larger, it still lags behind myopia. A cynic might conclude that research efforts have concentrated on myopia because most investigators who have a refractive error are myopic and the amount of myopia is directly correlated with intelligence. Does this mean that the smartest nearsighted investigators have been unleashed on this problem? The real answer lies in a combination of physiology, demographics, and economics. It is easier to flatten the cornea permanently for myopia than to steepen it centrally for hyperopia. The preoperative uncorrected vision plays a significant role in the motivation to undergo refractive surgery; a thirty-year-old myope is more likely to seek corrective surgery than 30-year-old three-diopter hyperope. In the last several years, the explosive growth of LASIK has led to a more intense interest in the treatment of hyperopia, hyperopic astigmatism, and presbyopia. This chapter will explore this recent work.

B. LASIK FOR HYPEROPIA

The early studies of the treatment of hyperopia with PRK were not encouraging. Maloney et al. (6) were unable to achieve a hyperopic correction using an erodible PMMA mask in experimental animals. Our group showed very limited success in reducing hyperopic shift after excimer PTK by attempting to steepen the peripheral corneal with an early prototype excimer laser (7). The use of automated lamellar keratoplasty (H-ALK) for hyperopia caused a deliberate corneal ectasia. The results of H-ALK were not satisfactory and produced irregular astigmatism as well as progressive ectasia in some patients (8). Other work showed significant regression and limited predictability. Ditzen and Nadimi demonstrated that it was possible to treat hyperopic refractive errors of more than 3 diopters. In a preliminary study, they reported more predictable results than with H-PRK (9). Condon reported another small series in 10 eyes ranging from +2 to +9 with an average correction at 6 months of +1.5 D (10). Other studies published at the same time also led investigators to modify and refine their techniques (11). The early encouraging results of myopic LASIK led surgeons to attempt LASIK for hyperopic errors. These initial studies pointed out that a number of technical challenges needed to be overcome before H-LASIK could be considered successful.

C. METHODS OF HYPEROPIC CORRECTION

In contrast to myopic correction, to achieve hyperopic change, one must permanently steepen the central cornea. A typical hyperopic profile, in this case from the VISX Star S2, is shown in Fig. 20.1. A comparison of the hyperopic profiles of ablation (2A) with those of myopic (2B) and astigmatic (2C and 2D) profiles is shown in Fig. 20.2.

Various laser systems accomplish this by different methods. The Summit Apex Plus laser utilizes an Axicon lens system to deliver most of the energy between 6.5 mm and out to 9.5 mm. The Axicon lens diverges the laser beam. The laser also uses an erodible disc, which absorbs laser energy so as to produce a smooth transition zone. The Chiron Technolas PlanoScan excimer laser (various models including the 117c and 217) delivers laser pulses (2 mm) at a relative high frequency (25 Hz) in a circular pattern over the cornea and optical zone of 6 to 9 mm (12). The VISX Star S2 laser utilizes a similar system, as pictured here (Figs. 20.3 and 20.4).

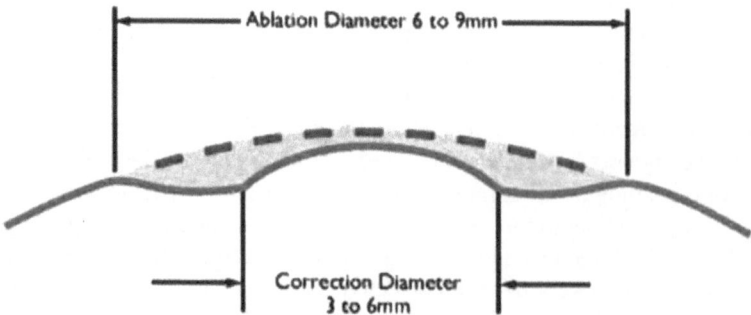

Figure 20.1   A typical hyperopic profile, in this case from the VISX Star S2 excimer laser. (Photo courtesy of Edward Manche, M.D., Palo Alto, CA.)

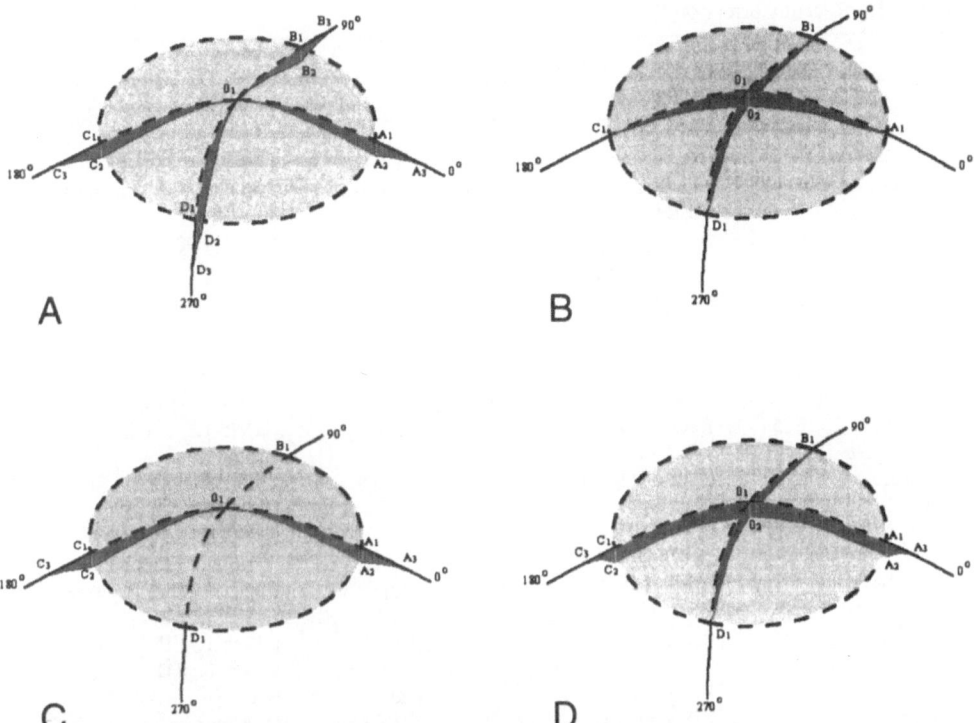

Figure 20.2   Ablation profiles of spherical hyperopia (A) results in twice the volume of tissue removal in hyperopic astigmatism (C). Myopic spherical treatments (B) result in approximately half the volume of tissue removed for the correction of myopic astigmatism (D).

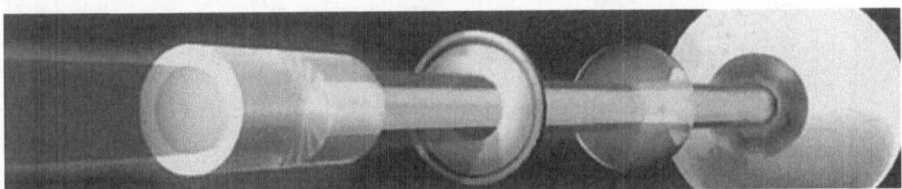

Figure 20.3   VISX STAR S2 laser, beam is subdivided into 7 beamlets. (Courtesy of VISX Inc.)

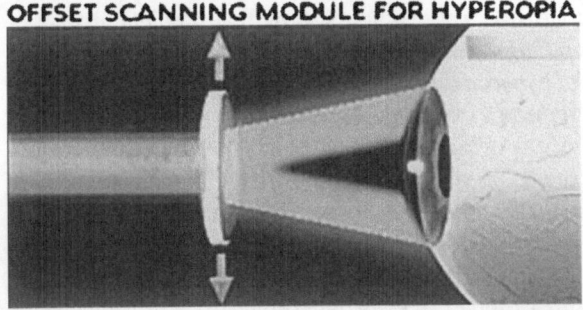

Figure 20.4   VISX STAR S2, laser beam offset scanning to achieve hyperopic ablation pattern.

Table 1 Recent Correction Studies

Study/year	# eyes	Laser/flap	Follow up (mos)	Treatment zone	Preop refractive error, range, SE	Postop refractive error, range, SE (D)
K. Ditzen et al., 1998	43	Aesculap-Meditec MEL 60	12	7.5 mm	2.50 ± 1.70 1 to 4 5.28 ± 1.92	0.33 ± 1.12 1.91 ± 1.83
S. Goker et al., 1998	54	Keracor 116	19	8.5 mm	6.5 ± 1.3	0.4 ± 1.9
C.J. Argento et al., 1998	203	Keracor 116/117 planoscan	6–12	8.1 to 9.5	1.68 ± 0.75 1.25 to 2.50 D	0.39 ± 0.70
CJ Argento et al., 1998	225	Same	6–12	Same	2.98 ± 0.44 D 2.25 ± 4.75 D	0.48 ± 0.75
CJ Argento et al., 1998	251	Same	6–12	Same	6.12 ± 1.71 D 5.59 ± 8.50 D	0.88 ± 0.96
M. Knorz, 1998	23	Keracor 117 C 8.5 mm flap		0 to 8.0 mm	NA D. Aron-rosa 5.1 to 10 D	
O. Ibrahim, 1998	58	Nidek EC 5000	6		3.75 D	2.25
D Aron-Rosa, 1999	20	Nidek EC-5000	3 to 6	5.25 to 8.25 mm	2.72 D 2 to 6.0 D	0.51 ± 0.87
	20	Nidek EC-5000	3 to 6	5.50 to 8.25 mm	2.75 2.00 to 6.0 D	−0.32 ± 1.42
D. Zadok, 2000	45	Nidek EC-5000	6	5.5 to 7.5 mm	2.02 ± 0.51	
D. Zadok, 2000	27	Nidek EC-5000	6	3.78 ± 0.57	1.09 ± 0.92	

Table 1 summarizes some of the recent studies (9,13–18) and shows encouraging results with several different excimer lasers. The studies show that the procedure is safe, having similar complications to myopic LASIK. These studies show that predictability after hyperopic LASIK is only moderate and lags behind myopic LASIK in predictability. One of the problems in assessing results in hyperopic surgery is the measurement uncorrected visual acuity. Unlike myopia, this parameter is very age dependent.

In the studies, which reported results in this manner, 67% to 100% achieved corrections within 1 D of the intended. In a small series of 14 eyes, Buzard and Fundingsland (19) found that 85% of eyes achieved a correction within 1 diopter. The predictability falls off sharply for higher hyperopic corrections. H-LASIK however was much better than some of the predecessor procedures such as ALK. For example, Manche (20) reported that only 41% of eyes achieved outcomes within 1 diopter in eyes undergoing ALK for hyperopia. Regression of effect was seen in a number of the reported series. The higher the attempted

Predictability			Loss of BCVA >2 lines	UCVA 20/40 or better	UCVA 20/20 or better	Retreatment	Complications	Comments
Within 0.5 D	Within 1.0 D	Within 2.0 D						
			5%		95		15% epithelial ingrowth, 7.5% haze interface 4.7% decent ration, 2.3% central island, 11.6% horizontal striae	
			4.3%		90			
	76%		6.8%					
	100			94.1			6.8% striae, decentration 3.5% free cap 2.9%	Complications of total series
	95.3			100				
	71.4			87.8				
100%	100%	100%						Spherical cases only
50%	67%	100%						
89%			0	96%	42%	20%		
52%			1.4%	78%	26%	33%		

hyperopic correction, the higher the regression. The mechanism of regression may be epithelial thickening. This was demonstrated by Reinstein et al. using high frequency ultrasound (21). This thickening begins at a point precisely coincident with the beginning of the donut-shaped zone of stromal tissue removal. It reverses the contouring effect of the laser ablation.

D. HYPEROPIC ASTIGMATISM

1. Earlier Work

The treatment of astigmatism with hyperopia presents the surgeon with an additional challenge. In myopia, the treatment of astigmatism involves flattening the steep meridian (Fig. 2D). Early studies by C. Barraquer showed poor results when this approach was used (22). In a subsequent study, C. Barraquer et al. attempted to steepen the flatter meridian (23). Using the Schwind-Keratom laser with a MultiScan system and active tracking, 111 eyes were treated. In this series, 54.5% of eyes were within ±0.5 D of emmetropia at 6 months for defects up to 9.75 D. The cylindrical component in steepening the flatter meridian was accurate to within ±0.50 D and with ±1.00 D in 90% of eyes.

Argento et al. reported another series in which steepening the flattest meridian was attempted by utilizing a variety of techniques utilizing the Keracor 116/117 laser (24). This technique produced a steepening in the flattest meridian, with almost no effect on the opposite meridian (Fig. 2C). The results with mixed astigmatism were quite good and better than simple astigmatism and compound astigmatism, although the degree of hyperopia was high in the latter group.

2. More Recent Work

The VISX STAR S2 laser corrects hyperopia and astigmatism using seven scanning beams over the cornea and offsetting them to effect an ablation out to 9.0 mm. Doane et al. (25) recently presented data on 100 eyes with hyperopia from 0.5 to 6.0 D (mean +2.08) and a cylinder from 0.5 to 4.0 (mean 0.74 D). They utilized the Hansatome and a 9.5 mm ring and an external fixation device to reduce decentration. The results were satisfactory with an effective reduction in hyperopic sphere and cylinder. The vast majority of eyes maintained, gained, or lost one line of best corrected visual acuity. In another study by Manche (20) using the same laser, good results were obtained with a mean pre and post of cycloplegic spherical equivalent of +3.23 and −0.21 D, respectively. There was a 70% reduction in mean astigmatism as measured by vector analysis and no loss of BCVA.

In another recent study, Ruiz (26) performed a study on 60 hyperopic eyes ranging from 4.0 to 6.75 D. The preoperative mean refraction was 5.24 D and the postoperative mean refraction was +0.46 D. The preoperative cylinder was 2.38 D and postoperatively it was 0.90 D. At one year, there was no loss of contrast sensitivity and a loss of 2 lines of BCVA in 2.4% of patients.

Azar and Primack's study of LASIK ablation profiles in hyperopic and mixed astigmatism showed that patients with compound hyperopic or mixed astigmatism may benefit from reduced ablation depths using hyperopic cylindrical and/or combined cylindrical treatments (27). In this study, the theoretical depths of tissue ablation during LASIK treatments of similar amounts of myopic spherical versus myopic cylindrical errors were compared. Similar comparisons of hyperopic spherical versus hyperopic cylindrical error were also performed. The depths of tissue ablation in the following four treatment approaches for both compound hyperopic astigmatism and mixed astigmatism were then compared. Figure 20.5 shows the patterns of ablation of correcting hyperopic with-the-rule astigmatism, and Fig. 20.6 shows the patterns of correcting mixed astigmatism.

In this study they demonstrate that the combined use of hyperopic spherical and myopic cylindrical corrections to treat hyperopic astigmatism or mixed astigmatism incurs the greatest amount of central and peripheral corneal tissue ablation and therefore may be the least optimal therapeutic alternative. Ironically, this treatment alternative was the only available laser surgical option for refractive surgeons in the United States to treat compound hyperopic or mixed astigmatism until October 2000. Although the final optical result may be the same, different strategies vary in the depth, profile, and amount of tissue ablation. Future studies comparing the visual outcomes of the above method of correcting hyperopic and mixed astigmatism should yield valuable clinical data that may strengthen these theoretical predictions.

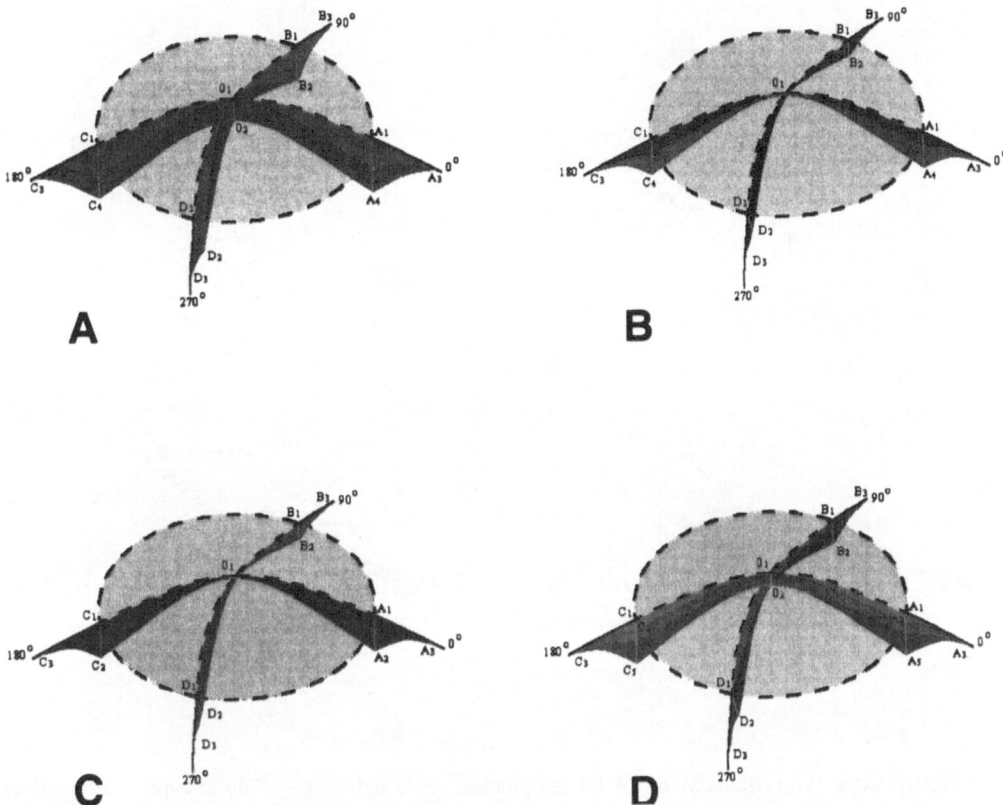

Figure 20.5 (A) (Azar) Hyperopic WTR astigmatism corrected with a +5.00 D hyperopic spherical (green) and a −3.00 D myopic cylindrical (blue) laser ablation pattern applied to the LASIK bed (resulting in greatest central ablation and volume of tissue removed). (B) (Azar) Hyperopic WTR astigmatism corrected with a +2.00 D hyperopic spherical (dark green) and +3.00 D hyperopic cylindrical (green) laser ablation pattern applied to the LASIK bed. Note absent ablation in central cornea. (C) (Azar) Hyperopic WTR astigmatism corrected with a +2.00 D × 180 (green) and =5.00 D × 90 (dark green) combined hyperopic cylindrical laser ablation pattern applied to the LASIK bed. Note absent ablation in central cornea. (D) (Azar) Hyperopic WTR astigmatism corrected with a combined cross-cylinder (+1.50 D × 90 [green] and −1.50 D × 180 [blue]) and +3.50 D SE (dark green) laser ablation pattern applied to the LASIK bed. Note intermediate depth and volume of ablation. [Color in original.]

E. H-LASIK IN APHAKIA

Ruiz also treated a series of aphakic patients (26) who could not undergo intraocular lens implantation. In 12 aphakic eyes, the preoperative average MR was +10.90 D and after surgery, at one year, it was 0.87 D. Centration and axis alignment are critical on these higher hyperopic cases, and Ruiz decenters the center of his ablation by 0.5 mm nasally.

F. LASIK AFTER PRIOR REFRACTIVE SURGERY

H-LASIK has been used for the treatment of consecutive hyperopia after RK, PRK, LTK, and myopic LASIK. Manche in the above series treated 29 eyes (12 post RK, 13 post

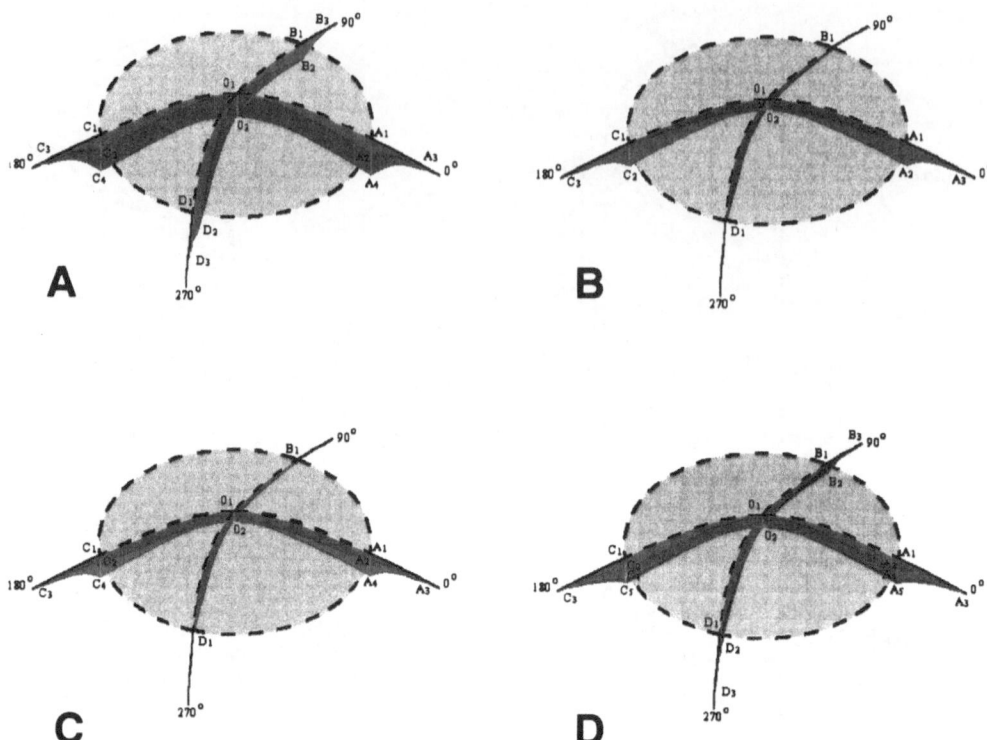

Figure 20.6 (A) (Azar) Mixed WTR astigmatism corrected with a +200 D hyperopic spherical (green) and a −3.00 D myopic cylindrical (blue) laser ablation pattern applied to the LASIK bed. Note greatest volume and depth of ablation. (B) (Azar) Mixed WTR astigmatism corrected with a −1.00 D myopic spherical (blue) and a +3.00 D hyperopic cylindrical (green) laser ablation pattern applied to the LASIK bed. (C) (Azar) Mixed WTR astigmatism corrected with combined −1.00 D myopic cylindrical (blue) and +2.00 D hyperopic cylindrical (green) laser ablation patterns applied to the LASIK bed. (D) (Azar) Mixed WTR astigmatism corrected with a combined cross-cylinder (+1.50 D × 90 [green] and −1.50 D × 180 [blue] and +0.50 D SE (dark green) laser ablation pattern applied to the LASIK bed. Note intermediate depth and volume of ablation. [Color in original.]

LASIK, 4 post PRK) for consecutive hyperopia with no difference in outcomes from the congenital hyperopia (astigmatism) group. A successful treatment for the growing number of consecutive hyperopia after RK has been elusive. Compression sutures, hyperopic PRK, and LTK have all been tried but not have had a high degree of success. Linebarger (28) has reported good success with LASIK post RK in 16 eyes with no increase in haze or loss of BCVA. There was one eye with epithelial ingrowth; see Figure 20.7). Portellinha et al. (29) and Attia et al. (30) reported good success after undercorrected hyperopia after LTK. The predictability was less than for primary H-LASIK.

G. COMPLICATIONS

In the early studies, the complication rates were relatively high, indicating a learning curve for the new LASIK procedure and keratomes that were not as reliable as the ones now available.

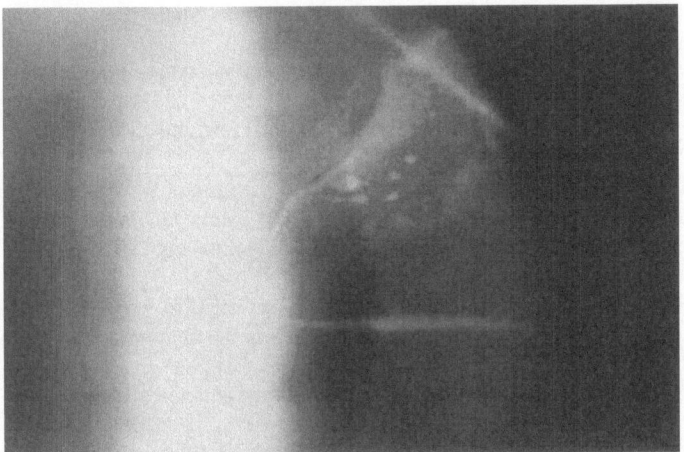

Figure 20.7   Epithelial ingrowth following H-LASIK for consecutive hyperopia after radial keratotomy. (Photo courtesy of Eric Linebarger, M.D., San Diego, CA.)

There were some complications that seemed to be higher in H-LASIK than in myopic LASIK. This included higher rates of decentration than in myopia. This resulted in loss of best corrected spectacle acuity. Probst et al. (31) and Ozdamar et al. (32) reported an epithelial pigmentation ring pattern, which they called a pseudo-Fleischer ring, after H-LASIK. A case of acute angle closure glaucoma after H-LASIK has been reported (33). Otherwise, the complications in H-LASIK were similar to those in myopia.

H.   PRESBYOPIC LASIK FOR PRESBYOPIA

With over 100,000,000 presbyopic individuals in the U.S. alone, the search for a successful correction of presbyopia has become the holy grail of refractive surgery. Research has centered on LASIK as well as scleral expansion techniques. The first description of presbyopic correction using the excimer laser was made by Anschutz in the early 1990s (34–36). Patients who are emmetropes or low hyperopes have the best results, while those with greater degrees of refractive error regress more. The principal problems experienced by most patients are a slight loss of uncorrected distance acuity and ghosting or double contours on images. This ghosting was typically worse at distance.

More recently, Bauerberg (37) described his results with an off-center ablation after LASIK to correct hyperopia and presbyopia. In a series of 16 eyes, all patients had a centered ablation in one eye and an inferior decentered ablation (1 mm) in the other eye. The patients with hyperopia that underwent inferior decentered ablation were able to read for a prolonged period of time, compared with eyes that had the conventional centered excimer laser ablation. Patients with steepened corneas in the inferior and eccentric zone ended up with better distance and near vision. There was no loss of best corrected spectacle acuity.

REFERENCES

1.   WL Basuk, M Zisman, GO Waring, LA Wilson, PS Binder, KP Thompson, HE Grossniklaus, RD Stulting. Complications of hexagonal keratotomy. Am J Ophthalmol 1994;117:37–49.

2. EE Manche, A Judge, RK Maloney. Lamellar keratoplasty for hyperopia. J Refract Surg 1996;12:42–49.
3. MH Friedlander, LF Rich, TP Werblin, HE Kaufman, N Granet. Keratophakia using preserved lenticules. Ophthalmology 1980;87:687–692.
4. RC Troutman, C Swinger. Refractive keratoplasty: keratophakia and keratomileusis. Trans Am Ophthal Soc 1978;76:329–339.
5. NA Sher, ed. Surgery of Hyperopia and Presbyopia. Baltimore: Williams and Wilkins, 1997.
6. RK Maloney, M Friedman, T Harmon, M Hayward, K Hagen, RP Gailitis, GO Waring III. A prototype erodible mask delivery system for the excimer laser. Ophthalmology 1993;100:542–549.
7. NA Sher, RA Bowers, RW Zabel, JM Frantz, RA Eiferman, DC Brown, JJ Rowsey, P Parker, V Chen, RL Lindstrom. Clinical use of the 193 nm excimer laser in the treatment of corneal scars. Arch Opthalmol 1991;109:491–498.
8. GM Kezirian, CM Gremillion. Automated lamellar keratoplasty for the correction of hyperopia. J Cataract Surg 1995;21:386–392.
9. K Ditzen, H Nadimi. Mid-summer symposium and scientific exhibition. International Society of Refractive Surgery, Minneapolis, MN, July 1996.
10. P Condon. Presented at the symposium on small incision cataract surgery, Rome 1996. Summarized in: HK Wu, VM Thompson, RF Steinert, SG Slade, PS Hersh. Refractive Surgery. New York: Thieme, 1999.
11. E Suarez, F Torres, M Duplessie. LASIK for correction of hyperopia and hyperopia with astigmatism. Int Ophthalmol Clin 1996;11:248–258.
12. MC Arbelaez. In Machat et al., eds. The Art of LASIK, 2d ed. New Jersey: Slack, 1999, pp 311–315.
13. S Goker, H Er, C Kahvecioglu. Laser in situ keratomileusis to correct hyperopia from +4.25 to +8.00 diopters. J Refract Surg 1998;14(1):26–30.
14. M Knorz, A Liemann, B Jendritza, P Hugger. LASIK for hyperopic astigmatism—results of a pilot study.
15. O Ibrahim. Laser in situ keratomileusis for hyperopia and hyperopic astigmatism. J Refract Surg 1998;14:S179–S182.
16. DS Aron-Rosa, JL Febbraro. Laser in situ keratomileusis for hyperopia. J Refract Surg 1999;15(suppl):S212–S215.
17. D Zadok, G Maskaleris, M Montes, S Shah, V Garcia, A Chayet. Hyperopic laser in situ keratomileusis with the Nidek EC-5000 excimer laser. Ophthalmology 2000;107(6):1132–1177.
18. CJ Argento, MJ Cosentino. Laser in situ keratomileusis for hyperopia. J Cataract Refract Surg 1998;24:1050–1058.
19. K Buzard, B Fundingsland. Excimer laser assisted in situ keratomileusis for hyperopia. J Cataract Refract Surg 1999;25:197–204.
20. EE Manche. Hyperopic LASIK for simple hyperopia and compound hyperopic using the VISX STAR S2 Smoothscan. Presented at American Society of Cataract and Refractive Surgery, April 1999.
21. DZ Reinstein, RH Silverman, HFS Sutton, DJ Coleman. Very high-frequency ultrasound corneal analysis identifies anatomic correlates of optical complications of lamellar refractive surgery. Ophthalmology 1999;106:474–482.
22. CC Barraquer. Laser in situ keratomileusis. In L Burrato, SF Brint, eds. LASIK; Principles and Techniques. Thorofare, NJ: Slack, 1998, pp 215–223.
23. CC Barraquer, M Gutierrez. Results of laser in situ keratomileusis in hyperopic compound astigmatism. J Cataract Refract Surg 1999;25:1198–1204.
24. CJ Argento, MD Cosentino, A Biondini. Treatment of hyperopic astigmatism. J Cataract Refract Surg 1997;23:1480–1490.
25. JF Doane, SB Morris, AD Border, J Denning. Presented at American Society of Cataract and Refractive Surgery, April 1999.

26. LA Ruiz. LASIK for hyperopic astigmatism. VisionQuest 2000, Chicago, IL, August 26, 2000.

27. DT Azar, JD Primack. Theoretical analysis of ablation depths and profiles in laser in situ keratomileusis for compound hyperopic and mixed astigmatism. J Cataract Refract Surg 2000;26:1123–1136.

28. EJ Linebarger. LASIK for the treatment of hyperopia after previous radial. Presented at American Society of Cataract and Refractive Surgery, April 1999.

29. W Portellinha, K Nakano, M Oliveira, R Simoceli. Laser in situ keratomileusis for hyperopia after thermal keratoplasty. J Refract Surg 1999;15(suppl):S218–S220.

30. W Attia, JJ Perez-Santonja, JL Alio. Laser in situ keratomileusis for recurrent hyperopia following laser thermal keratoplasty. J Refract Surg 2000;16:163–169.

31. LE Probst, MA Almasswary, J Bell. Pseudo-Fleischer ring after hyperopic laser in situ keratomileusis. J Cataract Refract Surg 1999;25(6):868–870.

32. A Ozdamar, C Aras, B Sener, M Karacorlu. Corneal iron ring after hyperopic laser-assisted in situ keratomileusis. Cornea 1999;18:243–245.

33. M Paciuc, CF Velasco, R Naanjo. Acute angle-closure glaucoma after hyperopic laser in situ keratomileusis. J Cataract Refract Surg 2000;26:620–623.

34. T Anschutz. Theoretic model of a combined presbyopia PRK. Presented at The European Excimer Laser Congress. Strasbourg, France, 1990.

35. T Anschutz. Multifocal excimer PRK combined myopia-presbyopia treatment (abstract). Am Soc Cataract Refract Surg May 1993, p 104.

36. T Anschutz. Presbyopic PRK. In: NA Sher, ed. Surgery of Hyperopia and Presbyopia. Baltimore: Williams and Wilkins, 1997, pp 63–77.

37. JM Bauerberg. Centered vs inferior off center ablation to correct hyperopia and presbyopia. J Refract Surg 1999;15:66–69.

21

LASIK Retreatments

AYMAN F. EL-SHIATY

*Cairo University, Cairo, Egypt, and Jules Stein Eye Institute at UCLA,
Los Angeles, California, U.S.A.*

BRIAN S. BOXER WACHLER

Jules Stein Eye Institute at UCLA, Los Angeles, California, U.S.A.

1. INTRODUCTION

The general aim of refractive surgery is an improvement in the uncorrected visual acuity (UCVA) so that daily life can be performed without optical aids. The hope is to achieve this goal by a single procedure. However, if this primary procedure does not reach the target, then a second procedure can be done. This is best called retreatment (1–6), although other terms such as enhancement (7–11), reoperation (12,13), and secondary treatment (14) have widely been used. The term LASIK retreatment may be applied for

1. A primary LASIK surgery followed by a secondary retreatment procedure, which may be LASIK, photorefractive keratectomy (PRK), incisional keratotomy, laser thermokeratoplasty (LTK), or intrastromal corneal segments (IN-TACS).
2. A secondary LASIK surgery following a primary corneal or intraocular surgery.

2. Indications

Although the predictability of excimer refractive surgery has improved over the years, retreatments of the primary procedure are still needed. Retreatments should not be performed before a stable refraction has been achieved after the primary procedure (12,15) and should be considered in terms of the benefit-to-risk ratio of further improving the uncorrected visual acuity (UCVA) versus compromising the best corrected visual acuity (BCVA) (7). Stability may be defined as a change in spherical equivalent of 0.50 D or less in three successive visits at least 1 month apart (2) or if history suggests stability. Retreatments are usually performed no sooner than 3 months postoperatively to allow for adequate healing and stability. Retreatments are usually indicated for errors of more than 0.75 D away from the target refraction (4,6,13) and UCVA of 20/40 or worse (2). Retreatment may be done for one of the following:

I.   Dissatisfied patient due to a residual error or an induced error. However, some patients (up to 24%) may be satisfied by a refractive outcome less than ideal and do not ask for retreatment or may not even come for follow-up (2,6,13). The retreatment rate and number of retreatments may be influenced by such subjective factors as patient expectations and demands (10). Presbyopic patients may well tolerate a small residual myopia.

    A.   The residual error may either be initial undercorrection or regression of the achieved effect over time.

        1.   Undercorrection may be defined as a residual spherical equivalent error of more than 0.75 D away from the target at the first postoperative week (5). Most factories used to configure excimer lasers to provide correction for PRK on the surface of the cornea, and a standard 10% reduction in programmed value was used for LASIK treatment. This standard reduction resulted in undercorrection, especially for high errors and when simultaneous astigmatic corrections are undertaken (16). LASIK nomograms with linear variability according to the attempted correction (Fig. 1) have decreased the incidence of undercorrection (13). Undercorrection may be induced intentionally in high myopia describing the golfing analogy to the patients. The first procedure will get them onto the green and the second procedure will putt them into the hole (8).

        2.   Regression is a less common problem in LASIK than in PRK (17). Although current laser algorithms aim at emmetropia, they do not allow for possible external and internal influences that may modulate the corneal healing process. So, following the excimer laser treat-

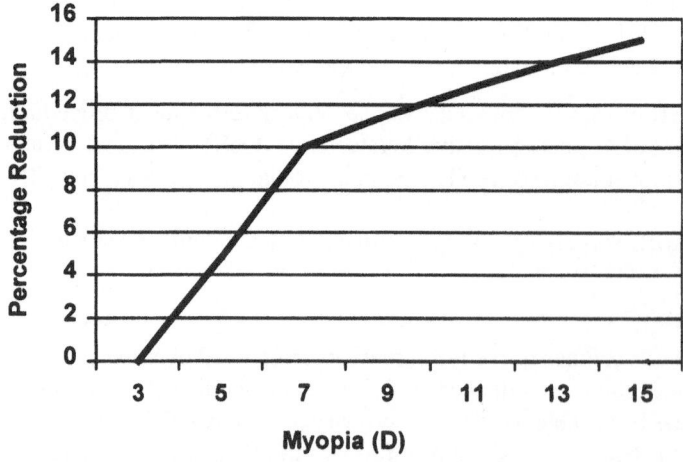

Figure 21.1   Percentage of reduction with the linearly changing LASIK nomogram. The reduction goes up to 10% for myopia ranging from −3.1 to −7.0 D and up to 15% for myopia ranging from −7.1 to −15.0 D. (From Ref. 13.)

ment, some regression of effect is typically seen. It is more significant in the first 6 weeks with smaller changes in the first several months (8,13,16). Regression may be defined as residual spherical equivalent error of more than 0.5 D away from the target with 0.25 D or more shift toward the original error between follow-up visits (5). Regression is the cause of retreatment in about 70% of cases (5).

B. The induced error may also be initial spherical overcorrection or induced astigmatism. Overcorrection is defined as spherical equivalent error of refraction 1 month postoperatively shifting away from the target refraction in the opposite direction of the original error.

II. Complications from the primary procedure as central islands (18–20), corneal haze (12,21), epithelial ingrowth (8,22,23), and corneal flap striae (8,24).

A. RETREATMENT PROCEDURES AFTER PRIMARY LASIK

Although the predictability of LASIK is higher than other refractive procedures, the nature of surgery upon living tissue is such that accurate prediction or refractive outcome is not entirely possible (25). As the field of refractive surgery continues to evolve, an increasing number of surgical options are available for LASIK retreatment. These allow refractive surgeons to treat a wider range of myopia, hyperopia, and astigmatism effectively with a history of LASIK even if multiple retreatments are required (4,5,7,11). The need for retreatment after primary LASIK surgery ranges from 0.7 to 36% (5–7,13,14,26,27). A higher retreatment rate was observed after astigmatic corrections than after spherical corrections (2). Retreatments after LASIK should not be performed earlier than 3 months after the primary procedure for myopia and 3 to 6 months for hyperopia and astigmatism, at which time the refraction has usually stabilized. Generally, retreatment for undercorrection, especially for lower degrees of original myopia, can be done earlier than that for regression or induced errors (8,21). However, some authors recommend waiting at least 3 months for any other ablation (6,7,9,18).

1. LASIK

Improvements in instruments and techniques allow for previous made LASIK flaps to be safely lifted for additional ablations even after several years (5,6,9,13). However, sufficient stromal bed thickness of 200 to 250 microns (4–6,8,14) or at least 30% of the total original thickness (18) left after retreatment is necessary to avoid subsequent ectasia. Laser retreatment is better avoided in eyes with less than 360 to 460 microns of total remaining corneal tissue after retreatment (4,9,12,14,20). When retreatment is for hyperopic correction, pachymetry should involve the 3 mm away from the corneal center (12). However, peripheral pachymetry after hyperopic LASIK may be misleading. Epithelial hyperplasia opposite the peripheral ablation gutter will overestimate the amount of remaining stromal tissue. Hence it is possible to induce peripheral ectasia after multiple hyperopic ablations. LASIK retreatment can be performed either by lifting the original flap or by creating a new keratectomy cut.

2. Lift Flap Retreatments

The procedure is done under topical anesthesia. The flap can be lifted rather than cut if the retreatment is performed before 6 to 18 months (8,12,13,17). The edge of the previous flap

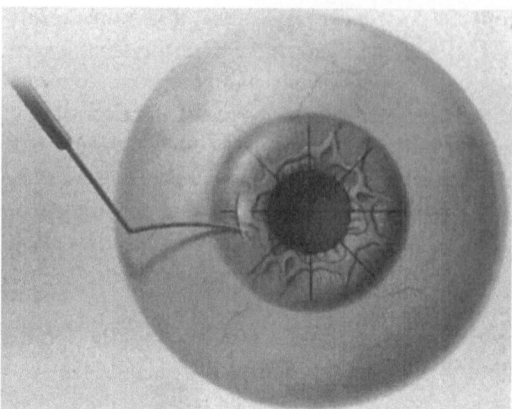

Figure 21.2 A Hunkeler hook is used to find the edge of the flap and free it for 3 to 4 hours. (From Ref. 28.)

is best identified on the slit lamp. Gentian violet may be used to mark the edge and the cylindrical axis (4,6,7). An 18-gauge needle (13) or a probe (23) may be used at the slit lamp at a point 180 degrees from the hinge to disengage the flap, with a lateral movement, from its bed along a short section of the flap. Alternatively, a Sinsky or Hunkeler hook can be used under the laser microscope to free the flap edge for 3 or 4 clock hours (Fig. 21.2). The Hunkeler hook has a round ball on the end and is less likely to cause corneal damage (28). The flap is then carefully dissected, under the laser microscope, with a tying forceps or a cyclodialysis spatula without allowing the spatula to exit the flap. The flap is gently lifted with the forceps and bent back (Fig. 21.3), creating a sharp demarcation along the epithelial edge in a technique similar to that used for capsulorhexis in cataract surgery (13) or with a slow and steady traction toward the hinge (8,23).

3. New Keratectomy

Flap recut may be resorted to when the initial flap is thin or irregular, or if there is difficulty in dissecting the original flap edge. Larger flaps (13), old flaps (6,13,14), and flaps with a

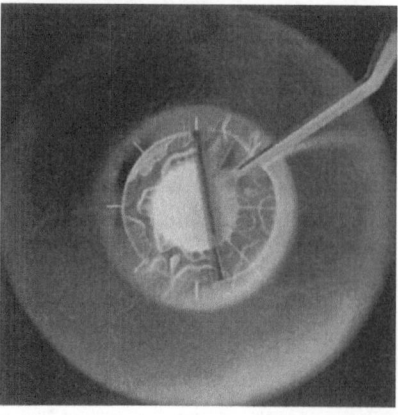

Figure 21.3 The flap is carefully lifted and reflected with nontoothed forceps. (From Ref. 28.)

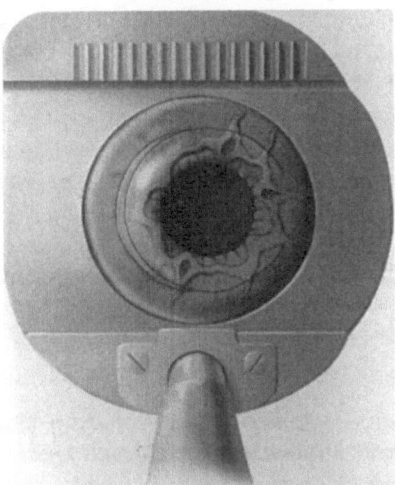

Figure 21.4   To perform a secondary keratectomy beneath the primary one, the suction ring is placed just temporal to the edge of the first keratectomy. (From Ref. 28.)

history of interface keratitis after the first LASIK (5) are more difficult to lift over time. Thin flaps need more care in handling (6). Intraoperative flap complications during a primary LASIK are best managed by realigning the flap edges as closely as possible and then recutting a new flap after at least 3 months (8). Also patients who have had previous incisional keratotomy or corneal transplantation may get torn flaps if blunt dissection is tried 2 months after LASIK (13). Hyperopia resulting from overcorrected myopic LASIK may need a larger flap (17), but since the degree of hyperopia is usually small, the original flap is sufficient in most cases. The technique for recutting involves decentering the suction ring 2 mm so that the new flap edge will be outside the edge of the first flap (Fig. 21.4). This decreases the chance of dislodging the original flap. The recut is usually done 20 microns deeper than the initial procedure (5). Ozdamar et al. (14) use the same microkeratome settings when more than 1 year has passed since the initial procedure and have not encountered any flap disconfiguration. Only two peripheral gray circular lines have been seen with small decentration of the suction ring. Peripheral epithelial ingrowth has also been noticed.

4.   Laser Ablation

Laser ablation may be performed according to the standard LASIK nomogram (4,13,26), reduced by a fixed percentage (7,8), or customized to each eye based on the response to the initial procedure (5). When working with a new laser, reducing the attempted correction is prudent, since most lasers incorporate a healing response that occurs only after primary excimer procedures and does not occur after retreatments. This protects against overcorrection from laser retreatment. As the UCVA is often better than the myopia measured after LASIK would suggest, 60 to 70% of the residual error may only be aimed at (8). In retreating astigmatism, some nomograms may take into consideration a 33% hyperopic shift as a result of toric ablation in the steep meridian (29). In retreating previous decentered ablation, the residual correction is made centered on the undilated pupil as the flap will smooth the edges of the two ablated areas (8). Central islands can be treated by using a double pretreatment in the 3 mm ablation zone and then performing half the refractive correction according to the Munnerlyn formula (depth of ablation = diameter^2 × height of the island/3) (30). This has been applied with both PRK and PTK modalities but with poor predictability (19).

A dry technique, in which the cul-de-sac is dried, the flap is lifted, the additional treatment is performed, and the flap is lowered before irrigation, may avoid introduction of any unwanted material underneath the flap (28). Any epithelial tissue detected at the flap edge should be pushed peripheral to the bed by a sponge (Fig. 21.5) (17,23,28). After the flap is reposited, a moistened sponge is used to roll back the epithelium into its original position (28). A soft contact lens can be put if epithelial defects are bothersome and to reduce the risk of epithelial ingrowth (23).

5. Results

The results of LASIK retreatment after primary LASIK in the literature are summarized in the table. The efficacy of the procedure can be demonstrated by the achieved UCVA. Thirty-one to 69 percent of eyes can achieve 20/20 or better (4–6,8,12,13,26), and 88 to 100% of eyes can achieve 20/40 or better UCVA (6,8,12,13,26).

The predictability can be estimated by the spherical equivalent refractive error achieved. Sixty to 92 percent of eyes may be within 0.5 D (5,6,8,13,26), and 64 to 100% may be within 1.0 D of target correction (4,5,7–9,13,26). However, 12% undercorrection of more than 2.0 D of myopia (9) and about 4% overcorrection of more than 1.0 D (4) have been reported. Retreatment for myopia is more predictable than that for hyperopia (12).

The safety of the procedure can be evaluated by the BCVA lost. Only 3 to 14% have been reported to lose one line of BCVA (8,13,26). On the other hand, 14 to 32% (6,8,12,13) have been reported to gain more than one line. LASIK retreatment has been found to improve decentration and night vision problems (4,7).

In terms of stability, significant refractive changes may occur in the first 3 months but is most unlikely after 6 months (6,8), although regression can develop up to 2 years after LASIK (5). It occurs in 10 to 18% of cases and is correlated to attempted correction, ablation depth, flat keratometry, and humidity (4,5). It may be caused by the molecular mem-

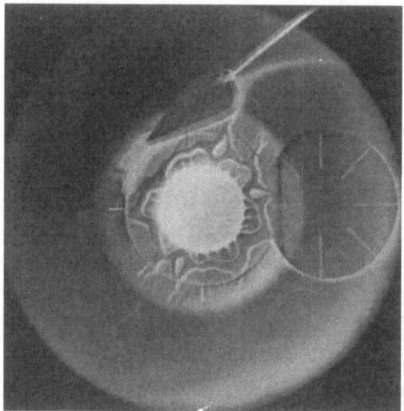

Figure 21.5 A sponge is used to reflect epithelial flaps out of host bed to decrease epithelial ingrowth. (From Ref. 28.)

Table 1 Results of Secondery LASIK Retreatment after Primary LASIK

Ref	Rate	Time	STL	≥20/20	≥20/40	≤0.5D	≤1.0D	BCVA Loss	BCVA Gain
5	0.7	3	250	68.8	98.1	81.5	97.5	1.3	
6	11	3	200	31.4	91.4	91.5			14.3
8			200	37.3	88.2	58.8	86.3	14	15
12			200	48.72	100	43.68	64.1	7.7	30.8
13	7.3	1.5			100	82	100	3	32
26	5.5		250	39.6	96.2	90.6	100	9.4	28.3

Ref = reference number, Rate = rate of retreatment in %, Time = duration between the primary and secondary procedures in months, STL = minimal stromal bed thickness left after retreatment in microns, ≥20/20 and ≥20/40 = % of eyes UCVA, ≤0.5 D and ≤1.0 D = % of eyes spherical equivalent away from the target, and BCVA loss and gain = % of eyes losing and gaining one line, respectively.

ory in the corneal collagen fibers, stromal remodeling, the effect of IOP on the thinned cornea, and epithelial hyperplasia in response to an excessively flattened corneal curvature (8).

6. Complications

Patients usually have worse UCVA in the first postoperative day than they had after the primary procedure (13). Discomfort, foreign body sensation, and excessive lacrimation also last longer than experienced after the primary LASIK. This is explained by the epithelial irregularity at the flap edge caused by surgical manipulations during lifting the flap, compared to the clear cut edge of the primary flap (6,8). Some complications have been encountered such as transient tear film disturbances (17%), interface deposits (8%), diminished night vision (5%), scarring at flap edge (5%), filamentary keratititis (3%) (6), diffuse lamellar keratitis (22), and keratectasia (31). The risk of epithelial ingrowth (3–30%) is higher than primary treatment due to the irregular flap edge (4,5,26,27). This risk increases with a history of interface inflammation and with the use of a spatula to break the interface by sweeping (17,23). The risk of flap melting (11%) and folds (2–5%) is also high due to poor flap adherence after repeated manipulations (4,5). Flap melting develops commonly on an epithelial ingrowth area on the peripheral flap edge not affecting visual acuity (4). Moderate haze has been recorded at the flap interface after retreatment (8). Other rare flap complications such as flap slippage and dislocation have been recorded (27). Recutting the corneal flap has the added risk of getting a centrally thin or perforated flap and the potential to generate a free corneal wedge of tissue where the two flaps intersect (8). A more meticulous surgical technique with a linear epithelial dissection, a copious irrigation of the interface for removing all implanted epithelial cells, and a strong adhesion with a minimal gap between the flap edge and the stromal bed may decrease the incidence of these complications (4,13,23). Although flap relifting is repeatable and has none of the added risks associated with recutting an already centrally flattened cornea, recutting the flap offers the advantage of a rapid visual rehabilitation without epithelial defects (8) but there is a risk of irregular cuts with free stromal pieces. The overall intraoperative complication rate is lower for enhancement than for primary procedures, while the postoperative complication rate is slightly higher (27).

7. Photorefractive Keratectomy (PRK)

Primary LASIK followed by second-stage PRK has been used to treat extremely high myopia either simultaneously (32) or with transepithelial PRK after LASIK (33). Transepithelial PRK can also be applied to correct small degrees of myopia due to regression after LASIK (17). Bond and Abell (34) described a technique of PRK over incomplete LASIK flaps. After the flap is replaced they use 180–220 phototherapeutic keratectomy (PTK) shots to go through the epithelium. A PRK is then performed as if the flap had never been created. Assuming that epithelial hyperplasia is the main cause of regression after LASIK, Guell et al. have described an intraepithelial photorefractive keratectomy for regression after LASIK. They use a PlanoScan mode, with the largest diameter zone possible, with an ablation depth not exceeding 50 microns for direct epithelial photoablation to avoid Bowman's membrane damage (35). Hyperopic PRK has also been used on the epithelial surface of the flap to treat myopic overcorrections (21). Although this is a simple, quick, and safe procedure, its efficacy (52%) is lower than a second LASIK and there is one-day discomfort and foreign body sensation due to punctate keratitis and tear film unstability. In addition, haze formation is significantly greater than that seen in primary PRK (8,21). This higher risk of haze is expected due to laser impact on the Bowman's membrane of a previously ablated cornea, which may not make PRK following LASIK a safe option.

8. Incisional Keratotomies

Eyes with iatrogenic or secondary ectasia may not be suitable for lamellar or further ablative surgery (12). Radial keratotomy (RK) was used for residual myopia after PRK (36) and can be used for residual undercorrected myopia of less than 3 D after primary LASIK when maximal stromal ablation has already been performed (8). However, the predictability is poor due to the previous flattening (21).

As most lasers ablate tissue along the steep meridian, they induce some hypermetropia. So, astigmatic keratotomy (AK) continues to play an important role in enhancement procedures for induced astigmatism, especially in cases of mixed and high astigmatism and when the spherical equivalent is near the target refraction. AK may be done underneath LASIK flap (11,21,22,27), or later over the flap (17), or outside the corneal flap (27). AK underneath the flap carries the risk of microperforation and the difficulty in obtaining flap adherence, increasing the risk of epithelial ingrowth (17,27). Limbal AK has an advantage over corneal AK of inducing less irregular astigmatism.

9. Laser Thermokeratoplasty (LTK)

Thermokeratoplasty by holmium laser has been proposed to correct low hyperopia by steepening the corneal center due to shrinkage of collagen in the midperipheral cornea. This effect is based on the ability of corneal collagen to shrink by 30 to 45% of its original length at temperatures ranging from 58 to 60°C (37). It has been found that corneal lamellar cutting 6 to 8 weeks before LTK with spots placed outside the previous lamellar cuts dramatically increases the efficacy of LTK with improvement in regression. This may be explained by the discontinuity and alteration of the integrity of Bowman's layer (38). This improved effect has also been noticed after PRK, suggesting that greater corneal thickness favors regression (39). Since, in LASIK, the Bowman's layer is interrupted and the corneal thickness is decreased, LTK can be used on the peripheral cornea with holmium laser 6 to 9 months after LASIK to treat under-corrected (40) or induced (21,41) hyperopia. LTK spots are applied first at 7.0 mm diameter regardless of the previous lamellar cut, but it is better to keep them outside the previous ablation zone if stromal haze is present, to avoid confluent haze. There is usually immediate postoperative myopic shift followed by stable emmetropic refraction in the following weeks with no later regression. The result of the operation is good with stable corneal flaps and no loss of BCVA (40,41). It is recommended to perform 50% of intended correction and use only a 6.0 mm ring to guard against overcorrection. A 7.0 mm ring may be used later if additional correction is needed.

10. Intrastromal Corneal Segments (INTACS)

Intrastromal corneal ring segments (INTACS) have demonstrated safety and efficacy for correction of myopia between −1.0 and −3.0 D with the advantage of removability. They have been recently used to correct residual myopia 10 months after LASIK (11,42). This option can be resorted to when the cornea has become too thin for further ablation. It can also be used as a method of monovision by undercorrecting the nondominant eye by two diopters using LASIK. Then INTACS are used to correct these two diopters until presbyopia develops when INTACS can be removed. The procedure is done using the standard nomogram for unoperated corneas, but intraoperative pachymetry in four quadrants at the 7.0 mm optical zone should be done to confirm thickness of at least 600 microns, to allow for 400 microns of corneal stroma overlying the segments after implantation. If the preceding LASIK was decentered to meet the pupillary center, INTACS may likewise be decentered as long as the segments do not impinge upon the limbus. The vertical incision at 12 o'clock may cross the LASIK flap edge (42).

We recommend waiting at least 6 months after LASIK to avoid flap slippage. If done earlier than 6 months, the lamellar dissection of the channel may cause the flap to torque with subsequent high astigmatism. If this occurs, the INTACS need to be removed followed by floating and reposition of the flap one week later.

11. Intraocular Lens Implantation

Since the number of LASIK procedures is expected to increase, an increasing volume of cataract surgeries after LASIK is anticipated. Therefore accurate IOL power prediction after LASIK is necessary. However, the change in corneal asphericity and in the ratio between the anterior and posterior corneal curvatures after LASIK leads to inaccurate determination of keratometric diopters. In addition, it is important to measure the stabilized refraction after LASIK before any myopic shift from nuclear sclerosis (43). If the refraction and keratometric diopters before LASIK are available to the cataract surgeon, the clinical history method should be applied (44). This involves subtracting the change in spherical equivalent refraction induced by LASIK from the keratometric diopters measured before LASIK. If these data are not available, the hard contact lens method is used, in which the difference between the manifest post-LASIK refraction with and without a plano RGP contact lens is determined and subtracted from the known contact lens base curve (power) (44). Keratometry = Basecurve of plano RGP(D) − (S.E. (spherical equivalent) MRx s̄ CTL − S.E. MRx CTL). Alternatively, the keratometric diopters of the anterior and posterior corneal curvature may be measured separately by a scanning slit topography and entered into an empirical quadratic regression formula (43).

12. Others

Homoplastic refractive keratomileusis and lamellar refractive keratoplasty may be used in cases of flap opacity in addition to the residual refractive error, as in cases of postoperative keratitis or stromal melting (12,21). Corneal flap striae can be treated by lifting the corneal flap and refloating it back into place during the first few postoperative days (8,24).

B. SECONDARY LASIK RETREATMENT AFTER OTHER PROCEDURES

1. Penetrating Keratoplasty (PKP)

The purpose of corneal and intraocular surgeries such as penetrating keratoplasty (PKP), cataract, and even traumatic corneal repair is to obtain an improved BCVA allowing the most possible visual function. In spite of the great advancement of these surgeries, the final refractive result may need to be refined after stable refraction for 6 months. Refractive unpredictability is common after PKP (45). Various refractive surgeries have been tried for patients with unsatisfactory spectacle or contact lens correction after PKP. PRK has been successful in the treatment of myopia and astigmatism but has a high incidence of complications including haze and scar formation leading to loss of BCVA (46). Since LASIK has the advantage of less loss of corneal sensation than PRK, it has been used to correct all refractive errors after PKP with more effective results in treating myopia than astigmatism (12,45,47). Secondary LASIK can be done 8 to 18 months (12,20,45,47,48) after PKP and 6 months after all sutures have been removed (12,20,45,47) or after topographic stability for at least 3 months following all suture removal (48). The flap diameter should equal to or larger than the PKP scar, unless the graft was decentered (12), with an attempt to avoid the temporal scar to allow the flap to drape over the wound, creating better wound apposition (45). The suction time should be minimized to avoid the risk of wound dehiscence (45,47) and retinal vascular or optic nerve compromise (49). More time is allowed for flap adherence before removing the speculum (45), and more postoperative corticosteroids are used than regular LASIK to avoid the risk of graft rejection (45,47). Predictability of 45% within 0.5 D (48), 63–73% within 1.0 D (45,48), and 88% within 2.0 D of target refraction (45) and efficacy of 36–55% within 20/40 UCVA (45,48) have been reported. Observations of 55–60% gain (45,47) and 9–12% loss (47,48) of more than one line of BCVA have been recorded. No graft rejection or loss of graft clarity has been documented (45,48,50). Flap complications such as paracentral perforation and dislocated flap (27,48) can occur. Results of LASIK treatment of postkeratoplasty high astigmatism may be improved by performing arcuate cuts in the stromal bed after laser ablation with the risk of perforation (47). Alternatively, LASIK can be repeated after elevating the original flap (50). It has also been advocated that making the flap first without ablation, rechecking refraction after some time and then elevating the flap for laser ablation may improve the predictability. LASIK with topographically guided customized ablation has been recently used successfully in the treatment of corneal irregularities following PKP and ocular trauma with significant improvement in corneal topography, astigmatism, and UCVA (20).

2. Intraocular Lenses (IOL)

Improvements in biometry or IOL power calculation have diminished, in most cases, the final refractive defect in cataract surgery as well as in phakic IOL implantation. The latter is becoming a popular technique having the possibility of changing the IOL if there is any postoperative gross refractive error. LASIK has been performed 3 months after phacoemulsification and after phakic IOLs instead of enlarging the wound to replace the IOL and to refine the residual astigmatism (12,51). LASIK treatment of high myopia results in thin corneas and small functional optical zones with compromised predictability and stability. Combined surgery to correct high myopia (>15.0 D) by performing phakic IOL implantation followed, 1 to 3 months later, by LASIK has been used effectively and called bioptics. This improves the predictability, as LASIK is more reliable to treat small residual errors and coexisting astigmatism (52,53). Adjustable refractive surgery (ARS) is a modification of this technique in which the lamellar microkeratome cut is done just before the lens implant surgery. The main advantage of this approach is to avoid the risk of endothelial-IOL touch during the microkeratome cut (54). Bioptics has given good results with 63–67% of eyes within 0.5 D and 85–100% of eyes within 1.0 D of emmetropia (52,53) and UCVA of 20/40 or better in 69% of eyes with no reported complications (52).

3. Radial Keratotomy (RK)

The need for retreatment after RK ranges from 30 to 33% of cases (55). Surface photoablation by PRK following RK is associated with a 5- to 10-fold increase in haze formation and at least a 20% reduction in refractive predictability (10). LASIK can be used to treat residual myopia and astigmatism as well as hyperopic shift one year following RK (10,12,56,57). A 0.5 D overcorrection may be aimed at preventing regression from occurring during the first week due to the healing process of the previous corneal incisions (10,57). A thorough preoperative slit-lamp microscopy must be performed to verify good incision healing. The presence of an epithelial cyst within an incision may indicate a predisposition to interface epithelial ingrowth. In such cases, debridement of the cyst associated with suturing of the incision may be important prior to LASIK (57).

A secondary LASIK after RK is better done by a new cut and not by flap dissection. It has been found to be safe to apply suction to these corneas (51). Alternatively, flap hydrodissection using a 27-gauge cannula placed under the flap near the hinge may be used (58). However, there is a slight risk of the old radial incisions coming apart either on the stromal bed (10) or on the flap during flap manipulation, increasing the risk of epithelial ingrowth adjacent to the incisions (12,35,57). So the flap and the pie-like pieces should be perfectly aligned (10).

Postoperative recurrent corneal erosions and slight daytime visual fluctuation may occur. UCVA of 20/20 is achievable in 29–56% (10,57) and 20/40 or better in 71% (57) of cases. Refraction within 0.5 D of emmetropia can be achieved in 57% of cases (57) with a 31% chance of gaining one line of BCVA (10). One line of BCVA may be lost in 7% of cases (57).

4. Astigmatic Keratotomy (AK)

The combined technique of keratomileusis in situ and AK has been described either simultaneously (59) outside or beneath the corneal flap (27) or sequentially (60) as a more effective method in the treatment of high astigmatism than each procedure alone (12,60,61). LASIK after AK has been used successfully to treat up to 6 D of astigmatism using the ARC-T nomogram (62) and Limbal AK nomogram (63). Four weeks after topographic and refractive stability of the cylinder, LASIK can be performed using a 6.0 mm optical zone with a peripheral treatment zone of 8.0 mm. Results of 54% within 0.5 D and 85% within 1.0 D of intended cylindrical correction have been encountered with 7% loss and 27% gain of one line of BCVA (60).

5. PRK

Retreatment after PRK may be required in 3.5–5% of cases of low myopia and 15–19% of cases of moderate and high myopia due to regression and haze (2,3). There is an effect of topical steroids in the treatment of regression and haze (11). PRK retreatment should not be attempted before 6 months of the primary PRK. It has been found to be less successful than the primary PRK (1,2,3) and can lead to a long-lasting fluctuation in vision and an increased incidence of haze, especially in eyes that experienced haze formation after the primary procedure (1,15,64). LASIK has been found to be as effective as PRK for residual myopia after PRK of up to −3.0 D and more effective in higher myopia (32,65). LASIK has a lower wound-healing response than PRK, which makes it possibly safer and more predictable. In addition, it avoids the possible influence of epithelial thickness, which tends to be nonuniform after PRK (20). However, since Bowman's layer is an important factor in maintaining the shape and stability of the cornea, adequate residual corneal thickness becomes more important in LASIK after PRK (66). Also, LASIK is only able to correct the residual refractive error and not the haze or irregular astigmatism (51). Nevertheless, the recent introduction of topographically guided (20) and wavefront-guided (67) customized ablation using the spot-scanning excimer lasers provides a potential platform to perform ablations of any shape. This may enable LASIK treatment of decentered and irregular ablations but not central islands (20). LASIK after PRK carries a higher risk of epithelial detachment at the site of the microkeratome (64). About 70% of eyes can achieve UCVA of 20/40 or better and only 2% may lose two lines of BCVA (25,64,65).

6. LTK

LASIK has been recently used 1.5 to 2.0 years after noncontact LTK as a retreatment for hyperopic regression (68,69). A corneal flap diameter of 8.5 mm can be fashioned after 6, 7, or 8 mm LTK rings. Ablation zone of 5.5–7.5 mm has been used. Although the efficacy and predictability are less than primary LASIK for hyperopia, the results are promising with regression of 26% after 6 months. There is a 72–91% chance of getting 20/40 or better and a 41% chance of getting 20/20 or better UCVA, with 42% of cases within 0.5 D and 60–67% within 1.0 D of target refraction. Seventeen to 34% of eyes can gain one or more lines of BCVA while 14–25% may lose one line and 16% two lines of BCVA. Interface epithelial ingrowth and confluent haze has been reported between previous LTK spots, especially when the LASIK flap cut coincides with the LTK spots, with no changes in the radial thermal scars (Fig. 21.6). It seems that excimer laser ablation induces activation of a wound-healing response in an area previously treated by LTK.

7. Others

If prior lamellar refractive surgery has been performed, such as epikeratophakia, keratophakia, keratomileusis, or ALK, retreatment should not be done before 1 year, and the lenticular diameter of the previous surgery should be estimated to avoid irregular cuts. In previous epikeratophakia, the flap diameter should be smaller than the zone where the pocket was made (12). Specifically in epikeratophakia for myopia, the previous lenticule should first be removed if there is irregular astigmatism.

C. CONCLUSION

LASIK is gaining popularity because it is both a patient-friendly and a doctor-friendly technique. The LASIK procedure allows for easy and accurate additional treatment to be done

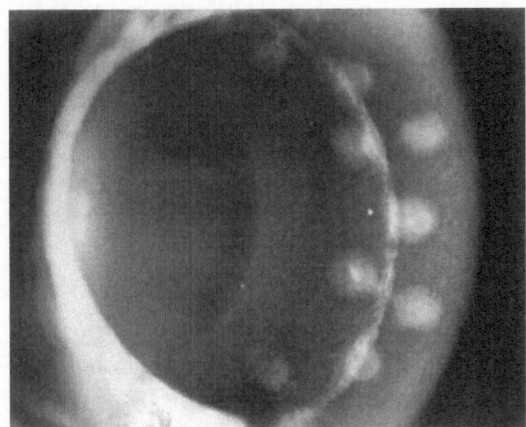

Figure 21.6 LASIK flap cut passing through LTK spots producing a ring-shaped haze. (From Ref. 66.)

without losing the advantages of fast visual recovery and minimal discomfort. The results of LASIK retreatment may suggest that equally small corrections can be treated as primary procedures with equal safety and predictability. High corrections can be treated conservatively, aiming at undercorrection for residual error to be retreated later, or, alternatively, nomograms can be directed toward achieving a plano result, since overcorrection can be equally treated. LASIK may be the procedure that can correct different refractive errors in different clinical situations with the ability to do additional surgery for residual or induced refractive errors.

REFERENCES

1. G Sutton, RS Kalski, MA Lawless, C Rogers. Excimer retreatment for scarring and regression after photorefractive keratectomy for myopia. Br J Ophthalmol 1995;79:756–759.
2. GR Snibson, CA McCarty, GF Aldred, B Bus, S Levin, HR Taylor. The Melbourne Excimer Laser Group. Retreatment after excimer laser photorefractive keratectomy. Am J Ophthalmol 1996;121:250–257.
3. EK Vorotnikova, VV Kourenkov, GS Plounin. Retreatment of regression after photorefractive keratectomy for myopia. J Refract Surg 1998;14(2 suppl):S197–S198.
4. JJ Perez-Santonja, MJ Ayala, HF Sakla, JM Ruiz-Moreno, JL Alio. Retreatment after laser in situ keratomileusis. Ophthalmology 1999;106:21–28.
5. WA Lyle, GJC Jin. Retreatment after initial laser in situ keratomileusis. J Cataract Refract Surg 2000;26:650–659.
6. KM Rashad. Laser in situ keratomileusis retreatment for residual myopia and astigmatism. J Refract Surg 2000;16:170–176.
7. E Martines, ME John. The Martines enhancement technique for correcting residual myopia following laser assisted in situ keratomileusis. Ophthalmic Surg Lasers 1996;27(5 suppl):S512–S516.
8. LE Probst, JJ Machat. LASIK enhancement techniques and results. In: L Burrato, SF Brint. LASIK Principles and Techniques. Thorofare NJ: SLACK, 1998, pp 325–338.
9. B Yang, J Chen, Z Wang. Enhancement ablation for the treatment of undercorrection after excimer laser in situ keratomileusis for correcting myopia. Chin Med J 1998;111:358–360.
10. L Yong, G Chen, W Li, J Chang, C Ngan, P Tong, C Qun. Laser in situ keratomileusis enhancement after radial keratotomy. J Refract Surg 2000;16:187–190.

11. DS Durrie, TL Vande Garde. LASIK enhancements. Int Ophthalmol Clin 2000;40:103–110.
12. AM Gutierrez. Reoperations with the excimer laser. In: L Burrato, SF Brint. LASIK Principles and Techniques. Thorofare NJ: SLACK, 1998, pp 339–350.
13. JL Febbraro, KA Buzard, MH Friedlander. Reoperations after myopic laser in situ keratomileusis. J Cataract Refract Surg 2000;26:41–48.
14. A Ozdamar, C Aras, H Bahcecioglu, B Sener. Secondary laser in situ keratomileusis 1 year after primary LASIK for high myopia. J Cataract Refract Surg 1999;25:383–388.
15. T Kohnen. Retreating residual refractive errors after excimer surgery of the cornea: PRK versus LASIK. J cataract Refract Surg 2000;(26):625–626.
16. RB Vajpayee, CA McCarty, GF Aldered, HR Taylor, the Excimer Laser Group. Undercorrection after excimer laser refractive surgery. Am J Ophthalmol 1996;122:801–807.
17. SE Wilson. LASIK: management of common complications. Cornea 1998;17:459–467.
18. PI Condon, M Mulhern, T Fulcher, A Foley-Nolan, M O'Keefe. Laser intrastromal keratomileusis for high myopia and myopic astigmatism. Br J Ophthalmol 1997;81:199–206.
19. EE Manche, RK Maloney, RJ Smith. Treatment of topographic central islands following refractive surgery. J Cataract Refract Surg 1998;24:464–470.
20. MC Knorz, B Jendritza. Topographically-guided laser in situ keratomileusis to treat corneal irregularities. Ophthalmology 2000;107:1138–1143.
21. L Burrato, S Brint, M Ferrari. Complications. In: L Burrato, SF Brint. LASIK Principles and Techniques. Thorofare NJ: SLACK, 1998, pp 113–132.
22. RJ Smith, RK Maloney. Diffuse lamellar keratitis: a new syndrome in lamellar refractive surgery. Ophthalmology 1998;105:1721–1726.
23. MB Walker, SE Wilson. Incidence and prevention of epithelial growth within the interface after laser in situ keratomileusis. Cornea 2000;19:170–173.
24. LE Probst, J Machat. Removal of flap striae following laser in situ keratomileusis. J Cataract Refract Surg 1998;24:153–155.
25. IG Pallikaris, DS Siganos. Laser in situ keratomileusis to treat myopia: early experience. J Cataract Refract Surg 1997;23:39–49.
26. D Zadok, G Maskaleris, V Garcia, S Shah, M Montes, A Chayet. Outcomes of retreatment after laser in situ keratomileusis. Ophthalmology 1999;106:2391–2394.
27. RD Stulting, JD Carr, KP Thompson, GO Waring III, WM Wiley, JG Walker. Complications of laser in situ keratomileusis for the correction of myopia. Ophthalmology 1999;106:13–20.
28. DS Durrie. LASIK retreatments and LASIK enhancements. Operative Tech Cataract Refract Surg 1998;1:21–25.
29. AS Chayet, R Magallanes, M Montes, S Chavez, N Robledo. Laser in situ keratomileusis for simple myopic, mixed, and simple hyperopic astigmatism. J Refract Surg 1998;14(suppl 2):S175–S176.
30. CR Munnerlyn, SJ Koons, J Marshall. Photorefractive keratectomy: a technique for laser refractive surgery. J Cataract Refract Surg 1988;14:46–52.
31. HS Geggel, AR Talley. Delayed onset keratectasia following laser in situ keratomileusis. J Cataract Refract Surg 1999;25:582–586.
32. IM Astudillo, CI Ortiz. Combined laser in situ keratomileusis and photorefractive keratectomy for extreme myopia. J Refract Surg 1999;15:58–60.
33. IG Pallikaris, DS Siganos. Excimer laser in situ keratomileusis and photorefractive keratectomy for correction of high myopia. J Refract Corneal Surg 1994;10:498–510.
34. WI Bond, T Abell. PRK over incomplete LASIK flap. J Refract Surg 2000;16:483.
35. JL Guell, CP Lohmann, FA Malecaze, J Junger, A Muller, S Deneuville. Intraepithelial photorefractive keratectomy for regression after laser in situ keratomileusis. J Cataract Refract Surg 1999;25:670–674.
36. AH Kolahdouz-Isfahani, FM Wu, JJ Salz. Refractive keratotomy after photorefractive keratectomy. J Refract Surg 1999;15:53–57.
37. T Seiler, M Matallana, T Bende. Laser thermokeratoplast by means of a pulsed holmium: YAG laser for hyperopic correction. Refract Corneal Surg 1990;6:335–339.

38. MM Ismail, JJ Perez-Santonja, JL Alio. Laser thermokeratoplasty after lamellar corneal cutting. J Cataract Refract Surg 1999;25:212–215.

39. CA Eggink, P Meurs, Y Bardak, AF Deutman. Holmium laser thermal keratoplasty for hyperopia and astigmatism after photorefractive keratectomy. J Refract Surg 2000;16:317–322.

40. K Ditzen. Laser thermal keratoplasty (Ho: YAG) application after hyperopic LASIK. J Refract Surg 1998;14(suppl 2):S204.

41. MM Ismail, JL Alio, JJ Perez-Santonja. Noncontact thermokeratoplasty to correct hyperopia induced by laser in situ keratomileusis. J Cataract Refract Surg 1998;24:1191–1194.

42. JF Fleming, CF Lovisolo. Intrastromal corneal ring segments in a patient with previous laser in situ keratomileusis. J Refract Surg 2000;16:365–367.

43. B Seitz, A Langenbucher. Intraocular lens power calculation in eyes after corneal refractive surgery. J Cataract Refract Surg 2000;16:349–361.

44. JT Holladay. Consultations in refractive surgery. Refract Corneal Surg 1989;5:203.

45. ED Donnenfeld, HS Kornstein, A Amin, MD Speaker, JA Seedor, PD Sforza, LM Landrio, HD Perry. Laser in situ keratomileusis for correction of myopia and astigmatism after penetrating keratoplasty. Ophthalmology 1999;106:1966–1975.

46. DR Lazzaro, DH Haight, SC Belmont, RP Gibralter, IM Aslanides, MG Odrich. Excimer laser keratectomy for astigmatism occurring after penetrating keratoplasty. Ophthalmology 1996;103:458–464.

47. SK Webber, MA Lawless, GL Sutton, CM Rogers. LASIK for post penetrating keratoplasty astigmatism and myopia. Br J Ophthalmol 1999;83:1013–1018.

48. AS Forseto, CM Francesconi, RAM Nose, W Nose. Laser in situ keratomileusis to correct refractive errors after keratoplasty. J Cataract Refract Surg 1999;25:479–485.

49. JH Talamo. Laser in situ keratomileusis for correction of myopia and astigmatism after penetrating keratoplasty: discussion. Ophthalmology 1999;106:1974–1975.

50. R Zaldivar, F Davidorf, S Oscherow. LASIK for myopia and astigmatism after penetrating keratoplasty. J Refract Surg 1997;13:501.

51. JL Guell, O Gris, A de Muller, B Corcostegui. LASIK for the correction of residual refractive errors from previous surgical procedures. Ophthalmic Surg Lasers 1999;30:341–349.

52. R Zaldivar, JM Davidorf, S Oscherow, G Ricur, V Piezzi. Combined posterior chamber phakic intraocular lens and laser in situ keratomileusis: bioptics for extreme myopia. J Refract Surg 1999;15:299–308.

53. JL Guell, M Vazquez, O Gris, A DeMuller, F Manero. Combined surgery to correct high myopia: iris claw phakic intraocular lens and laser in situ keratomileusis. J Refract Surg 1999;15:529–537.

54. JL Guell. The adjustable refractive surgery concept (ARS). J Refract Surg 1998;14:271.

55. JL Gayton, M VanDerKarr, V Sanders. Radial keratotomy enhancements for residual myopia. J Refract Surg 1997;13:374–381.

56. HD Gimbel. Photorefractive keratectomy and laser in situ keratomileusis hyperopic correction of overcorrected radial keratotomy. J Refract Surg 1998;14(2 suppl):205–206.

57. AS Forseto, RAM Nose, CM Francesconi, W Nose. Laser in situ keratomileusis for undercorrection after radial keratotomy. J Refract Surg 1999;15:424–428.

58. V Thompson. Flap management during LASIK after radial keratotomy. J Refract Surg 1997;13:128.

59. EE Manche, RK Maloney. Astigmatic keratotomy combined with myopic keratomileusis in situ for compound myopic astigmatism. Am J Ophthalmol 1996;122:18–28.

60. JL Guell, M Vazquez. Correction of high astigmatism with astigmatic keratotomy combined with laser in situ keratomileusis. J Cataract Refract Surg 2000;26:960–966.

61. C Argento, JF Mendy, MJ Cosentino. Laser in situ keratomileusis versus arcuate keratotomy to treat astigmatism. J Cataract Refract Surg 1999;25:374–382.

62. FW Price, RB Grene, RG Marks, JS Gonzales, ARC-T Study Group. Astigmatism reduction clinical trial: a multicenter prospective evaluation of the predictability of arcuate keratotomy. Arch Opthalmol 1995;113:277–282.

63. K Budak, NJ Friedman, DD Koch. Limbal relaxing incisions with cataract surgery. J Cataract Refract Surg 1998;24:503–508.

64. A Ozdamar, B Sener, C Aras, R Aktunc. Laser in situ keratomileusis after photorefractive keratectomy for myopic regression. J Cataract Refract Surg 1998;24:1208–1211.

65. TE Dias-Martines, VM Sheludchenko, VV Kurenkov. Comparative results evaluation of residual myopia and astigmatism correction after radial keratotomy by photorefraction keratectomy and laser specialized keratomileusis. Vestn Oftalmol 1999;115:38–41.

66. Y Sakarya, EC Isik, SS Ermis. LASIK after PRK for myopic regression. J Cataract Refract Surg 1999;25:879.

67. M Mrochen, M Kaemmerer, T Seiler. Wavefront-guided laser in situ keratomileusis: early results in three eyes. J Refract Surg 2000;16:116–121.

68. W Attia, JJ Perez-Santonja, JL Alio. Laser in situ keratomileusis for recurrent hyperopia following laser thermal keratoplasty. J Refract Surg 2000;16:163–169.

69. W Portellinha, K Nakano, M Oliveira, R Simoceli. Laser in situ keratomileusis for hyperopia after thermal keratoplasty. Refract Surg 1999;15(suppl):S218–S220.

22

LASIK Following Radial Keratotomy and Photorefractive Keratectomy

NATALIE A. AFSHARI

Duke University Eye Center, Durham, North Carolina, U.S.A.

DIMITRI T. AZAR

Massachusetts Eye and Ear Infirmary, Schepens Eye Research Institute, and Harvard Medical School, Boston, Massachusetts, U.S.A.

Corneal refractive procedures change the corneal curvature in an attempt to correct myopia or hyperopia. Radial keratotomy (RK) flattens the center of the cornea through peripheral corneal incisions. Photorefractive keratectomy (PRK) reduces or increases corneal curvature by direct photoablation of the corneal stroma, while laser assisted in situ keratomileusis (LASIK) performs the same task after a flap is created and is lifted up.

Patient satisfaction following a refractive surgery procedure is the ultimate goal of any refractive surgeon. Many patients require enhancement following their initial procedure to reach their expected visual outcome.

This enhancement rate has been reported to be about 30% in patients who have undergone radial keratotomy (1,2). The Prospective Evaluation of Radial Keratotomy (PERK) study reported that 25% to 30% of patients who had undergone RK were hyperopes 10 years after treatment and as many as 43% of post RK patients had hyperopic shift of 1.00 D or more (3). The same study revealed that 17% of eyes had a residual myopia of greater than 1.00 D.

Undercorrection and regression following myopic PRK is dependent on the primary magnitude of the refractive error. Regression is the most common complication of PRK (4,5). Undercorrection of more than 1.00 D has been reported in only 2.7% of eyes with myopia of up to 6.00 D but in 42.8% of eyes with myopia of more than 10.00 D (6).

A. MANAGEMENT OF RESIDUAL REFRACTIVE ERRORS AFTER RADIAL KERATOTOMY AND PHOTOREFRACTIVE KERATECTOMY

1. Management of Refractive Errors After Radial Keratotomy

a. Residual Myopia

Spectacles, contact lenses, and reoperations including adding incisions, deepening incisions, reducing the clear zone, or performing another keratorefractive procedure such as PRK or LASIK have all been attempted in order to correct residual refractive error following RK (1). Sanders and coauthors reported that clear zone size is the most important factor affecting refractive change after primary RK (7). However, for optimal optical effect, there are limitations in the reduction of the size of the clear zone. Recent advances in excimer laser technology and its ease of use give the possibility of utilizing PRK and LASIK for enhancement after other refractive surgeries. Radial keratotomy works on the periphery of the cornea, while PRK flattens its central aspect. Thus the two can easily have additive effect. Yet studies have shown lower predictability of the refractive results in patients who have undergone PRK after RK compared to those with no previous surgical procedure (8–14). PRK following RK has been reported to lead to haze formation (5 to 10 times increase) and a significant (20%) reduction in refractive predictability. Azar and colleagues in a large multicenter retrospective study of PRK after RK reported that 11.1% of eyes lost 2 or more lines of BCVA at 12 months postoperatively (15). They also noted that patients with lower original and residual myopia after RK had better visual outcome after PRK compared to those patients with higher myopia. These results leave the surgeon with the most common procedure currently performed in the United States or LASIK as an enhancement tool.

Enhancement after refractive surgery brings out the important issue of the integrity of the eye after procedure. It is well known that radial keratotomy weakens the eye significantly, and more so than laser refractive surgery. Thus a thorough preoperative evaluation prior to any attempt at enhancement is required for optimal outcome.

b. Residual Hyperopia

Hyperopic treatment in these patients can be done through placement of peripheral circumferential compression sutures. Unfortunately, the refractive results from these procedures are unpredictable and surgeon dependent. Additionally, the effect of these sutures can decrease over time. LASIK is again an optimal procedure for enhancement in patients with hyperopia after PRK (16,17).

2. Management of Refractive Errors After Photorefractive Keratectomy

Photorefractive keratectomy as a measure to treat regression following primary PRK has been studied and found to have a lower success rate than the primary procedure. LASIK, a procedure with better refractive results, more postoperative comfort, and faster recovery of vision, has gradually replaced PRK in patients with high myopia. Additionally, LASIK can be used to treat residual myopia after PRK.

a. Outcomes

Published studies of LASIK after radial keratotomy and photorefractive keratectomy are listed in Tables 1 and 2.

Table 1 Results of LASIK after RK

Author	Eyes	Laser	Keratome	F/U	Preop	Postop
Forseto	14	VISX 20/20B	ACS	12.64 ± 5.02	−3.48 ± 3.52	−0.04 ± 0.87
Li Yong	16	Chiron 217	ACS	8.3	−3.14 ± 3.04	+0.16 ± 0.68
Viggiano	13	NA	NA	NA	+2.96 SE	+1.00
	7	NA	NA	NA		
Albon	8	Visx Star Smooth Scan	Moria LSK	3	+1.50	−0.75
De Wit	15	Chiron 217 Technolas	Hansatome	6	−0.25 to −10.0 sph −0.25 to −6 cyl	−0.74

F/U = mean follow-up in months; preop RE = mean spherical equivalent of preoperative refractive error in diopters; postop myopia = mean spherical equivalent of postoperative refractive error in diopters; cyl = cylinder in diopters; sph = sphere in diopters; ACS = Automated Corneal Shaper (Chiron vision); NA = not available.

b. LASIK After Radial Keratotomy

Forseto and colleagues performed LASIK for undercorrection after RK on 14 eyes with the VISX 20/20B excimer laser. Spherical equivalent decreased from −3.48 ± 3.52 D preoperatively to −0.04 ± 0.87 D postoperatively with an average follow-up of 12.64 ± 5.02 months (18).

Yong and colleagues reported 16 eyes of 10 patients that underwent LASIK enhancement with the Chiron 217 excimer laser following radial keratotomy. The mean spherical equivalent dropped from −3.14 ± 3.04 D preoperatively to +0.16 ± 0.68 D at a mean follow-up of 8.3 months (19).

Viggiano and colleagues reported 13 eyes that had LASIK after radial keratotomy for overcorrection with an average refractive error of +2.96 D and an average astigmatism of −4.00 D. Postoperatively the refractive error decreased to +1.00 D sphere and −1.04 D cylinder.

Alban and colleagues treated 8 eyes with consecutive hyperopia from prior corneal surgeries (RK, PRK, and/or LASIK). Mean spherical equivalent was +1.50 preoperatively and −0.75 3 months postoperatively (21).

De Wit and colleagues compared two groups of patients who underwent LASIK. The first group consisted of 15 eyes that underwent LASIK with the 217 Chiron Technolas excimer laser for residual myopia after RK ranging from −0.25 to −10.0 spherical and from

Table 2 Results of LASIK after PRK

Author	Eyes	Laser	Keratome	F/U (mon)	Preop (D)	Postop (D)
Ozdaman	45	Chiron Keracor 116	ACS	78.5 ± 8.12	5.96 ± 3.06	−0.67 ± 0.77
Kontos	35	VISX Star S-2	NA	12	1.87 (1.10 cyl)	0.3 (0.23 cyl)

PRK = photorefractive keratectomy; F/U = mean follow up in months; preop = mean spherical equivalent of refractive error in diopters before LASIK; postop = mean spherical equivalent of refractive error in diopters after LASIK; cyl = cylinder in diopters; ACS = Automated Corneal Shaper; mon = months; D = diopters; NA = not available.

−0.25 to −6.0 cylinder diopters (22). The second group consisted of 15 eyes with a similar refractive range but no previous RK. Six months postoperatively, group 1 had a mean spherical equivalent of 0.74, and group 2 had a mean spherical equivalent of −0.72. Mean anterior elevation, pachymetry, and keratometry were similar in both groups.

c.   LASIK After Photorefractive Keratectomy

Ozdamar and colleagues evaluated 45 eyes of 25 patients that had LASIK with the Chiron Keracor 116 excimer laser at a mean of 18.50 ± 8.12 months after photorefractive keratectomy for myopic regression. The mean spherical equivalent decreased from −5.95 ± 3.06 to −0.67 ± 0.77 D 6 months postoperatively (23).

Kontos reported 35 eyes that underwent LASIK using the VISX Star S-2 after PRK with a spherical reduction from 1.87 to 0.3 and average cylindrical reduction from 1.10 to 0.23 (24).

3.   Complications

a.   LASIK After Radial Keratotomy

Complications were rare in the reported series. A major concern in LASIK after RK is incisional dehiscence. Other complications include epithelial ingrowth, flap tear or dislocation, interface wrinkling or haze, infection, and central islands. A thorough preoperative evaluation including slit lamp examination and corneal topography is required to select patient candidates. Epithelial plugs within the RK incisions, which can lead to epithelial ingrowth, can be detected by slit lamp examination preoperatively. The time between primary RK and LASIK enhancement should be noted, and the integrity of the wound should be estimated preoperatively to avoid the "pizza pie" effect while creating a LASIK flap.

Forseto and colleagues reported epithelial ingrowth in one eye out of 14 eyes that had undergone LASIK for undercorrection after radial and arcuate keratotomy (18).

Yong and colleagues reported an intraoperative complication in two eyes out of the sixteen eyes in their series (19). The two eyes of one patient had their RK incision on the stromal bed partially opened when the corneal flap was lifted even though 10 years had elapsed from the time of the initial RK procedure. The flap was realigned and allowed to heal. Corneal incisions healed well without epithelial ingrowth, and emmetropia was noted 3 months postoperatively. Another patient in this series had a dislocated flap secondary to lid trichiasis. The eyelash was removed, the flap was revised, and a bandage contact lens was placed. The cornea remained clear postoperatively.

Viggiano and colleagues also reported opening of one inferior RK incision out of the 20 eyes that were treated with LASIK for myopia or hyperopia after RK (20).

b.   LASIK After Photorefractive Keratectomy

Ozdamar and colleagues in a study of 45 eyes that had LASIK after PRK for myopic regression reported no statistically significant difference in corneal haze before and after LASIK (23).

Kontos in a study of 35 eyes that had LASIK for residual refractive errors following PRK with the VISX Star S-2 laser noted 10% epithelial defects at the time of surgery and concluded that there was an increased risk of developing epithelial defects in patients undergoing LASIK following PRK (24).

B. SUMMARY

The PERK study has revealed that many patients have residual errors following radial keratotmy. Also, regression and undercorrection occurs in many patients who have undergone PRK for high myopia. Several options are available to correct these residual errors. Laser assisted in situ keratomileusis, by having a good refractive predictability, a low incidence of haze compared to PRK, and a fast visual recovery, can be a safe procedure for enhancement. A thorough preoperative evaluation is required for the best outcome.

REFERENCES

1. JL Gayton, M Van der Karr, V Sanders. Radial keratotomy enhancements for residual myopia. J Refract Surg 1997;13:374–381.
2. TP Werblin, GM Stafford. The Casebeer system for predictable keratorefractive surgery: one-year evaluation of 205 consecutive eyes. Ophthalmology 1993;100:1095–1102.
3. GO Waring, J Lynn, PJ McDonnell. Results of the prospective evaluation of radial keratotomy (PERK) study 10 years after surgery. Arch Ophthalmol 1994;112:1298–1308.
4. JH Kim, WJ Sah, CK Park, TW Hahn, MS Kim. Myopic regression after photorefractive keratectomy. Ophthalmic Surg Lasers 1996;27(suppl):S435–S439.
5. RB Vajpayee, CA McCarty, GF Aldred, HR Taylor. Undercorrection after excimer laser refractive surgery. Am J Ophthalmol 1996;122:801–807.
6. T Seiler, B Jean. Photorefractive keratectomy as a second attempt to correct myopia after radial keratotmy. Refract Corneal Surg 1992;8:211–214.
7. DR Sanders, MR Deitz, D Gallagher. Factors affecting predictability of radial keratotomy. Ophthalmology 1985;92:1237–1243.
8. RK Maloney, WK Chan, R Steinert, P Hersh, M O'Connell. A multicenter trial of photorefractive keratectomy for residual myopia after previous ocular surgery. Ophthalmology 1995;102:1042–1052.
9. PS Binder. Discussion. Ophthalmology 1995;102:1052–1053.
10. JC Ribeiro, MB McDonald, MM Lemos, JJ Salz, JV Della Russo, JV Aquavella, CA Swinger. Excimer laser photorefractive keratectomy after radial keratotomy. J Refract Surg 1995;11:165–169.
11. PJ McDonnell, JJ Garbus, JJ Salz. Excimer laser myopic photorefractive keratectomy after undercorrected radial keratotomy. Refract Corneal Surg 1991;7:146–150.
12. TW Hahn, JH Kim, YC Lee. Excimer laser photorefractive keratectomy to correct residual myopia after radial keratotomy. Refract Corneal Surg 1993;9(suppl);S25–S29.
13. DS Durrie, DJ Schumer, TB Cavanaugh. Photorefractive keratectomy for residual myopia after previous refractive keratotomy. J Refract Corneal Surg 1994;10:S235–S238.
14. J Meza, JJ Perez-Santonja, E Morena, MA Zato. Photorefractive keratectomy after radial keratotomy. J Cataract Refract Surg 1994;20:485–489.
15. DT Azar, S Tuli, RA Benson, DR Hardten. Photorefractive keratectomy for residual myopia after radial keratotomy. J Cataract Refract Surg 1998;303–311.
16. RL Lindstrom, DR Hardten, DM Houtman, YR Chu, EJ Linebarger. Six-month results of hyperopic and astigmatic LASIK in eyes with primary and secondary hyperopia. Trans Am Ophthalmol Soc 1999;97:241–255.
17. Linebarger EJ, Hardten DR, Lindstrom RL. Laser-assisted in situ keratomileusis for correction of secondary hyperopia after radial keratotomy. Int Ophthalmol Clin 2000;40:125–132.
18. AS Forseto, RA Nose, CM Francesconi, W Nose. Laser in situ keratomileusis for undercorrection after radial keratotomy. J Refract Surg 1999;15:424–428.
19. L Yong, G Chen, W Li, J Chang, C Ngan, P Tong, C Qun. Laser in situ keratomileusis enhancement after radial keratotomy. J Refract Surg 2000;16:187–190.

20. D Viggiano, O Baca, R Velasco, L Lopez. Photorefractive keratectomy and laser in situ keratomileusis (LASIK) after radial keratotomy. ARVO 2000.

21. T Alban, BD Soloway, R Maw. Hyperopic LASIK results in patients with consecutive hyperopia. ASCRS 2000.

22. G de Wit, R Malvaiz, E Hernandez, G Palacios, A Nino, R Naranjo. LASIK after RK: refractive and elevation topography results. ASCRS 2000.

23. A Ozdamar, B Sener, C Aras, R Aktunc. Laser in situ keratomileusis after photorefractive keratectomy for myopic regression. J Cataract Refract Surg 1998;24:1208–1211.

24. MA Kantos. LASIK using Visx Star S-2 for the treatment of residual refractive errors after PRK. ASCRS 2000.

23

LASIK After Penetrating Keratoplasty

GLENN C. COCKERHAM

Allegheny Ophthalmology and Orbital Associates, Pittsburgh, Pennsylvania, U.S.A.

NATALIE A. AFSHARI

Duke University Eye Center, Durham, North Carolina, U.S.A.

A. INTRODUCTION

Full-thickness penetrating keratoplasty (PK) is a common ocular surgery, in which recipient cornea is removed and replaced with tissue obtained from a cadaveric donor. This surgery is useful in a variety of conditions that result in corneal opacification, edema, scarring, irregularity, or thinning. An estimated 41,000 PKs are performed in the United States each year (1). A variety of factors may influence postoperative refractive error and astigmatism. The antemortem curvature and cylinder of the donor cornea will affect the final result; this information, however, is not available to the surgeon. Thinning of the recipient cornea, as in keratoconus, has been reported to lead to increased cylinder after PK (2). Trephination technique and graft sizing also may affect postoperative refractive error; enhanced effect of suture tension on the central cornea should theoretically occur in smaller grafts.

Sutures exert a profound influence on the sphericity of the transplanted corneal button. Radial sutures cause flattening of the central cornea, with tighter and longer sutures creating more effect. Plus cylinder is induced in the axis of tight sutures. Techniques to minimize astigmatism include placement of a single or double continuous running suture. Qualitative or quantitative keratometry may allow dynamic intraoperative adjustment of suture tension if epithelium is present on the donor button. Adjustment of continuous suture tension based on keratometry or topographic analysis may be beneficial in the immediate postoperative period. Selective removal of tight interrupted sutures beginning several weeks after surgery will also modify postoperative astigmatism. Even in the hands of experienced surgeons, residual refractive errors, including high amounts of astigmatism, are common after PK. Most studies report average postkeratoplasty astigmatism of 4 to 5 diopters (D) (2). Kirkness and associates reported that 20% of patients required refractive surgery for astigmatism after successful PK (3).

B. EVALUATION OF ASTIGMATISM

Postkeratoplasty astigmatism is measured after final stabilization of the cornea. This requires an interval of 4 to 6 months after removal of all sutures. Using a common methodology allows investigators to compare results across different studies. The advantages of standard office keratometry include widespread availability and familiarity by clinicians, as well as ease of calibration. The main disadvantage is limitation of measurement to the central anterior corneal surface, encompassing an area with a diameter of approximately 3 mm. Central keratometry does not evaluate the status of the peripheral graft surfaces. Unlike naturally occurring orthogonal astigmatism, peripheral curvatures and cylinder after keratoplasty may not correlate well with central measurements. Computerized videokeratography, or topographic analysis, projects a Placido disk image onto the anterior corneal surface and interprets the reflected pattern. Topography provides a representation of the surfaces of peripheral graft and recipient cornea, allowing estimation of degree and direction of vector forces acting upon the transplanted tissue. Current programs permit comparison of serial images and provide subtraction analysis of interim changes, which is useful as sutures are removed and postoperative corneal healing and remodeling occur. Analysis of posterior corneal surfaces is now possible by technology that interprets optical sections by a scanning slit beam.

C. MANAGEMENT OF POSTKERATOPLASTY ASTIGMATISM

1. Refractive aids

Spectacles are helpful in some postkeratoplasty patients, but their use is limited by image disparity caused by anisometropia. Tilt and optical aberrations from spectacle correction of high amounts of astigmatism may be difficult to adapt to, especially in older patients. Finally, spectacles cannot correct irregular astigmatism. Rigid gas permeable lenses create less object minification or magnification than spectacles and thereby reduce anisometropia. Additionally, they provide a smooth anterior surface and effectively reduce both regular and irregular astigmatism. Postkeratoplasty astigmatism as high as 17 D has been managed with rigid gas permeable lenses (4). Contact lens fitting in the postkeratoplasty patient may be difficult and time-consuming. Altered corneal topography at the graft–host interface may complicate lens wear. Lens wear may stimulate corneal neovascularization, with increased potential for graft rejection. Wearing rigid lenses in a setting of high myopia and astigmatism is difficult; in a study of postkeratoplasty patients, 13 percent of patients discontinued rigid gas permeable lenses owing to intolerance (4).

2. Incisional Surgical Procedures

a. Radial Keratotomy

Radial keratotomy (RK) has been used to reduce postkeratoplasty myopia, allowing the wearing of spectacles (5). RK is not effective for reducing postkeratoplasty astigmatism.

Potential problems with RK after PK include permanent structural weakening of the cornea, induction of irregular astigmatism, and neovascular ingrowth along the radial cuts. The use of RK for correction of myopia has decreased with the introduction of the excimer laser.

b. Corneal Relaxing Incisions

Troutman described the basic concepts of corneal relaxing incisions (6). Incisions placed in the cornea cause relaxation of tissue, effectively adding tissue to the area incised. Transverse incisions placed in the steep meridian cause reduction of astigmatism. Factors influencing the magnitude of cylinder reduction include distance of the cut from the optical center and the length and depth of the incision. Relaxing incisions in general do not change the spherical power of the cornea; thus they may reduce astigmatism but not myopia. Arcuate incisions provide a longer chord length than linear incisions. Relaxing incisions may be combined with compression sutures of polypropylene placed through the graft–host interface in the flat meridian, allowing some titration of effect by postoperative suture adjustment or removal. Average keratometric reduction of cylinder of 7.95 D has been reported (7). Arffa reported a 77% reduction in mean astigmatism in six patients treated with relaxing incisions and compression sutures, with a minimum time of 8 months after penetrating keratoplasty (8). Complications of relaxing incisions include corneal perforation, infection, graft rejection, and over- or undercorrection (Figure 23.1).

3. Excimer laser

Precise ablation of a desired amount of corneal tissue is possible using the excimer laser at a wavelength of 193 nm. The excimer laser has the ability surgically to correct myopia, hyperopia, and astigmatism, depending on the laser system and profile chosen. Correction of myopia and myopic astigmatism is possible using an expanding slit diaphragm, as in the VISX laser delivery systems. Simultaneous treatment of myopia and cylinder is possible by expanding the circular and slit diaphragms concurrently; however, with this method the amount of astigmatism corrected cannot exceed the spherical component. Sequential expansion of the circular and slit diaphragms allows correction of more astigmatism than myopia. An undesired hyperopic shift of the spherical equivalent is prevented by limiting the width of the slit to 80% of the length (9).

Scanning laser technology uses a smaller beam for photoablation. Astigmatism is corrected by additional treatment in a specific meridian. Both myopic and hyperopic astigmatism can be corrected. However, because of the smaller beam size, more time is required for treatment, and a reliable eye tracking mechanism is necessary for precise treatment.

An ablatable mask allows transference of the anterior curvature of the mask onto the anterior surface of the cornea, theoretically allowing a precise ablation of any profile, including myopia, myopic astigmatism, hyperopia, hyperopic astigmatism, and irregular astigmatism (9). Several laser systems use variations of this principle to achieve a desired refractive effect. Nonorthogonal, or irregular, astigmatism is often present after PK. Simple geometric profiles will not reduce this surface irregularity. Gibralter and Trokel have described a customized ablation using circles of varying sizes to create a more regular optical surface (10). Linkage of a scanning laser to a topographic map holds promise for individualized treatment of irregular corneas.

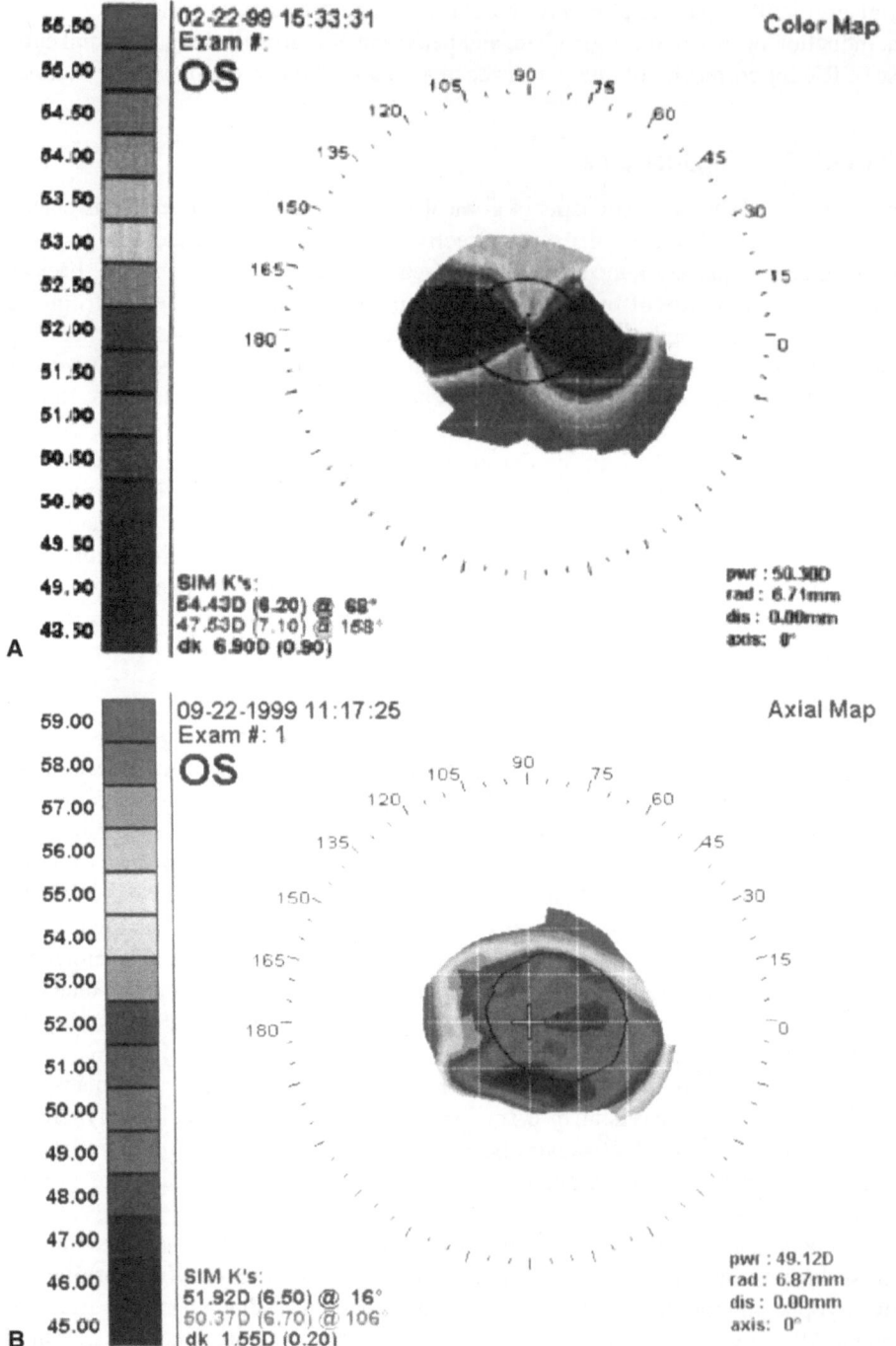

A

B

Table 1 Results of PRK After Penetrating Keratoplasty

Author	Eyes	Laser	Mode	Int PK (min) (mo)	F/U (min) (mo)	Preop myopia (D)	Postop myopia (D)	Preop cyl (D)	Postop cyl (D)
John	3	Summit	PRK	NA	6 to 11	8.83	5.37	NA	NA
Campos	12	VISX 20/20	PARK	NA	6	7.4	3.3	7.0	4.3
Nordan	5	VISX 20/20	PRK	15	6	5.9	2.6	3.05	1.30
Tuunanen	10	VISX 20/20	PARK	12	12	2.89	0.56	5.98	3.36
Lazzaro	7	VISX	PARK	24	12	5.9	2.52 @ 6 mo	5.32	2.79
Amm	13	Aesculap	PARK	18	6	NA	NA	5.7	3.6

PRK = photorefractive keratectomy; Int PK = minimal interval after previous penetrating keratoplasty in months before PRK; F/U = minimal follow-up in months; preop myopia = mean spherical equivalent of myopia in diopters before PRK; postop myopia = mean spherical equivalent of myopia in diopters after PRK; preop cyl = mean cylinder in diopters before PRK; postop cyl = mean cylinder in diopters after PRK; PARK = photoastigmatic refractive keratectomy; mo = months; D = diopters; NA = not available. [Color in original.]

4. Photorefractive Keratectomy (PRK) After PK

Treatment of the anterior corneal surface by PRK has been employed for the correction of myopia and myopic astigmatism after penetrating keratoplasty. Results of published studies are listed in Table 1. John and colleagues treated three PK patients for myopia, with initial improvement in all (11). Amm and associates used an Aesculap Meditec MEL excimer laser with a rotating mask system for correction of postkeratoplasty cylinder in 16 eyes. The mean preoperative cylinder of 5.7 D was reduced by 2.8 D with 6 months follow-up (12). Campos and associates performed toric ablations on 12 patients with disabling astigmatism after PK. Mean reduction of astigmatism was 38% with a minimum follow-up of 6 months (13). Nordan and associates reported a mean reduction in cylinder of 45% in five PK patients followed for at least 6 months (14). Tuunanen and associates studied ten eyes of nine patients treated 4 months or later after suture removal. The preoperative astigmatism ranged from 3.5 to 11.25 D (mean 5.98); net corneal astigmatism was reduced 48% with a minimum follow-up of 12 months (15). In a series by Lazzaro and colleagues, an average

Figure 23.1 Corneal topography of a 35-year-old man who presented 5 years status after keratoplasty and 3 years status after astigmatic keratectomy with high astigmatism in the operated left eye. His visual acuity was 20/30 in the unoperated right eye and he counted fingers at 5 feet in the left eye. Manifest refraction OD was plano-2.00 × 95 and OS −4.50−8.00 × 167. Patient underwent a LASIK flap cut with Hansatome microkeratome initially without any laser treatment. On postoperative day 7, his manifest refraction OS had stabilized to the preoperative measurement of −4.50−8.75 × 155. Subsequently, the flap was lifted and the patient underwent partial treatment of the refractive error. The laser was programmed with −1.8−3.75 × 170 and his 2 weeks postoperative refraction improved to −4.25−3.00 × 155. Three months later the flap was lifted and the patient was given the rest of the treatment as the laser was programmed with −3.00−3.75 × 155. Two months later, the patient's manifest refraction had stabilized to +0.25−2.50 × 47. The pre-LASIK corneal topography is shown in A and the final corneal topography is shown in B.

reduction of astigmatism by 48% was found in seven eyes after treatment with a minimum follow-up of 12 months (16).

Problems were encountered with PRK after previous PK. John et al. reported substantial regression in three of three patients, with significant haze in one (11). Campos et al. found a mean shift in axis of 58 degrees, with astigmatic overcorrections in four patients (13). Significant haze and regression were encountered in some cases. Tuunanen et al. noted regression as late as 7 to 8 months postoperatively; in their series four patients developed significant haze and scarring (15). Lazzaro et al. reported that one eye developed dense haze with scar formation (16).

Single case reports raise the possibility of increased risk of graft rejection after surface ablation with an excimer laser. An endothelial rejection occurred 2 weeks after phototherapeutic keratectomy for recurrent lattice corneal dystrophy in a six-year-old graft (17); in another case endothelial rejection was diagnosed 5 days after PRK for myopia and astigmatism in a three-year-old graft, despite postoperative use of 0.1% fluomethalone (18). These cases suggest a temporal association of an immune response to surface ablation by an excimer laser. Possible catalysts include mechanical epithelial debridement, ultraviolet radiation emission by the excimer laser, or postoperative epithelial defect.

D. LASER-ASSISTED IN-SITU KERATOMILEUSIS (LASIK)

1. Introduction

LASIK offers refractive ablation under a hinged flap of epithelium, Bowman's layer, and anterior stromal tissue. Replacement of this flap after the procedure lessens postoperative pain and reduces wound remodeling, haze, and regression. The association of potentially severe haze and regression with PRK after PK has led to increased interest in LASIK as the preferred refractive method for correction of postkeratoplasty astigmatism and myopia. In all instances, surgery was performed in patients who were intolerant of both spectacle and contact lens wear.

A Chiron Vision Automated Corneal Shaper microkeratome was used in all published reports to date. This microkeratome makes about an 8.5 mm flap with a nasal hinge, depending on the corneal curvature. In one series an attempt was made to avoid initiating a microkeratome cut at the graft–host interface (19). Kritzinger and Probst described a sequenced LASIK technique in which the suction ring is applied and the flap created. However, the flap is left undisturbed for 2 to 3 weeks. Preoperative assessment is repeated; the refraction changes in about half of eyes, especially the amount and orientation of cylinder. Using the new parameters, the flap is lifted and treatment performed. Kritzinger and Probst speculate that the dynamic forces acting upon a postkeratoplasty donor cornea are altered by the LASIK cut (20). Standard LASIK nomograms were utilized in these studies. A variation of this technique with sequential laser correction has also proven successful (Fig 23.1).

2. Results of Published Studies

Published studies of LASIK after penetrating keratoplasty are listed in Table 2. Arenas and Maglione performed LASIK on four eyes from 1.7 to 9 years after PK with a Technolas Keracor 116 excimer laser to correct myopia and astigmatism. Mean spherical equivalent decreased from -10.75 to -2.37 D after surgery with a mean follow-up of 7 months. However, mean astigmatism increased after surgery from 2.87 to 3.50 D (21). Parisi and associates described LASIK in a case 2 years after PK. A Chiron Vision Keracor 117

Table 2 Results of LASIK After Penetrating Keratoplasty

Author	Eyes	Laser	Keratome	F/U (min) (mo)	Int PK (min) (mo)	Int PK (mean) (mo)	Preop myop (D)	Postop myop (D)	Preop cyl (D)	Postop cyl (D)	TIA (D)	SIA (D)
Forseto	22	VISX 20/20	ACS	6	18	63	4.55	0.67	4.24	1.79	NA	NA
Webber	26	Summit Apex	ACS	6	23	107	5.2	1.31	8.67	2.92	5.91	3.88
Parisi	1	Chiron Keracor	ACS	11	24	24	7.67	0.67 (Hyper)	1.25	0.75	NA	NA
Koay	8	Chiron Technolas	ACS	6	24	71	6.79	0.64	6.79	1.93	6.79	5.5
Arenas	4	Chiron Technolas	ACS	6	19	NA	10.75	2.37	2.87	3.5	NA	NA
Donnenfeld	23	VISX	ACS	1	8	44	7.58	1.09	3.64	1.98	NA	NA
Spadea	4	VISX 20/20	ACS	12	20	25	9.31	1.13	4.87	1.5	NA	NA

F/U (min) = minimal follow up in months; Int PK (min) = minimal interval in months between penetrating keratoplasty and LASIK; Int PK (mean) = mean interval in months between penetrating keratoplasty and LASIK; Preop myop = mean spherical equivalent of preoperative myopia in diopters; Postop myop = mean spherical equivalent of postoperative myopia in diopters; Preop cyl = mean preoperative cylinder in diopters; Postop cyl = postoperative cylinder in diopters; TIA = target induced astigmatism (attempted reduction of astigmatism); SIA = surgically induced astigmatism; ACS = automated corneal shaper (Chiron Vision); mo = months; D = diopters; NA = not available.

excimer laser was used. Refraction changed from -7.00-1.25×60 to $+1.00$-0.75×80 after 11 months of follow-up (22).

Forseta and colleagues performed LASIK on 22 eyes with a VISX 20/20 excimer laser with a mean interval after PK of 5.3 years. Spherical equivalent decreased from -4.55 to -0.67 D after LASIK with at least 6 months follow-up. There was no statistically significant difference between 1-month and 6-month values. Mean preoperative cylinder decreased from 4.24 to 1.79 D after surgery (23). In a series by Donnenfeld and associates, 23 eyes underwent LASIK with a VISX Star excimer laser with a mean time of 44 months after PK and 35.3 months after suture removal. The mean spherical equivalent was reduced from -7.58 preoperatively to -0.79 D (22 eyes) at 3 months postoperatively. Mean cylinder decreased from 3.64 preoperatively to 1.64 D (22 eyes) at 3 months (19).

Koay and colleagues evaluated eight eyes that received LASIK with a Technolas 217 excimer laser after a mean 71 months after PK and several months after suture removal. The mean spherical equivalent dropped from-6.79 preoperatively to -1.93 D at 6 months follow-up. The mean cylinder changed from 6.79 to 1.93 D at 6 months follow-up (24).

Spadea and associates reported four eyes that underwent LASIK after a mean interval of 24.75 months after PK. In all cases a VISX 20/20 B excimer laser was used. The mean spherical equivalent changed from -9.31 preoperatively to -1.13 D at 3 months postoperatively (25).

Webber and associates reported a series of 26 eyes undergoing LASIK after PK with a Summit Apex Plus excimer laser. Fourteen eyes with higher degrees of cylinder also received arcuate cuts in the stromal bed with a guarded diamond knife set at 360 µm. The mean interval between PK and LASIK was 8 years and 11 months. Sutures had been removed at least 10 months before LASIK. The mean preoperative spherical equivalent of -5.20 D was reduced to -0.24 at 1 month. The mean preoperative cylinder of 8.67 D was reduced to 2.48 D at 1 month. At 1 month the mean surgically induced astigmatism (SIA) was 7.04 D for the entire group. SIA was 8.86 D for the group with arcuate incisions, and 4.86 D for the group without incisions (26).

3. Complications

Complications were rare in the reported series. A major concern in LASIK after PK is wound dehiscence from the high intraocular pressure achieved during application of suction. Internal ocular pressure is documented to be over 65 mm Hg with the Barraquer tonometer; however, pneumotonometry often reveals pressures over 100 mm Hg. For this reason, wound healing of the graft–host interface was allowed for several years before LASIK in most of the previous studies. In general, LASIK after PK should be performed by experienced surgeons to minimize total time of suction.

Abnormality or loss of endothelial cells as a consequence of elevated intraocular pressure is another potential complication of LASIK. Several studies suggest that short-term loss of endothelium is minimal after LASIK in corneas without previous surgery. Fresh cadaver globes were treated for up to 25 D of myopia with LASIK; after organ culture for 1 week the endothelial cells were stained and evaluated with fluorescence microscopy. There were no significant differences between treated eyes and untreated control globes (27). Specular microscopy of the corneal endothelium after LASIK has revealed no significant differences between preoperative values and postoperative intervals of 3 and 6 months (28). Previous ocular surgery changes the pace of endothelial dropout. Corneal transplantation leads to accelerated endothelial cell loss for at least 5 years. Bourne reported that mean endothelial cell density declined at a rate of 7.8% per year from 3 to 5 years after PK, compared with approximately 0.5% per year in the same time interval in unoperated normal corneas. The mean cell loss at 5 years after keratoplasty was 59% compared with preoperative values (29). The long-term response of the endothelium to superimposed LASIK on a previous keratoplasty is unknown; however, no significant differences were noted in preoperative and postoperative central endothelial cell counts of 22 eyes undergoing LASIK after PK with a minimal follow-up of 6 months (23).

A long interval between PK and LASIK also allows reestablishment of corneal sensation. Theoretically, there is less loss of sensation with LASIK than with PRK, because the hinge area contains intact superficial nerve fibers. Sterile ulceration and intractable dry eye have not been reported in this setting.

Endothelial rejection of a donor graft after LASIK is a cause of concern and may arise either from flap creation or handling, or from the ultraviolet radiation of excimer laser treatment. However, none has been reported during the study interval of these series. Possibly the maintenance of an epithelial cap diminishes immunostimula tion by cytokines produced from a wounded corneal surface. Postoperative use of topical steroids may also exert a protective effect.

E. SUMMARY

Despite modern instrumentation and techniques to minimize tissue disparity and unequal suturing, ametropia, including high astigmatism, remains a common problem after penetrating keratoplasty. Anisometropia leads to spectacle intolerance. Rigid contact lenses are very beneficial in the postkeratoplasty setting, but satisfactory wear is not possible in all patients. Incisional refractive techniques have been utilized with some successes. Arcuate cuts to reduce cylinder are useful, and may be combined with excimer laser surgery for higher amounts of astigmatism. The excimer laser is a tool capable of precise tissue modeling. PRK has demonstrated significant reductions in myopia and astigmatism, but unacceptable haze and regression reduce its effectiveness. LASIK has also proven useful in reducing postkeratoplasty myopia and astigmatism, with few complications. Prerequisites for LASIK after penetrating keratoplasty include adequate healing and wound strength of the graft–host interface, corneal and refractive stabilization after removal of all sutures, and, in principle, spectacle and contact lens intolerance. The long-term effects of LASIK on the corneal endothelium and graft longevity remain to be determined, but early results are promising. LASIK provides the corneal surgeon with a means of rehabilitating this group of patients with clear grafts and disabling refractive consequences.

REFERENCES

1. DD Verdier. Penetrating keratoplasty. In: JH Krachmer, MJ Mannis, EJ Holland, eds. Cornea: Surgery of the Cornea and Conjunctiva. Vol III. St Louis: Mosby, 1997, pp 1581–1592.
2. CS Reing, MG Speaker. Postkeratoplasty astigmatism. In: JH Krachmer, MJ Mannis, EJ Holland, eds. Cornea: Surgery of the Cornea and Conjunctiva. Vol III. St. Louis: Mosby, 1997, pp 1675–1686.
3. CM Kirkness, LA Ficker, AD Steele, NS Rice. Refractive surgery for graft-induced astigmatism after penetrating keratoplasty for keratoconus. Ophthalmology 1991;98:1786–1792.
4. GI Genvert, EJ Cohen, JJ Arentsen, PR Laibson. Fitting gas-permeable contact lenses after penetrating keratoplasty. Am J Ophthalmol 1985;99:511–514.
5. MB Shapiro, DA Harrison. Radial keratotomy for intolerable myopia after penetrating keratoplasty. Am J Ophthalmol 1993;115:327–331.
6. RC Troutman. Corneal wedge resections and relaxing incisions for postkeratoplasty astigmatism. Int Ophthalmol Clin 1983;23:161–168.
7. DL McCartney, LE Whitney, WJ Stark, SK Wong, DA Bernitsky. Refractive keratoplasty for disabling astigmatism after penetrating keratoplasty. Arch Ophthalmol 1987;105:954–957.
8. RC Arffa. Results of a graded relaxing incision technique for postkeratoplasty astigmatism. Ophthalmic Surg 1988;19:624–628.
9. A Poon, HR Taylor. Astigmatic photorefractive keratectomy. In: HK Wu, VM Thompson, RF Steinert, SG Slade, PS Hersh, eds. Refractive surgery. New York: Thieme, 1999, pp 307–318.
10. R Gibralter, SL Trokel. Correction of irregular astigmatism with the excimer laser. Ophthalmology 1994;101:1310–1315.
11. ME John, E Martines, T Cvintal, AM Filho, F Soter, MC Barbosa, KL Boleyn, C Ballew. Photorefractive keratectomy following penetrating keratoplasty. J Cataract Corneal Surg 1994;10:S206–S210.
12. M Amm, GI Duncker, E Schroeder. Excimer laser correction of high astigmatism after keratoplasty. J Cataract Refract Surg 1996;22:313–317.
13. M Campos, L Hertzog, J Garbus, M Lee, PJ McDonnell. Photorefractive keratectomy for severe postkeratoplasty astigmatism. Am J Ophthalmol 1992;114:429–436.
14. LT Nordan, PS Binder, BS Kassar, J Heitzmann. Photorefractive keratectomy to treat myopia and astigmatism after radial keratotomy and penetrating keratoplasty. J Cataract Refract Surg 1995;21:268–273.
15. TH Tuunanen, PJ Ruusuvaara, RJ Uusitalo, TM Tervo. Photoastigmatic keratectomy for correction of astigmatism in corneal grafts. Cornea 1997;16:48–53.
16. DR Lazzaro, DH Haight, SC Belmont, RP Gibralter, AM Aslanides, MG Odrich. Excimer laser keratectomy for astigmatism occurring after penetrating keratoplasty. Ophthalmology 1996;103:458–464.
17. PS Hersh, AJ Jordan, M Mayers. Corneal graft rejection episode after excimer laser phototherapeutic keratectomy (letter). Arch Ophthalmol 1993;111:735–736.

18. RJ Epstein, JB Robin. Corneal graft rejection after excimer laser phototherapeutic keratectomy (letter). Arch Ophthalmol 1994;112:157.

19. ER Donnenfeld, HS Kornstein, A Amin, MD Speaker, JA Seedor, PD Sforza, LM Landrio, HD Perry. Laser in situ keratomileusis for correction of myopia and astigmatism after penetrating keratoplasty. Ophthalmology 1999;106:1966–1975.

20. M Kritzinger, LE Probst. LASIK after penetrating keratoplasty. In: JJ Machat, SG Slade, LE Probst, eds. The Art of LASIK. Thorofare, NJ: Slack, 1998, pp 325–327.

21. E Arenas, A Maglione. Laser in situ keratomileusis for astigmatism and myopia after penetrating keratoplasty. J Refract Surg 1997;13:27–32.

22. A Parisi, DJ Salchow, ME Zirm, C Stieldorf. Laser in situ keratomileusis after automated lamellar keratoplasty and penetrating keratoplasty. J Cataract Refract Surg 1997;23:1114–1118.

23. AS Forsetto, CM Francesconi, RAM Nose, W Nose. Laser in situ keratomileusis to correct refractive errors after keratoplasty. J Cataract Refract Surg 1999;25:479–485.

24. PYP Koay, CNJ McGhee, KH Weed, JP Craig. Laser in situ keratomileusis for ametropia after penetrating keratoplasty. J Refract Surg 2000;16:140–147.

25. L Spadea, L Mosca, E Balestrazzi. Effectiveness of LASIK to correct refractive error after penetrating keratoplasty. Ophthalmic Surg Lasers 2000;31:111–120.

26. SK Webber, MA Lawless, GL Sutton, CM Rogers. LASIK for post penetrating keratoplasty astigmatism and myopia. Br J Ophthalmol 1999;83:1013–1018.

27. DG Kent, KD Solomon, Q Peng, SB Whiteside, SJ Brown, DJ Apple. Effect of surface photorefractive keratectomy and laser in situ keratomileusis on the corneal endothelium. J Cataract Refract Surg 1997;23:386–397.

28. JJ Perez-Santonja, HF Sakla, F Gobbi, JL Alio. Corneal endothelium changes after laser in situ keratomileusis. J Cataract Refract Surg 1997;23:177–183.

29. WM Bourne, DO Hodge, LR Nelson. Corneal endothelium five years after transplantation. Am J Ophthalmol 1994;118:185–196.

24

Bioptics
Combined LASIK and Phakic Intraocular Lens Surgery

**JOSÉ L. GÜELL, MERCEDES VÁZQUEZ, FORTINO VELASCO,
and FELICIDAD MANERO**

Instituto de Microcirugía Ocular, Barcelona, Spain

A. INTRODUCTION

Bioptics is the combination of two refractive procedures: (1) an intraocular procedure, especially a phakic intraocular lens (ph-IOL) implantation, and (2) a corneal procedure such as laser in situ keratomileusis (LASIK), intracorneal ring segments (ICRS) implantation, or, in the near future, intracorneal lens implantation. The primary goal is to correct high degrees of refractive errors within safe limits and with the best quality of vision.

The bioptics concept, first described by Zaldivar et al. (1,2) was born from the need to correct the residual myopia that could not be completely corrected with the implantation of a posterior chamber ph-IOL. The risk of implanting lenses with powers higher than −20.00 diopters (D), even though in the anterior or posterior chamber, was the original reason for performing a combined surgery.

With the goal of working with the largest possible optical zone in both the ph-IOL and LASIK, we started using bioptics in most corrections greater than −15.00 D. We intended to correct up to −15.00 D with the IOL and correct the rest of the myopic and/or cylindrical residual defect with LASIK in a second surgery, maintaining a 6 mm minimal optical zone in both procedures (3).

B. ADJUSTABLE REFRACTIVE SURGERY (ARS)

The adjustable refractive surgery (ARS) concept (3,4) applied to this combination procedure introduced the innovation of performing the flap during but immediately before the IOL implantation (first procedure).

329

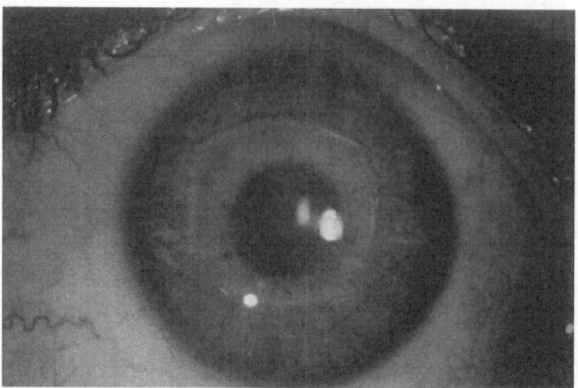

Figure 24.1 Artisan™ lens implantations plus LASIK in a patient with −18.00 D of myopia.

The first procedure, the intraocular surgery, is performed under topical or peribulbar anesthesia depending on the IOL style and the surgeon's preference. The lamellar cut is made, we check for any irregularity, and the interface is cleaned with balanced salt solution (BSS), being then replaced again and its border dried. Immediately after, implantation is done as usual (5). We have been using the Artisan™ lens (Figs. 24.1, 24.2), an iris-fixed IOL that allows the maintenance of a 6 mm optical zone up to −15.00 D of power. Other advantages are a safer distance to the endothelium compared with angle-supported lenses, no contact with posterior chamber structures, and, most important in our opinion, a surgeon-dependent centration and fixation. The main disadvantage of this PMMA lens is its size. Although an iridectomy is probably not necessary in most cases, because they are quite far from the iris to induce a pupillary block, we do regularly perform a slit peripheral iridotomy.

After all suture removal under videokeratographic control and cylinder stabilization, LASIK is performed, as in any other LASIK enhancement, 2 to 5 months after the ph-IOL implantation. A 6 mm minimal optical zone is also maintained in this second procedure.

Some of the advantages of the ARS approach are larger optical zones compared to LASIK or ph-IOL implantation alone and higher predictability (6). In addition to the pos-

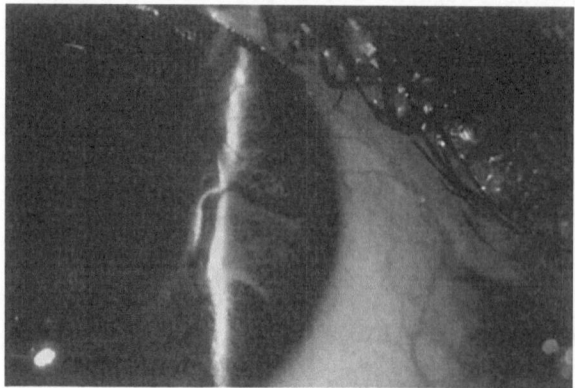

Figure 24.2 Iris grasped with both "claws."

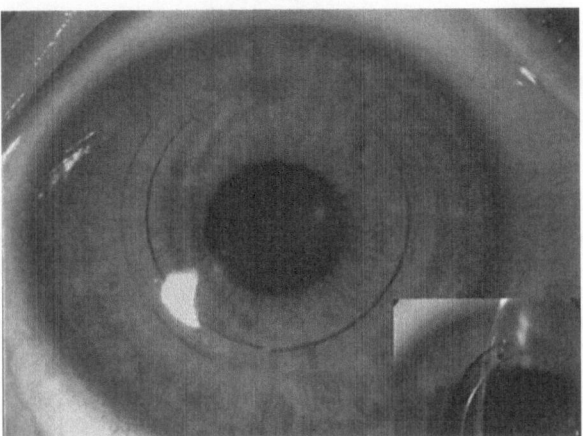

Figure 24.3   Iris on a post LASIK eye.

sible complications associated with each of the procedures, an increased rate of epithelial ingrowth has been reported in some LASIK enhancement series (7), but we did not see this in our series (4).

C.   POSSIBLE COMBINATIONS IN BIOPTICS

Several combinations of procedures to perform bioptics are available. Each surgeon must choose the combination most appropriate for each patient.

For safety reasons it is not possible to correct high ametropias with a 6 mm optical zone ph-IOL. The higher the ametropia to be corrected, the thicker will be the ph-IOL, in the center in lenses for hyperopia correction and in the periphery in lenses for myopia correction. Obviously, the main concern is corneal endothelium–IOL touch with phakic anterior chamber IOLs and pigmentary dispersion with or without glaucoma and cataract induction with phakic posterior chamber IOLs.

The standard alternative to reducing the IOL thickness is to reduce its optical zone, but this will also reduce the quality of vision, especially under dim illumination conditions.

In high myopic or hyperopic patients submitted for lens surgery with or without cataract, a bioptics procedure used to be a good option if the desired postoperative result is emmetropia; even with the new formulas and technology improvements there are still difficulties in calculating the exact IOL dioptric power in these cases. On the other hand, it is usually easier to titrate the final ideal refraction for each patient, once they are close to emmetropia after the intraocular surgery.

Possible bioptics combinations that have improved our results within safety conditions are as follows:

1.   Phakic IOL implantation plus LASIK or ICRS implantation. Anterior chamber ph-IOLs: angle-fixated IOLs (MA20 Nu Vita™ IOL, Bausch & Lomb Surgical/Chiron Vision, Irvine, CA, USA; Phakic 6 Model 130, Ophthalmic Innovations International Inc., CA, USA; Morcher Model 93[a], Morcher GMBH, Stuttgart, Germany; iris-fixed IOLs, Artisan™ IOL, Ophthec, Groningen, Netherlands. Posterior ph-IOLs: silicone lenses (Fyodorov style, Chiron-Adatomed, Munich, Germany; International Vision Medenium posterior chamber phakic refractive lens; or collagen lenses, hydrogel-collagen IOL, Collamer Implantable Contact Lens™, STAAR Surgical AG, Nidau, Switzerland.

2. Clear or semiclear lens extraction plus LASIK or ICRS implantation.
3. Cataract surgery plus LASIK or ICRS implantation.
4. Other combinations, not strictly considered within the bioptics concept but extremely helpful in some clinical settings, are arcuate keratotomy with LASIK (8) and LASIK with ICRS (9) (Fig. 24.3).

D. PREOPERATIVE EXAMINATION

As in any refractive procedure, the preoperative examination must include

1. Uncorrected and best corrected visual acuity (UCVA/BCVA). We suggest obtaining BCVA with spectacles (BSCVA) and also over rigid gas-permeable contact lenses with residual refractive error of less than −4.00 D of myopia.
2. Manifest and cycloplegic refraction, measured at the spectacle plane.
3. Pupil size under photopic and scotopic conditions. It is very important to warn patients with large pupils that they might suffer from glare and halos after the surgery. Most high-risk patients for halo have already had this experience with their contact lenses.
4. Corneal topography will identify any possible corneal problem, such as keratoconus.
5. Central and midperipheral corneal pachymetry will allow calculation of the safety range of corneal laser ablation and determine the depth at which ICRS must be implanted.
6. Axial length and anterior chamber depth map (central and peripheral) are essential when a ph-IOL will be implanted, especially in cases where the final option is an anterior chamber model.
7. Endothelial cell count and morphologic examination are indispensable for assessing the long-term safety of phakic anterior chamber IOL implantation.
8. Contrast sensitivity is a complementary exam to evaluate objectively the quality of vision. We, as do many other groups, perform several other procedures (front wave analysis) to evaluate the optical performance of the eye (v.gr. OQAS, Optical Quality Analysis System—Politecnica University of Catalunya. Optical Development Department).
9. Indirect and direct ophthalmoscopy are especially important to evaluate the peripheral retina and posterior pole. If prophylactic laser retinal treatment is needed, it should be performed and controlled before any refractive surgery.
10. Other standard examinations are applanation tonometry and Javal keratometry readings. Javal or topographic keratometry will also indicate the best suction ring size for performing the flap or the intrastromal channels to position the ICRS.

E. INDICATIONS AND CONTRAINDICATIONS

High myopic or hyperopic patients older than 30 years with medium or large size pupils are the best candidates for bioptics. Contraindications for ph-IOL implantation are central anterior chamber depth less than 3 mm or less than 2.6 mm at the enclavation area especially in myopes, endothelial cell counts below 2,000 cells/mm^3, and any lens opacity or anterior segment pathology. Relative contraindications for LASIK are corneal pachymetry less than 450 μm, irregular topography, and keratometry readings less than 41 D, depending, of course, on the degree of myopia to be corrected.

F. OVERVIEW OF REPORTED RESULTS

Zaldivar et al. first described bioptics (1) for the correction of residual refractive error that could not be corrected with posterior chamber ph-IOL implantation. In their series of extreme myopes, the optical zone of the phakic lens was always less than 4.5 mm.

Later, the same authors reported on a group of 67 myopic eyes subjected to bioptics; the mean postoperative spherical equivalent and cylinder after LASIK were -0.20 ± 0.90 and 0.50 ± 0.50 D, respectively (2). Eighty-five percent (57 eyes) were within ± 1.00 D, and 67% (45 eyes) were within ± 0.50 D of emmetropia. The most serious complications were cataract formation (one eye) and macular hemorrhage (one eye).

Cataract formation is the main concern with posterior chamber ph-IOLs (10,11); possible explanations are mechanical irritation of the anterior lens capsule and the obstruction of aqueous circulation to the anterior lens crystalline, causing metabolic changes. No visually significant LASIK-related complications were detected in this study. Twenty-six of 18 patients with a preoperative spherical equivalent of -16.00–23.00 were subjected to the ARS approach, and the mean postoperative spherical equivalent and cylinder after LASIK were -0.38 ± 0.65 and -0.66 ± 0.66 D, respectively. All of the eyes were within ± 1.00 D and 80.7% were within ± 0.50 D of emmetropia. An outstanding finding in this series is that there were no changes in contrast sensitivity values; only two patients complained of mild visual disturbances at night. The larger the optical zone used in a refractive procedure, the better are the optical performance results, and vice versa; with the ARS approach an effective 6 mm optical zone is usually maintained. We decided to work with the Artisan™ lens due to its location in the eye, far from the corneal endothelium and avoiding the posterior chamber; for this reason it can be built with larger optical zones than other ph-IOLs for the same range of correction. On the other hand, centration over the pupil is dependent on the surgeon's ability rather than on the angle situation or white-to-white measurements as with other ph-IOLs (angle-supported or posterior chamber lenses, respectively). Decentered pupils are a common finding in high myopic patients; with the Artisan™ lens the surgeon may center the IOL over the decentered pupil. The main disadvantage of this lens is that its implantation requires a long incision (6.2 mm), but we have not found any significant astigmatic changes after all the sutures have been removed.

The main concern with anterior chamber IOLs is endothelial cell count with time (12,13). Our results (4) with the ARS approach showed a 0.61% mean loss during the first 12 months and 0.60% loss during the next 16 months. Our results doing a complete LASIK after implanting an Artisan™ show no statistical differences with the ARS at 4 years. It seems that the suction and microkeratome pass do not affect endothelial cell population as we initially suspected. However, a careful long-term follow-up (at least 10 years) must be carried out to determine the stability of the endothelial cell count in these patients. Today, ARS that is to perform the flap before the ablation makes sense only for LASIK after penetrating keratoplasty and, from our point of view, for LASIK in front of any customized (topographically or front wave guided) ablation.

G. CONCLUSIONS

Currently, the limits of LASIK have been significantly lowered (6). It is acceptable to perform this procedure up to $-8.00/-12.00$ D considering, of course, each patient as an individual case. In myopia higher than -12.00 D, ph-IOL implantation or clear lens extraction with IOL implantation are better options. In patients with myopia higher than −15.00 D, especially with medium or large pupils (6 mm or more), a combination procedure is a much better choice.

It is possible to correct myopia higher than −15.00 D with one procedure but at the expense of a reduction in the optical zone. As a consequence, a reduced quality of vision, especially under dim illumination conditions, and glare and halo problems will be common complaints, objectively evidenced as reduced contrast sensitivity values, and by other visual quality tests. Bioptics, by combining intraocular and corneal surgeries, maintains larger optical zones with better objective and subjective results. We hope that in the future, technology and a better knowledge of the optical properties of the eye will provide new biomaterials with higher refractive indexes and/or new optical surface designs to produce lenses with very large optical zones but thin enough to be compatible with the anterior or posterior segment anatomy.

REFERENCES

1. R Zaldivar, JM Davidorf, S Oscherow, G Ricur, V Piezzi. Combined posterior chamber phakic intraocular lens and laser in situ keratomileusis: bioptics for extreme myopia. J Refract Surg 1999;15:299–308.
2. R Zaldivar, JM Davidorf, S Oscherow. Posterior chamber phakic intraocular lens for myopia of −8 to −19 diopters. J Refract Surg 1998;14:294–305.
3. J Güell. The adjustable refractive surgery concept (ARS) (letter to the editor). J Refract Surg 1998;14:271.
4. JL Güell, M Vázquez. ARS (adjustable refractive surgery): 6 mm Artisan™ lens plus LASIK for the correction of high myopia. Ophthalmology, in press.
5. JL Güell, M Vázquez, O Gris, A deMuller, F Manero. Combined surgery to correct high myopia: iris claw phakic intraocular lens and laser in situ keratomileusis. J Refract Surg 1999;15:529–537.
6. JL Güell. The correction limits with LASIK. In: IG Pallikaris. LASIK. Thorofare, NJ: Slack, 1997, pp 183–185.
7. JJ Pérez-Santonja, MJ Ayala, HF Sakla, JM Ruíz-Moreno, JJ Alio. Retreatment after laser in situ keratomileusis. Ophthalmology 1999;106:21–28.
8. JL Güell, M Vázquez. Correction of high astigmatism with astigmatic keratotomy combined with laser in situ keratomileusis. J Cataract Refract Surg 2000;26:960–966.
9. JL Güell, M Vázquez. Intracorneal ring segments (ICRS) after LASIK: a preliminary report. J Cataract Refract Surg, in press.
10. F Trindade, F Pereira. Cataract formation after posterior chamber phakic intraocular lens implantation. J Cataract Refract Surg 1998;24:1661–1663.
11. PH Brauweiler, T Wehler, Busin M. High incidence of cataract formation after implantation of a silicone posterior chamber lens in phakic, highly myopic eyes. Ophthalmology 1999;106:1651–1655.
12. JL Alio, F de la Hoz, JJ Pérez-Santonja, JM Ruíz-Moreno, JA Quesada. Phakic anterior chamber lenses for the correction of myopia: a 7-year cumulative analysis of complications in 263 cases. Ophthalmology 1999;106:458–466.
13. S Leroux-les-Jardins, M Ullern, AL Werthel. Implants myopiques en P.M.M.A de chambre antérieure: bilan à 8 ans. [Myopic anterior chamber intraocular lens implantation: evaluation at 8 years]. J Fr Ophtalmol 1999;22:323–327.

25

LASIK and Intrastromal Corneal Ring Segments (ICRS)

JONATHAN D. PRIMACK and SAMIR G. FARAH

Massachusetts Eye and Ear Infirmary, Boston, Massachusetts, U.S.A.

DIMITRI T. AZAR

*Massachusetts Eye and Ear Infirmary, Schepens Eye Research Institute,
and Harvard Medical School, Boston, Massachusetts, U.S.A.*

A. INTRODUCTION

Both laser in situ keratomileusis (LASIK) and intrastromal corneal ring segments (ICRS) are effective surgical techniques for the treatment of myopia (1–6). LASIK corrects low to moderately high levels of myopia [<10 diopters (D)] and myopic astigmatism (up to 5 D). In contrast, ICRS are designed to treat only low levels of nearsightedness (up to 3 D) without clinically significant astigmatism. The procedure's effect results from two arc-shaped, intralamellar polymethylmethacrylate (PMMA) spacers that shorten the central corneal arc length. In this chapter we present data comparing LASIK to ICRS for low myopia and we explore the potential benefit of both as either simultaneous or sequential procedures in high myopia. Advantages of combined LASIK and ICRS surgery include an expanded range of myopic correction and the potential to adjust refractions months to years postoperatively.

B. INTRASTROMAL CORNEAL RING SEGMENTS

The current form of ICRS evolved from a prototype ring design first envisioned by A. E. Reynolds (6). In 1987, he and his colleagues demonstrated in rabbits that an expanded 360 degree PMMA ring placed in the peripheral cornea could produce central corneal flattening (7). Further investigations revealed that the refractive effect did not result from the device's circular conformation but rather from its thickness. Greater hyperopic shifts

Table 1 Predicted Dioptric Correction
for the Intrastromal Corneal Ring
Segments by Thickness: Refined
Nomogram—Phase II Study Results

Thickness (mm)	Predicted average correction (D)
0.25	−1.30
0.30	−2.00
0.35	−2.70
0.40	−3.40
0.45	−4.10

mm—Millimeters; D—Diopters. Source:
Ref. 3.

could be produced by rings of progressively increasing girth (8,9). Clinical studies involving human eyes began in the early 1990s and demonstrated that the technique produced only small (several diopters) myopic corrections (10–12). A change in product design occurred when researchers observed that similar refractive outcomes could be achieved using separate ring segments instead of a complete ring insert (13,14). This modification allowed for a technically easier implantation and eliminated PMMA at the incision site, which had previously contributed to healing difficulties. Table 1 illustrates the expected dioptric correction by ICRS thickness as determined by the USFDA phase II trials (3). The nomogram predicts an estimated increase of 0.7 D of hyperopic shift per 0.05 mm increase in ring thickness.

The commercially marketed form of ICRS is called Intacs (Kera Vision, Inc., Fremont, CA) and consists of two 150 degree PMMA segments available in several widths (0.25, 0.30, and 0.35 mm) depending on the degree of myopic correction (Fig. 25). Twa and colleagues (4) recently reported the one-year follow-up of patients participating in the USFDA phase III clinical trials of Intacs. Ninety-nine percent of 90 patients with low myopia had an UCVA (uncorrected visual acuity) of 20/40 or better and 92% of eyes were ± 1.00 D of their intended correction. In April 1999, the USFDA (United States Food and Drug Administration) approved Intacs for the treatment of low myopia (1 to 3 D) with 1 D or less of astigmatism.

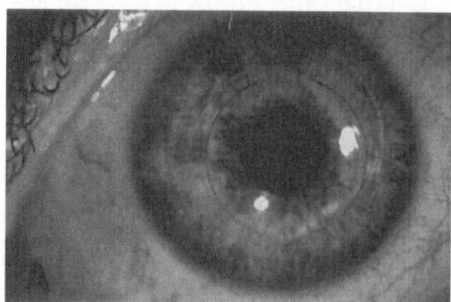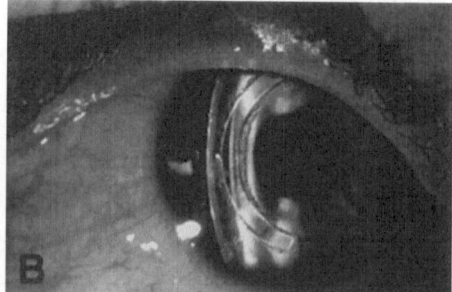

Figure 25.1 (A) Photograph of eye after ICRS implantation (Intacs). (B) Slit lamp photograph showing ICRS at 2/3 stromal depth.

C. LASIK VS. ICRS: EFFICACY AND SAFETY FOR LOW MYOPIA

A comparison of LASIK and ICRS would help assess the efficacy and safety of the two techniques and allow better counseling of low myopes. For this purpose, we reviewed the recent literature addressing LASIK for the correction of low myopia and compared it with the ICRS data submitted to the USFDA (15).

We identified pertinent articles published in peer-reviewed journals through a multi-staged systematic approach. In the first stage, we performed a computerized Medline search from 1990 to 1999 databases to identify all articles about the efficacy and safety of LASIK. The search terms were laser in situ keratomileusis, keratomileusis, and LASIK.

In the second stage, the abstracts were scanned to identify articles, written in English, that reported the results of a clinical series. Copies of these articles were obtained. Articles describing series with a spherical equivalent (SE) of −4 D were retained and their reference lists searched for additional articles. All identified journals were manually searched through the July 1999 issues using the same search guidelines.

In the third stage, articles were reviewed and analyzed in relation to preoperative and postoperative SE, follow-up (F/U), final UCVA, predictability, and safety. Results were used to calculate the weighted mean of each category.

In a fourth stage, the means were compared to those of similar categories of the USFDA submitted data for the ICRS. The Student t test, the Z test, and Fisher's exact test were used for statistical comparison.

The peer-reviewed reports about LASIK for low myopia were published after January 1997. Table 2 summarizes the reports on the efficacy and safety of LASIK for low myopia; Table 3 compares the LASIK and ICRS data. In the LASIK reports, the total number of eyes was 1125 compared to 410 in the ICRS document (15–23). F/U for LASIK reports ranged between 1 and 12 months with a mean of 4.5 months; in the ICRS document the F/U was 24 months with an emphasis on the 12-months results.

LASIK and ICRS procedures seem to have comparable safety for low myopia (≤ -4 D). The ICRS procedure seems to have a better visual outcome although LASIK has a better predictability (% within 0.5 diopters). The better UCVA with ICRS may be due to the nonalteration of the optical zone with subsequent less loss of contrast sensitivity, less irregularity of the central corneal surface, and less induced irregular astigmatism.

1. Advantages and Disadvantages of LASIK in Low Myopia

With current techniques and equipment, LASIK has proven to be a good procedure for all ranges of myopia (17,22,23). The advantages of LASIK include fast clinical and functional visual rehabilitation, minimal postoperative pain, avoidance of epithelial stromal interactions, reduced need for steroids, minimal regression or progression of the refractive change, the possibility of simultaneous treatment, the ease of reoperation, and the fact that a single technique works for all levels of myopia. The disadvantages of LASIK include the expense and complexity of the microkeratome and the excimer laser devices, the lack of standardized nomograms for tissue ablation, the steep learning curve, the increased risk of overcorrection in the low myopia range, and the relative weakening of the corneal wall.

2. Advantages and Disadvantages of ICRS in Low Myopia

The advantages of the ICRS procedure include the reversibility of the procedure with return to the preoperative refractive baseline, the ease of replacing or removing the rings in

Table 2 Efficacy and Safety of LASIK for low Myopia

First Autor (ref. no.)	Number of eyes	Follow-up (months)	Preoperative	Postoperative	Postop UCVA >20/40 (%)	Postop UCVA >20/20 (%)	% within ±1 (%)	% within ±0.5 (%)	Loss >2 lines (%)
Wang (16)	103	12	— (1.25 to −6)	—	91	83	89	71	1
Salchow (17)	28	6	−3.14 ± 1.28 (−1.5 to −5.5)	−0.1 ± 0.5 (−1 to +2)	100	51.90	96.40	92.80	10.70
El Danasoury (18)	24	12	−3.44 ± 0.72 (−2 to −5.5)	−0.14 ± 0.31	100	79.20	100	87.50	0
Pirzada (19)	85	6	−2.09 (−1 to −3.5)	—	93	—	—	—	—
Casebeer (20)	260 sum	3	— (−1 to −4)	−0.3 ± 0.51	93	39	91	78	0
	208 Visx			−0.42 ± 0.46	90	46	89	73	0
Montes (21)	168	6	−3.6 ± 1.27 (−1.5 to −6)	−0.12 ± 0.31 (−1 to +0.5)	100	81	100	94	0
Davidorf (22)	81	3	−3.62 ± 1.55 (−0.75 to −5.87) ast: −1.57 ± 1.27	−0.03 ± 0.43 ast: −0.3 ± 0.51	91	43	—	—	0
Lindstrom (23)	103	1	−3.6 ± −1.24 (−0.5 to −6) ast <1	−0.0 ± 0.62 (−2.25 to +1.63)	94	60	93	—	
	65	1	−3.7 ± 1.13 (−0.5 to −6) ast >1	+0.06 ± 0.78	91	37	87	—	0
Total Mean	1125	4.46	−3.64 ± 1.28	−0.2 ± 0.46	93.50	55.10	92.25	80	0.39

SE = spherical equivalent; UCVA = uncorrected visual acuity; Sum = Summit; () = range; ast = astigmatism; — = Not available.

Table 3 Efficacy and Safety of LASIK and ICRS for Low Myopia

	LASIK	ICR	
No. of eyes	1125	410	
F/U (months)	4.46	12	
Preop SE	−3.4 ± 1.28	−2.24 ± 0.69	
Postop UCVA >20/40 (%)	93.50	97	$P = 0.0069, Z = 2.7$
Postop UCVA >20/20 (%)	55.10	74	$P < 0.0001, Z = 6.6$
% within ±0.5 (%)	80	69	$P < 0.0001, Z = 4.2$
% within ±1 (%)	92.25	92	$P = 0.8338, Z = 0.21$
Loss >2 lines (%)	0.39	1	$P = 0.233$

F/U = follow-up; SE = spherical equivalent; UCVA = uncorrected visual acuity.

case of an emerging cataract or of over- or undercorrection, the low cost of the instruments as compared to LASIK, the nonalteration of the optical zone, and the faster clinical and functional rehabilitation (absence of central corneal wound healing). The disadvantages of the ICRS procedure include the inability to treat the astigmatism, the steep learning curve, the decline in efficacy with thicker rings, the introduction of a foreign body inside the cornea, and the fact that the surgeon has to master both techniques: ICRS for low myopia and LASIK for moderate and high myopia.

3. ICRS Complications

Intra- and postoperative complications have been described with ICRS (3–6,12,14,24). A 2% incidence of serious complications was observed among the 452 patients enrolled in the USFDA phase II and III studies. Adverse events such as perforation through the posterior cornea into the anterior chamber (2 eyes), anterior corneal perforation (3 eyes), significant decentration of segments requiring removal or repositioning (5 eyes), and infectious keratitis (1 eye) underscore the need for meticulous surgical technique (5). Interestingly, all of these eyes regained their preoperative best corrected visual acuity (BCVA) over the following 6 months. Less serious events have included undercorrection and overcorrection (amenable to segment exchange), glare, halos, induced astigmatism, decreased corneal sensation, stromal thinning, and corneal neovascularization. Epithelial cysts or gape can occur at the incision if the site is not sutured leading to incomplete wound healing that could affect the final refraction. Diurnal variation in keratometry and refraction following ICRS has been described, but the etiology remains unclear (4,25).

Non–clinically significant observations associated with ICRS include epithelial iron lines, intrachannel opacification, and crystalline deposits (Figs. 25.2–25.5) (3,12,26–29). These findings do not affect visual acuity.

4. Summary of Comparative Analysis

Taking into consideration the recent introduction of the ICRS procedure and the nonavailability of long F/U studies on LASIK for low myopia, we cannot present the results of paired series. We believe that, with the earlier stabilization of refraction and the comanagement option, there is a loss of patient F/U several weeks postoperatively. Furthermore, in the ICRS document the preoperative SE was −2.24 ± 0.69 diopters (range, −0.75 to −4.125 D) with a sphere ranging between −1 D and −4.5 D and a cylinder ±1 D. In the

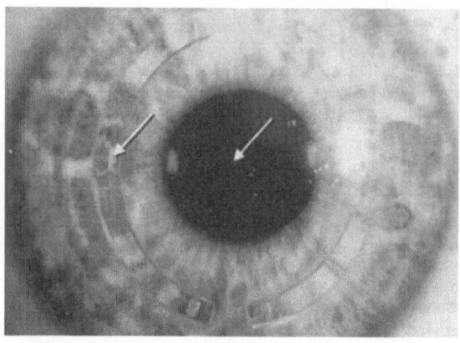
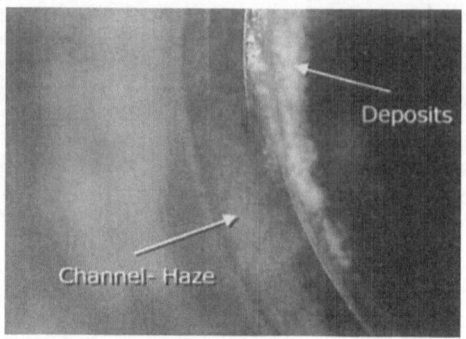

A   B

Figure 25.2   Photograph of ICRS. (A) Arrows indicate location of ICRS in relation to the center of the pupil. The peripheral arrow also indicates lamellar channel deposits. (From Ref. 29.) (B) Different eye with magnified view of channel hazed lamellar channel deposits. These deposits are incidental and without clinical significance. (From Ref. 28.)

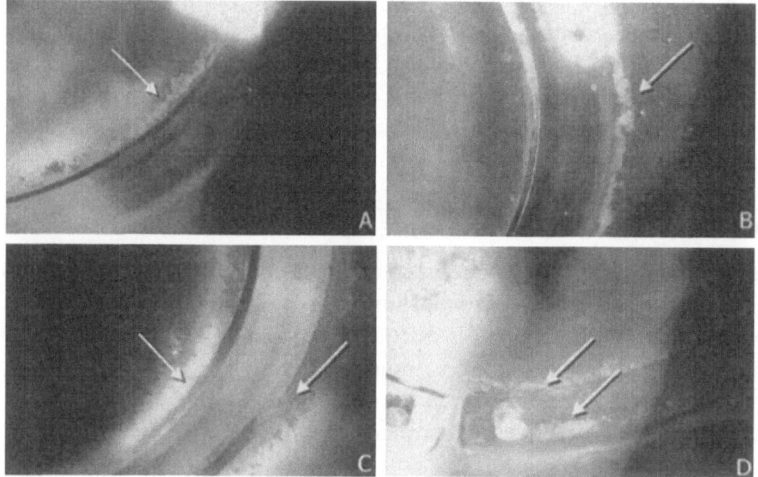

Figure 25.3   (Ruckhofer) Location of deposits. (A) Along the inside of the segment curvature. (B) Along the outside of the segment curvature. (C) Along the inside and outside of the segment curvature. (D) Along the inside of the curvature and anterior to the segment. (From Ref. 28.)

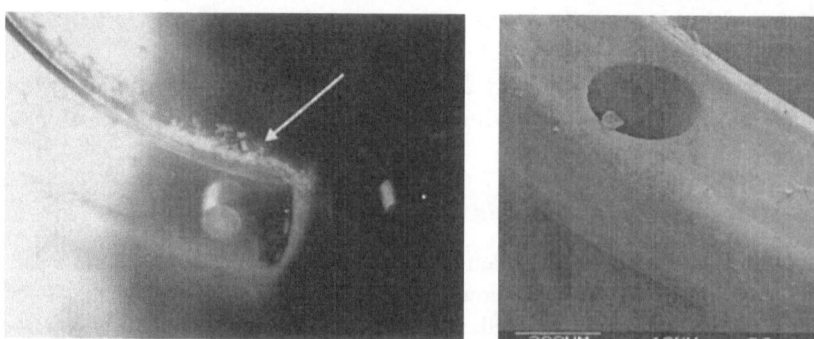

B

Figure 25.4   ICRS segment in the stroma. Arrow indicates lamellar channel deposits visualized by slit lamp biomicroscopy (A) and scanning electron microscopy (B) showing the positioning hole of the ICRS. (From Ref. 28.)

LASIK reports the preoperative SE was -3.64 ± 1.28 D with a sphere of -0.5 to -6 D and a cylinder reaching 3.75 D. The statistical difference in the preoperative SE [$t(409) = 20.52$, $P < 0.0001$] may cause some bias in the interpretation and comparison of the visual outcomes, especially since the LASIK reports included high amounts of cylinder.

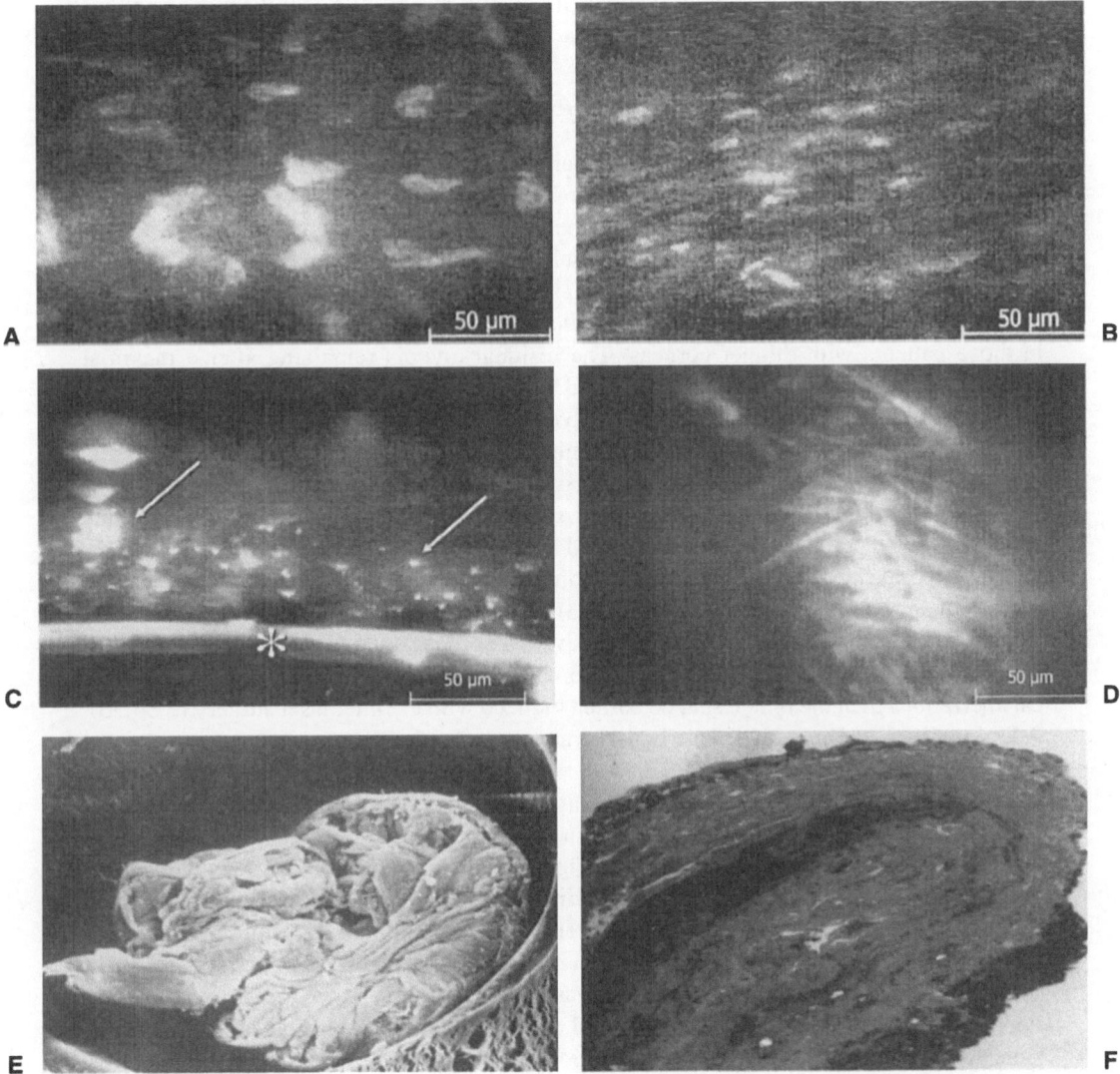

Figure 25.5 Confocal images of the posterior stroma. (A) A compound stromal layer around the ICRS. (B) Confocal microscopy of lamellar channel deposits. (C) With * pointing at edge of ICRS and arrows pointing at deposits of different sizes. Confocal microscopy of fibrosis adjacent to ICRS. (D) Scanning electron micrographs of a deposit in the suture hole of an ICRS. Note the convoluted lamellar appearance of the tissue (From Ref. 29.) (E) Transmission electron micrograph of a section through another deposit located in an ICRS suture hole. (F) The deposit consists of an amorphous core with cellular constituents that have a curved appearance. (From Ref. 27.)

In conclusion, both the LASIK and the ICRS procedures seem to be equally safe for low myopia, and ICRS has the advantages of being less expensive and having a better visual outcome. Keeping in mind that the refractive outcome declines with thicker rings, the ICRS seems a plausible procedure for very low myopia (-1 to -2.5 D), especially when there is no astigmatism.

We believe that more prospective, randomized studies with longer F/U are needed to determine better the visual outcomes and establish the indications of each procedure in low myopia. Although ICRS is simpler than LASIK, it still has its own complications and limitations.

D. LASIK COMBINED WITH ICRS FOR HIGH MYOPIA

The correction of high myopia remains a challenge. LASIK alone has been shown to provide satisfactory results, but limitations exist (23,30,31). Higher levels of myopia cannot be treated with deeper excimer laser ablations because a sufficient amount of corneal stromal tissue must remain to guard against potential keratectasia and refractive instability (32). Current recommendations suggest a minimal residual stromal bed thickness of approximately 250 microns. This precludes the application of highly myopic ablations, especially in those patients with thinner corneas. The residual myopia remaining after a maximal LASIK treatment could possibly be corrected by combining LASIK with another refractive procedure such as ICRS that does not involve the removal of stromal tissue. Their union may offer the refractive surgeon the opportunity to treat safely an additional 3 D of myopia.

ICRS possess specific qualities that make it a potentially valuable adjunct to LASIK. First, the technique spares the visual axis of surgical manipulation. The PMMA segments are placed in the peripheral cornea and would not be expected to interfere with the centrally located corneal flap. Second, the effect is adjustable, and the final refractive result can be titrated by exchanging the ring segments (33). If the patient is dissatisfied, they can be removed altogether with an almost complete reversal of the refractive effect (3,4). ICRS also maintains the natural prolate shape of the cornea, which may be associated with less optical aberrations than the oblate shaped cornea induced with excimer laser surgery (5,34,35). Additionally, LASIK and ICRS are both extraocular procedures, so intraocular surgery and its attendant risks are avoided.

In patients with high myopia, LASIK and ICRS treatments may be performed simultaneously. Table 4 describes three different surgical approaches (A–C) from which to choose when performing the techniques together. Figure 25.6 schematically illustrates method A. The implantation of ICRS may be performed in a laser suite setting. Topical anesthetic drops and antibiotics are administered preoperatively. Peri- or retrobulbar anesthesia is unnecessary and could interfere with patient fixation if concomitant LASIK were also planned.

The surgical procedure is straightforward but does require some unique instrumentation. The center of the cornea is located and an Incision and Placement Marker (Kera Vision, Inc., Fremont, CA) is applied to indicate where the PMMA inserts and superior, radial incision will ultimately lie. Ultrasonic pachymetry is performed at the 12 o'clock incision site and an approximately 1 mm incision of 68% corneal thickness is created with a calibrated diamond knife. A modified Suarez spreader may be used to perform a small lamellar dissection at the base of the incision, so as to create an entry pocket on either side. Next, a Vacuum Centering Guide (Kera Vision, Inc., Fremont, CA) is positioned on the globe and stabilized under high suction. Specially designed dissectors measuring 0.9 mm are then introduced through the incision (clockwise and counterclockwise) to

Table 4   Surgical Approaches for Combined LASIK and ICRS for High Myopia

Method	Step 1—Form stromal channels and LASIK flap	Step 2—Perform LASIK ablation (% of maximally safe ablation)	Step 3—Place ICRS segments into channels	Expected residual error	Secondary procedure (1–5 weeks)
A	+	100	+	Minimal	Remove or exchange ICRS
B	+	0	+	2–3 D less than preoperative refractive error	Perform LASIK ablation
C	+	70–80	+	2–3 D	LASIK ablation to correct residual error

LASIK—Laser in situ keratomileusis; ICRS—intrastromal corneal ring segments; D—Diopters.

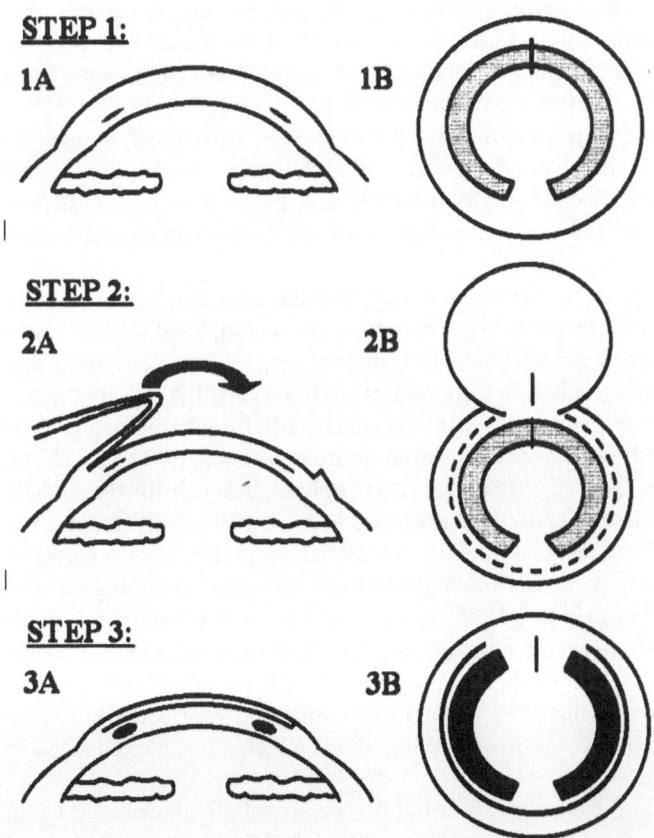

STEP 1:

1A   **1B**

STEP 2:

2A   **2B**

STEP 3:

3A   **3B**

Figure 25.6   Surgical steps of Method A summarized in Table 4.

create stromal tunnels by blunt dissection. Ideally, the channels are located at two-thirds of the corneal depth. Suction is then released and the centering guide removed.

Once the channels have been created, a microkeratome is used to create a corneal flap. Based on the patient's intraoperative pachymetry value, the maximal excimer laser ablation considered to be safe is performed. Subsequently, the flap is refloated into place. Using forceps, the PMMA segments are introduced into the channels. In their final position, the segments are located 3 mm apart superiorly. If necessary, the flap could be refloated to eliminate any iatrogenically induced wrinkles. The incision site may be hydrated, or, alternatively, closed with 10-0 nylon sutures. Postoperatively, if the patient possesses mild ametropia or later desires undercorrection to ameliorate presbyopic symptoms, the ICRS may be exchanged.

The presence of empty intralamellar channels in the corneal periphery should not interfere with performing LASIK. This becomes evident when one considers the spatial relationships between the channels, hinged corneal flap, and excimer laser optical zone (OZ). The Intacs segments lie at two-thirds stromal depth and have an inner diameter of 6.9 mm and an outer diameter greater than 8 mm. A hinged corneal flap of 8.5 to 10.0 mm would cover the tunnels, but its anterior location would make intersection extremely unlikely. The flap could incur a small, full thickness defect where the microkeratome crosses the superior incision site, but that is of negligible clinical significance.

For illustrative purposes, let us consider a cornea with a peripheral thickness of 700 μm at the Intacs incision site and a central thickness of 550 μm. The empty tunnels (following explantation) are located at 466 μm from the surface (2/3 the depth of 700 μm). An 8.5 mm wide flap measuring 160 μm thick would leave 306 μm of tissue that would have to be ablated from the stromal bed before the channels were penetrated [466 μm − 160 μm (flap) = 306 μm]. This is a not a concern clinically for two reasons. First, most myopic excimer laser ablations have a 6.5 mm OZ, which is central to the more peripherally located tunnels (inner diameter 6.9 mm). Second, if larger optical zones were used, concerns over adequate residual central corneal thickness would preclude ablations deep enough to encounter the peripherally located tunnels.

Methods B and C are similar to method A except that the laser ablation is initially withheld or is partially performed, respectively. The remainder is completed later as a secondary procedure. An advantage of these techniques is that the surgeon can incorporate any ICRS induced refractive changes (including astigmatism) into the final LASIK ablation.

Patients with a moderate degree of myopia could also benefit from combined LASIK and ICRS surgery. Although these patients can often be treated successfully by LASIK alone, potential safety concerns exist. Myopic LASIK ablates tissue from the central cornea, and although the thickness of residual corneal bed necessary to avoid ectasia is not known, most surgeons agree that a residual thickness of 250 μm or greater is safe. Cases of keratectasia occurring in patients who were thought to have adequate remaining corneal thickness have been reported (36). Up to 3 D of myopia could be treated with ICRS, sparing precious central stroma and improving corneal stability. Another advantage of this procedure is that surgeons could easily exchange ring segments, with a resultant myopic shift if patients decided postoperatively that they wanted to become undercorrected to reduce presbyopic symptoms. If this change was dissatisfying, the ICRS could be reexchanged to restore the previous refraction.

As in the previous section, the surgeries could be performed simultaneously using multiple approaches (Table 5). In method A, a 70% to 80% LASIK ablation is performed (depending on intended final refraction) followed by ICRS implantation. Once the refrac-

Table 5 Surgical Approaches for Combined LASIK and ICRS for Moderate Myopia

Method	Step 1—Form stromal channels and LASIK flap	Step 2—Perform LASIK ablation (% of maximally safe ablation)	Step 3—Place ICRS segments into channels	Expected residual error	Secondary procedure (1–5 weeks)
A	+	70–80	+	Minimal	ICRS exchange or LASIK
B	+	0	+	3 D less than preoperative refractive error	LASIK for remaining myopia
C	+	70–80	−	2–3 D	ICRS placement

LASIK—Laser in situ keratomileusis; ICRS—Intrastromal corneal ring segments; D—diopters.

tion has stabilized, either the ring segments can be exchanged or the LASIK treatment enhanced by relifting the flap. Alternatively, in method B, only the ICRS are put into place initially. The LASIK ablation follows as a secondary procedure after the corneal curvature stabilizes. Another approach (method C) is to perform 70% to 80% of the LASIK ablation initially followed by ICRS implantation 1 week postoperatively to correct residual myopia. This technique may be less desirable as the ring segments may induce astigmatism that could require a third surgical visit for LASIK enhancement.

E. ICRS AFTER LASIK

The opportunity to implant ICRS in an eye that has previously undergone LASIK may arise if the ablation was deep enough to preclude the safe application of further excimer laser. Patients corresponding to this profile usually include high myopes and patients with thin corneas. Potential candidates should understand that the hyperopic shift expected following ICRS would be no more than approximately 3 D.

It would seem that the technical challenge underlying ICRS implantation following LASIK would be to form the intraamellar channels without disturbing the corneal flap. As discussed earlier, this process requires a suction ring that could, theoretically, compromise the flap, resulting in wrinkles, dislocation, or potentially avulsion. Preliminary reports of this procedure, however, have been without complications. Fleming and Lovisolo (37) reported a patient who received ICRS 10 months following LASIK that left a residual SE of −3.375 D. Four months after ICRS placement, the patient had an UCVA of 20/20. No flap complications occurred. Lovisolo (30) also presented a series of 15 eyes at the American Society of Cataract and Refractive Surgery (ASCRS) 2000 meeting that underwent Intacs implantation following LASIK. Patients had received their LASIK 6 to 11 months previously and had residual myopia ranging from a SE of −2.75 to −4.75 D. Eight months following ICRS placement, all eyes had an UCVA of 20/25. Once again, no flap complications were observed. ICRS may be a safe procedure following LASIK if enough time is allowed between procedures to ensure adequate corneal flap healing.

F. LASIK AFTER ICRS

1. Following Explantation

If a patient becomes dissatisfied with ICRS, the PMMA segments may be removed and the resultant ametropia treated with LASIK. Intacs patients represent a population with low myopia in which LASIK has been demonstrated to be effective. Lindstrom and colleagues (23) reported that after treating 101 eyes with low myopia (mean SE -4.16 ± 1.41 D), 90% had an UCVA of 20/40 or better 1 month postoperatively. Pirzada and Kalaawry (19) reported similar success after 85 eyes underwent LASIK for -1.00 to -3.50 D of myopia. Ninety-three percent of these eyes had an UCVA of 20/30 or better by 6 months.

Once the ICRS have been explanted, the surgeon must allow for the cornea to reassume its natural curvature. Immediately performing LASIK with the original pre-ICRS implantation refraction may not provide full correction as eyes tend to return to refractive errors similar, but not necessarily identical to, their preoperative values (3,4). After spacer removal, one or two 10-0 nylon sutures may be placed at the incision site to promote proper healing. These may be removed 2 to 3 weeks later. The patient's refraction and topography should be monitored after suture removal to document stability before treating with LASIK.

Complications could arise with LASIK after ICRS explantation. If the Intacs were removed because their initial placement was incorrect (i.e., too anteriorly), the LASIK flap could intersect the channels, resulting in an irregular stromal bed and/or irregular ablation. Additionally, the superior incision site could open during flap formation, resulting in a full thickness 1–2 mm flap defect. This compromise in tissue integrity is probably inconsequential. Barring these concerns, the patient is at no greater risk for the documented complications of LASIK than any other patient (32).

Few reports of refractive surgery following ICRS explantation have been written given its recent USFDA approval. Asbell and associates (40) reported a patient who received a photorefractive keratectomy (PRK) 10 months following Intacs removal for complaints of glare and halos. The patient's manifest refraction stabilized within $\pm$ 0.50 D of his original manifest refraction by 1 month after explantation. PRK has demonstrated equivalent results compared to LASIK for the treatment of low myopia (18). However, it has been demonstrated that patients prefer LASIK over PRK, given the fast, almost painless recovery. Eight months following PRK, this patient had a BSCVA of 20/16. Ucakhan and colleagues (41) presented an abstract at the 1999 Association for Research in Vision and Ophthalmology meeting (ARVO) which described ten patients who received LASIK following ICRS explantation. No complications were reported. Gomez and Chayet (42) reported at the 2000 ARVO meeting on eight patients who had their ICRS removed between 5 and 24 months after implantation and subsequently underwent LASIK. All patients achieved an UCVA of 20/20 or better after 6 to 15 months of follow-up. Davis and colleagues (43) reported on five patients who received LASIK following ICRS explantation for induced astigmatism and intraoperative complications. All patients experienced uneventful LASIK.

2. Following Implantation

Patients may develop refractive errors after the placement of ICRS. If, over time, a patient with Intacs develops additional nearsightedness, the PMMA spacers may be exchanged for a different thickness to treat up to 3 D of myopia. However, if the error exceeds -3 D or requires cylindrical correction, the patient must consider other refractive modalities. LASIK may be an appropriate option for treating such conditions.

The surgeon must anticipate the potential influence of ICRS when performing LASIK. ICRS and LASIK can coexist on a cornea without interference, but the presence of previously placed PMMA spacers could theoretically disrupt proper flap formation. The ICRS could cause tissue distortion that prevents adequate suction or tissue distribution during the microkeratome pass, resulting in an irregular stromal bed surface. At this time it is unclear what effect ICRS have on LASIK flap formation and which approach is safer, as no reports have yet been published. To avoid potential problems, the surgeon may wish to explant preoperatively the ICRS and then perform LASIK. As discussed in the previous section, the excimer laser ablation will not penetrate deeply enough to affect the channels holding the Intacs segments. Once LASIK has been performed, subsequent changes in refraction could be addressed by simply relifting the flap and ablating further stromal tissue. Any patient who experiences progressive refractive shifts should be thoroughly examined for other pathology, with special attention aimed at detecting subtle lenticular changes.

G. CONCLUSIONS

LASIK and ICRS are two techniques that when used in combination, may benefit high and moderate myopes. The combination of these two procedures may be especially valuable for patients with relatively thin corneas. Early reports of their use together are promising, but further studies are necessary to establish efficacy, stability, and safety of these surgical procedures.

REFERENCES

1. T Salah, GO Waring III, A El Maghraby, K Moadel, SB Grimm. Excimer laser in situ keratomileusis under a corneal flap for myopia 2 to 20 diopters. Am J Ophthalmol 1996;121:143–155.
2. SG Farah, DT Azar, C Gurdal, J Wong. Laser in situ keratomileusis: literature review of a developing technique. J Cataract Refract Surg 1998;24:989–1006.
3. DJ Schanzlin, PA Asbell, TE Burris, DS Durrie. The intrastromal corneal ring segments: phase II results for the correction of myopia. Ophthalmology 1997;104:1067–1078.
4. MD Twa, PM Karpecki, BJ King, SH Linn, DS Durrie, DJ Schanzlin. One year results from the phase III investigation of the keravision intacs. J Am Optom Assoc 1999;70(8):515–524.
5. EJ Linebarger, D Song, J Ruckhofer, DJ Schanzlin. Intacs: the intrastromal corneal ring. Int Ophthalmol Clin 2000;40(3):199–208.
6. DJ Schanzlin. Studies of intrastromal corneal ring segments for the correction of low to moderate myopic refractive errors. Tr Am Ophth Soc 1999;97:815–890.
7. JF Fleming, AE Reynolds, L Kilmer, TE Burris, RL Abbot, DJ Schanzlin. The intrastromal corneal ring: two cases in rabbits. J Refract Surg 1987;3(6):227–232.
8. TE Burris, CT Ayer, DA Evensen, JM Davenport. Effects of intrastromal corneal rings size and thickness on corneal flattening in human eyes. Refract and Corneal Surg 1991;7:46–50.
9. TE Burris, PC Baker, CT Ayer, BE Loomas, ML Mathis, TA Silvestrini. Flattening of central corneal curvature with intrastromal corneal rings of increasing thickness: an eye bank study. J Cataract Refract Surg 1993;19:182–187.
10. W Nose, RA Neves, DJ Schanzlin, R Belfort. Intrastromal corneal ring—one-year results of first implants in human: a preliminary nonfunctional eye study. Refract Corneal Surg 1993;9:452–458.

11. KK Assil, AM Barrett, BD Fouraker, DJ Schanzlin. One year results of the intrastromal corneal ring in nonfunctional human eyes. Arch Ophthalmol 1995;113:159–167.

12. W Nose, RA Neves, TE Burris, DJ Schanzlin, R Belfort Jr. Intrastromal corneal ring: 12 month sighted myopic eyes. J Refract Surg 1996;12:20–28.

13. RR Krueger, TE Burris. Intrastromal corneal ring technology. Int Ophthalmol Clin 1996;4:89–106.

14. TE Burris. Intrastromal corneal ring technology: results and indications. Curr Opin Ophthalmol 1998;9:9–14.

15. Professional Use Information Manual for Correction of Myopia with Keravision Intacs. Physician Booklet.

16. Z Wang, J Chen, B Yang. Comparison of laser in situ keratomileusis and photorefractive keratectomy to correct myopia from −1.25 to −6.00 diopters. J Refract Surg 1997;13:528–534.

17. DJ Salchow, ME Zirm, C Stieldorf, A Parisi. Laser in situ keratomileusis for myopia and myopic astigmatism. J Cataract Refract Surg 1998;24:175–182.

18. MA El Danasoury, A El Maghraby, SD Klyce, K Mehrez. Comparison of photorefractive keratectomy with excimer laser in situ keratomileusis in correcting low myopia (from −2.00 to −5.50 diopters)—a randomized study. Ophthalmology 1999;106(2):411–420.

19. WA Pirzada, H Kalaawry. Laser in situ keratomileusis for myopia −1 to −3.50 diopters. J Refract Surg 1997;13:S425–S426.

20. Casebeer JC, Kezirian GM. Outcomes of spherocylinder treatments in the comprehensive refractive surgery LASIK study. Semin Ophthalmol 1998;13:71–78.

21. M Montes, A Chayet, L Gómez, R Magallanes, N Robledo. Laser in situ keratomileusis for myopia of −1.50 to −6.00 diopters. J Refract Surg 1999;15:106–110.

22. JM Davidorf, R Zaldivar, S Oscherow. Results and complications of laser in situ keratomileusis by experienced surgeons. J Refract Surg 1998;14:114–122.

23. RL Lindstrom, DR Hardten, YR Chu. Laser in situ keratomileusis for the treatment of low, moderate, and high myopia. Trans Am Ophthalmol Soc 1997;95:285–296.

24. T Kohnen. Consultation section: refractive surgical problem. J Cataract Refract Surg 2000;26:799–802.

25. G Baikoff, N Maia, D Poulhalec, A Fontaine, B Giusiano. Diurnal variations in keratometry and refraction with intracorneal ring segments. J Cataract Refract Surg 1999;25:1056–1061.

26. AM Fink, C Gore, ES Rosen. Corneal changes associated with intrastromal corneal ring segments. Arch Ophthalmol 1999;117:282.

27. AJ Quantock, KK Assil, DJ Schanzlin. Electron microscopic evaluation of intrastromal corneal rings explanted from nonfunctional human eyes. J Refract Corneal Surg 1994;10:142–148.

28. J Ruckhofer, MD Twa, DJ Schanzlin. Clinical characteristics of lamellar channel deposits after implantation of Intacs. J Cataract Refract Surg 2000;26:473–1479.

29. J Ruckhofer, M Bohnke, E Alzner, G Grabner. Confocal microscopy after implantation of intrastromal corneal ring segments. Ophthalmology 2000;107:2144–2151.

30. GM Kawesch, GM Kezirian. Laser in situ keratomileusis for high myopia with the VISX star laser. Ophthalmology 2000;107(4):653–661.

31. MC Knorz, B Wiesinger, A Liermann, V Seiberth, H Liesenhoff. Laser in situ keratomileusis for moderate and high myopia and myopic astigmatism. Ophthalmology 1998;105(5):932–940.

32. SD McLeod, TA Kisla, NC Caro, TT McMahon. Iatrogenic keratoconus: corneal ectasia following laser in situ keratomileusis for myopia. Arch Ophthalmol 2000;118(2):282–284.

33. PA Asbell, OO Ucakhan, DS Durrie, RL Lindstrom. Adjustability of refractive effect for corneal ring segments. J Refract Surg 1999;15:627–631.

34. DK Holmes-Higgin, PC Baker, TE Burris, TA Silvestrini. Characterization of the aspheric corneal surface with intrastromal corneal ring segments. J Refract Surg 1999;15:520–528.

35. DK Holmes-Higgin, TE Burris, and Intacs study group. Corneal surface topography and associated visual performance with Intacs for myopia: phase III clinical trial results. Ophthalmology 2000;107:2061–2071.

36. Amoils SP, Deist MB, P Gous, PM Amoils. Iatrogenic keratectasia after laser in situ keratomileusis for less than −4.0 to −7.0 diopters of myopia. J Cataract Refract Surg 2000;26: 967–977.
37. JF Fleming, CF Lovisolo. Intrastromal corneal ring segments in a patient with previous laser in situ keratomileusis. J Refract Surg 2000;16:365–367.
38. CF Lovisolo. Intac ring segments and LASIK: better quality vision for high myopia; removal option for prepresbyopic patients (abstr.). American Society of Cataract and Refractive Surgery (ASCRS) Meeting. Abstract 763, 2000.
39. NG Iskander, NT Peters, EA Penno, HV Gimbel. Postoperative complications in laser in situ keratomileusis. Curr Opin Ophthalmol 2000;11(4):273–279.
40. PA Asbell, OO Ucakhan, M Odrich. Photorefractive keratectomy after intrastromal corneal ring segment explantation. Am J Ophthalmol 1999;128:755–756.
41. OO Ucakhan, SBL Thompson, DS Durrie, M Odrich, PA Asbell. Refractive surgery following ICRS removal (abstr). Invest Ophthalmol Vis Sci. 1999;40(4):B525. Abstract nr. 565.
42. L Gomez, A Chayet. 6 month LASIK results after removal of intracorneal ring segments (abstr.). Invest Ophthalmol Vis Sci. 2000;41(4):B827. Abstract nr. 4880.
43. EA Davis, DR Hardten, RL Lindstrom. Laser in situ keratomileusis after intracorneal rings—report of five cases. J Cataract Refract Surg 2000;26(12):1733–1741.

26

Intraoperative Complications

LI WANG, MANJULA MISRA, and DOUGLAS D. KOCH

Cullen Eye Institute, Baylor College of Medicine, Houston, Texas, U.S.A.

A basic medical tenet is that it is better to prevent a complication than it is to treat it. This is perhaps magnified with LASIK, the elective nature of which makes even the slightest deviation from a perfect outcome a potential disappointment for both surgeon and patient. The intraoperative complication rate for LASIK is reportedly between 0.7% and 6.6% (1–6). Most of these complications have been found to occur as a result of creating the keratectomy with the microkeratome (7,8).

As will be reviewed in this chapter, the preoperative examination is critical to identify risk factors for specific intraoperative complications. Surgeon experience is a vital factor as well: several studies have documented the steep learning curve associated with the performance of LASIK (1,2,6,7,9–12). A sharp decline in the number of complications is expected after sufficient surgical and medical experience has been gained in the management of laser refractive patients. Preparation and attention to detail with each procedure are fundamental, as are familiarity with all equipment and instrumentation by surgeon and assistant alike. Cooperation between all members of the surgical team, with clearly identified roles for each individual, and development of an unvarying, efficient routine that incorporates redundant safety measures will also help to minimize intraoperative complications. Finally, proper management and counselling of the patient who experiences a complication will maximize the likelihood of a positive outcome for all concerned.

A. MICROKERATOME-RELATED FLAP COMPLICATIONS

Each surgeon's microkeratome complication rate and profile will vary with the model of instrument used, individual ocular anatomy, and surgeon experience.

Microkeratome: The incidences of various LASIK complication rates vary with the model of microkeratome used. For example, complication rates have been reported to be significantly lower overall with the Bausch & Lomb Hansatome™ compared to the Automated Corneal Shaper™ (ACS) (8,13–14). There is a complicated sequence of steps required for the assembly of the former, and failure to insert the footplate can cause the devastating complication of corneal perforation. This problem has been eliminated in almost all of the newer microkeratomes, which incorporate the depth plate into the body of the head. As another example of instrument-specific complications, microkeratomes that promote advancement of the blade at a constant speed may minimize the creation of irregular flaps, especially in the hands of less experienced surgeons. Some devices now provide clear applanation plates that give a view of the anticipated flap and hinge sizes, which may reduce the risk of free caps in eyes predisposed to this problem.

Ocular anatomy: The preoperative examination will allow the surgeon to determine the patient's relative risk for a number of intraoperative complications. Palpebral fissure width and orbital anatomy determine the ease of accessibility of the microkeratome to the cornea. Epithelial integrity is assessed by careful screening for signs of epithelial basement membrane dystrophy and by considering the patient's age and history of corneal trauma or diabetes mellitus. Eyelid retraction with poor blinking or lagophthalmos will heighten epithelial vulnerability to intraoperative and postoperative problems. Corneal topography will reveal excessively steep or flat corneal curvatures that can predispose to free caps and buttonholes, respectively. Eyes having undergone previous surgery such as penetrating keratoplasty and scleral buckle repair of retinal detachment are also more likely to develop a flap buttonhole. All anatomic factors considered as a whole will allow the surgeon to choose the appropriate flap width and thickness, and in certain cases, the placement of the hinge as well.

Surgeon experience: As would be expected with any surgical procedure, increasing experience performing LASIK leads to a reduction in the rate of complications (2,5,7,12,15,16). Some authors have noted the rate to decrease significantly after 500 to 1000 cases have been performed (1,12). The number of cases required to complete the learning curve can also be compressed with prior experience performing other corneal refractive procedures such as myopic keratomileusis, epikeratophakia, and automated lamellar keratoplasty (2). Fellowship training or an extended proctorship is certainly invaluable to condense the time required to gain the necessary expertise (17).

Microkeratome-related flap complications can be categorized as thin flaps or buttonholes, free caps, incomplete or irregular flaps, and corneal perforations. When properly managed, poor keratectomies will rarely result in significant visual loss (12,13), even when the edge of the flap crosses the visual axis. In a retrospective review of 3998 eyes that underwent LASIK by Tham and Maloney, only 1 of 27 eyes that experienced flap complications had a decrease in BSCVA of greater than 2 lines (12). However, 12 of 27 eyes (41%) did lose one line of BSCVA, and it should also be considered that BSCVA may not adequately characterize the consequences of the poor keratectomy on the quality of vision, which is best quantified by measurements of contrast sensitivity, glare, and optical aberrations, in addition to BSCVA.

With poor keratectomies in general, laser treatment should be deferred if any part of the ablation would not be applied to the stroma of the keratectomy bed. One exception to this guideline is hyperopic treatments in which the bed is minimally smaller than the treatment zone and only the extreme periphery of the well-centered ablation would be applied to epithelium. Unsatisfactory flaps should not be lifted or manipulated beyond light irrigation and/or placement of a bandage contact lens as required. The patient should be informed of the complication while still under the laser; however extensive counselling should be reserved for later examinations. When laser ablation is not performed, no significant change in refractive error is expected. In the authors' experience, most patients will return to preoperative refractive status within one week, if not within one day. Tham and Maloney reported that 18 or 19 eyes experiencing a flap complication and in whom laser ablation was not performed returned to a spherical equivalent within 1 D of the preoperative value, and 16 or 19 eyes reached a cylinder within 1 D of the preoperative amount (12). It is considered safe to repeat the procedure a minimum of three months later (7,18) with a new microkeratome pass using a thicker plate when possible, although the complication rate reportedly will remain higher at 12.5% than the 0.66% complication rate associated with primary flaps (12). This 20-fold increase most likely is because in many cases there is a particular feature of the patient's anatomy that predisposed to the original flap complication.

1. Flap Buttonhole

Among the various possible flap complications, buttonholes are particularly undesirable, as they are more likely to cause visual symptoms than free or incomplete flaps (2). This may be due to the greater area of stromal irregularity that involves the visual axis. These thin flaps are also more difficult to handle and position intraoperatively and are more likely to wrinkle postoperatively (19).

The mechanism of buttonhole formation appears to be buckling of the cornea during the passage of the microkeratome blade (14). Buttonholes occur predominantly in eyes with excessively steep corneas, including those following penetrating keratoplasty. In addition, a number of surgeons have reported average keratometry readings of 44.23 to 50.00 D in eyes that experience this complication, with readings as low as 42.94 D. Thus keratometry readings alone do not fully predict which eyes are at increased risk of experiencing this complication. Buttonholes may also occur owing to one of the following: (1) loss of suction during the passage of the microkeratome, (2) a defective blade, (3) irregular advancement of a manual microkeratome, and (4) abnormal function of the motor of an automated microkeratome, resulting in abnormal advancement or oscillations of the blade (20). Lam et al. reported the latter aetiology after investigating a temporal cluster of six cases of buttonholes, experiencing an immediate drop in the rate of this complication upon servicing of the motor unit of the microkeratome (21).

When a cornea is felt to be at risk for a buttonhole owing to high keratometry readings or the occurrence of the same complication in the fellow eye, a smaller diameter suction ring and thicker depth plate may be chosen, and adequate intraocular pressure should be carefully verified prior to passage of the blade. Relatively low intraocular pressures may result in unsatisfactory applanation of the cornea by the depth plate and consequently allow inward dimpling of the cornea during passage of the blade (7,13). Loss of vision alone may not ensure a satisfactory intraocular pressure: using a Langhans tonometer, Gimbel et al. have noted that intraocular pressure can rapidly decrease during the early phase of suction prior to passage of the microkeratome blade (7). They have postulated this to be the result of either retraction of the eye or inadvertent lifting of the suction ring. After adopting their "pressure pass technique," they reported no buttonholes in over 1600 consecutive procedures. The pressure pass technique requires the application of additional manual pressure to the suction ring as the blade is being passed to ensure proper applanation of the cornea. Conjunctival scarring as a result of previous surgery can cause a falsely high intraocular pressure reading in the presence of inadequate intraocular pressure during the keratectomy. This may have predisposed to the buttonhole reported by Stulting et al. in an eye with a scleral buckle (2).

In general, laser ablation is best abandoned when buttonhole keratectomies are created (2), allowing a recut and ablation a minimum of 3 months later. In some eyes, central haze and/or irregular astigmatism may occur, which can lead to visual loss. Wilson has recommended the use of a combination of PTK and PRK early in the postoperative period to eliminate the irregular tissue (13). It is a mixed blessing that there are insufficient numbers of buttonholes to conduct a study that would properly compare approaches to management.

2. Free Cap

Free caps are caused by the inadequate tissue captured in the suction ring relative to the excursion of the blade. In general, they may occur more frequently in flat corneas (<40 D) owing to reduced protrusion of tissue above the plate of the suction ring. With the Hansatome, for example, they occur more commonly when the 8.5 mm ring (vs. the 9.5 mm ring) is used on flat corneas. Free caps may occur with the Automated Corneal Shaper due to inadvertent omission or misinsertion of the stopper (6). Other purported mechanisms include insufficient suction and loss of suction during the pass of the microkeratome, with a reported incidence of 0.7% to 5.9% (1,4–6). Some surgeons have also suggested an increase in the incidence of free caps when nasally hinged flaps are made in patients with with-the-rule astigmatism; this again implicates the flat cornea, since the hinge is created along the flat meridian. Finally, with the Moria microkeratomes, they may occur when a thin suction ring is used on a steep cornea.

To prevent the creation of free caps, the surgeon should select the optimal combination of microkeratome components (e.g., use of a larger ring as noted above). Microkeratomes with adjustable stops can be set for a larger hinge, or the physician may manually stop the blade prior to completion of the pass, a process that is presumably facilitated by the use of a microkeratome with a clear applanation plate. However, this challenging technique requires further validation.

Experience with myopic keratomileusis suggests that the occurrence of a free cap need not be considered a surgical complication, as long as the cap itself is retrieved in reasonable condition. Depending on the design of the instrument, the cap may remain lodged within the head of the microkeratome following keratectomy, and careful disassembly of the unit may be required to retrieve the lenticule. Unlike the situation with buttonholes, when free caps occur, it is best not to postpone the laser treatment, since attempting a new microkeratome pass for a later ablation puts the eye at risk of complications related to disruption of the free cap.

The ablation may be performed while the cap is stored in an antidessication chamber or placed epithelial side down on the conjunctival (18). To prevent postoperative regular and irregular astigmatism, the surgeon should use the surface markings as a guide to orient the cap properly as it is replaced on the keratectomy bed. Surface markings are not necessary for reorientation when the cap has an irregular shape, since this easily allows for correct orientation within the stromal bed. Reattachment is achieved by air-drying the cap for a minimum of 3 to 5 minutes. Even if it is damaged, it is advantageous to salvage the cap whenever possible. In the rare situations where the cap is lost or unusable, the eye should be treated as though a photorefractive keratectomy had been performed. Patients are at risk for increased amounts of haze, but on occasion surprisingly good results can be achieved. Later surface ablation could also be considered, once all haze has resolved.

3. Incomplete, Short, or Irregular Flaps

These types of flaps usually occur when there is inadequate suction or a microkeratome malfunction. The reported incidence of incomplete flaps is 0.7% to 6.6% (1,4). A common cause of inadequate suction with a falsely normal pressure reading is conjunctival aspiration into the suction ring, one sign of which is subtle rotation of the cornea during the buildup of suction. Excessive upward lifting of the suction ring may be a contributing factor as well. Microkeratome malfunctioning can also result in an irregular or incomplete flap; potential causes include inadequate or irregular speed of advancement of the blade with manually advanced microkeratomes, corrosion of gears, electrical failure, obstruction of the blade or gears by lashes, drape, or eyelids (1), and poor blade quality. Metallic blades vary in surface quality, and therefore each blade should be inspected prior to use. Balanced salt solution should never be used intraoperatively to avoid mineral deposition in the motor spindle that can cause friction and malfunction (22). The microkeratome should be cleaned according to the manufacturer's instructions, and proper functioning should be verified in both forward and reverse directions prior to each microkeratome pass (18).

To insure that the intraocular pressure is adequate prior to initiating the keratectomy, three signs should be noted: (1) pupillary dilation, (2) patient confirmation of loss of vision, and (3) tactile or tonometric evidence of high intraocular pressure. The use of a pneumotonometer has been advocated by some (8,13), since this may be the most reliable means of quantifying intraocular pressure values that exceed 75 mmHg. With a Hansatome and other microkeratomes that "ramp up" to the target pressure, it is important to allow a few seconds for the pressure to build prior to passing the blade across the cornea. In this respect, use of a tonometer serves a second role: in the process of checking the pressure, additional time elapses during which suction is allowed to build.

At the first hint of inadequate suction, the machine should be turned off and the suction ring repositioned. If necessary, redundant conjunctiva can be stretched towards the fornices by repositioning the eyelid speculum. Mild conjunctival chemosis is diminished by gently stroking the conjunctiva centrifugally with wet and dry Merocel sponges. When the suction ring is reapplied, it is helpful to apply firm pressure on both sides of the section ring for 10 to 15 seconds prior to activating suction. This helps to express fluid from beneath the suction ring, which increases the likelihood of obtaining adequate suction. If adequate suction is not obtained after two or three attempts, then the case should be postponed for an hour or longer in order to await resolution of conjunctival chemosis. In rare instances, it may be necessary to defer surgery for a day or two.

If an incomplete or short flap is created, we recommend that the flap be minimally manipulated, that no attempts be made manually to extend the flap, and that laser treatment be deferred. If a smaller optical zone is appropriate and would fit in the keratectomy bed, ablation may still be performed; otherwise ablations should be postponed for a minimum of 3 months before the flap is recut (1,2,7,18). Laser treatment to a partially exposed stromal bed or manual dissection of the flap may result in highly irregular astigmatism (23), while PRK to the surface of an incomplete flap predisposes to the development of visually significant haze. A contact lens may be placed on the eye and the patient briefly counselled while on the table. More detailed counselling should be given shortly afterwards once the patient is out of the laser room, as well as on subsequent days. If the complication arises in the first eye, the procedure on the fellow eye should be deferred as well (23).

Allowing the flap to heal for at least 3 months is the recommended course of action when a flap complication occurs. The patient will usually regain the preoperative BSCVA within a few days of the surgery. Even when the edge of the flap abuts the visual axis, patients tend to remain surprisingly asymptomatic. Postoperatively, the patient should be carefully monitored for epithelial ingrowth, the incidence of which may be higher with short flaps and buttonholes due to the irregular, thin flap edge that allows epithelium to remain in contact with the interface (24). The flap should be allowed to heal for at least 3 months, until refractive and topographic stability are confirmed, prior to proceeding with a recut and subsequent laser ablation. At the stage of refractive and topographic stability, the flap is assumed to be well enough adherent to the stromal bed to withstand the rigors of a new, deeper microkeratome pass. Although such stability may be attained as early as 1 month in some patients (25), it is generally expected to have been achieved by 3 months postoperatively (2,13,15,26), and waiting even longer may further minimize the risks of reoperating.

4. Corneal Perforation

This devastating complication has been reported to arise with the Automated Corneal Shaper in the event of misinsertion or failure to insert the depth plate (13,27,28). Damage to anterior segment structures as well as vitreous loss and expulsive hemorrhage have occurred due to corneal perforation under high intraocular pressure, necessitating surgical repair (29). By incorporating the depth plate into the body of the microkeratome, most current microkeratomes avoid this potential complication. If perforation is noted with extrusion of aqueous fluid, suction should be immediately deactivated and the microkeratome removed from the eye while avoiding the exertion of any pressure on the globe. Surgical repair using sterile technique is then indicated.

Corneal perforation during the actual laser ablation has been reported in two patients as well (30). In one of these patients, the management of excessive limbal bleeding resulted in extreme stromal dehydration with subsequent overcorrection during laser ablation. Presumably a microperforation could go unnoticed following flap replacement and then lead to endophthalmitis, as was reported by Mulhern et al. (31). This case illustrates three fundamentals related to corneal tissue. First, excess corneal tissue removal can leave insufficient support tissue in the keratectomy bed, which can predispose to keratectasia or even perforation during laser ablation. Second, stromal exposure leads to dehydration and subsequent overcorrection by the laser beam. Finally, flap thicknesses vary even in the absence of microkeratome malfunction or blade defects (32), and this variability must be accounted for when calculating available tissue for removal.

B. POOR ACCESS TO THE CORNEA

Adequate exposure of the globe is essential for the application of the keratome/suction ring assembly. This can be limited in patients with deep-set eyes, blepharospasm, or small palpebral fissures (8,18). In these eyes, it is helpful to have more than one type of lid speculum available. For the lid squeezer, it may be preferable to use a locking speculum with a posteriorly angulated hinge. The authors often prefer a flexible speculum that can be opened as needed by the fingers and the pressure of the microkeratome. Careful draping of the eyelids is important to prevent lashes from interfering with the microkeratome. Turning the patient's head slightly to the opposite side will position the cornea in a wider section of the palpebral fissure and will help to reduce interference by the eyelid speculum. Elevation of the patient's chin to center the cornea within the palpebral fissure is another valuable maneuver. To increase exposure, the globe should also be proptosed by pressing down on the eyelid speculum and/or pulling up slightly on the suction ring, once engaged. One common error is to open the locking speculum to the width of the orbital rim, allowing the globe to fall back. Rather, the speculum should be kept moderately open and pressed into the orbit in order to proptose the globe.

In patients with very tight palpebral fissures, the keratectomy can be performed without using an eyelid speculum. Another option is a lateral canthotomy (16), which provides excellent access to the eye; the canthotomy can be repaired with a single suture. Although a light retrobulbar block may be administered to proptose the globe (11,18), this option introduces the risk of additional sight-threatening complications, may eliminate the patient's ability to fixate during the procedure, and, by causing a poor blink reflex, predisposes to corneal dryness postoperatively. For these reasons we do not recommend retrobulbar blocks. Due consideration should always be given to aborting the procedure or to performing an alternative procedure when access to the globe is at issue.

C. CORNEAL EPITHELIAL DEFECT

Intraoperative epithelial defects can be surprisingly troublesome because, depending on their size and location, they can predispose to delayed healing, diffuse lamellar keratitis (33), and epithelial ingrowth (1), especially when the defect is at the edge of the flap. Epithelial defects may also lead to regression, haze, and flap striae. Importantly, they cause patient discomfort and can require additional postoperative follow-up visits.

Careful preoperative screening for any signs of epithelial basement membrane dystrophy (EBMD), however subtle, will unfortunately not reveal all cases of loosely adherent epithelium. Other risk factors include older age, prior corneal trauma, and diabetes mellitus. When any signs of EBMD are present, careful consideration should be given to performing PRK instead of LASIK, as the extent of observable pathology will not reliably predict the amount of epithelium that will slide (34). Specific informed consent, possibly with the use of special consent forms, should be obtained from the patient in this regard.

As discussed earlier, certain types of microkeratomes, such as the Hansatome, appear to be associated with a higher incidence of epithelial defects. Defects may also be created during placement and removal of the eyelid speculum as well as during flap relifts for enhancements. In all patients, preoperative inspection of the blade, sparing use of topical anaesthetics, which destabilize the epithelium (16), and generous lubrication of the corneal surface prior to the passage of the blade will minimize epithelial disruption. Experienced surgeons using the Hansatome may employ alternative techniques such as removal of the entire blade-suction ring assembly from the eye at the conclusion of the forward pass (33).

Epithelial defects are frequently noted at the conclusion of the keratectomy and can vary in extent and severity. Relatively small defects are not considered a contraindication for proceeding with laser treatment. Following laser ablation and replacement of the flap, the dislodged epithelium should be repositioned as well as possible using dry Merocel sponges or forceps. Larger defects (>1 mm) usually require a bandage contact lens (35), and the patient should be counselled accordingly about expected postoperative recovery. Smaller defects that spare the visual axis often heal without the support of a bandage lens. In questionable cases, careful slit lamp inspection of the loose tag of epithelium for movement with blinks will dictate the need for a bandage lens. When large epithelial defects are created, treatment of the fellow eye should be performed at the surgeon's discretion, taking into account the patient's personality and expectations, as well as the prospects for performing PRK in the fellow eye.

D. WOUND DEHISCENCE

Wound dehiscence during LASIK can occur in two situations: after penetrating keratoplasties and after incisional refractive procedures. Dehiscence of the graft–host junction in patients that have undergone penetrating keratoplasty can rarely occur during passage of the microkeratome blade. At present there is no consensus as to the ideal timing of LASIK following penetrating keratoplasty. However, reasonable indicators that the wound will successfully resist the suction forces of the microkeratome ring include waiting at least 6 months after all sutures have been removed, ensuring the presence of a good wound scar, and confirming topographic stability.

In patients that have undergone incisional refractive procedures, cysts in the incisions and wound gape are the clues to poor healing of the cuts. Corneas with T-cuts or hexagonal keratotomies are at risk of developing holes in the flaps corresponding to the rectangular cuts; this likelihood is even greater in eyes with intersecting incisions. In such patients, it may advisable to recommend against LASIK and consider other options such as PRK or a phakic IOL. Many surgeons have recommended against the use of PRK in these patients owing to the risk of excessive postoperative haze formation. However, the authors have performed both myopic and hyperopic PRK in approximately 20 patients, and none have developed any sight-threatening haze.

Intraoperative steps to minimize incisional dehiscence include use of the thickest depth plate feasible and elevation of the flap by gently inserting a spatula, rather than lifting with forceps. In the event that the keratotomy incisions begin to separate intraoperatively, laser treatment may still be performed, the interface irrigated, and the segments of the flap carefully repositioned. There is much greater risk of epithelial ingrowth through these dehisced incisions, and this can even occur with incisions that appear normal preoperatively and remain intact during the procedure. Fortunately, this ingrowth is usually self-limited and typically requires no additional treatment.

Retreatments in these eyes are more difficult owing to the risk of incisional separation as the flap is dissected free. As a result, the authors counsel these patients about the increased risks associated with both primary treatment and enhancements.

E. LIMBAL BLEEDING

Blood vessels can be transected in two instances: when a corneal pannus is present, as is common in contact lens wearers, and when an inappropriately sized or positioned suction ring results in passage of the blade over limbal and conjunctival vessels. Managing corneal bleeding can significantly prolong the time required to complete the procedure. This may concern the patient, especially when surgery takes longer in one eye than another. Therefore, whenever corneal bleeding is anticipated, specific preoperative counselling should be done in order to manage patient expectations regarding the length of time that the procedure will take in each eye.

Preoperative examination of the cornea is again critical to identify risk factors for this complication. Occasionally ghost vessels emanating from a small pannus will refill and bleed when sheared. In some patients it is not possible to avoid these vessels. The choice of suction ring size, where applicable, is based on the size as well as the steepness of the cornea, and it should be kept in mind when making the choice that the actual flap size is usually smaller than the diameter of the suction ring chosen.

Corneal bleeding is rarely of any consequence, as long as the surgeon assures that it does not interfere with any critical steps of the surgery. It is sometimes helpful to attempt to control the bleeding before lifting the flap prior to performing the ablation. Gentle pressure is applied on the oozing vessels or on their limbal feeders with a dry or slightly moistened Merocel sponge. Alternatively, pressure may be applied with a dry Merocel sponge through a fold of conjunctiva that is pushed over the limbal feeders.

Blood in the interface is a physical barrier to the laser and will interfere with the ablation. Therefore, any blood that oozes onto the ablation zone of the stromal bed must be removed. If blood persists in oozing onto the peripheral stroma during laser treatment, it can be left alone as long as it does not encroach upon the ablation zone. Not removing every drop of blood from the peripheral stroma during the laser treatment will allow the surgeon to concentrate on the important tasks of monitoring centration, focus, and patient fixation, while removing blood and other debris from the stromal bed as required. At the conclusion of the ablation, the flap should be replaced prior to attending to the bleeding, again in order to employ the flap as an additional tamponade for the cut vessels. Phenylephrine 2.5% may be used at this stage to constrict the blood vessels and reduce the flow of blood. It should not be used prior to laser treatment, as uneven pupillary dilation will change the center of the pupil and thus eliminate the key landmark for the centration of the ablation.

In general, small amounts of blood in the stromal interface are well tolerated and cause no complications. There has been one report of diffuse lamellar keratitis that occurred in an area of interface blood. In some patients, it is not possible to remove all of the blood from the interface without using excessive irrigation. It is generally preferable to minimize the irrigation to prevent overhydration of the flap, which can lead to flap striae and flap slippage.

F. FLAP WRINKLING AND DISLOCATION

Intraoperative factors leading to flap wrinkling are flap hydration from excessive irrigation of the stromal interface (36,37), decentration of the flap within the keratectomy bed, and flap dislocation caused by squeezing of the eyelids. The ultimate goal of intraoperative flap management is a clear interface with a small gutter, as large gutters reflect shrinkage of the flap as a result of excess hydration.

Irrigation should be performed with a brief, high-pressure burst of fluid. One helpful option is to place a fiberoptic endoilluminator at the limbus in order to retroilluminate the cornea and allow identification of fine striae and interface debris, thus allowing the surgeon to minimize the amount of fluid delivered to the interface.

Although flap dislocation is not strictly an intraoperative complication, most dislocations occur within the first few hours of surgery (38,39). Excessive dryness of the surface of the flap may be one predisposing factor, as it can predispose to excessive friction with the lid during blinking. The authors have found it helpful to administer artificial tears several times in the first 30 minutes postoperatively and to encourage patients to close their eyes for the first few hours. Gimbel et al. reported a significant decrease in the number of flap dislocations since they instituted postoperative use of clear plastic moisture chambers with their patients (7).

G. SKIN LACERATION

This can occur when using the Hansatome in patients with narrow palpebral fissures or deep-set eyes. Careful attention to the eyelids while placing the suction ring will avoid entrapment of skin or drape material and eliminate this complication. It is often helpful to have the surgical assistant retract the lower lid and watch it to ensure that it is not caught beneath the microkeratome. At most, the skin will be lightly nicked. Bleeding can be controlled by light pressure with a dry Merocel sponge and local postoperative application of phenylephrine drops.

H. VASOVAGAL OR OCULOCARDIAC REFLEX

The oculocardiac reflex is commonly defined as a 10% decrease in heart rate resulting from external pressure on the eye. In the case of LASIK, this pressure results from the suction ring acting on the eye. A study of 20 patients who underwent LASIK reported that 20% had a heart rate drop of more than 10% at the time of suction; an additional 20% had a heart rate increase of more than 20% from baseline at the time of positioning under the laser (40). The same team subsequently repeated the study using sedation to eliminate the effect of stress and found that the oculocardiac reflex occurs more frequently in sedated patients: 14 of 30 patients had a heart rate decrease of at least 10% at the time of suction, while 2 of 30 patients had an increase in heart rate of greater than 10% (41).

During preoperative evaluation, patients should be questioned for a history of syncope, cardiac disease, and cerebrovascular disease. Patients considered to be at risk may benefit by not receiving perioperative sedatives. Surgeons should always remain in verbal communication with the patient during the procedure, since an intraoperative syncopal episode can be otherwise difficult to recognize. It is actually more common for the vasovagal reaction to occur postoperatively as the patient sits up or walks to the slit lamp. Therefore patients should be moved slowly after surgery, and a staff member should always remain close to the patient during the first minute of ambulation.

I. INTERFACE DEBRIS

Interface debris is commonly seen in corneas that have undergone LASIK. There are numerous sources of interface debris, including meibomian gland secretions, particles from sponges and instruments, talc from gloves, particles in the air, metallic fragments from the blades, blood cells, epithelial cells, and debris from within the tear film (42). Excess irrigation can itself draw debris from the fornices into the interface, especially when an aspirating speculum is not used (7,33). The use of an aspirating speculum (13) and nonfragmenting sponges, operating in a lint-free environment, careful draping of lashes and eyelids, and most important, judicious irrigation of the interface will help to limit the amount of debris present (18). A perilimbal sponge, such as the Chayet LASIK Eye Drain (BD Ophthalmic, Franklin Lakes, NJ) can be helpful as well to protect the interface from debris (43).

As discussed above, the ideal interface is a pristine one, but achieving this goal must be balanced against the adverse effects of excess irrigation of the interface. With rare exceptions, interface debris is well tolerated and creates no complications. However, there are rare reports of infectious keratitis (44) or irregular astigmatism that were attributed to interface debris (45,46). In addition, in some instances, interlamellar debris may stimulate a localized inflammatory response. This usually responds to increased treatment with topical corticosteroids (47); however, if the inflammation is excessive (e.g., involves full thickness of the flap), then irrigation may be indicated. When examining patients immediately following the surgery, the authors' preference is to irrigate only debris that is sufficiently large to pose a potential threat, e.g., a fiber of ≥2 mm in length.

Occasionally, significant amounts of lipid are drawn into the interface and noted on the postoperative slit lamp examination. Eyelid squeezing by the patient may cause the bottom of the flap to briefly lift up and draw tears into the interface by capillary action. This lifting effect may also occur when the very edge of the flap is stroked too hard with the wet Merocel sponge. This lipid can be observed without intervention if there is no effect on vision and no associated inflammation.

J. RETINAL AND CHOROIDAL COMPLICATIONS

There are rare reports of intraoperative retinochoroidal and optic nerve complications. Luna and colleagues reported bilateral macular hemorrhages following LASIK in a high myope (<−16 D) with no preexisting myopic degeneration; the pathogenesis was presumably a break in Bruch's membrane in the fovea, but no preoperative lacquer cracks or macular hemorrhages were noted (48). Risk factors for choroidal rupture may include preexisting lacquer cracks, choroidal neovascularization, Fuchs' spots, and high axial myopia. Lee and colleagues reported four cases of optic neuropathy following LASIK (49). The etiology is unknown but may be related to the marked increase in intraocular pressure that occurs during the microkeratome portion of the procedure.

K. MANAGEMENT OF THE PATIENT WITH AN INTRAOPERATIVE FLAP COMPLICATION

Although each patient who undergoes LASIK does so having given informed consent, an intraoperative flap complication is nonetheless a devastating event for surgeon and patient alike. When a significant intraoperative complication is encountered, the first step for the surgeon is to abandon the procedure and inform the patient of the complication while the patient is still lying on the table. A matter of fact tone should be used, and the problem explained honestly in as simple and few words as possible. At this stage the patient is usually in a state of disbelief and is unable to absorb the meaning of what he or she is told. There usually develops such a fear of permanent loss of vision that the patient becomes unable to take in any meaningful information. If the complication occurs on the first eye, surgery on the second eye should be postponed. Gentle reassurance should be repeatedly given as the postoperative examination and treatment are completed.

A more detailed explanation of the complication and prognosis should be reserved for later on in the day in the presence of friends or family members, or the following day. The patient should be told what happened and what is expected to occur. Even when no loss of vision is expected, it can be quite disquieting for patients to not have the procedure performed, and they should be given every opportunity to express their feelings about the event. The surgeon should make himself or herself available to the patient and devote as much time as the patient needs during each visit in the early postoperative period. It is natural for the surgeon to experience guilt over the event and to want to apologize; however, it is important to remember that a complication is not the same thing as negligence or lack of surgical skill. Complications arise even when correct procedures are followed, and the complication rate never drops to zero, regardless of the extent of surgeon skill and training. The vast majority of properly informed patients understand the risks when they elect to undergo the procedure.

Honesty, compassion, and communication are the keys to management of patients with LASIK complications. In some instances, patients are more dissatisfied with their postoperative treatment by the surgeon and his or her team rather than with the complication itself. Appropriate care of these patients is a critical element of their postoperative recovery and of their maintenance of trust in the surgical team.

REFERENCES

1. RT Lin, RK Maloney. Flap complications associated with lamellar refractive surgery. Am J Ophthalmol 1999;127:129–136.
2. RD Stulting, JD Carr, KP Thompson, GO Waring III, WM Wiley, JG Walker. Complications of laser in situ keratomileusis for the correction of myopia. Ophthalmology 1999;106:13–20.
3. RD Stulting, K Balch, JD Carr, K Walter, KP Thompson, GO Waring III. Complications of LASIK. Invest Ophthalmol Vis Sci 1997;38:S231.
4. MC Knorz, A Lierman, V Seiberth, H Steiner, B Wiesinger. Laser in situ keratomileusis to correct myopia of −6.00 to −29.00 diopters. J Refract Surg 1996;12:575–584.
5. JJ Perez-Santonja, MJ Ayala, HF Sakla, JM Ruiz-Moreno, JL Alio. Retreatment after laser in situ keratomileusis. Ophthalmology 1999;106:21–28.
6. A Marinho, MC Pinto, R Pinto, F Vaz, MC Neves. LASIK for high myopia: one-year experience. Ophthalmic Surg Lasers 1996;27(5 suppl):S517–S520.
7. HV Gimbel, EEA Penno, JA van Westenbrugge, M Ferensowicz, M Furlong. Incidence and management of intraoperative and early postoperative complications in 1000 consecutive laser in situ keratomileusis cases. Ophthalmology 1998;105:1839–1847.
8. ON Serdarevic. Avoidance of complications related to microkeratome use in LASIK. Ophthalmic Practice 1998;16(2):68–72.
9. AM Bas, R Onnis. Excimer laser in situ keratomileusis for myopia. J Refract Surg 1995;11(3 suppl):229.
10. HV Gimbel, S Basti, GB Kaye, M Ferensowicz. Experience during the learning curve of laser in situ keratomileusis. J Cataract Refract Surg 1996;22:542–550.
11. JM Davidorf, R Zaldivar, S Oscherow. Results and complications of laser in situ keratomileusis by experienced surgeons. J Refract Surg 1998;14:114–122.
12. VM Tham, RK Maloney. Microkeratome complications of laser in situ keratomileusis. Ophthalmology 2000;107:920–924.
13. SE Wilson. LASIK: management of common complications. Cornea 1998;17:459–467.
14. MB Walker, SE Wilson. Lower intraoperative flap complication rate with the Hansatome microkeratome compared to the Automated Corneal Shaper. J Refract Surg 2000;16:79–82.
15. SG Farah, DT Azar, C Gurdal, J Wong. Laser in situ keratomileusis: literature review of a developing technique. J Cataract Refract Surg 1998;24:989–996.
16. HV Gimbel, SG Levy. Indications, results, and complications of LASIK. Curr Opin Ophthalmol 1998;9(IV):3–8.
17. C Yo, C Vroman, S Ma, L Chao, PJ McDonnell. Surgical outcomes of photoreactive keratectomy and laser in situ keratomileusis by inexperienced surgeons. J Cataract Refract Surg 2000;26:510–515.
18. EA Davis, DR Hardten, RL Lindstrom. LASIK complications. Int Ophthalmol Clin 2000;40(3):67–75.
19. L Burrato, M Ferrari, C Genisi. Myopic keratomileusis with the excimer laser: one year follow-up. Refract Corneal Surg 1993;9:12–19.

20. ATS Leung, SK Rao, ACK Cheng, EWY Yu, DSP Fan, DSC Lam. Pathogenesis and management of laser in situ keratomileusis flap buttonhole. J Cataract Refract Surg 2000;26:358–362.

21. DS Lam, AC Cheng, AT Leung. LASIK complications. Ophthalmology 1999;106(8): 1455–1457.

22. TB Clinch. Discussion of article: HV Gimbel, EEA Penno, JA van Westenbrugge, M Ferensowicz, M Furlong. Incidence and management of intraoperative and early postoperative complications in 1000 consecutive laser in situ keratomileusis cases. Ophthalmology 1998;105: 1847–1848.

23. SP Holland, S Srivannaboon, DZ Reinstein. Avoiding serious corneal complications of laser assisted in situ keratomileusis and photorefractive keratectomy. Ophthalmology 2000;107:640–652.

24. NG Iskander, NT Peters, EA Penno, HV Gimbel. Postoperative complications in laser in situ keratomileusis. Current Opinion in Ophthalmology 2000;11:273–279.

25. SK Rao, P Padmanabhan, F Sitalakshmi, R Rajagopal, DSC Lam. Timing of retreatment after a partial flap during laser in situ keratomileusis (letter). J Cataract Refract Surg 1999;25:1424.

26. HV Gimbel. Flap complications of lamellar refractive surgery. Am J Ophthalmol 1999;127(2): 202–204.

27. SF Brint, M Ostrick, C Fisher, C Fisher, SG Slade, RK Maloney, R Epstein, RD Stulting, KP Thompson. Six-month results of the multicenter phase 1 study of excimer laser myopia keratomileusis. J Cataract Refract Surg 1994;20:610–615.

28. IG Pallikaris, DS Siganos. Excimer laser in situ keratomileusis and phtotrefractive keratectomy for correction of high myopia. J Refract Corneal Surg 1994;10:498–510.

29. IG Pallikaris, DS Siganos. Laser in situ keratomileusis to treat myopia: early experience. J Cataract Refract Surg 1997;23:39–49.

30. CK Joo, TG Kim. Corneal perforation during laser in situ keratomileusis. J Cataract Refract Surg 1999;25(8):1165–1167.

31. MG Mulhern, PI Condon, M O'Keefe. Endophthalmitis after laser in situ keratomileusis. J Cataract Refract Surg 1997;23:948–950.

32. BJ Jacobs, TA Deutsch, JB Rubenstein. Reproducibility of corneal flap thickness in LASIK. Ophthalmic Surg Lasers 1999;30:350–353.

33. MN Shah, M Misra, KR Wilhelmus, DD Koch. Diffuse lamellar keratitis associated with epithelial defects after laser in situ keratomileusis. J Cataract Refract Surg 2000;26(9):1312–1318.

34. KA Dastgheib, TE Clinch, EE Manche, P Hersh, J Ramsey. Sloughing of corneal epithelium and wound healing complications associated with laser in situ keratomileusis in patients with epithelial basement membrane dystrophy. Am J Ophthalmol 2000;130(3):297–303.

35. EF Carpel, KH Carlson, S Shannon. Folds and striae in laser in situ keratomileusis flaps. J Refract Surg 1999;15:687–690.

36. GO Waring III, JD Carr, RD Stulting, KP Thompson, W Wiley. Prospective randomized comparison of simultaneous and sequential bilateral laser in situ keratomileusis for the correction of myopia. Ophthalmology 1999;106:732–738.

37. DSC Lam, ATS Leung, JT Wu, ACK Cheng, DSP Fan, SK Rao, JH Talamo, C Barraquer. Management of severe flap wrinkling or dislodgement after laser in situ keratomileusis. J Cataract Refract Surg 1999;25:1441–1447.

38. LE Probst, J Machat. Removal of flap striae following laser in situ keratomileusis. J Cataract Refract Surg 1998;24:153–155.

39. OF Recep, N Cagil, H Hasiripi. Outcome of flap subluxation after laser in situ keratomileusis: results of 6-month follow-up. J Cataract Refract Surg 2000;26:1158–1162.

40. M Paciuc, G Mendieta, R Naranjo. Oculocardiac reflex during laser in situ keratomileusis. J Cataract Refract Surg 1998;24(10):1317–1319.

41. M Paciuc, G Mendieta, R Naranjo, E Angel, E Reyes. Oculocardiac reflex in sedated patients having laser in situ keratomileusis. J Cataract Refract Surg 1999;25(10):1341–1343.

42. LW Hirst, KW Vandeleur. Laser in situ keratomileusis interface deposits. J Refract Surg 1998;14:653–654.

43. M Montes, A Chayet, L Gomez, R Magallenes, N Robledo. Laser in situ keratomileusis for myopia of −1.50 to −6.00 diopters. J Refract Surg 1999;15:106–110.

44. SG Slade. LASIK complications and their management. In: JJ Machat, ed. Excimer laser Refractive Surgery. Practice and Principles. Thorofare, NJ: SLACK, 1996, pp 360–368.

45. M Campos, MJ Carvalho, M Scarpi, W Chamon. Excimer laser intrastromal keratomileusis (LASIK): a clinical follow-up. Ophthalmic Surg Lasers. 1996,27(suppl):S534.

46. RK Maloney. Epithelial ingrowth after lamellar refractive surgery (suppl). Ophthalmic Surgery and Lasers 1996;27:S534.

47. MC Helena, DM Meisler, SE Wilson. Epithelial growth within the lamellar interface following laser in situ keratomileusis (LASIK). Cornea 1997;16:300–305.

48. JD Luna, VE Reviglio, CP Juarez. Bilateral macular hemorrhage after laser in situ keratomileusis. Graefes Arch Clin Exp Ophthalmol 1999;237:611–613.

49. AG Lee, T Kohnen, R Ebner, JL Bennett, NR Miller, TJ Carlow, DD Koch. Optic neuropathy associated with laser in situ keratomileusis. J Cataract Refract Surg 2000;26(11):1581–1584.

27

Postoperative Complications of LASIK

SAMIR G. FARAH

Massachusetts Eye and Ear Infirmary, Boston, Massachusetts, U.S.A.

JAE BUM LEE and DIMITRI T. AZAR

Massachusetts Eye and Ear Infirmary, Schepens Eye Research Institute, and Harvard Medical School, Boston, Massachusetts U.S.A.

This chapter will cover LASIK postoperative complications. It is not uncommon that these complications arise from preoperative and intraoperative complications as discussed in Chap. 15 and 26 (Figures 26.1–26.3). Although several studies have focused on these complications (1–34), most studies included a relatively small number of patients and reported a relatively small number of complications. In a study (2) on 1026 eyes that underwent LASIK, the rate of postoperative complications averaged 3.1%.

A. EARLY POSTOPERATIVE COMPLICATIONS (Figures 27.4–27.8)

1. Overcorrection and Undercorrection

Undercorrection is the most frequent complication after primary LASIK (11,17,20). It is usually diagnosed in the first few weeks postoperatively, and the refractive error stabilizes early thereafter. The presence of punctate keratopathy (Figure 27.4), epithelial ingrowth (Figure 27.5, 27.6) and irregularities (Figure 27.7), however, may delay the diagnosis.

Overcorrection is most often seen after retreatments (32) and in elderly patients (>50 years). In the currently used myopic nomograms and laser algorithms, undercorrection is intentionally considered, thus decreasing to a minimum the risk of overcorrection, which is extremely unappreciated by myopes. On the other hand, overcorrection is considered in the hyperopic nomograms, because hyperopes may appreciate better being overcorrected than undercorrected.

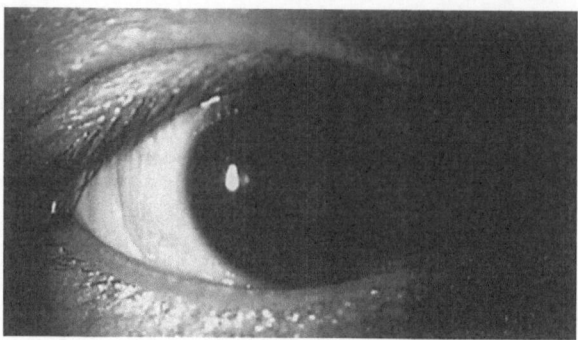

Figure 27.1 Redundant conjunctiva may cause inadequate suction when suction ring is applied.

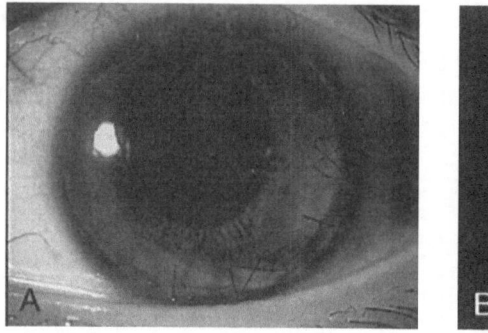 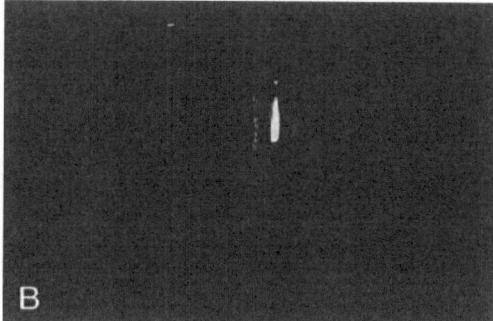

Figure 27.2 (A) Corneal perforation occurred during the laser ablation; several sutures were used just after LASIK to prevent further keratoectasia. (B) Slit beam view of the same patient.

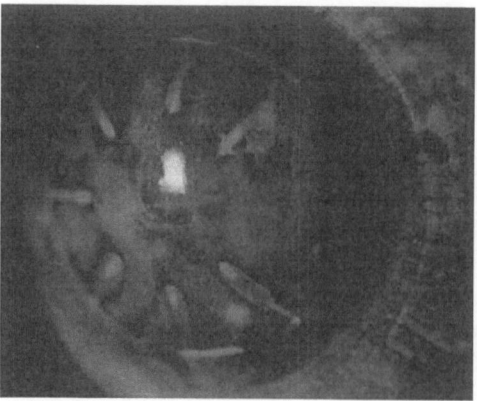

Figure 27.3 Radial corneal staining due to corneal marker can be seen following the day of surgery. Minimal marker is needed to avoid corneal epithelial toxicity after LASIK.

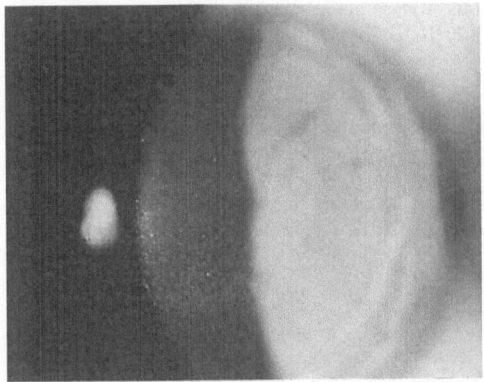

Figure 27.4 Multiple tiny superficial punctate keratopathy can be seen in the interpalpebral fissure zone of the cornea 1 month after LASIK. This is commonly seen in patients with dry eye disease. It is difficult to refract patients suffering from this condition, which contributes to fluctuating refractive errors.

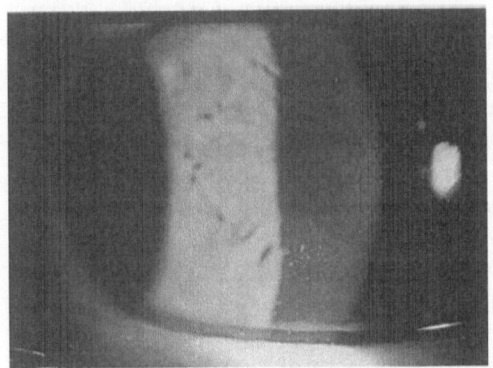

Figure 27.5 Epithelial ingrowth with fine epithelial nests can be seen 15 days after LASIK.

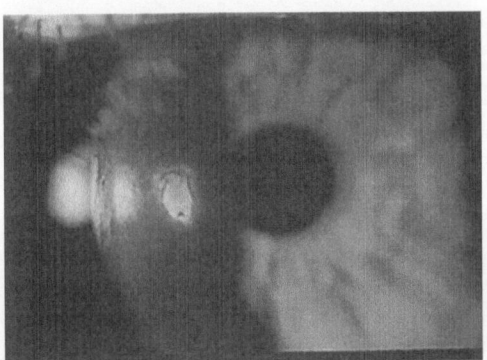

Figure 27.6 Large epithelial nest can be seen near the papillary area 2 months after LASIK.

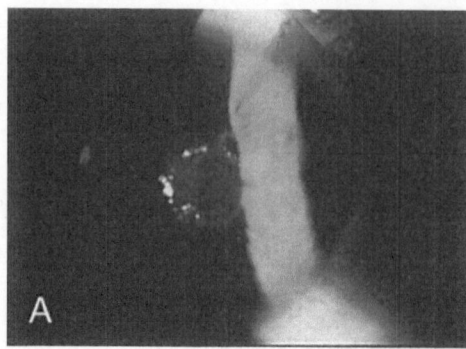 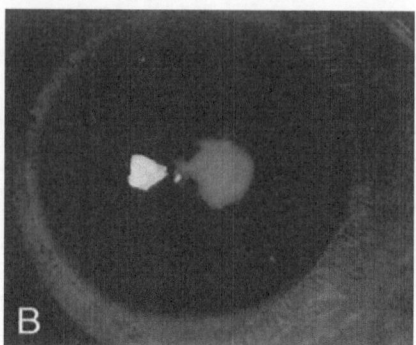

Figure 27.7 (A) Geographic pattern of herpetic corneal ulceration following LASIK. (B) Fluore-scien staining in the same patient.

Under- and overcorrection are related to the ablation algorithm, the nonaccurate nomograms, the age, and the amount of myopia, astigmatism, or hyperopia to be corrected (33,34). Several factors determine the maximum correction possible for high myopia patients, including the total corneal thickness (4,20) (flap and residual bed thickness) and the diameter of the optical zone (20). Often the full correction is not possible, which explains the undercorrected results in many high myopia groups (see Chapter 10).

Overcorrection is disappointingly common after LASIK, especially in the hands of aggressive surgeons, who are still adjusting their nomograms. Luckily, many of these cases will have regression during the first year after surgery. Thus patients are best monitored for at least 6 to 12 months postoperatively. Some cases, however, will be permanently over-corrected to clinically significant hyperopia.

With LASIK, a tendency toward mild overcorrection was noted in Fiander and Tay-four's series (10). An undercorrection greater than 1.5 D was present in 15.2% of eyes, and an overcorrection greater than 1 D occurred in 17.3% of eyes 6 months after LASIK (9). In Salah et al.'s series (12) there was a trend toward overcorrection at 3 weeks postoperatively, with a mean refraction of +0.79 D. Thirty-two percent were overcorrected by more than +1.0 D, and 6.0% were undercorrected by more than −1.0 D (12). By 5 months postoper-

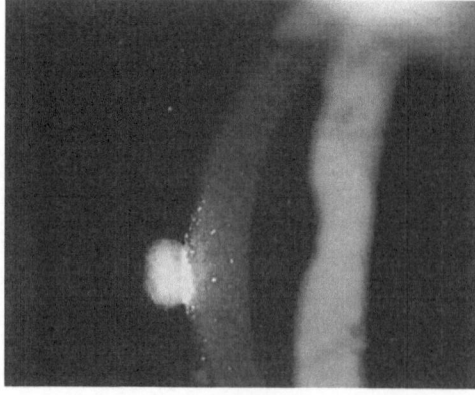

Figure 27.8 Wrinkling of the flap seen 2 days after LASIK.

Table 1 Postoperative Flap Dislocation

Etiology
(1) Excessive lid squeezing, (2) rubbing the operated eye, (3) excessively dry eye, (4) reduced blinking, (5) anesthesia from lateral canthotomy, (6) poor wetting of the eye, (7) from eyelid anomalies (lagophthalmous), (8) from orbit anomalies (exophthalmous), (9) incorrect use of fluids during the operation, (10) poor adhesion of the flap, (11) due to disruption of the epithelium, (12) due to poor intraoperative repositioning, (12) due to excessive irrigation with edema of the flap and the stromal bed, (13) postoperative trauma.
Results
(1) Repositioning is required, (2) risk of flap edema, (3) risk of abrasion, (4) risk of epithelial ingrown, (5) risk of striae, (6) risk of infection, (7) sutures may be required.
Prevention
(1) Pay attention to anatomic abnormalities of the eyelids and orbit, (2) check adhesion of the flap after repositioning, (3) remind the patient not to rub the eye, not to squeeze, and to wear a Fox shield for the first 24 hours and every night for the first week.
Treatment
(1) Carefully reposition the flap, (2) equally distend the flap in the event of folds and striae, (3) use sutures in the event of persistent folds, prolonged epithelial defects, or if the flap had to be repositioned intraoperatively, (4) keep the flap lubricated with nonpreserved artificial tears.

atively, the mean refraction decreased to $+0.22$ D, with 17.0% overcorrected by more than $+1.0$ D and 11.4% undercorrected by more than -1.0 D (12). Guell and Muller (11) did not report any overcorrection. The retreatment rate reached up to 17% (5,7,11,17,20,35).

2. Sliding or Dislodged Flap (8,9,36) (Table 1)

It may be caused by rubbing of the eyes in the immediate postoperative period or by the posterior edge of the eyelid catching the edge of the flap and flipping it out of position, or by surgeon error in allowing insufficient time for the flap to adhere to the bed during surgery (Figure 27.8).

This complication has tremendously decreased with the concept of down–up flap. Flap displacement occurs most commonly in the first 24 hours after LASIK, before the epithelium has had time to heal over the lamellar entry site. The appropriate time to allow for flap adhesion intraoperatively is still debatable; recommended times vary between 3 and 5 minutes. Whatever the waiting time is, performing the flap striae maneuver at the end is recommended. In this maneuver, a dry merocel is used to indent the cornea just outside the flap edge. If the striae generated are seen in the flap too, this is a sign of good adhesion at that site. The maneuver is repeated in all four quadrants.

3. Flap Wrinkles (5,9,20,27,36,37) (Table 2)

They may be due to missed intraoperative wrinkles caused by flap swelling or malpositioning. Although minimally noticeable on the slit lamp exam, these wrinkles may cause postoperative irregular astigmatism and loss of BCVA (Figure 27.8).

These flap wrinkles are not detected until after 24 hours of LASIK and are presumably due to pressure patching, eye rubbing, pressure on the eye while sleeping without a protective shield, or the eyelid pressure partially dislodging the flap.

Table 2   Flap Wrinkling and Traction Folds

Etiology

(1) Poot distention and repositioning of the flap/cap at the end of the operation, (2) partial postoperative displacement of the flap, (3) deep, highly myopic ablation with a relatively reduced optic zone, (4) areas of greater traction (interrupted sutures).

Results

(1) Irritating glare, (2) image distortion, (3) poor quality vision.

Prevention

(1) LASIK with superior hinge, (2) examine the flap carefully at the end of the operation for symmetry and gutter alignment, and refloat immediately if necessary.

Treatment

(1) Spontaneous resolution some weeks after suture removal.

---

4.   Superficial Epithelial Abrasions

These are sometimes noticed on the slit lamp in the immediate postoperative or the next day. These abrasions take the shape of the marking surface of the marker used (Figure 27.3). In the case of an RK marker they appear linear and radial. These abrasions denote corneal epithelial toxicity to the marking dye. These can also result from flap complications or HSV keratitis (Figure 27.7 A and B).

5.   Diffuse Lamellar Keratitis or the Shifting Sands of the Sahara (Table 3)

Diffuse lamellar keratitis (DLK) is a diffuse inflammation in the interface without microbial cause. This sterile inflammation may appear within 24 hours or be delayed a few days

Table 3   Diffuse Lamellar Keratitis

Etiology

(1) Toxic reaction, (2) immunological reaction, (3) idiosyncratic reaction from secretions from Meibomian glands, exotoxins from gram-negative bacteria, staphylococcal blepharitis, material that has accumulated in the cannulas, betadine, ethylene oxide residue, residue from cleaning solutions, gentian violet, residue of Merocel sponges, red blood cells under the flap, debris from the eyelid margin, rust from the microkeratome or blade, oil from the microkeratome gears or oil residue on the blade or from the motor, (4) thermal lesions, (5) toxicity from UV light, (6) interaction between the laser and debris.

Symptoms

(1) Decrease in visual acuity (including hyperopic shift), (2) discomfort, (3) stromal melting with induced hyperopia, (4) alterations in the corneal topography.

Prevention

(1) Careful cleaning of the cannulas and syringes, (2) careful cleaning of the microkeratome and suction ring, (3) maintenance to the microkeratome by the manufacturer every 3 to 4 months, (4) avoid cleaning the instruments with ultrasound, (5) use topical steroid for 4 to 5 days after the LASIK operation, (6) preoperative treatment of blepharitis, (7) protection of the cornea from excess heat and UV damage: use cold BSS to cool the cornea, check the laser's internal optics (UV filter), interrupt the ablation to allow the cornea to cool.

Treatment

(1) Potent, frequent steroid drops, (2) antibiotic prophylaxis, (3) raising and cleaning the flaps for grades 3 and 4 (controversy in timing and steroid drop usage among various surgeons).

---

after surgery. It has a diffuse white granular appearance that may cover the entire interface, with waves of increased density giving an appearance of shifting sand dunes in the Sahara, or it may appear as a focal crescentic or numular opacity near the edge of the flap (38,39). Direct cultures from the interface after lifting the flap show no growth of bacteria or fungi. The course of this disorder can be highly variable, gradually disappearing, persisting, or increasing (see Chapter 34).

DLK typically presents within the first week after LASIK with a foreign body sensation, photophobia, and decreased or cloudy vision (40). The symptoms may be mild or severe. Examination reveals diffuse or multifocal fine granular inflammation that is confined to the interface. The eye is surprisingly white and quiet for the amount of corneal inflammation. Anterior chamber cell and flare are occasionally present.

Careful inspection by day one is crucial in identifying DLK, as the cellular reaction will almost always be present in the first 24 hours. Once identified, a staging of severity and location is made. Several stages have been described:

Stage I: presence of white granular cells in the periphery of the interface, with sparing of the visual axis. This is the most common presentation at day one.

Stage II: diffuse presence of the white granular cells in the interface. Frequently seen on day 2 or 3.

Stage III: central aggregation of the dense white and clumped cells, with relative clearing in the periphery of the interface. Subtle decline in the visual acuity and subjective description of haze are often present.

Stage IV is the rare end result of DLK with stromal melting, permanent scarring, and associated visual morbidity. The aggregation of inflammatory cells and release of collagenases result in fluid collection in the central lamellae, with stromal volume loss.

The cells in DLK should be carefully distinguished from epithelial surface abnormalities, such as punctate epithelial keratitis, epithelial edema, and tear film debris. These cells should also be distinguished from meibomian gland debris in the interface, which has a glistening, oily appearance (see Chapter 34 for more details).

DLK is distinguished from infectious keratitis by the absence of an epithelial defect, and the absence of extension into the posterior stroma or into the flap.

DLK appears to be caused by an inflammation to some unknown antigen. Possible antigens include blood from neovascular vessels, various drops used, microkeratome blade debris or fluids (41), various bacterial toxins from the lids, or sebaceous debris found within the fornices. The inciting cause seems to be multifactorial.

Although more common following primary LASIK, this complication can develop following LASIK retreatments where a new cut was not made, but the original corneal flap has only been lifted (40).

Although typically unilateral, DLK has been described to occur bilaterally. It is the opinion of many surgeons that the incidence is rising and approaching about 0.2%. One study (13) reported an incidence of 3.1% on 679 eyes operated on with H-LASIK.

When the surgeon is in doubt between DLK and bacterial keratitis, a culture taken from the interface after lifting the flap is highly recommended. Scrapings of the interface material have demonstrated neutrophils, but no bacteria.

6. Infectious Keratitis (Tables 4 and 5)

Bacterial infection under a LASIK flap is rarely reported but remains one of the most vision threatening complications. LASIK carries a significant risk of infection because the

Table 4 Infectious Keratitis

Etiology
(1) Bacterial, (2) viral.
Symptoms
(1) Pain, (2) photophobia, (3) blurring of vision.
Prevention
(1) Cleaning, adequate sterilization of the instruments: cannulas, syringes, microkeratome, (2) preoperative treatment of blepharitis, (3) use a sterile surgical technique, (4) avoid excessive intraoperative irrigation, (5) postoperative antibiotic prophyaxis, (6) avoid swimming and eye makeup for 2 weeks postoperatively, (7) avoid complications that will encourage infection: dislocated flap, lost flap, preforated flap, epithelial ingrowth, melting, debris in the interface.
Treatment
(1) Diligent follow-up, (2) antibiotic treatment, (3) treatment with NSAIDs.

corneal stroma can be exposed to infective agents during lamellar surgery. Eyelashes, conjunctiva, drapes, the speculum, the microkeratome, and the surrounding atmosphere are all sources of infection (see Chapter 34).

There are several reports in the literature detailing culture positive infective keratitis associated with LASIK (42–48). The symptoms include lid swelling, eye discharge, pain, photophobia, and blurred vision. On slit lamp exam there is a ciliary injection, stromal infiltrates or abscess in a single or multiple pattern, anterior chamber reaction, flap swelling with overlying epithelial defect, and probable flap necrosis.

Although complications such as epithelial ingrowth and interface inflammation can cause similar symptoms, we believe that a high index of suspicion should be maintained for infections, and that the patient should be treated accordingly.

The risk factors include epithelial defects, exogenous and endogenous sources of infection, dry eyes, and prolonged use of corticosteroids postoperatively (Figure 27.7A, B).

The bacteria isolated in the cases reported were *Staphylococcus aureus* (42,43,45), *Streptococcus viridans* (44), *Mycobacterium chelonae* (46), *Nocardia asteroides* (47), *Streptococcus pneumoniae,* (48) and culture negative interface abscess (49).

When faced with this problem, the most important considerations are the need for early diagnosis, adequate microbiologic sampling, and appropriate treatment. Lifting the

Table 5 Differential Diagnosis

Infectious keratitis	Sands of the Sahara syndrome
Appears after 24 or 48 hours	Appears after 12 or 24 hours
Pain	Absence of or minimal pain
Globe is soft to touch	Globe has normal consistency
Marked decrease in vision	Slight decrease in vision
Objective findings related to	Objective findings not related
Symptoms and appearance	to symptoms, even at stage 4
Treatment response to antibiotics	Treatment response to steroids

flap for a culture scrape and debulking and cleaning of the interface and irrigation with antibiotics has a diagnostic and therapeutic effect. Corneal scraping through the flap may result in loss of the flap.

Most of the reported cases had a final BCVA of 20/40 or better. It is reassuring to note that it is possible for these patients to attain an unaided acuity and final refraction compatible with an uncomplicated LASIK procedure. However, other patients have not fared well, with two having lost the flap (45,48) and another requiring a penetrating keratoplasty (46). Only one case (45) did have a bilateral corneal infection, yet other reported cases were done simultaneously (42,43,46).

Bacterial keratitis is one of the major concerns that the surgeon should consider and inform the patient about when deciding on simultaneous or sequential surgery. The augmented risk of bilateral simultaneous LASIK compared with sequential LASIK appears to be low (50). It would appear that there is as yet insufficient evidence to compel surgeons to perform sequential rather than simultaneous surgery. But on the other hand, LASIK should be performed under sterile operative conditions, as one would expect for intraocular surgery. A number of very prominent surgeons do not use gloves during LASIK and do not report infection as a complication. Despite this the standard should be to wear powder-free surgical gloves. Typically fluoroquinolone antibiotic is applied QID per day for 5 to 7 days after surgery.

7. Corneal Haze (Table 6)

Haze after LASIK is minimal or absent (15,22,23,25,27,51).

The most probable causes are the absence of interaction between the epithelium and the stroma in LASIK and the minimal collagen production during wound healing (52–54). In one study (6), all treated eyes had a minimal degree of haze after LASIK. Haze was less than that reported after PRK and rapidly regressed between the first and third months after the operation (6,23). Six to 24 months postoperatively, there was no haze (6).

8. Anterior Chamber Reaction

The blood–aqueous barrier seems to be altered in LASIK, most probably owing to the flap manipulation and photoablation. The anterior chamber reaction is minimal and in correlation with the depth of the stromal photoablation (55,56).

Table 6 Stromal Clouding and Haze in the Interface

Etiology
(1) Correction of high refractive errors, (2) intrastromal edema from direct photoablation, (3) intrastromal edema as a toxic reaction to substances used during the operation, (4) intrastromal edema as a toxic reaction to debris in the interface.
Results
(1) Reduced visual acuity, (2) visual disturbances.
Prevention
(1) Thoroughly clean instruments to remove any chemical residues.
Treatment
(1) Transitory phenomenon, (2) topical steroid treatment for 2 to 3 weeks.

Table 7 Epithelial Ingrowth

Etiology

(1) Poor adhesion of the flap edges, (2) epithelial abrasions at the flap margins, (3) poor flap alignment, (4) perforated buttonholed flap, (5) free cap, (6) ablation at the edges of the stromal bed or beyond (especially hyperopic ablation), (7) epithelial irregularities at the edge of the flap (particularly with enhancement), (8) accidental introduction of epithelial cells during the cut with the microkeratome, (9) manipulation of the intrastromal surfaces, (10) introduction of cells following insertion of instruments in the interface (e.g., cannulas, spatulas), (11) the cap folds over on itself during the operation, (12) inadequate irrigation and cleaning of the surfaces involved, (13) previous radial keratotomy, especially with epithelial plugs and incisions.

Results

(1) Reduced visual acuity, (2) irregular astigmatism, (3) discomfort (irregularity of the surface), (4) risk of stromal melting.

Prevention

(1) Be gentle to the epithelium, (2) replace all torn epithelium to the edges of the flap, (3) remove epithelial cells and debris from the stromal bed prior to repositioning the flap, (4) avoid wide ablation zones on small beds and protect the area around the hinge if necessary.

Treatment

(1) Nonprogressive epithelial nests that do not affect vision, observe, (2) if progression, lift flap and scrape.

---

9. Epithelial Ingrowth (Table 7)

The prevalence after LASIK varies from 0 to 20% (6–9,11,20,25,27,51). Most surgeons agree that it is increasing in prevalence, especially in reoperation cases.

Two types of epithelial ingrowth are identified. The epithelium may be introduced into the interface at the time the lamellar cut is performed and may not always grow in from the peripheral surface epithelium. If the epithelial tissue contains viable cells, then these cells may proliferate and produce a nest of tissue within the interface (Figure 27.6). These cells usually have limited proliferative potential, and if so, a nest of cells may appear, stop expanding, and remain stable within the interface for years. Occasionally, the nest of cells will continue to expand and may produce more significant complications. In other cases, it is clear from a visible track of cells that epithelium grew into the interface from the periphery (Figure 27.5). In such cases the following principles are identified (58): (1) The ingrowth is not caused by epithelial cell implantation during surgery but by epithelial growth under the edge of a poorly adherent flap. (2) It is more likely to occur if an epithelial defect was created during the procedure. (3) Fluorescein pooling on the edge of the flap or fluorescein tracking under the flap on the first postoperative day predicts epithelial ingrowth later. Finally, the epithelium may grow from a central defect in the flap or cap.

The clinical signs are epithelial pearls or a sharply demarcated area of interface lucency. Epithelial ingrowth can cause irregular astigmatism, loss of BCVA, and corneal flap melt (59).

The theoretical mechanisms (59) for epithelial ingrowth are dragging of the cells by the microkeratome blade, fluid backflow during stromal bed irrigation, outgrowth from epithelial plugs in eyes that had previous RK, and growth into the lamellar interface at the junction of the flap.

The main risk factor for epithelial ingrowth is a deficient technique that results in a peripheral epithelial defect, poor flap adhesion, or a perforated corneal flap.

The frequency of this complication appears to be highly variable. It was 0.5% in one report (60). LASIK retreatments (61) may be associated with a higher risk of interface epithelial growth, especially if a spatula is inserted through the epithelium and used to break open the interface by sweeping. The epithelial tissue may adhere to the spatula and be transferred into the interface using this approach. It may be preferable to break open the interface temporally or inferiorly with a probe, grasp the temporal or inferior edge of the flap with a 0.12 forceps, and gently peel the flap back.

The treatment is dependent on the extent and location of the ectopic epithelial tissue. A small nest of epithelium that is present in the periphery can be left alone if it does not progress or affect visual acuity.

10. Flap Melt (Table 8)

In all reported cases, flap melting always developed over an area of epithelial ingrowth (9,62). When epithelial ingrowth is progressive it is more likely to develop a stromal melt at the edge of the flap. The edges become blunt and eroded. The eye becomes photophobic, injected with foreign body sensation. The vision becomes blurred.

The pathogenesis of this complication is not clearly understood. One theory is that stromal necrosis can occur when sandwiched between epithelium within the interface and on the surface, causing a nutritional deficit of glucose, which is mandatory to the keratocytes and which is supplied by facilitated diffusion from the aqueous humor. Another theory is that after a complicated LASIK procedure, cytokines released by the epithelial cells could activate more epithelial cells and corneal fibroblasts to produce plasminogen, collagenases, or other proteases in a significant amount to cause lysis of the flap. A combined nutritional and inflammatory mechanism is the most probable (62).

Flap thickness was not found to correlate with flap melt (9).

The incidence can be decreased by careful keratectomy with no epithelial damage, good irrigation of the stromal bed, ensuring strong adhesion with minimal gap between flap edge and stromal bed, and early epithelial cell debridement, when significant areas of ingrowth are present or progression or melt are observed. If a spontaneous epithelial defect occurs on the surface above a nest of epithelium, the ectopic epithelium should be removed.

Table 8 Flap Melting

Etiology
(1) Poor hydration by the lacrimal film with a consequent reduction in oxygen supply, (2) epithelial ingrowth, (3) reduced blinking, (4) lacrimal film pathologies, (5) thin flap.
Results
(1) Patient discomfort, (2) reduced visual acuity, (3) loss of the flap.
Prevention
(1) Copious lubrication, (2) aggressive treatment of epithelial ingrowth.
Treatment
(1) Lift the flap, (2) clean the interface, (3) use a bandage contact lens, (4) use topical antibiotic and lubricant treatment, (5) carefully monitor, (6) perform a homoplastic lamellar transplant as a last resort.

B. LATE POSTOPERATIVE COMPLICATIONS

1. Regression

Regression is a documented return in the direction of the original refractive error, recorded over several visits, 3 to 6 months after LASIK. Regression appears to be minimal after LASIK, but long-term studies should be done. Regression after LASIK is related to the amount of correction attempted (11,63).

Some studies (23,25) mention that the spherical equivalent seems to stabilize from very early postoperative, with minor changes between 3 and 6 months.

In one study (9), there was a significant regression of effect (0.53 D) between 1 and 3 months, but no significant regression between 3 and 6 months. Another study (11) showed that changes between ±0.5 D occurred in 90.38% of moderate myopes (7–12 D) and 80.9% of high myopes (12–18.5 D) between 1 and 6 months postoperatively. Pallikaris and Siganos (6) found that the refraction stabilized soon after surgery (at 1 month). The mean regression between 1 and 12 months was less than 1.5 D in most of the cases (6). In Knorz et al.'s series (7), the mean regression of myopia was 0.2 D between the 4 to 8 week period and the 4 to 6 month period. Salah et al. (12) found a myopic change of −0.61 D in the manifest spherical equivalent (MSE) refraction between 3 weeks and 5 months after LASIK for the correction of a preoperative MSE of −8.24 D. Chayet et al. (63) observed an early postoperative regression of effect that stabilized between 3 and 6 months after treatment. At 3 months, the mean refractive regression was −1.07 D (63).

Regression is reported to be more pronounced after hyperopic than in myopic LASIK (64). The profile and size of the ablation and transition zone are incriminated. As the epithelium grows from the periphery, it encounters the sudden depression and will try to fill this depression via a hyperplastic response. This process reduces the power of the positive lens shape created by ablation and leads to regression and loss of effect.

Regression after LASIK was associated with increased corneal thickness and increased corneal steepening (63). Potential mechanisms for regression of the refractive effect include nuclear sclerosis, stromal synthesis (wound healing) (65), compensatory epithelial hyperplasia (CEH), and iatrogenic keratectasia.

Some investigators argue that owing to the absence of haze and the minimal formation of collagen after LASIK (52), CEH appears to be the key mechanism in refractive regression (63). This concept is endorsed by postoperative ultrasound corneal epithelial thickness measurements, which were found to be increased, and which correlated highly with the postoperative regression (66).

2. Induced Regular and Irregular Astigmatism

Irregular astigmatism may be induced by minimal laser beam decentration, central islands, variations in flap wound healing, epithelial ingrowth, flap irregularities (irregular cut, thin, wrinkled, misaligned, sutured), interface debris, and surface irregularities caused by the microkeratome cut or by the laser ablation (beam heterogeneity) (20,67,68).

Regular astigmatism may be induced when the laser treatment deviates from the corneal astigmatic axis to be treated. Such cases occur when there is a discrepancy between the topographic and the refractive axes of the astigmatism, when the posterior curvature of the cornea does not follow the anterior curvature, and in cases of uncompensated positional eye cyclotorsion under the laser.

In some studies, induced astigmatism was a rare complication of LASIK using a sutureless technique, with occurrences as low as 1.1% (4,6,25,69). Other studies (8,10,15,20,22,27) report higher rates.

Pallikaris and Siganos (23) found that postoperative astigmatism was minimally influenced by the surgical creation of a corneal flap. Topographic data in another study (9) showed no difference between pre- and postoperative corneal astigmatism, proving that creating the corneal flap does not affect corneal astigmatism.

Some studies (4,15) reported irregular astigmatism 3 to 6 months after LASIK, while others (11,70) found none. Pallikaris and Siganos (6) followed astigmatic changes after LASIK to study the effect of ablation center deviation and the corneal flap healing. The authors (6) found that the mean preoperative and postoperative astigmatism were the same, but the cylinder axis changed with time, denoting continuing cornea healing even during the last follow-up visit at 24 months. Hersh et al. (71) did not find a statistical difference between the LASIK and PRK groups studied regarding axis or magnitude of induced astigmatism. Yet the mean induced astigmatism in the LASIK group was lower than in the PRK group, and the axis of the induced astigmatism in the LASIK group was random, suggesting that the lamellar corneal flap may mask induced stromal changes (71).

3. Endothelial Cell Loss

One safety concern about LASIK is its effect on the corneal endothelium. This issue is raised because of the relative proximity of the treatment area to the endothelium, unlike with PRK. Kent et al. (72) examined short- to intermediate-term in vitro endothelial cell toxicity after -10.0 D PRK and -10.0, -15.0, -20.0, and -25.0 D LASIK treatments in fresh human autopsy eyes. The authors (72) used fluorescent vital dyes, which allowed them to count the cells and assess their viability. No significant difference between treated and control corneas was noticed after 7 days in corneal organ culture.

Pérez-Santonja and coauthors (73,74) performed preoperative and postoperative central endothelial specular microscopy, assessing cell density, coefficient of variation in cell size, and hexagonality. After LASIK, the number of cells per square millimeter increased, the difference among cell sizes was smaller, and the cells tended to become more hexagonal. The authors believed this was the result of contact lens discontinuation after the procedure, leading to a rearrangement of the endothelial pattern (73,74). They suggested that LASIK does not cause significant observable damage to the central corneal endothelium up to 1 year after surgery.

Pallikaris and Siganos (23) described an 8.67% reduction in the endothelial cell count 1 year after LASIK, and they recommend that this should be considered cautiously as an "acceptable range." Guell and Muller (11) described a reduction in endothelial cells similar to a physiological change 6 months after surgery. In their second study, Pallikaris and Siganos (6) indicated that the higher the attempted correction, the greater the endothelial cell loss, as seen by the higher cell loss in one group (correction of -15.0 to -25.0 D). The 12 month postoperative loss was 3.79% and 4.11% in the two other groups. The authors believe that some endothelial cell loss is unavoidable because of the shock waves of the excimer ablation and the corneal manipulation during keratomileusis. The loss seemed to stabilize at 12 months and even to regress somewhat thereafter (6). In other studies (24,75), the correction of up to 29 diopters of myopia did not cause any clinically significant effect on the corneal endothelial cell density or morphology after LASIK. However, long-term follow-up studies are needed to confirm endothelial safety at 5 and 10 years.

Table 9 Corneal Ectasia and Iatrogenic Keratoconus

Etiology
(1) Excessively deep central ablation, (2) thickness of residual stroma less than 250 microns, (3) thickness of residual stromal less than 30% of the initial corneal thickness.
Results
(1) Significant and progressive reduction of vision.
Prevention
(1) Avoid ablations that are excessively deep, (2) leave at least 250 microns of residual stroma under the flap, (3) total thickness of residual stroma must be at least 30% of the initial corneal thickness.
Treatment
(1) Contact lens, (2) lamellar keratoplasty, (3) penetrating keratoplasty.

---

4. Induced or Iatrogenic Keratectasia (76,77) (Table 9)

Iatrogenic keratectasia is a vision threatening complication after LASIK. It is related to the weakening of the cornea's mechanical strength (see Chapter 10).

The corneal flap does not contribute to the biomechanics of the cornea. Most of the corneal stress is withstood by the residual thickness of the stromal bed only. Therefore the question of a minimal thickness of the residual stroma arises. It is related to the upper limits of myopia correction by means of LASIK. The minimal thickness of residual stroma to withstand progressive ectasia has been derived from biomechanical measurements to be 250 μ or 30% of the original thickness.

Clinically there is a progressive deterioration in UCVA with a regression of the refractive effect (progressive myopic shift) and possible identification of the keratectasia on slit lamp biomicroscopy.

Serial corneal topographies show progressive steepening of the central cornea.

Most reported cases (76–79) had thin corneas on preoperative pachymetry, high myopia (>10 D), and a residual postoperative stromal thickness of less than 250 μ. Preoperative corneal pachymetry is mandatory on each case, in order to make individual decisions about the ablation depth and subsequently the amount of myopia that could be corrected (80). Even with adequate corneal thickness, this complication still may arise, because of the inconsistencies in flap thickness with the current microkeratomes, leading to deeper ablations than anticipated (Figure 27.2A, B).

During the early postoperative period, it is not easy to differentiate topographically between a conventional central island that resulted from the ablation and a central keratectasia. The temporal evolution, however, will determine the nature of the central steep zone. The conventional central steep island tends to disappear within several months after surgery, whereas the central keratectasia shows progression on topography.

5. Night Vision Problems and Glare (Table 10)

Distortion of vision in the form of glare and halos is one of the major concerns after LASIK. Glare and halo symptoms typically become worse at night when the pupil dilates and more peripheral light rays enter the eye from the untreated zone. The major contributor to glare and halo symptoms is the effective spherical aberration of the centrally flattened cornea (81).

Decentered ablations, small treatment zones, newly formed cataracts, and induced astigmatism are other important causes of night glare after LASIK.

Guell and Muller (11) reported that night vision was slightly impaired in 23.0% of cases 6 months after LASIK. Pérez-Santonja et al. (9) reported that night halos and starbursts occurred in 29.0% and 31.5% of eyes, respectively, at 6 months. The night halos were related to small ablation diameters and improved with time. Two percent of patients had night vision problems in a series of Buratto and coauthors (22). Sixteen percent of Kremer and Dufek's (25) patients had transient halos around lights at night. In Kim and Jung's series (69), 55.6% of eyes had night halos 6 months postoperatively. El Danasoury et al. (82) reported a low incidence of permanent night glare in 7% of their series. They attributed this to the relatively large transition zone that they used.

With current LASIK techniques, patients with pupillary diameters larger than 6 mm in scotopic conditions and those with high myopia will be the most affected. These patients should be warned of this potential complication. In the early postoperative period, when in doubt about the cause of glare in the presence of wound healing and flap complications, the decrease or disappearance of glare in the affected eye while shining the pen light in the contralateral eye is a pathognomonic sign. Luckily, the majority of patients improve with time. With bilateral treatment, the patient usually learns to ignore optical aberrations as a result of cortical integration (83).

6. Contrast Sensitivity

Functional vision changes do occur following LASIK. They are due to changes in the optical quality of the cornea. Optical quality changes can be due to surface microirregularities or to shape changes in the cornea (84).

Snellen visual acuity measurements are of limited value and do not describe visual performance for a variety of spacial frequencies and contrasts (85).

Contrast sensitivity testing expands on the information gained from Snellen acuity testing by determining the resolving power of the eye over a spectrum of target sizes. Contrast sensitivity testing maps the resolving sensitivity of the eye over a much broader area than Snellen acuity testing, which represents only the high-contrast end of the contrast curve (86).

Visual performance after LASIK is commonly evaluated by UCVA, BCVA, and number of Snellen lines gained or lost (87).

Light scatter from the interface or from the flap edge in LASIK may degrade visual acuity, increase glare, reduce vision at night, or decrease object contrast. Contrast sensitiv-

Table 10 Night Glare and Halos

Etiology
(1) Optic zones that are smaller than the scotopic pupil diameter (spherical aberration), (2) subjects with unusually large scotopic pupil size, (3) severe myopia, (4) symptoms are aggravated by residual refractive errors.
Results
(1) Disturbances of visual function, (2) night myopia.
Prevention
(1) New ablation algorithms with large transition zones, (2) multizone technique or aspheric profile, (3) central pretreatment.
Treatment
(1) Symptomatic improvement with time and bilateral treatment (cortex integration), (2) the patient learns to disregard the problem.

ity, a more sensitive measure of visual function than Snellen acuity, is important to evaluate because LASIK can produce subtle changes in the optical media that theoretically may affect visual function only under conditions of reduced contrast, glare, or both. Holladay et al. (84) noticed that none of the visual function parameters measured in darkness returned to normal 6 months after surgery. The lower the contrast of the object and the larger the pupil, the more significant was the reduction in visual performance (84). The aspheric change in the cornea was suggested to be the predominant factor in limiting the visual performance and not the surface microirregularities (84). On the other hand, another report (88) studying the contrast sensitivity after LASIK found that it decreased 1 month after surgery and returned to preoperative levels at 3 months. Higher values at 6 months than preoperatively were noticed although they are not significantly different (but they suggest that LASIK can improve the quality of vision in moderate and high myopia).

7. Retinal Detachment

Retinal detachments after LASIK were often thought to be caused by missed peripheral holes outside or within areas of lattice degeneration in the extreme retinal periphery. Such peripheral changes are known to be commonly associated with high myopia. A good fundus exam with peripheral retinal indentation is a must in LASIK patients, especially the high myopes.

Recently, mechanical stretch on the vitreous base was incriminated in the pathogenesis of peripheral retinal tears during the sudden change in IOP while activating or releasing the suction ring (89). The excimer laser induced shock wave also has been incriminated in the occurrence of the peripheral retinal breaks.

C. INTRAOCULAR PRESSURE MONITORING AFTER LASIK

The results of Goldmann tonometry are influenced by corneal thickness (90,91) and to a lesser extent by corneal curvature (92) and corneal astigmatism (93).

Central corneal thickness is the major factor in the decreased intraocular pressure after photorefractive ablative procedure.

Intraocular pressure decrease after LASIK was found to correlate significantly with central corneal thickness decrease (94). The difference between the mean pre- and post-LASIK measurements of applanation intraocular pressure was significant (94,95). The decrease in intraocular pressure was in the range of 1 mmHg per 37.8 μ reduction in central corneal thickness (94). In other terms, each diopter of refractive correction is expected to decrease the intraocular pressure by 0.3 to 0.4 mmHg.

In another study (96), mean drop in IOP at 1 month after LASIK was 1.9 ± 2.9 mmHg (range -9.0 to $+6.0$ mmHg). No significant correlations were found between the change in IOP and the change in spherical equivalent, preoperative spherical equivalent, age, change in keratometric astigmatism number of laser pulses, duration of ablation, ablation depth, or suction time during the lamellar cut (96). A change in the aqueous dynamics was thought to be responsible together with the corneal changes for the decline in IOP after LASIK. The drop in pressure after LASIK remained constant during the 6 months follow-up (96).

Central corneal thickness is an important variable in the evaluation of applanation intraocular pressure and should be included in the assessment of any case of potential glaucoma or ocular hypertension, particularly in eyes with previous photoablative refractive surgery and in LASIK patients treated with steroids for DLK who may have increased IOP masquarading as DLK (97).

REFERENCES

1. V Filatov, JS Vidaurri-Leal, JH Talamo. Selected complications of radial keratotomy, photorefractive keratectomy, and laser in situ keratomileusis. Int Ophthalmol Clin 1997;37(1): 123–148.
2. RD Stulting, JD Carr, KP Thompson, GO Waring III, WM Wiley, JG Walker. Complications of Laser in situ keratomileusis for the correction of myopia. Ophthalmology 1999;106:13–20.
3. L Buratto, M Ferrari. Indications, techniques, results, limits and complications of laser in situ keratomileusis. Curr Opin Ophthalmol 1997;8(4):59–66.
4. AM Bas, R Onnis. Excimer laser in situ keratomileusis for myopia. J Refract Surg 1995;11 (suppl):S229–S233.
5. HV Gimbel, S Basti, GB Kaye, M Ferensowicz. Experience during the learning curve of laser in situ keratomileusis. J Cataract Refract Surg 1996;22:542–550.
6. IG Pallikaris, DS Siganos. Laser in situ keratomileusis to treat myopia: early experience. J Cataract Refract Surg 1997;23:39–49.
7. MC Knorz, A Liermann, V Seiberth, H Steiner, B Wiesinger. Laser in situ keratomileusis to correct myopia of −6.00 to −29.00 diopters. J Refract Surg 1996;12:575–584.
8. A Marinho, MC Pinto, R Pinto, F Vaz, MC Neves. LASIK For high myopia: one year experience. Ophthalmic Surg Lasers 1996;27(suppl):S517–S520.
9. JJ Pérez-Santonja, J Bellot, P Claramonte, MM Ismail, JL Alio. Laser in situ keratomileusis to correct high myopia. J Cataract Refract Surg 1997;23:372–385.
10. DC Fiander, F Tayfour. Excimer laser in situ keratomileusis in 124 myopic eyes. J Refract Surg 1995;11(suppl):S234–S238.
11. JL Guell, A Muller. Laser in situ keratomileusis (LASIK) for myopia from −7 to −18 diopters. J Refract Surg 1996;12:222–228.
12. T Salah, GO Waring III, A El-Maghraby, K Moadel, SB Grimm. Excimer laser in situ keratomileusis under a corneal flap for myopia of 2 to 20 diopters. Am J Ophthalmol 1996;121: 143–155.
13. CJ Argento, MJ Cosentino. Laser in situ keratomileusis for hyperopia. J Cataract Refract Surg 1998;24:1050–1058.
14. YH Kim, JS Choi, HJ Chun, CK Joo. Effect of resection velocity and suction ring on corneal flap formation in laser in situ keratomileusis. J Cataract Refract Surg 1999;25(11): 1448–1455.
15. SF Brint, DM Ostrick, C Fisher, SG Slade, RK Maloney, R Epstein, RD Stulting, KP Thompson. Six-months results of the Multicenter Phase I Study of excimer laser myopic keratomileusis. J Cataract Refract Surg 1994;20:610–615.
16. M Gomes. Laser in situ keratomileusis for myopia using manual dissection. J Refract Surg 1995;11(suppl):S239–S243.
17. R Zaldivar, JM Davidorf, S Oscherow. Laser in situ keratomileusis for myopia from −5.5 to −11.5 diopters with astigmatism. J Refract Surg 1998;14:19–25.
18. J Davidorf, R Zaldivar, S Oscherow. Results and complications of laser in situ keratomileusis by experienced surgeons. J Refract Surg 1998;14:114–122.
19. AS Forseto, CM Francesconi, RAM Nose, W Nose. Laser in situ keratomileusis to correct refractive errors after keratoplasty. J Cataract Refract Surg 1999;25:479–485.
20. PI Condon, M Mulhern, T Fulcher, A Foley-Nolan, M O'Keeffe. Laser intrastromal keratomileusis for high myopia and myopic astigmatism. Br J Ophthalmol 1997;81:199–206.
21. MG Mulhern, A Foley-Nolan, M O'Keefe, PI Condon. Topographical analysis of ablation centration after excimer laser photorefractive keratectomy and laser in situ keratomileusis for high myopia. J Cataract Refract Surg 1997;23:488–494.
22. L Buratto, M Ferrari, C Genisi. Keratomileusis for myopia with the excimer laser (Buratto technique): short term results. Refract Corneal Surg 1993;9(suppl):S130–S133.
23. IG Pallikaris, DS Siganos. Excimer laser in situ keratomileusis and photorefractive keratectomy for correction of high myopia. J Refract Corneal Surg 1994;10:498–510.

24. MC Knorz, B Wiesinger, A Lierman, V Seiberth, H Liesenhoff. Laser in situ keratomileusis for moderate and high myopia and myopic astigmatism. Ophthalmology 1998;105:932–940.

25. FB Kremer, M Dufek. Excimer laser in situ keratomileusis. J Refract Surg 1995; 11(suppl): S244–S247.

26. YS Rabinowitz, K Rasheed. Fluorescein test for the detection of striae in the corneal flap after laser in situ keratomileusis. Am J Ophthalmol 1999;127(6):717–718.

27. I Kremer, M Blumenthal. Myopic keratomileusis in situ combined with VISX 20/20 photorefractive keratectomy. J Cataract Refract Surg 1995;21:508–511.

28. LW Hirst, KW Vandeleur. Laser in situ keratomileusis interface deposits. J Refract Surg 1998;14:653–654.

29. HM Stein. Powder-free gloves for ophthalmic surgery. J Cataract Refract Surg 1997;23: 714–717.

30. M Paciuc, G Mendieta, R Naranjo. Oculocardiac reflex during laser in situ keratomileusis. J Cataract Refract Surg 1998;24:1317–1319.

31. M Paciuc, G Mendieta, R Naranjo, E Angel, E Reyes. Oculocardiac reflex in sedated patients having laser in situ keratomileusis. J Cataract Refract Surg 1999;25(10):1341–1343.

32. A Ozdamar, B Sener, C Aras, R Aktunc. Laser in situ keratomileusis after photorefractive keratectomy for myopic regression. J Cataract Refract Surg 1998;24:1208–1211.

33. D Huang, RD Stulting, JD Carr, KP Thompson, GO Waring III. Multiple regression and vector analyses of laser in situ keratomileusis for myopia and astigmatism. J Refract Surg 1999;15(5): 538–549.

34. K Ditzen, A Handzel, S Pieger. Laser in situ keratomileusis nomogram development. J Refract Surg 1999;15(2 suppl):S197–S201.

35. D Zadok, G Maskaleris, V Garcia, S Shah, M Montes, A Chayet. Outcomes of retreatment after laser in situ keratomileusis. Ophthalmology 1999;106(12):2391–2394.

36. DS Lam, AT Leung, JT Wu, AC Cheng, DS Fan, SK Rao, JH Talamo, C Barraquer. Management of severe flap wrinkling or dislodgment after laser in situ keratomileusis. J Cataract Refract Surg 1999;25(11):1441–1447.

37. L Buratto, M Ferrari, C Genisi. Myopic keratomileusis with the excimer laser: one year follow up. Refract Corneal Surg 1993;9:12–19.

38. WW Haw, EE Manche. Sterile peripheral keratitis following laser in situ keratomileusis. J Refract Surg 1999;15:61–63.

39. GE Fraenkel, PR Cohen, GL Sutton, MA Lawless, CM Rogers. Central focal interface opacity after laser in situ keratomleusis. J Refract Surg 1998;14:571–575.

40. RJ Smith, RK Maloney. Diffuse lamellar keratitis. A new syndrome in lamellar refractive surgery. Ophthalmology 1998;105(9):1721–1726.

41. SC Kaufman, DY Maitchouk, AGY Chiou, RW Beuerman. Interface inflammation after laser in situ keratomileusis. Sands of the Sahara syndrome. J Cataract Refract Surg 1998;24: 1589–1593.

42. SK Webber, MA Lawless, GL Sutton, CM Rogers. Staphylococcal infection under a LASIK flap. Cornea 1999;18:361–365.

43. M Al-Reefy. Bacterial keratitis following laser in situ keratomileusis for hyperopia. J Refract Surg 1999;15:S216–S217.

44. H-M Kim, J-S Song, H-S Han, H-R Jung. Streptococcal keratitis after myopic laser in situ keratomileusis. Korean J Ophthalmol 1998;12:108–111.

45. H Watanabe, S Sato, M Maeda, Y Inoue, Y Shimomura, Y Tano. Bilateral corneal infection as a complication of laser in situ keratomileusis. Arch Ophthalmol 1997;115:1593–1594.

46. V Reviglio, ML Rodriguez, GS Picotti, M Paradello, JD Luna, CP Juàrez. Mycobacterium chelonae keratitis following laser in situ keratomileusis. J Refract Surg 1998;14:357–360.

47. JJ Pérez-Santonja, HF Sakla, JL Abad, A Zorraquino, J Esteban, JL Alió. Nocardial keratitis after laser in situ keratomileusis. J Refract Surg 1997;13:314–317.

48. MG Mulhern, PI Condon, M O'Keefe. Endophthalmitis after astigmatic myopic laser in situ keratomileusis. J Cataract Refract Surg 1997;23:948–950.

49. C Aras, A Ozdamar, H Bahçecioglu, B Sener. Corneal interface abscess after excimer laser in situ keratomileusis. J Refract Surg 1998;14:156–157.

50. GO Waring III, JD Carr, RD Stulting, KP Thompson, W Wiley. Prospective randomized comparison of simultaneous and sequential bilateral laser in situ keratomileusis for the correction of myopia. Ophthalmology 1999;106(4):732–738.

51. SA Helmy, A Salah, T Badawy, AN Sidky. Photorefractive keratectomy and laser in situ keratomileusis for myopia between 6.00 and 10.00 diopters. J Refract Surg 1996;12:417–421.

52. CK Park, JH Kim. Comparison of wound healing after photorefractive keratectomy and laser in situ keratomileusis. J Cataract Refract Surg 1999;25:842–850.

53. M Amm, W Wetzel, M Winter, D Uthoff, GI Dunker. Histopathological comparison of photorefractive keratectomy and laser in situ keratomileusis in rabbits. J Refract Surg 1996; 12:758–766.

54. SW Chang, A Benson, DT Azar. Corneal light scattering with stromal reformation after laser in situ keratomileusis and photorefractive keratectomy. J Cataract Refract Surg 1998;24(8): 1064–1069.

55. PJ Pisella, C Albou-Ganem, JL Bourges, C Debbasch, S Limon. Evaluation of anterior chamber inflammation after corneal refractive surgery. Cornea 1999;18:302–305.

56. R Vita, M Campos, R Belfort Jr, ER Paiva. Alterations in blood–aqueous barrier after corneal refractive surgery. Cornea 1998;17:158–162.

57. K Ditzen, H Huscka, S Pieger. Laser in situ keratomileusis for hyperopia. J Cataract Refract Surg 1998;24:42–47.

58. RK Maloney. Epithelial ingrowth after lamellar refractive surgery (abstract). Opthalmic Surg lasers 1996;7(suppl):S535.

59. MC Helena, D Meisler, SE Wilson. Epithelial growth within the lamellar interface after laser in situ keratomileusis (LASIK). Cornea 1997;16:300–305.

60. SE Wilson. LASIK: management of common complication. Cornea 1998;17:459–467.

61. JJ Perez-Santonja, MJ Ayala, HF Sakla, JM Ruiz-Moreno, JL Alio. Retreatment after laser in situ keratomileusis. Ophthalmology 1999;106(1):21–28.

62. A Castillio, D Diaz-Valle, AR Gutierrez, N Toledano, F Romero. Peripheral melt of flap after laser in situ keratomileusis. J Refract Surg 1998;14:61–63.

63. AS Chayet, KK Assil, M Montes, M Espinosa-Lagana, A Castellanos, G Tsioulias. Regression and its mechanisms after laser in situ keratomileusis in moderate and high myopia. Ophthalmology 1998;105:1194–1199.

64. O Ibrahim. Laser in situ keratomileusis for hyperopia and hyperopic astigmatism. J Refract Surg 1998;14:S179–S182.

65. MC Helena, F Baerveldt, W-J Kim, SE Wilson. Keratocyte apoptosis after corneal surgery. Invest Ophthalmol Vis Sci 1998;39:276–283.

66. CP Lohmann, JL Guell. Regression after LASIK for the treatment of myopia: the role of the corneal epithelium. Semin Ophthalmol 1998;13:79–82.

67. P Vinciguerra, M Azzolini, P Airaghi, P Radice, V De Molfetta. Effect of decreasing surface and interface irregularities after photorefractive keratectomy and laser in situ keratomileusis on optical and functional outcomes. J Refract Surg 1998;14:S199–S203.

68. P Vinciguerra, M Azzolini, P Radice, M Sborgia, V De Molfetta. A method for examining surface and interface irregularities after photorefractive keratectomy and laser in situ keratomileusis: predictor of optical and functional outcomes. J Refract Surg 1998;14:S204–S206.

69. H-M Kim, HR Jung. Laser assisted in situ keratomileusis for high myopia. Ophthalmic Surg Lasers 1996;27(suppl):S508–S511.

70. L Ruiz, SG Slade, SA Updegraff. Excimer myopic kreratomileusis: Bogota experience. In: JJ Salz, ed. Corneal Laser Surgery. St Louis, MO: Mosby, 1995, pp 195.

71. PS Hersh, R Abbassi, Summit PRK-LASIK Study Group. Surgically induced astigmatism after photorefractive keratectomy and laser in situ keratomileusis. J Cataract Refract Surg 1999;25:389–398.

72. DG Kent, KD Solomon, Q Peng, SB Whiteside, SJ Brown, DJ Apple. Effect of surface photorefractive keratectomy and laser in situ keratomileusis on the corneal endothelium. J Cataract Refract Surg 1997;23:386–397.

73. JJ Pérez-Santonja, HF Sakla, F Gobbi, JL Alio. Corneal endothelial changes after laser in situ keratomileusis. J Cataract Refract Surg 1997;23:177–183.

74. JJ Pérez-Santonja, HF Sakla, JL Alio. Evaluation of endothelial cell changes 1 year after excimer laser in situ keratomileusis. Arch Ophthalmol 1997;115:841–846.

75. SS Jones, R Azar, SM Cristol, DH Geroski, GO Waring III, RD Stulting, KP Thompson, HF Edelhauser. Effects of laser in situ keratomileusis (LASIK) on the corneal endothelium. Am J Ophthalmol 1998;125:465–471.

76. T Seiler, K Koufala, G Richter. Iatrogenic keratectasia after laser in situ keratomileusis. J Refract Surg 1998;14:312–317.

77. T Seiler, AW Quurke. Iatrogenic keratectasia after LASIK in a case of forme fruste keratoconus. J Cataract Refract Surg 1998;24:1007–1009.

78. Z Wang, J Chen, B Yang. Posterior corneal surface topographic changes after laser in situ keratomileusis are related to residual corneal bed thickness. Ophthalmology 1999;106:406–410.

79. HS Geggel, AR Talley. Delayed onset keratectasia following laser in situ keratomileusis. J Cataract Refract Surg 1999;25:582–586.

80. FW Price Jr, DL Koller, MO Price. Central corneal pachymetry in patients undergoing laser in situ keratomileusis. Ophthalmology 1999;106(11):2216–2220.

81. MA el Danasoury. Prospective bilateral study of night glare after laser in situ keratomileusis with single zone and transition zone ablation. J Refract Surg 1998;14:512–516.

82. MA el Danasoury, GO Waring III, A El Maghraby, K Mehrez. Excimer laser in situ keratomileusis to correct compound myopic astigmatism. J Refract Surg 1997;13:511–520.

83. L Buratto, S Brint. Complications of LASIK. In: L Buratto, S Brint, eds. LASIK: Surgical Techniques and Complications. New Jersey: Slack, pp 177–264.

84. JT Holladay, DR Dudeja, J Chang. Functional vision and corneal changes after laser in situ keratomileusis determined by contrast sensitivity, glare testing and corneal topography. J Cataract Refract Surg 1999;25:663–669.

85. LF Jindra, V Zemon. Contrast sensitivity testing: a more complete assessment of vision. J Cataract Refract Surg 1989;15:141–148.

86. D Miller. Glare and contrast sensitivity testing. In: W Tasman, EA Jaeger, eds. Duane's Clinical Ophthalmology. Philadelphia, PA: Lippincott–Raven, 1992, Chap. 35.

87. MJ Lynn, GO Waring III, JT Carter. Combining refractive error and uncorrected visual acuity to assess the effectiveness of refractive corneal surgery. Refract Corneal Surg 1990;6:103–109.

88. JJ Pérez-Santonja, HF Sakla, JL Alio. Contrast sensitivity after laser in situ keratomileusis. J Cataract Refract Surg 1998;24:183–189.

89. A Ozdamar, C Aras, B Sener, M Oncel, M Karacorlu. Bilateral retinal detachment associated with giant retinal tear after laser-assisted in situ keratomileusis. Retina 1998;18:176–177.

90. RC Wolfs, CC Klaver, JR Vingerling, DE Grobbee, A Hofman, PT deJong. Distribution of central corneal thickness and its association with intraocular pressure: the Rotterdam study. Am J Ophthalmol 1997;123:767–772.

91. MM Whitacre, RA Stein, K Hassanein. The effect of corneal thickness on applanation tonometry. Am J Ophthalmol 1993;115:592–596.

92. M Kohlhass, R-C Lerche, J Draeger. The influence of corneal thickness and corneal curvature on tonometry readings after corneal refractive surgery. Eur J Implant Refract Surg 1995;7:84–88.

93. JT Holladay, ME Allison, TC Prager. Goldmann applanation tonometry in patients with regular corneal astigmatism. Am J Ophthalmol 1983;96:90–93.

94. B Emara, LE Probst, DP Tingey, DW Kennedy, LJ Willms, J Machat. Correlation of intaocular pressure and central corneal thickness in normal myopic eyes and after laser in situ keratomileusis. J Cataract Refract Surg 1998;24:1320–1325.

95. D Zadok, DB Tran, M Twa, M Carpenter, DJ Schanzlin. Pneumotonometry versus Goldmann tonometry after laser in situ keratomileusis for myopia. J Cataract Refract Surg 1999;25(10): 1344–1348.

96. AV Fournier, M Podtetenev, J Lemire, P Thompson, R Duchesne, C Perreault, N Chehade, P Blondeau. Intraocular pressure change measured by Goldmann tonometry after laser in situ keratomileusis. J Cataract Refract Surg 1998;24:905–910.

97. S Hannush. DLK-masquarade syndrome after LASIK. American Society of Cataract and Refractive Surgery meeting, Philadeplphia, 2002.

98. SA Melki, DT Azar. LASIK Complications. Survey Ophthalmol 2001.

28

Optical Aberrations After LASIK

SAMIR A. MELKI and CINTHIA E. PROANO

*Massachusetts Eye and Ear Infirmary and Harvard Medical School,
Boston, Massachusetts, U.S.A.*

DIMITRI T. AZAR

*Massachusetts Eye and Ear Infirmary, Schepens Eye Research Institute,
and Harvard Medical School, Boston, Massachusetts, U.S.A.*

A. INTRODUCTION

Success after refractive surgery is not limited to the patients' performance in identifying optotypes on Snellen charts in dim examination rooms. In addition to the loss of best corrected visual acuity (BCVA), the quality of vision can be affected by loss of contrast sensitivity, glare, halos and other optical abberations (1). The effect of LASIK surgery on light transmission through the corneal tissue is not limited to changes in corneal curvature. Other effects include decreased corneal sensation, epithelial irregularities, flap wrinkling, interface inflammation, epithelial ingrowth, and corneal ectasia (2,3). The quality of vision after LASIK may also be reduced as a result of decentration, irregular astigmatism, regression, and keratoconjunctivitis sicca (4).

B. HALOS, GLARE, AND LOSS OF CONTRAST SENSITIVITY

Night glare and halos are reported by many patients after LASIK and have multiple etiologies. The negative clearance phenomenon is mainly responsible for abberations resulting from pupils larger than the optical zone, especially under mesopic conditions. This occurs when rays of light refracted by the untreated cornea gain access through the entrance pupil and result in retinal blur circles. We believe that these symptoms are more pronounced af-

Adapted from: SA Melki, CE Proano, DT Azar. Int Ophthalmol Clin 2000;40:45–56.

ter treatment of cylindrical errors due to the oval area of laser treatment with inherently smaller optical zone in the steep meridian. In addition, correction of higher refractive errors is associated with increased abberrations due to the larger refractive differential between the ablated and the intact cornea. El Danasoury conducted a prospective bilateral study showing that a peripheral transition 1.0 mm diameter larger than the 5.5 mm ablation zone significantly decreased night glare after LASIK (5). Holladay et al. (6) recently showed worsening in functional vision as the target contrast diminishes and the pupil size increases. They concluded that the oblate shape of the cornea following LASIK is the predominant factor in the functional vision decrease. On the other hand, Perez-Santonja et al. reported improvement in contrast sensitivity at certain frequencies 6 months after LASIK in eyes with moderate to high myopia (7). Other factors such as dry eyes with irregular epithelium, irregular astigmatism due to flap folds, topographic abnormalities, or simply residual myopia can also contribute to these symptoms.

Most patients report improvement in night glare and halos few months after the surgery. It is not clear to what extent this improvement is due to patient adaptation or to actual resolution of optical abberations. A small subset reports no significant improvement and can be substantially incapacitated. Detection of patients with widely dilating pupils is an essential component of preoperative screening. Pupil size can be gauged using a Rosenbaum near card scale or an infrared Colvard pupillometer (8). Room lights should be dimmed in both situations to replicate mesopic conditions encountered by the patient at night. Patients with pupil diameter of more than 6.0 mm should be informed of the significant risk of night vision disturbances after LASIK. Postoperatively, strategies designed to minimize these symptoms include miotics, surface lubrication for dry eyes, tinted contact lenses with artificial pupils, and yellow-tinted eyeglasses. Prescribing correcting spectacles can sometimes be the easiest solution to relieve poor night vision if it is due to residual myopia.

C. REFRACTIVE SURPRISES AND INDUCED ABERRATIONS

Several factors may alter the predictability of LASIK surgery. These include surgeon and refraction errors, interindividual variations in corneal healing, and alterations of atmospheric pressure and ambient temperature. Patients with residual near-sightedness can suffer from night myopia. Myopic patients with a hyperopic result can suffer from quite unsatisfactory UCVA, both at near and distance, especially if they are in the presbyopic age group.

Undercorrected myopic refractions are often easily addressed with LASIK enhancement, but treating overcorrected patients is associated with greater unpredictability and greater chance of induced aberrations. The degree of induced spherical and astigmatic aberrations and the efficacy of using hyperopic LASIK to reverse refractive surgery-induced hyperopia is not known. Laser thermokeratoplasty (LTK) is a promising alternative to treat patients with this problem. In a study of 13 overcorrected eyes after LASIK, Ismail et al. (9) reported a mean increase of 4.1 D in central keratometric power using the noncontact holmuim:YAG (Ho:YAG) LTK (18 months follow-up). However, the authors did not report the consequences of the retreatment on the postoperative quality of vision.

Strategies to prevent large postoperative refractive surprises have been discussed in previous chapters. They include meticulous refractions, ensuring stable refractions (especially in rigid contact lens wearers) and a conservative approach in treating planocylindrical errors. It is likely that careful periodic review of surgical results can lead to the development of surgeon-specific nomograms that may narrow the window of refractive uncertainty after LASIK surgery.

D. IRREGULAR ASTIGMATISM, CENTRAL ISLANDS, AND DECENTRATION

Perhaps the most frustrating symptoms in patients experiencing "uneventful" LASIK surgery are those related to central islands and irregular astigmatism. These include blurred vision, marked visual fluctuations, ghost images, and monocular diplopia. Both uncorrected and best corrected vision are impacted; miotics are rarely helpful, and hard contact lenses may be the only means of regaining lost visual acuity. Multiple theories exist regarding the etiology of central islands (10,11). It must be kept in mind that the incidence of this complication depends on factors such as laser software, pattern of laser ablation, and surgical technique. Central islands after PRK have a better chance of resolving spontaneously, probably as a result of more extensive epithelial remodeling. Wilson reports a higher incidence of central islands with LASIK than with PRK (12). The incidence of central islands has diminished since the introduction of specific ablation software by some excimer laser manufacturers. Treatment of persistent islands and irregular astigmatism might not be as easy as predicted by developers of topography-linked lasers. Custom ablations solely based on videokeratography data might erroneously treat areas of overlying epithelial hyperplasia over areas of stromal depression not achieving the intended stromal smoothness (13). Manche et al. (14) described a specific technique for treating central islands after LASIK but cautioned against its associated hyperopic shift. Rachid et al. also reported improvement of visual outcomes after surgical correction of central islands following PRK (15,16).

The optical sequelae of decentered laser ablation during LASIK are related to uneven ablation within the pupillary axis with resultant irregular astigmatism causing glare, monocular, iplopia, and halos. Decentration is best measured with tangantial topography (10,17,18). Less than 0.3 mm of decentration is rarely visually significant. Decentration may be due to treatment displacement or to intraoperative drift, the latter being due to involuntary eye movement during treatment or to an intraoperative correctional effort by the surgeon to salvage a decentered ablation (18). Once the patient's symptoms have been determined to be the result of a decentered ablation, a recentering procedure can be attempted, especially if other strategies, including the administration of miotics to restrict the visual axis to the central smooth ablation in cases of mild to moderate decentration or hard contact lens fitting, were not successful. Surgical management involves lifting the corneal flap, decentering the laser ablation in the opposite direction, and applying a masking agent to the already ablated area. This technique is easier performed after PRK, as the epithelium can be used as the masking medium. Improvement in centration and visual outcomes were reported by Rachid et al. using the latter technique (15,16).

E. CORNEAL ECTASIA AFTER LASIK

There is no published data regarding which residual thickness of the corneal bed is proven to be safe. A minimum of 250 μm is currently accepted by the ophthalmic community as a safe level. Barraquer has recommended a minimal thickness of 300 μm of stress-bearing corneal stroma (19). Seiler et al. reported three patients who developed a delayed central island with progression after LASIK (26). The presumed residual stromal bed thickness was less than 250 μm in all cases. He later reported another case of iatrogenic keratectasia in a patient with forme fruste keratoconus and presumed residual stromal bed thickness of 260 μm (21). Another report by Geggel and Talley (22) describes iatrogenic corneal ectasia after LASIK for a correction as low as 6.6 D of myopia, but preoperative pachymetry was not available. Light microscopy of the button obtained at the time of penetrating keratoplasty revealed no underlying inflammation, suggesting biomechanical corneal weakening as the cause of the ectasia. Optical abberations in these patients would mimic those of patients with keratoconus mainly secondary to steep corneas and irregular astigmatism (see Chapter 10).

Specific precautions can be taken to avoid this devastating complication. Calculations should be made prior to surgery to determine if a safe corneal bed thickness can be achieved. It must be stressed that there can be considerable variation in the actual flap thickness compared to the expected one (from the microkeratome footplate) (23). In borderline cases, pachymetry should be performed on the stromal bed after lifting the flap. This can guide the surgeon later if enhancement is necessary. Safeguarding 250 μm of stromal bed is the current standard of care but could be proven inadequate when longer follow-up on well-documented cases becomes available. Preoperatively, keratoconus suspects should be approached carefully. Orbscan topography (Orbtek Inc., Salt Lake City, UT) can provide information on posterior corneal curvature before and after refractive surgery (24) and detailed pachymetry that can help detect forme fruste keratoconus. High-frequency ultrasound corneal analysis may be able to resolve flap from residual stromal bed with a 2 micron precision (13,25). This could turn out to be a highly useful tool in the analysis of cases with poor postoperative optical quality or unexpected ectasia.

F. OPTICAL ABERRATIONS FOLLOWING DIFFUSE LAMELLAR KERATITIS, EPITHELIAL INGROWTH, AND FLAP-RELATED COMPLICATIONS

Diffuse lamellar keratitis (DLK) and epithelial ingrowth are perhaps among the most feared LASIK complications, in part because corneal stromal melting may occur following these conditions. In DLK, melting is usually limited to the central cornea, resulting in optical aberrations, hyperopia, or hyperopic astigmatism. Epithelial ingrowth is more likely to induce melting in the overlying flap, inducing irregular astigmatism and hyperopic shift. Additional symptoms can include glare, halos, polyopia, and loss of BCVA.

DLK or sands of the Sahara syndrome is a recently described syndrome of unknown incidence characterized by proliferation of presumably inflammatory cells at the LASIK interface (26). It has been reported to occur sporadically or in clusters with primary procedures or in cases of LASIK enhancement. Cultures taken from the interface are typically negative for microorganisms. No single agent has been demonstrated to be responsible for this rare complication. Its incidence is about 1.8% (27). Current recommended management is through an intensive steroid and/or antibiotics regimen. Early flap lift and scraping is essential if any signs of melting are noted (see Fig. 17.5 and Chapter 34).

Epithelial ingrowth is characterized by a collection of epithelial cells with a pearly appearance under the LASIK flap. More concerning is epithelial ingrowth that is contiguous with the flap edge. This can progress to involve the visual axis with irregular astigmatism and possible surrounding stromal melting. The extent of the ingrowth is often more extensive than appreciated with slit-lamp examination. A low threshold for intervention should be maintained as connection to the outside epithelium or extension into the visual axis might be imperceptible at the slit-lamp (see Fig. 17.6 and Chapter 33).

Epithelial ingrowth is more common after enhancement procedures, as the lifting of the flap can induce adjacent epithelial abrasions with increased cell proliferation. Perez-Santonja reported 31% epithelial ingrowth and 10.9% flap melting after LASIK enhancement (series of 59 eyes) (28). This is in contrast to Stutling's 3.2% rate after enhancement (series of 283 eyes) (29). Waring et al (30) reported higher incidence of ingrowth with simultaneous than with sequential bilateral LASIK. Buttonholed flaps are also vulnerable to epithelial infiltration at the edges of the perforation. Flap folds are another source of epithelial cell infiltration and should be addressed promptly, especially if they extend towards the edge of the flap.

Management of epithelial ingrowth involves lifting the flap and thoroughly debriding both the stromal bed and the back of the flap from any detectable cells. This can be achieved mechanically such as with a #64 blade or with dedicated instruments such as the Yaghouti LASIK Sander. Excimer laser bursts in PTK mode can be applied to remove any remaining cells (31). Early management can lead to a sharp reduction in optical disturbances, preventing lasting abberations.

It has been our experience that low myopes who develop flap wrinkle folds report a certain degree of blur and haziness in their vision after surgery, which may or may not be associated with Snellen acuity loss (BCVA). Tissue folds observed after LASIK are mostly detected in the early period after surgery. They adversely affect the visual outcome of the procedure by induced irregular astigmatism. Reported symptoms include the starburst effect around lighting at night and the loss of BCVA or UCVA. A linear fold or multiple parallel folds may induce streaking of light in a manner similar to that observed with a Bagolini lens (Azar, unpublished data).

Flap folds occur from uneven realignment of the flap at the time of surgery or from postoperative displacement. In eyes with high myopia and deeper ablations, flaps are repositioned on a bed with significant loss of convexity and support. This may be inevitable in some patients and may lead to redundant flap tissue that can wrinkle despite adequate edge positioning.

The earlier a fold is attended to the easier it is to flatten. Longer standing flaps can become quite resistant to stretching presumably from epithelial hyperplasia in the fold's crevices. Small folds in the early postoperative period can be smoothed at the slit-lamp with dedicated instruments (such as a Pineda iron) or a methylcellulose sponge. Probst and Machat (32) described a method to flatten LASIK flap folds using the red reflex better to detect subtle irregularities. More recalcitrant and/or longer standing folds usually require lifting and refloating of the flap. Using 60 to 80% saline to hydrate the flap has also been described. We have used it successfully in recalcitrant folds. If it is unsuccessful, placement of sutures to stretch the flap or epithelial debridement over the wrinkled area has been advocated. The latter is thought to be beneficial, as epithelial hyperplasia possibly develops in the crevices of longer standing flaps, preventing adequate stretching. We prefer using a soft contact lens after refloating and flap ironing. Most patients report significant improvement in their visual disturbances and even in Snellen acuity after resolution of the surface folds.

Corneal light scattering can occur because of interface debris, cells, or irregular collagen deposition. Interface debris should be distinguished from inflammatory or infectious reactions. This distinction is difficult at times. As a rule, debris is usually inert, having no progression or effects on vision unless present in large quantity. Nevertheless, some patients may be more susceptible than others and may present with optical disturbances and inflammatory response to a variety of debris. Sources of debris include mettalic shatter from the keratome blade, meibomian gland secretions, glove powder, lint fibers from surrounding clothes, and surgical gauze. Hirst and Vandeleur (33) showed that dry methylcellulose sponges used to protect the flap during laser ablation are the source of brown interface deposits at the LASIK interface. The light scattering effect from the various kinds of debris is enough to make it visible but most often with little impact on the quality of vision. Braunstein et al. described a reliable method of measuring corneal light scattering after refractive surgery (34).

If an inflammatory reaction is suspected secondary to interface debris, the flap should be lifted and copious irrigation applied using powder-free gloves, draping the lashes and applying a moist methylcellulose (Chayet) ring around the limbus to provide a barrier from surrounding ocular secretions. This has significantly reduced the presence of any debris at the LASIK interface at our center. Vinciguerra et al. (35) proposed a PTK-style smoothing technique after the refractive ablation to decrease interface irregularities and improve refractive and optical outcomes.

Chang et al. (36) has demonstrated a statistically significant positive correlation between the objective light scattering index and the thickness of new collagen formation after LASIK. Corneal light scattering was significantly lower after LASIK than after PRK (37). This may be related to differential expression of matrix metalloproteinases after wounding (38,39). Further studies are needed to correlate these measurements with patients' symptoms.

Epithelial cell implantation at the LASIK interface occurs with seeding during surgery either by the keratome blade or the surgical instruments in contact with both epithelial and stromal aspects of the cornea. Cells migrating in the interface may have deleterious effects on the overlying stroma, presumably by the production of the matrix metalloproteinases and gelatinase B (40). Most isolated nests of cells will disappear without consequences. The significance of their light-scattering effect is similar to that of inert debris.

A LASIK flap can get displaced early (24 h) or later, after the procedure. Early displacement can result from spontaneous slippage or mechanical disruption such as blinking or eye rubbing. The incidence of this complication was reported to be 1.2% (out of 1000 eyes) by Gimbel et al. (41), 2.0% (out of 1017 eyes) by Lin and Maloney (27), and 1.1% (out of 1062 eyes) by Stulting et al. (29) in the largest series of complications in the peer-reviewed literature. All studies show no loss of BCVA worse than two lines of visual acuity due to flap dehiscence. Later, more severe trauma can detach the flap from its bed despite apparent healing. Although traumatic flap displacement has been anecdotally reported as long as 8 months after the procedure, no clear incidence has yet emerged. Chaudhry and Smiddy (42) reported dislocation of a LASIK flap with epithelial debridement at the time of pars plana vitrectomy 4 months after LASIK.

A displaced or subluxed flap is an emergency (43). It should be repositioned as soon as possible to prevent fixed folds and epithelial ingrowth. The flap should first be reflected and the interface (stromal bed and stromal aspect of the flap) carefully examined for epithelial cells and debris. If present, they should be aggressively scraped prior to repositioning the flap. A contact lens can be applied to provide added protection from further displacement. Techniques concerning management of associated folds and epithelial ingrowth are discussed in their respective sections. If a flap is totally detached from its bed, repositioning in the proper orientation becomes quite difficult after the loss of surgical marks. This can result in irregular astigmatism and loss of BCVA. A bandage contact lens could be tried to hold it in place; otherwise suturing might be necessary. If the flap is lost, the epithelium is allowed to heal as in a PRK situation, usually leading to significant flattening and hyperopic shift.

We routinely advise patients to wear a hard shield for eye protection when asleep in the first two weeks after the procedure. Patients should also be informed of the flap vulnerability to trauma even months after the surgery. Occupational hazards (e.g., contact sports) should be considered a factor in the decision process to undergo refractive surgery, namely LASIK vs. PRK.

According to a review of complications in a series of 1062 eyes, Stulting et al. (29) reported that flap buttonholes were more likely to cause loss of BCVA than free or incomplete flaps. A buttonhole occurs when the keratome blade emerges from the interface in mid-incision and immediately reenters, leaving a central area of uncut epithelium. Steeper corneas (12,41) and eyes that underwent previous surgeries (29) have been implicated in this complication. Deeper microkeratome footplates should be used in these situations to try to avert this complication.

A buttonholed flap is best managed by proper repositioning and deferring the procedure to a later date (2–3 months) when a deeper cut can be safely performed. These patients should be carefully monitored for epithelial infiltration centrally. It is unclear if buttonholed flaps without subsequent epithelial ingrowth are more prone to degradation of visual quality. Treatment with transepithelial PRK is to be cautioned, considering the risks of associated haze.

G. SURFACE LIGHT SCATTERING WITH DRY EYES

A significant number of patients complain of dry eye symptoms after LASIK. It is not known whether patients report these symptoms as frequently after PRK. Symptoms usually include burning, foreign body sensation, and occasionally eye pain. Many patients with dry eyes after LASIK will experience visual fluctuations as well as visual aberrations such as glare and halos at night (3). It can also result in temporary loss of UCVA and BCVA. Many patients report improvement in the quality of vision immediately after blinking or in the morning hours prior to day-long exposure to surface evaporation. This can be confirmed by an improvement in visual acuity immediately after the application of artificial tears. A hard contact lens refraction can also be performed to confirm the implication of surface irregularity in visual impairment (18,42). The most common finding on examination is superficial punctate keratopathy. The mires with keratoscopy are often not sharply delineated and may or may not be irregular. It is not known whether the surface irregularity results from forward scattering of light (34). Artificial tears and punctal plugs will usually relieve this condition. We favor tapering the postoperative topical steroid over a 4 week period to help alleviate some of the symptoms. Most patients note improvement in their symptoms a few weeks after the procedure.

There are two theories regarding the etiology of dry eyes after LASIK. The first is related to the decreased blinking rate secondary to decreased corneal sensation. Kim and Kim (2) report persistent impairment in corneal sensation 6 months after the surgery, while Linna et al. (45) measured a return to preoperative values at the same time period. The second theory relates to damage to perilimbal goblet cells from the application of the suction ring. Lenton and Albietz showed faster improvement in symptoms, tear breakup time, and rose bengal staining with carmellose-based artificial tears as compared to balanced salt solution (46). They also report a greater restoration of mean goblet cell density at 1 month after LASIK.

REFERENCES

1. IG Pallikaris. Quality of vision in refractive surgery. J Refract Surg 1998;14:551–558.
2. WS Kim, JS Kim. Change in corneal sensitivity following laser in situ keratomileusis. J Cataract Refract Surg 1999;25:368–373.

3. SG Farah, DT Azar, C Gurdal, J Wong. Laser in situ keratomileusis: literature review of a developing technique. J Cataract Refract Surg 1998;24:989–1006.

4. SA Melki, CE Proano, DT Azar. Optical disturbances and their management after myopic laser in situ keratomileusis. IOC 2000;40:45–56.

5. MA el Danasoury. Prospective bilateral study of night glare after laser in situ keratomileusis with single zone and transition zone ablation. J Refract Surg 1998;14:512–516.

6. JT Holladay, DR Dudeja, J Chang. Functional vision and corneal changes after laser in situ keratomileusis determined by contrast sensitivity, glare testing, and corneal topography [in process citation]. J Cataract Refract Surg 1999;25:663–669.

7. JJ Perez-Santonja, HF Sakla, JL Alio. Contrast sensitivity after laser in situ keratomileusis. J Cataract Refract Surg 1998;24:183–189.

8. M Colvard. Preoperative measurement of scotopic pupil dilation using an office pupillometer. J Cataract Refract Surg 1998;24:1594–1597.

9. MM Ismail, JL Alio, JJ Perez-Santonja. Noncontact thermokeratoplasty to correct hyperopia induced by laser in situ keratomileusis. J Cataract Refract Surg 1998;24:1191–1194.

10. TK Chan, DT Azar. Photorefractive keratectomy (PRK) outcomes and complications. In: DT Azar et al., eds. Phototherapeutic Keratectomy, Management of Scars, Dystrophies, and PRK Complications. Baltimore: Williams & Wilkins, 1997, pp 157–174.

11. RR Krueger, NF Saedy, PJ McDonnell. Clinical analysis of steep central islands after excimer laser photorefractive keratectomy. Arch Ophthalmol 1996;114:377–381.

12. SE Wilson. LASIK: management of common complications. Laser in situ keratomileusis. Cornea 1998;17:459–467.

13. DZ Reinstein, RH Silverman, HF Sutton, DJ Coleman. Very high-frequency ultrasound corneal analysis identifies anatomic correlates of optical complications of lamellar refractive surgery: anatomic diagnosis in lamellar surgery. Ophthalmology 1999;106:474–482.

14. EE Manche, RK Maloney, RJ Smith. Treatment of topographic central islands following refractive surgery. J Cataract Refract Surg 1998;24:464–470.

15. MD Rachid, SH Yoo, DT Azar. Excimer laser retreatment for the management of PRK decentration and central islands. New Orleans: American Academy of Ophthalmology, Annual Meeting, 1998.

16. MD Rachid, SY Yoo, DT Azar. Phototherapeutic keratectomy for decentration and central islands after photorefractive keratectomy. Ophthalmology 2001;108:545–552.

17. L Strauss, D Azar. Optics rediscovered for the keratorefractive surgeon. In DT Azar, ed. Refractive Surgery. Stamford: Appelton & Lange, 1997, pp 113–124.

18. DT Azar, PC Yeh. Corneal topographic evaluation of decentration in photorefractive keratectomy: treatment displacement vs. intraoperative drift. Am J Ophthalmol 1997;124:312–320.

19. J Barraquer. Querato Mileusis y Queratofaquia. Bogota: Instituto Barraquer de America, 1980, p 342.

20. T Seiler, K Koufala, G Richter. Iatrogenic keratectasia after laser in situ keratomileusis. J Refract Surg 1998;14:312–317.

21. T Seiler, AW Quurke. Iatrogenic keratectasia after LASIK in a case of forme fruste keratoconus. J Cataract Refract Surg 1998;24:1007–1009.

22. HS Geggel, AR Talley. Delayed onset keratectasia following laser in situ keratomileusis [in process citation]. J Cataract Refract Surg 1999;25:582–586.

23. PS Binder, M Moore, RW Lambert, DM Seagrist. Comparison of two microkeratome systems. J Refract Surg 1997;13:142–153.

24. Z Wang, J Chen, B Yang. Posterior corneal surface topographic changes after laser in situ keratomileusis are related to residual corneal bed thickness. Ophthalmology 1999;106:406–409; discussion 409–410.

25. N Allemann, W Chamon, RH Silverman, DT Azar, DZ Reinstein, WJ Stark, DJ Coleman. High-frequency ultrasound quantitative analyses of corneal scarring following excimer laser keratectomy. Arch Ophthalmol 1993;111:968–973.

26. RJ Smith, RK Maloney. Diffuse lamellar keratitis. A new syndrome in lamellar refractive surgery. Ophthalmology 1998;105:1721–1726.

27. RT Lin, RK Maloney. Flap complications associated with lamellar refractive surgery [see comments]. Am J Ophthalmol 1999;127:129–136.

28. JJ Perez-Santonja, MJ Ayala, HF Sakla, JM Ruiz-Moreno, JL Alio. Retreatment after laser in situ keratomileusis. Ophthalmology 1999;106:21–28.

29. RD Stulting, JD Carr, KP Thompson, GO Waring III, WM Wiley, JG Walker. Complications of laser in situ keratomileusis for the correction of myopia. Ophthalmology 1999;106:13–20.

30. GO Waring III, JD Carr, RD Stulting, KP Thompson, W Wiley. Prospective randomized comparison of simultaneous and sequential bilateral laser in situ keratomileusis for the correction of myopia. Ophthalmology 1999;106:732–738.

31. MC Helena, D Meisler, SE Wilson. Epithelial growth within the lamellar interface after laser in situ keratomileusis (LASIK) [see comments]. Cornea 1997;16:300–305.

32. LE Probst, J Machat. Removal of flap striae following laser in situ keratomileusis. J Cataract Refract Surg 1998;24:153–155.

33. LW Hirst, KW Vandeleur, Jr. Laser in situ keratomileusis interface deposits. J Refract Surg 1998;14:653–654.

34. RE Braunstein, S Jain, RL McCally, WJ Stark, PJ Connolly, DT Azar. Objective measurement of corneal light scattering after excimer laser keratectomy. Ophthalmology 1996;103:439–443.

35. P Vinciguerra, M Azzolini, P Airaghi, P Radice, V De Molfetta. Effect of decreasing surface and interface irregularities after photorefractive keratectomy and laser in situ keratomileusis on optical and functional outcomes. J Refract Surg 1998;14:S199–S203.

36. SW Chang, A Benson, DT Azar. Corneal light scattering with stromal reformation after laser in situ keratomileusis and photorefractive keratectomy. J Cataract Refract Surg 1998;24: 1064–1069.

37. S Jain, JM Khoury, W Chamon, DT Azar. Corneal light scattering after laser in situ keratomileusis and photorefractive keratectomy. Am J Ophthalmol 1995;120:532–534.

38. DT Azar, D Pluznik, S Jain, JM Khoury. Gelatinase B and A expression after laser in situ keratomileusis and photorefractive keratectomy. Arch Ophthalmol 1998;116:1206–1208.

39. HQ Ye, DT Azar. Expression of gelatinases A and B, and TIMPs 1 and 2 during corneal wound healing. Invest Ophthalmol Vis Sci 1998;39:913–921.

40. M Maeda, BD Vanlandingham, H Ye, PC Lu, DT Azar. Immunoconfocal localization of gelatinase B expressed by migrating intrastromal epithelial cells after deep annular excimer keratectomy. Curr Eye Res 1998;17:836–843.

41. HV Gimbel, EE Penno, JA van Westenbrugge, M Ferensowicz, MT Furlong. Incidence and management of intraoperative and early postoperative complications in 1000 consecutive laser in situ keratomileusis cases. Ophthalmology 1998;105:1839–1847; discussion 1847–1848.

42. NA Chaudhry, WE Smiddy. Displacement of corneal cap during vitrectomy in a post-LASIK eye. Retina 1998;18:554–555.

43. SA Melki, JH Talamo, A Demetriades, NS Jabbur, JP Essepian, TP O'Brien, DT Azar. Late traumatic dislocation of laser in situ keratomileusis corneal flaps. Ophthalmology 2000;107:2136–2139.

44. DT Azar, RF Steinert. PTK in the management of PRK complications. In: Azar et al., eds. Phototherapeutic Keratectomy, Management of Scars, Dystrophies, and PRK Complications. Baltimore: Williams & Wilkins, 1997, pp 175–188.

45. TU Linna, JJ Perez-Santonja, KM Tervo, HF Sakla, JL Alio y Sanz, TM Tervo. Recovery of corneal nerve morphology following laser in situ keratomileusis. Exp Eye Res 1998;66: 755–763.

46. LM Lenton, JM Albietz. Effect of carmellose-based artificial tears on the ocular surface in eyes after laser in situ keratomileusis [in process citation]. J Refract Surg 1999;15:S227–S231.

29

Posterior Segment Complications of LASIK

RON AFSHARI ADELMAN

Massachusetts Eye and Ear Infirmary, Boston, Massachusetts, and Yale University Eye Center, New Haven, Connecticut, U.S.A.

NATALIE A. AFSHARI

Duke University Eye Center, Durham, North Carolina, U.S.A.

Posterior segment complications of LASIK are rare but visually significant. Myopes have a tendency to develop lattice degeneration, early posterior vitreous detachment, retinal breaks, and retinal detachment. Between 1.5% and 14% of myopic eyes may need some form of treatment for vitreoretinal pathologies before LASIK (1–3). In a retrospective study of about 30,000 eyes after LASIK, vitreoretinal complications were noted only in 0.06% of the eyes (2). However, in a prospective study, new vitreoretinal pathology after LASIK was reported in 2.5% of the eyes (3).

Posterior segment complications of LASIK include:

Retinal tears and detachment
Vitreous loss
Macular hemorrhage
Choroidal neovascularization
Subhyaloid hemorrhage
Possible retinal nerve fiber layer changes

Additionally, cystoid macular edema has been reported after excimer laser photorefractive keratectomy (4). Prompt diagnosis and management of these complications may help to prevent irreversible visual loss. Preoperative dilated fundus examination with scleral depression may be useful in recognizing posterior segment pathologies that need to be addressed prior to LASIK.

A. EFFECT OF EXCIMER LASER ON THE OCULAR ELECTROPHYSIOLOGY

Spadea et al. studied the effects of excimer laser photorefractive keratectomy on the electrophysiologic function of the retina and the optic nerve in 25 patients (5). Pattern electroretinograms and pattern visual evoked potentials were performed prior to laser vision correction, and 3, 6, 12, and 18 months after the procedure. In each patient the fellow eye served as the control. There were no statistically significant differences between the treated and the control eyes, or between treated eyes preoperatively and postoperatively. Therefore there is no evidence that excimer laser photorefractive keratectomy alters the electrophysiological function of the retina and optic nerve. However, the electrophysiological effects of the mechanical pressure of the microkeratome plus the excimer laser during LASIK are not known.

B. RETINAL TEARS AND DETACHMENT

Retinal detachment is a recognized complication of almost any type of refractive surgery. Charteris and coworkers were the first to describe an association between retinal detachment and previous excimer laser treatment (6). They reported retinal detachment in 11 eyes of 10 myopic patients who had undergone photorefractive keratectomy (PRK) or phototherapeutic keratectomy (PTK) by excimer laser. The interval between PRK/PTK and the diagnosis of retinal detachment ranged from 1 to 20 months. Barraquer et al. studied incidence of retinal detachment following clear-lens extraction in 165 myopic eyes and found retinal detachment in 12 (7.3%) eyes (7). Ruiz-Moreno and coworkers reported retinal detachment in eight (4.8%) of 166 eyes that underwent phakic anterior chamber intraocular lens implantation to correct myopia (8). Rodriguez and Camacho reported seven cases of retinal detachment following radial keratotomy, and another seven cases of retinal detachment following keratomileusis (9).

In 1998 Ozdamar and coworkers reported a case of bilateral retinal detachment associated with bilateral giant retinal tears two months after the LASIK procedure (10). Since then several case reports and case series of retinal detachment following LASIK have been published (1,2,11–14).

The mechanism of retinal detachment after LASIK is not fully understood. The microkeratome produces a uniform and appropriate flap, when the intraocular pressure exceeds 65 mmHg (11). Ozdamer et al. (10) and Aras et al. (11) proposed that sudden increase and decrease of the intraocular pressure during suction or release of the suction ring may cause a mechanical stretch on the vitreous base. Additionally, the excimer laser results in an acoustic shock wave. The laser-induced shock wave produces a pressure of up to 100 atm. This shock wave may cause posterior vitreous detachment and might contribute to the development of retinal detachment in an eye with predisposing vitreoretinal lesions (11).

Arevalo and coworkers in a multicenter retrospective study reviewed vitreoretinal pathologies in 29,916 eyes after LASIK (2). Twenty eyes (0.06%) of 17 patients developed vitreoretinal complications. Rhegmatogenous retinal detachments were seen in 14 eyes. Two eyes had corneoscleral laceration with the microkeratome; one developed retinal detachment and the other had vitreous hemorrhage. Four eyes had retinal tears without retinal detachment, and one eye developed choroidal neovascular membrane. These authors attributed their low incidence of vitreoretinal complications after LASIK to very thorough dilated fundus examination with scleral depression prior to LASIK. They estimate that about 1.5% of eyes in their series required some form of treatment for predisposing retinal pathologies before LASIK.

To investigate the incidence of retinal complications of LASIK, Nassaralla performed a prospective study examining 200 myopic eyes before and after LASIK (3). Prior to LASIK peripheral retinal changes were noted in 61% of eyes, including lattice degeneration (28%), round holes (4%), white without pressure (5%), and oral chorioretinal degeneration (23%). After LASIK the eyes were examined at 1 week and at 1, 3, and 12 months. New retinal problems were noted in five (2.5%) eyes. These included small peripheral holes in three (1.5%) eyes and lattice degeneration in two (1%) eyes. In this study, with prompt diagnosis and management, vision was not affected by the peripheral holes.

Management of retinal tears and detachments after LASIK include laser retinopexy, cryotherapy, pneumatic retinopexy, vitrectomy, and scleral buckle. The advantage of vitrectomy over scleral buckle is that the length of the globe remains unchanged (2,12). Therefore some authors avoid encircling buckles whenever possible. Rodriguez and Camacho suggested the following management when refractive errors have occurred after buckling procedures (9):

> Wait for possible spontaneous improvement
> In the meantime, correct refractive errors with glasses or contact lenses. It should be noted that in general the fitting of contact lenses after scleral buckling procedures is difficult because of conjunctival scarring secondary to 360 degree peritomy.
> Remove the scleral buckle after making sure that all breaks have sealed and that no retinal detachment is present in the fundus. However, removing the scleral buckle is an additional surgery and may result in recurrence of the detachment.
> Consider additional refractive surgery. This may be difficult for the patient to accept.

C. VITREOUS LOSS

Corneoscleral perforation is a well recognized complication of LASIK and may result in vitreous loss and hemorrhage. Arevalo et al. reported a myopic patient who had ocular perforation, loss of crystalline lens, vitreous loss, and vitreous hemorrhage during LASIK (2). The refractive surgeon had omitted placing a spacing plate into the microkeratome. It should be emphasized that patients with vitreous loss have a high incidence of retinal tears, retinal detachments, and cystoid macular edema. Therefore these patients should be followed carefully.

D. MACULAR HEMORRHAGE AND CHOROIDAL NEOVASCULARIZATION

Macular hemorrhage following LASIK is rare. Review of literature reveals seven cases of macular hemorrhage after LASIK (15–19) and four cases following photorefractive keratectomy (PRK) (15,19,20). Shock waves produced by the excimer laser and mechanical pressure during LASIK may result in alteration in fragile subretinal vessels, Bruch's membrane, and retinal pigment epithelium. These alterations may contribute to macular hemorrhage and cystoid macular edema (4,16). Luna and coworkers reported a case of bilateral macular hemorrhage after bilateral LASIK for the correction of high myopia (16). Dilated fundus examination demonstrated multifocal subretinal macular and posterior pole hemorrhages, and fluorescein angiogram showed macular lesions compatible with lacquer cracks. Ellies et al. reported two women with high myopia who developed macular hemorrhage after LASIK (15). The first patient noticed severe loss of vision 4 days after LASIK, and in fundus examination submacular hemorrhage was noted. The second patient had a Fuchs' spot without hemorrhage below the fovea that was noted during the preop examination. One day after LASIK the patient had severe loss of vision and a retinal hemorrhage. Fluorescein angiogram showed choroidal neovascularization at the site of a previous pigmented lesion. Ellies recommends (15)

> A careful examination of the fundus should be conducted before performing LASIK surgery on highly myopic patients. In case of similar macular pathology, fluorescein angiography should be done before LASIK. Preexisting macular pathology, such as choroidal neovascularization and lacquer cracks, could be a new contraindication to LASIK for high myopia.

E. SUBHYALOID HEMORRHAGE

Mansour and Ojeimi reported a case of premacular subhyaloid hemorrhage following LASIK in a moderately myopic patient who did not have any predisposing factor for subhyaloid hemorrhage (22) The subhyaloid hemorrhage did not resolve spontaneously over 1 month of observation. Therefore YAG laser posterior hyaloidotomy was performed, which resulted in immediate improvement in visual acuity to 20/200. Mansour and Ojeimi speculate that subhyaloid hemorrhage resulted from the sudden release of vacuum pump pressure from 65 mmHg to 0. They advise the use of newer generations of microkeratomes that allow gradual release of the vacuum pressure based on the hypothesis that it would decrease the chance of fundus hemorrhage (22).

F. LASIK AND THE RETINAL NERVE FIBER LAYER THICKNESS

The effect of LASIK on the nerve fiber layer of retina is controversial. Yavitz reported that the nerve fiber layer had decreased 5% to 10% following LASIK and proposed that elevated intraocular pressure during LASIK causes hypoxia and apoptosis of the retinal nerve fiber layer (23). Yavitz recommended administration of topical brimonidine starting 3 days prior to LASIK and continuing until 1 week after LASIK. On the other hand, Nath suggested that LASIK does not have a damaging effect on the nerve fiber layer (24). Tsai and Lin studied retinal nerve fiber layer thickness in 35 eyes of 20 patients before and 1 month after LASIK (25). They found that LASIK significantly decreased retinal nerve fiber layer thickness determined by scanning laser polarimetry. However it should be noted that measurement of the retinal nerve fiber layer by laser polarimetry depends on a corneal compensator inherent in the instrument. Therefore LASIK may affect scanning laser polarimetry measurements (26).

G. SUMMARY

Posterior segment complications of LASIK are rare. Refractive surgeons should be aware of the risk of retinal detachment and macular hemorrhage. In pre-LASIK evaluation, dilated fundus examination with special attention to lacquer cracks and Fuchs' spots in the macula and scleral depression for peripheral pathologies is recommended. Consultation with a retina specialist prior to LASIK in cases with significant macular or peripheral pathologies will help to prevent some of these complications. If a patient needs photocoagulation for retinal tears, waiting at least 15 days between photocoagulation and LASIK is recommended. Routine post-LASIK dilated fundus examination is helpful in diagnosis of posterior segment complications. In evaluation of patients with poor vision after LASIK, macular complications should be ruled out.

REFERENCES

1. JM Ruiz-Moreno, JJ Perez-Santonja, JL Alio. Retinal detachment in myopic eyes after laser in situ keratomileusis. Am J Ophthalmol 1999;128:588–594.
2. JF Arevalo, E Ramirez, E Suarez, J Morales-Stopello, R Cortez, G Ramirez, G Antzoulatas, J Tugues, J Rodriguez, D Fuenmayor-Rivera. Incidence of vitreoretinal pathologic conditions within 24 months after laser in situ keratomileusis. Ophthalmology 2000;107:258–262.
3. JJ Nassarralla. LASIK may not raise risk of retinal complications. Ophthalmol Times 2000; 25(15):27.
4. P Janknecht, JM Soriano, LL Hansen. Cystoid macular edema after excimer laser photorefractive keratectomy. Br J Ophthalmol 1993;77:681.
5. L Spadea, T Dragani, R Magni, G Rinaldi, E Balestrazzi. Effect of myopic excimer laser photorefractive keratectomy on the electrophysiologic function of the retina and optic nerve. J Cataract Refract Surg 1996;22:906–909.
6. DG Charteris, RJ Cooling, MJ Lavin, D McLeod. Retinal detachment following excimer laser. Br J Ophthalmol 1997;81:759–761.
7. C Barraquer, C Cavelier, LF Mejia. Incidence of retinal detachment following clear lens extraction in myopic patients. Arch Ophthalmol 1994;112:336–339.
8. JM Ruiz-Moreno, JL Alio, JJ Perez-Santonja, F de la Hoz. Retinal detachment in phakic eyes with anterior chamber intraocular lenses to correct myopia. Am J Ophthalmol 1999;127: 270–275.
9. A Rodriguez, H Camacho. Retinal detachment after refractive surgery for myopia. Retina 1992;12:S46–S50.
10. A Ozdamar, C Aras, B Sener, M Oncel, M Karacorlu. Bilateral retinal detachment associated with giant retinal tear after laser-assisted in situ keratomileusis. Retina 1998;18:176–177.
11. C Aras, A Ozdamar, M Karacorlu, B Sener, H Bahcecioglu. Retinal detachment following laser in situ keratomileusis. Ophthalmic Surg Lasers 2000;31:121–125.
12. JF Arevalo, E Ramirez, E Suarez, G Antzoulatos, F Torres, R Cortez, J Morales-Stopello, G Ramirez. Rhegmatogenous retinal detachment after laser-assisted in situ keratomileusis (LASIK) for the correction of myopia. Retina 2000;20:338–341.
13. RD Stulting, JD Carr, KP Thompson, GO Waring III, WM Wiley, JG Walker. Complications of laser in situ keratomileusis for the correction of myopia. Ophthalmology 1999;106:13–20.
14. DG Charteris. Retinal detachment associated with excimer laser. Curr Opin Ophthalmol 1999;10:173–176.
15. P Ellies, D Pietrini, L Lumbroso, DA Lebuisson. Macular hemorrhage after laser in situ keratomileusis for high myopia. J Cataract Refract 2000;26:922–924.
16. JD Luna, VE Reviglio, CP Juarez. Bilateral macular hemorrhage after laser in situ keratomileusis. Graefe's Arch Clin Exp Ophthalmol 1999;237:611–613.
17. HM Kim, HR Jung. Laser assisted in situ keratomileusis for high myopia. Ophthalmic Surg Lasers 1996;27:S508–S511.
18. T Salah, GO Waring III, A el Maghraby, K Moadel, SB Grimm. Excimer laser in situ keratomileusis under a corneal flap for myopia of 2 to 20 diopters. Am J Ophthalmol 1996;121: 143–155.

19. IG Pallikaris, DS Siganos. Laser in situ keratomileusis to treat myopia: early experience. J Cataract Refract Surg 1997;23:39–49.
20. I Toda, Y Yagi, S Hata, S Itoh, K Tsubota. Excimer laser photorefractive keratectomy for patients with contact lens intolerance caused by dry eyes. Br J Ophthalmol 1996;80:604–609.
21. A Loewenstein, I Lipshitz, D Varssano, M Lazar. Macular hemorrhage after excimer laser photorefractive keratectomy. J Cataract Refract Surg 1997;23:808–810.
22. AM Mansour, GK Ojeimi. Premacular subhyaloid hemorrhage following laser in situ keratomileusis. J Refract Surg 2000;16:371–372.
23. E Yavitz. LASIK study shows brimonidine provides neuroprotective effect. Ocular Surg News 1999;10:48.
24. S Nath. Study shows NFL safe after LASIK. Ocular Surg News 2000;11:35.
25. YY Tsai, JM Lin. Effect of laser-assisted in situ keratomileusis on the retinal nerve fiber layer. Retina 2000;20:342–345.
26. R Gurses-Ozden, ME Pons, C Barbieri, H Ishikawa, DF Buxton, JM Liebmann, R Ritch. Scanning laser polarimetry measurements after laser-assisted in situ keratomileusis. Am J Ophthalmol 2000;129:461–464.

30

Management of Topographical Irregularities Following LASIK

JEFFREY JOHNSON

*Massachusetts Eye and Ear Infirmary and Harvard Medical School,
Boston, Massachusetts, U.S.A.*

ROSELYN JEUN

Massachusetts Eye and Ear Infirmary, Boston, Massachusetts, U.S.A.

DIMITRI T. AZAR

*Massachusetts Eye and Ear Infirmary, Schepens Eye Research Institute,
and Harvard Medical School, Boston, Massachusetts, U.S.A.*

The importance of computerized corneal videokeratography in the evaluation and management of laser in situ keratomileusis (LASIK) patients cannot be overstated. While corneal topography is important in the preoperative stages of refractive surgery as a screening device for corneal irregularities, including contact lens warpage and keratoconus, it is also necessary postoperatively, as mild corneal irregularities can often be detected only through topographical analysis. These corneal irregularities include central islands, ablation decentration, corneal ectasia, and other forms of irregular astigmatism. Despite their low incidence, these complications can lead to patient dissatisfaction, as image quality can be adversely affected. As frustrating as these cases can be to patients, they can be equally frustrating to the refractive surgeon. Not all surgically induced topographical irregularities following LASIK are amenable to further treatment, and depending upon the type of irregularity found, treatment options often vary considerably. Therefore, these complications must be approached cautiously, and a thorough understanding of the treatment options and the likelihood of success is essential.

A. CENTRAL ISLANDS

Central islands were first described following automated lamellar keratoplasty (ALK) and occur in varying frequency following PRK and LASIK (1–7). Kreuger and colleagues described central islands following excimer laser ablation as central areas of steepness at least

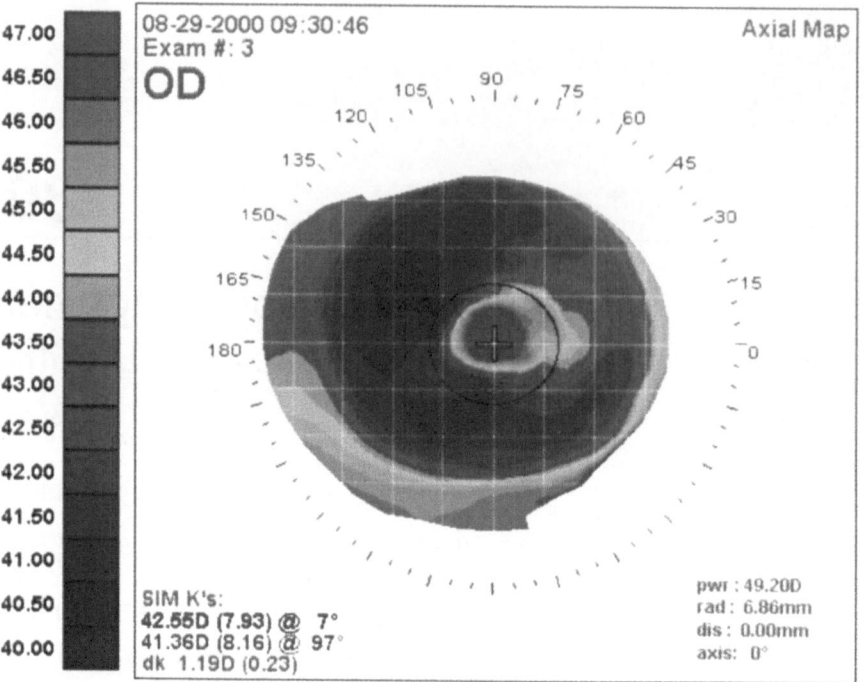

Figure 30.1   Central island occurring after LASIK.

1.5 mm in diameter and 3.0 diopters in height noted with corneal topography (8). The definition has changed over the years and we now understand that any central area of steepening may induce irregular astigmatism and interfere with visual acuity (Fig. 30.1).

While central islands tend to resolve in most patients following PRK (9,10), they may be more likely to persist following LASIK (11,12). One recent review showed an incidence of central islands of 5.7% following LASIK, and only 25% of those resolved over a 6 month period (13). Because of the limited regression that may occur in these patients, surgical intervention is often required.

1. Nonsurgical Management

Prior to attempting surgical intervention, monitoring the patient for 6 months may be valuable to determine if regression or progression of the central island has occurred. Partial improvement in symptoms (shadows, double vision, decreased contract sensitivity, etc.), uncorrected visual acuity (UCVA), best spectacle corrected visual acuity (BSCVA), and topographical appearance (Figs. 30.2A and 30.2B) are all signs that further monitoring may be required. It is often difficult to differentiate between a true central island and corneal ectasia. The latter is less likely to show substantial improvement with time. In fact, corneal ectasia is often a progressive condition that may worsen if retreatment is attempted. Therefore if improvement in symptoms and central island appearance occur during this follow-up period, it is more likely the patient has a true central island as opposed to a psuedo–central island caused by corneal ectasia.

During this follow-up period, patient education regarding the occurrence and natural progression of central islands is critical in alleviating the frustration resulting from reduced quality of vision. After PRK, epithelial hyperplasia in the mid-peripheral area surrounding the central island and epithelial thinning overlying the central island may lead to complete topographical and visual improvement (10,14). Furthermore, treatment of residual central islands after PRK is less likely to induce corneal ectasia because of the greater residual stromal thickness present following PRK. Because LASIK is associated with a decreased epithelial healing response as compared to PRK, central island regression after LASIK may occur more slowly and retreatment may carry greater risk, especially if the residual stromal bed is relatively thin.

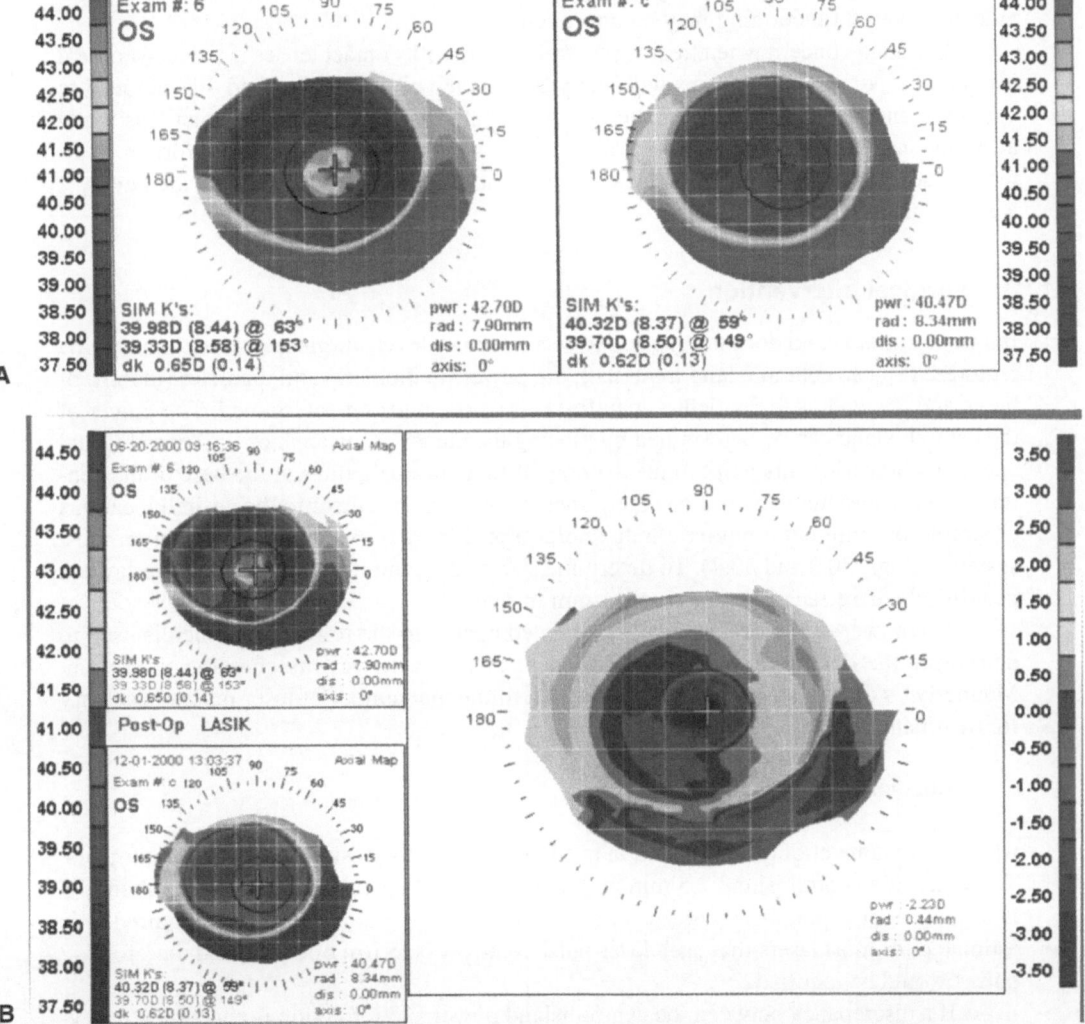

Figure 30.2 Improvement of central island over time. (A) Central island occurring immediately following LASIK with topographical improvement 6 months later. (B) Difference map showing regression of central island over the 6 month period.

During this time, the patient may benefit from wearing a contact lens to improve visual functioning. Often a rigid gas permeable contact lens is required. Standard design RGPs may be adequate with a base curve chosen slightly steeper than the postoperative central corneal curve (15). This will likely yield a fluorescein pattern with mild central pooling and mid-peripheral alignment (15–17). Mid-peripheral alignment should be the goal when fitting these lenses, as this will be the area of the cornea supporting the contact lens. If a satisfactory fit is not achieved due to the corneal shape change induced by LASIK, then specialty RGP designs may be required. Reverse geometry lenses, in which the central base curve is flatter than the surrounding steeper peripheral curves, are available (18).

If the patient is intolerant to RGP contact lenses, a soft toric contact lens may be tried (19). A careful refraction is necessary to detect fully the amount of astigmatism that these central islands can create. Correcting a significant portion of this astigmatism in a soft toric contact lens may not provide the crisp, consistent visual acuity that an RGP lens could provide, but overall functioning may be improved.

The main concern when treating central islands with contact lenses is induced corneal irregularity. A rigid contact lens will likely bear on the central island, and this can lead to curvature and elevation changes. Therefore, if a patient is fitted with a contact lens while awaiting surgical intervention, removal of the lens for 2 to 4 weeks prior to further treatment is advisable. Serial topographies and repeat refractions should be performed every 2 weeks until stability is confirmed.

2. Surgical Intervention

If a true central island does not regress to a satisfactory level, surgical intervention may be required. Prior to central island treatment, the power (in diopters) and diameter (in mm) of the island, as well as the patient's manifest refraction, must be determined. The power of the central island can be determined by placing the cursor at the apex of the central island and then comparing this point to the average of four cardinal points at the base of the central island. These numbers can be determined by moving the cursor to the desired locations or simply printing out a numeric map and/or a profile map (which are available on most systems) (Figs. 30.3 and 30.4). To determine size of the central island, the grid overlay can be utilized where each box represents 1 mm in size.

The power of the central island is then compared to the refraction, which is used to determine the desired correction. If the central island power matches the refraction, Munnerlyn's equation (20) can be used to determine the number of laser pulses necessary for treatment:

$$\text{Ablation depth} = \frac{S^2 * D}{3}$$

where S = diameter of central island in millimeters and D = desired correction in diopters. Therefore, if a central island 2.5 mm in diameter and 5 diopters in height has resulted in 5 D of induced myopia, then 10.41 μm ($2.5^2 * (5/3)$) of tissue ablation will be required. It is estimated for most lasers that each laser pulse removes 0.25 μm of tissue, and therefore 42 pulses would be required.

If a discrepancy between the central island power and refraction is encountered, several authors have advocated using the central island power instead of refraction and overcompensating for the estimated height of the central island when using Munnerlyn's equation (i.e., multiply the central island height D by 1.5). This would be done in order to avoid

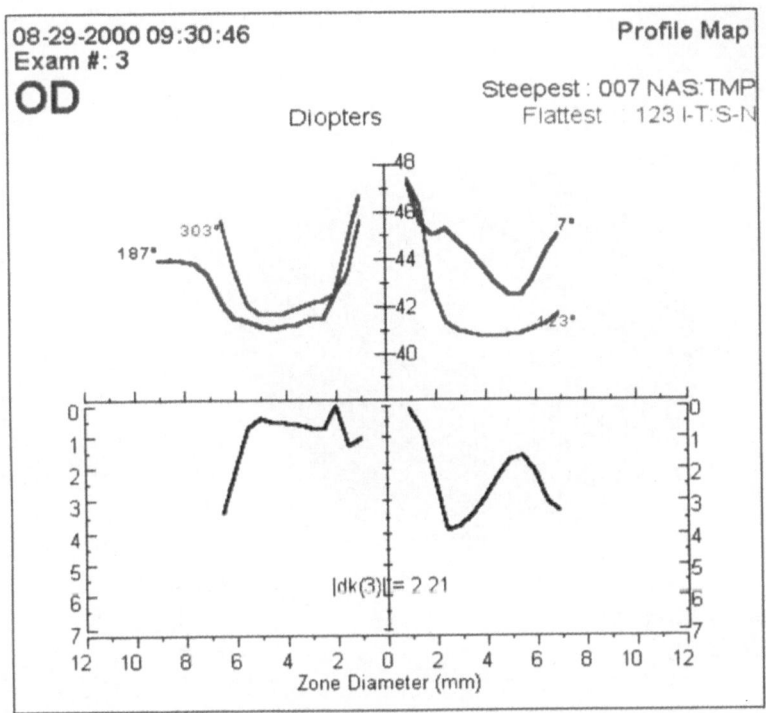

Figure 30.3　Profile map showing a 5–6 diopter (approximately) central island.

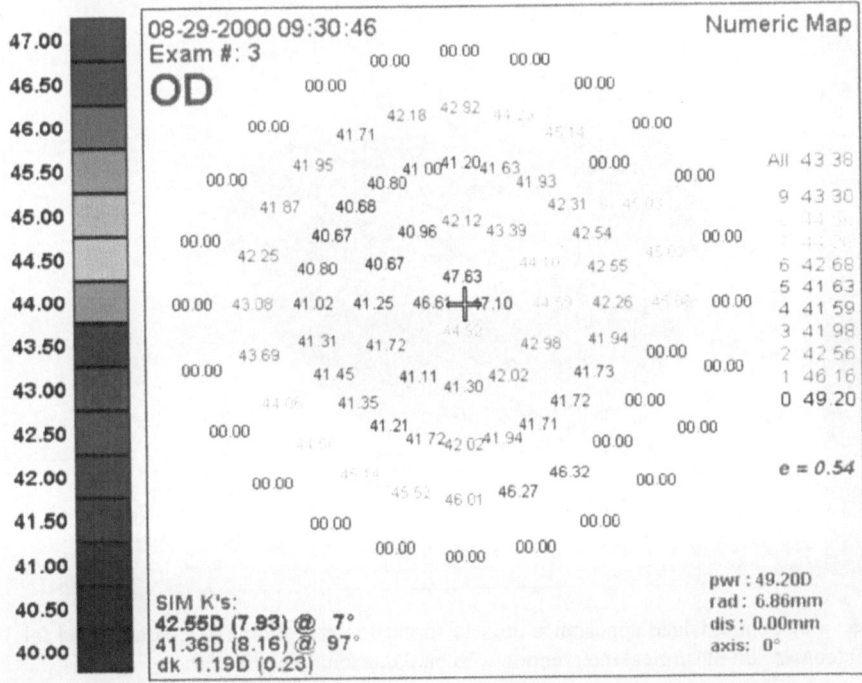

Figure 30.4　Numeric map showing same central island as in Fig. 3, confirming approximate height of 5 diopters.

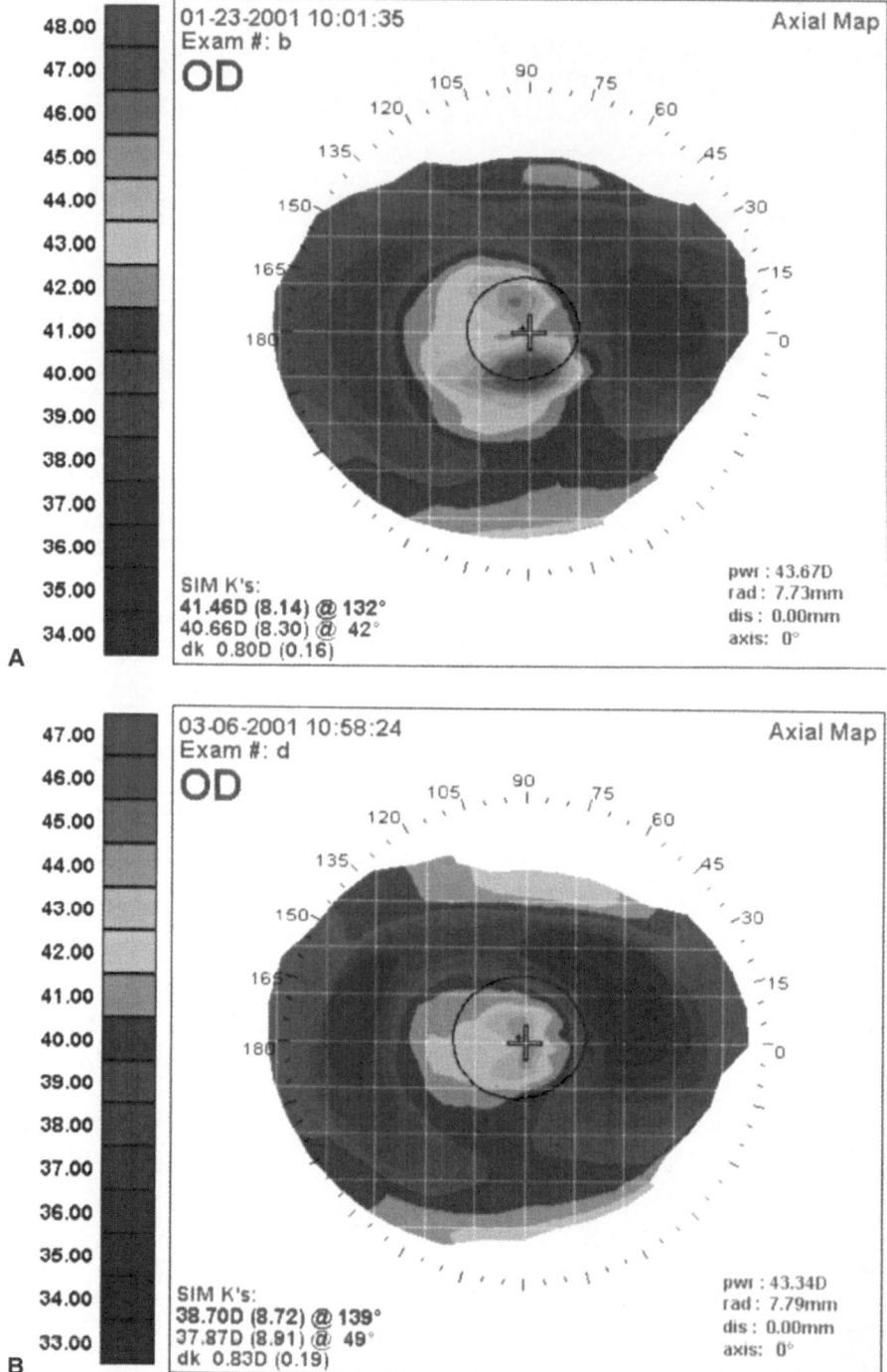

Figure 30.5 (A) Central island appearance prior to surgical intervention. (B) Central island following initial (conservative) surgical intervention with partial resolution of island.

undercorrection (21,22) and the laser would be set to PTK mode. In the example above, the number of laser pulses would increase from 42 to 63. While this is only a minor increase in the number of pulses, our strategy is to approach these cases in a conservative manner and limit treatment to PRK mode based upon reproducible refraction, if available. Further CI treatment can be applied in the future if undercorrection of the island occurs (Fig. 30.5A and 30.5B).

Several caveats must be considered when determining the required refractive correction. If the central island is visible on elevation-based topography and the estimated number of pulses determined using Munnerlyn's equation correlates with the manifest refraction, then eliminating the central island may lead to satisfactory improvement of UCVA after a single treatment. More likely, the irregular astigmatism and decreased BSCVA associated with the CI may have created a variable refraction that is not extremely accurate. If the central island's power and diameter predicts a significantly different number of laser pulses as compared to the manifest refraction, then the treatment may require a two-step approach. The central island should be treated based upon the refractive data and the prescription monitored during follow-up visits. If this process topographically eliminates the central island, yet a refractive error still exists, then further ablation may be required after corneal stabilization is established 3 to 6 months later.

Again, these ablations should be performed in PRK mode owing to the smooth ablation profile that PRK creates. While PTK allows for the ablation zone diameter to be programmed in 0.1 mm steps from 2.0 to 6.5 mm, it may create abrupt treatment edges. In PRK mode, the treatment should be halted when the ablation diameter reaches the predetermined diameter of the central island (which is determined by monitoring the number of pulses using a wide area ablation laser).

In the future, topography-linked lasers may lead to improved outcomes when treating central islands (23,24). The ability to link the topographical data directly to a scanning spot laser may eliminate or reduce the estimation errors that can occur with current treatment equations. Furthermore, a topography-linked system could aid in centering the treatment directly over the central island. Ideally, such treatments would allow for topographical analysis to be performed once the LASIK flap has been retracted, so that the true curvature of the stromal bed could be obtained (25). Trials are currently underway utilizing topography-linked laser treatments, although early results have been somewhat equivocal (26).

Wave front analysis will also become more important in the future when assessing central island position and optical effect. Currently, a patient with a central island is monitored based upon subjective symptoms and elevation-based topographical analysis. As wave front technology becomes more commonplace, we will be able to understand better the amount of distortion that a specific central island is creating. This may allow for improved monitoring of the patient, as it is a further objective measurement of possible regression of the central island.

3. Prevention

While no single etiology has been proven, several preventative strategies for central islands do exist. First, newer laser ablation profiles (scanning lasers) seem to have reduced the incidence of central islands (27). Secondly, many laser companies have developed algorithms in which a series of laser pulses is initially applied to the central stromal bed. These pulses are applied just prior to the actual prescriptive ablation and can be performed in PRK or PTK mode. This anti-island software is available on all of today's commercially available wide-area ablation excimer lasers. Also, when performing highly myopic treatments, intraoperative wiping of the stromal bed is often recommended to reduce the risk of fluid and cellular debris accumulation. This buildup can adversely affect the uniformity of the laser ablation and has been implicated in the formation of central islands. Minimizing the time between flap creation and laser treatment is also important in order to prevent localized differences in stromal bed hydration levels. Finally, proper laser maintenance and strict adherence to calibration will help prevent equipment errors that may be contributing to this problem.

B. DECENTRATION

Ablation decentration can occur following LASIK owing to misalignment of the laser treatment over the patient's entrance pupil or from involuntary eye movement of the patient during laser treatment (Fig. 30.6) (28,29). Decentration can lead to patient symptoms of monocular diplopia, shadows, glare, and reduced contrast sensitivity (both high and low contrast) (30). These complications are often due to induced irregular astigmatism and are associated with a loss of best spectacle corrected visual acuity. While slight decentration typically will cause no patient complaints (31), significant decentration can be problematical.

Ablation decentration should be differentiated from intraoperative treatment drift, a complication that can occur if the surgeon attempts to compensate intraoperatively for an observed decentration (Fig. 30.7) (31). Treatment drift can result in an uneven ablation profile with a flatter treatment zone shifted peripherally. If the treatment drift is due to

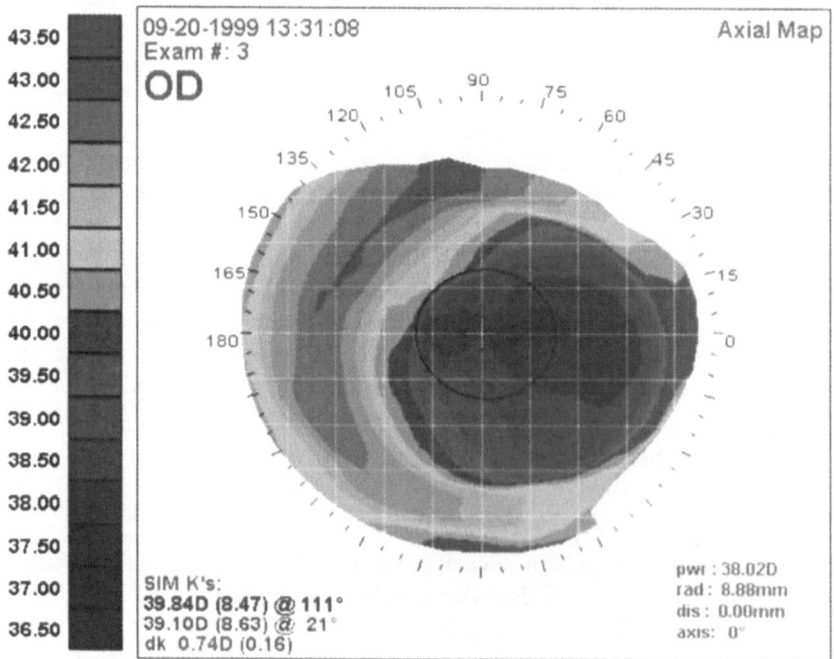

Figure 30.6 Nasal decentration of ablation following LASIK.

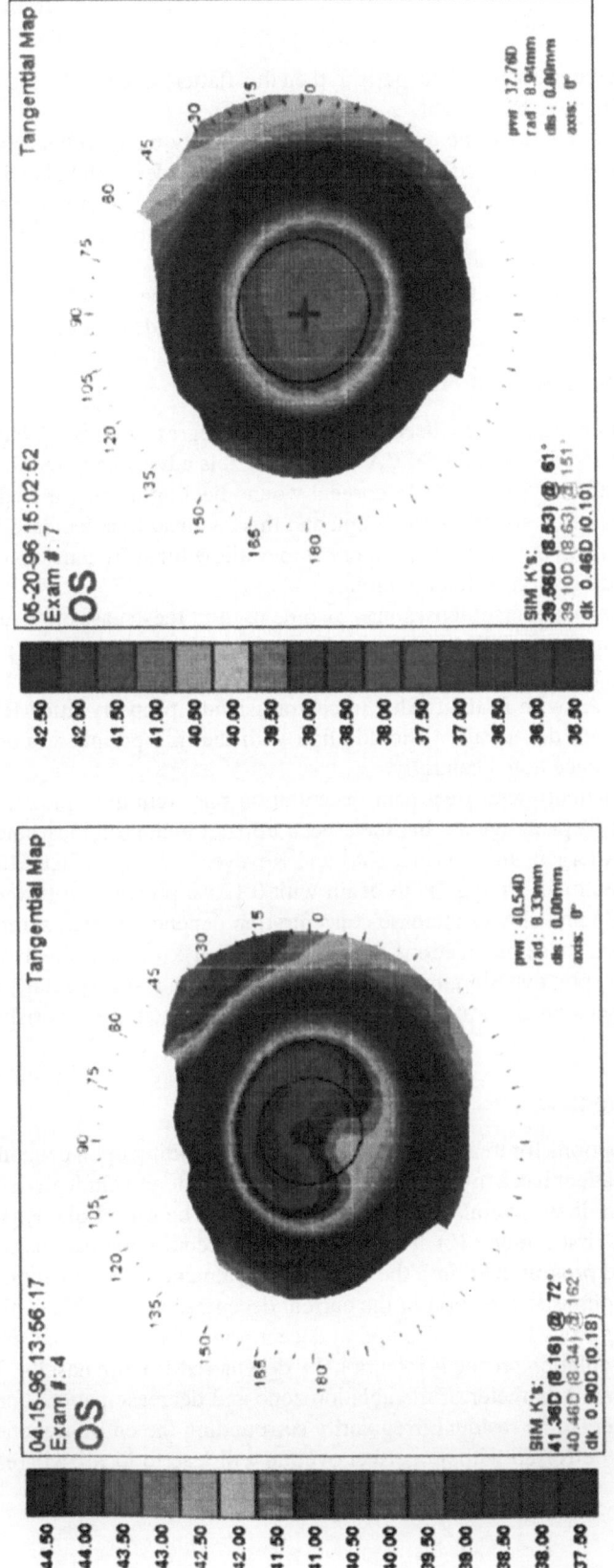

Figure 30.7 Treatment drift is illustrated (left) with a contrasting illustration of a centered laser treatment after PRK (right). The two patients were treated with similar number of pulses for similar preoperative refractive errors, but ended with different topographical maps. The phenomenon of intraoperative treatment drift is best illustrated with tangential topography and is best avoided using a tracking laser. (From Ref. 31.)

involuntary eye movements made by the patient, then this flatter zone will be located in the direction opposite to the eye movement.

Treatment decentration can be evaluated topographically using either axial or tangential maps. As has been discussed elsewhere, axial data provides a global estimation of the corneal curvature while tangential data provides a more precise estimation of each point on the corneal surface. Therefore, it is recommended that tangential maps be utilized to monitor treatment decentration and drift (31).

Although ablation decentration and laser drift can be difficult to manage, a similar general management approach as was discussed with central islands applies to these cases.

1. Nonsurgical Management

Unlike some cases of central islands, decentration will not regress with time. However, if irregular astigmatism and decreased BSCVA are present, it is advisable to monitor the patient for a minimum of 3 to 6 months. As corneal wound healing occurs, the edge of the treatment zone may become slightly less abrupt, and this can lead to a decrease in patient complaints. While this will not solve the problem, it may allow for sufficient subjective improvement, thus avoiding surgical intervention.

Rigid gas permeable contact lenses may also be used in these cases to decrease patient complaints and increase BCVA. The anterior surface of the contact lens provides a smooth refracting surface, while the posterior curvature allows for tear neutralization of the corneal irregularities. As with RGPs fit due to central islands, properly fitted RGPs on a post-LASIK patient with decentration should align with the mid-peripheral cornea with mild to moderate clearance noted centrally.

Finally, some patients with treatment decentration may require topical miotics to eliminate complaints. Topical agents that have been utilized include pilocarpine, Alphagan® (brimonidine, Allergan, Inc., Irvine, CA) and Reveyes® (dapiprazolen HCl 0.5%). Our recommended treatment strategy is to begin with 0.125% pilocarpine (titrated down from the available 1%) and slowly increase concentration depending upon symptomatology. Keep in mind that these medications do carry a small risk of side effects including stinging and irritation upon insertion, browache, accommodative loss (especially in young patients) and retinal detachment. Patients need to be fully informed of these risks prior to initiating use.

2. Surgical Intervention

The current surgical options for treating decentration vary depending upon concomitant refractive error. If the patient has a myopic residual refractive error and clinically significant treatment decentration, then several treatment options exist. The use of diametrically opposed ablations is the first option (32). To perform this procedure, the residual refractive error is calculated and programmed into the laser. The treatment is then intentionally decentered in the exact opposite direction of the current decentration (Fig. 30.8). For example, if a patient suffers from 1.5 mm of temporal decentration, then the enhancement procedure with a myopic ablation profile is intentionally decentered 1.5 mm nasally. This may act to increase the overall diameter of the ablation zone and decrease patient complaints. There will be, however, some residual irregularity surrounding the entire treatment zone, as two laser ablations delivered without perfect overlap will lead to localized areas of differing curvature.

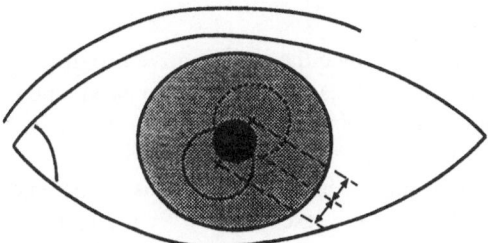

Figure 30.8   Diametral ablation. (From Ref. 32.)

The second option is to mask the original ablation zone and apply further laser pulses to the surrounding tissue in an attempt to increase overall ablation zone diameter. Rachid et al. have recently shown improvement in decentration following PRK by using the epithelium as a masking agent with a transepithelial ablation. The treatments were guided by epithelial fluorescence in PTK mode and resulted in significant improvement in ablation centration (33). Talamo et al. described a similar technique following PRK (34), but the ablation zone was masked with a modulating agent instead of the corneal epithelium. This use of a modulating agent can be modified slightly for decentration following LASIK. Following flap retraction, fluid is added to the area of the original ablation and a murocel sponge is used to provide further protection to this area of the stromal bed. Reablation is then performed in a direction exactly opposite to the original ablation. The excimer pulses are therefore applied to the surrounding stromal bed that was not ablated during the original treatment. By masking the original ablation zone with a modulating agent, less refractive effect will be induced as compared to the procedure described above. Therefore, this technique is recommended when only minimal to no residual refractive error remains following the initial treatment.

A further option that is currently under investigation is to obtain elevation based topography and/or wave front analysis to guide the laser ablation (26). As has been discussed, these techniques produce variable results, and deferring a retreatment procedure in a severely decentered eye until advanced techniques are available may be the best option at this time.

Myopic ablation decentration with a residual hyperopic refractive error (overcorrection) can be more difficult to treat surgically. In this case, the central ablation zone is already flatter than it should be for the patient's specific refractive error. Any further tissue removal will result in increased overcorrection and further hyperopia. This situation requires a two-step treatment process in which the first step is similar to those discussed above. The ablation decentration is recentered using a modulating agent and peripheral laser pulses. Once the ablation has been recentered, the patient is monitored for several months while the refractive error stabilizes. Once refractive stability is achieved, a hyperopic enhancement procedure can be performed to address refractive needs.

Alternatively, the sequence may be reversed, in which a hyperopic treatment is performed in order to correct the residual refractive error. This hyperopic ablation expands the peripheral optical zone and may, in itself, alleviate patient complaints. If clinically significant decentration is still noted following hyperopic ablation, correction of this decentration may be attempted utilizing the techniques discussed above.

3. Prevention

The incidence of treatment decentration has decreased since the preoperative use of pilo-carpine has been discontinued. Pilocarpine causes a nasal displacement of the pupil, and if the laser ablation is centered over this pharmacologically displaced pupil, decentration will occur. When the pupil returns to normal position and size, a treatment that was perfectly centered intraoperatively is now considered displaced. Decentration also tends to decrease as surgeon experience increases. Consistently aligning the laser beam over the entrance pupil prior to beginning the ablation process is key to avoiding such a complication. Providing the patient feedback throughout the treatment is also important in preventing involuntary eye movements. Furthermore, if a small amount of decentration is noted intraoperatively, it is best to not make corrective movements (31). This can create laser drift, which can also induce irregular astigmatism. If significant decentration is noted intraoperatively, realignment may be necessary.

Finally, eye trackers are becoming more prevalent and will likely become standard in the future. These systems employ either laser or video monitoring of the pupillary margin and allow the laser to adjust position in conjunction with any eye movements. While sampling rates of up to 4,000 Hz have been achieved with the LADARVision® laser eye tracking system by Alcon-Summit-Autonomous, true response rates are slower in both laser and video systems. Studies have shown that patients' eye movements average 0.4 mm with passive fixation, and this amount may be reduced to 0.1 mm or less with the use of an active eye tracker (35). Therefore this technology will provide further protection against decentration-induced loss of BSCVA and the various symptoms that coincide with this complication.

C. IRREGULAR ASTIGMATISM

There are numerous etiologies of irregular astigmatism in patients after LASIK. The possible explanations can be broken down into three broad categories: preoperative/preexisting irregular astigmatism, intraoperative/induced irregular astigmatism, and postoperative irregular astigmatism. Preoperative irregular astigmatism can be noted in several situations including keratoconus, high myopia, and generalized preexisting irregular astigmatism. Intraoperative causes of irregular astigmatism include poor laser optics, nonuniform stromal bed hydration, irregular flap creation (including flap buttonholes, thin flaps, lost flap, etc.), and irregular corneal wound healing. Central islands and ablation decentration are two forms of intraoperative irregular astigmatism that have been discussed previously. Postoperative irregular astigmatism can be noted following flap displacement (including flap folds and wrinkles) or in the context of progressive corneal ectasia.

Preoperative irregular astigmatism should generally be approached in a conservative manner, surgery being deferred at this time. With current laser technology, treatment of an irregular surface will likely transfer this irregularity to a lower depth within the cornea. Topography-linked and wave front–linked laser treatments utilizing a scanning-spot beam profile may allow for the treatment of such irregular astigmatism in the future, but these studies are only recently underway.

The current treatment options for induced irregular astigmatism are limited. The best option may also be to defer a retreatment procedure until topography-linked or wave front-linked treatments become standard. Consideration should be given to rigid gas permeable contact lens wear pending such laser advances. As discussed previously, some specific forms of induced irregular astigmatism such as central islands and ablation decentration may be amenable to further treatment with current laser technology, but these results are often variable.

Posterior corneal ectasia can cause irregular astigmatism, as is evident in keratoconus and other ectactic corneal disorders. Following LASIK, if irregular astigmatism is noted, posterior ectasia must be suspected, and this problem would only be exacerbated with further laser treatment. Therefore, prior to attempting surgical treatment of irregular astigmatism, residual corneal thickness needs to be considered. The current assumption is that a residual stromal bed of 250 μm or more should prevent corneal ectasia following refractive surgery. Several case reports have been published, however, showing corneal ectasia in patients with a residual stromal bed measurement of greater than 250 μm (36–38). Furthermore, Buzard et al. have recently shown that LASIK performed on ectactic eyes (keratoconus) often will cause progression to the point of requiring penetrating keratoplasty (39). Because of this, when the 250 μm limit is approached and irregular astigmatism is present, posterior corneal ectasia should be suspected. The only way in which the residual stromal bed thickness can be known is if pachymetry measurements are taken preoperatively and intraoperatively. Flap thickness can vary significantly between patients even when the same depth plates are used on the same microkeratome. Therefore, following flap dissection, stromal bed thickness should be measured utilizing a high-frequency ultrasound pachymeter prior to laser ablation. The depth of ablation can then simply be subtracted from this measurement to determine the residual stromal bed thickness.

Regardless of residual stromal bed thickness, posterior corneal ectasia can also be evaluated using the Orbscan corneal topographer. While the optical pachymetry reading generated by this system will give an overall thickness of the cornea, it will not differentiate residual stromal bed and overlying flap thickness. Therefore the overall residual corneal thickness and depth plate used to create the corneal flap can be used to estimate residual stromal bed thickness but will not give a definitive measurement. Posterior corneal elevation can also be observed with the Orbscan, and this aids in the diagnosis of posterior corneal ectasia. If the posterior elevation map shows a forward bowing of the posterior corneal surface, then posterior ectasia may be present and further laser ablation would be contraindicated (Figs. 30.9A and 30.9B).

Once posterior corneal ectasia is ruled out as a possible explanation for postoperative irregular astigmatism, regularity of the flap should be closely evaluated. Small flap striae, no matter how mild, can induce irregular astigmatism. The flap should be carefully inspected under high illumination and with retroillumination through a dilated pupil (Fig. 30.10). If striae are present, even mild, they should be attended to prior to any laser ablation. When attempting to treat flap striae, a two-step approach should be considered.

The first step is accomplished by lifting the corneal flap in an effort to smooth any irregularity. The flap is hydrated with a relatively hypotonic solution to cause mild edema prior to repositioning of the flap. This slight swelling of the flap may help to eliminate any striae present. Once the flap has been repositioned, the second step involves scraping the overlying epithelium in an attempt to eliminate any fixed folds. When folds and striae occur, overlying epithelial extension may occur, leading to an anchoring of these folds in a fixed position. By scraping the overlying epithelium, the tension created by this anchoring is released and can aid in the elimination of these folds or striae. Following epithelial scraping, flap ironing should be performed in a direction perpendicular to the folds. Instruments

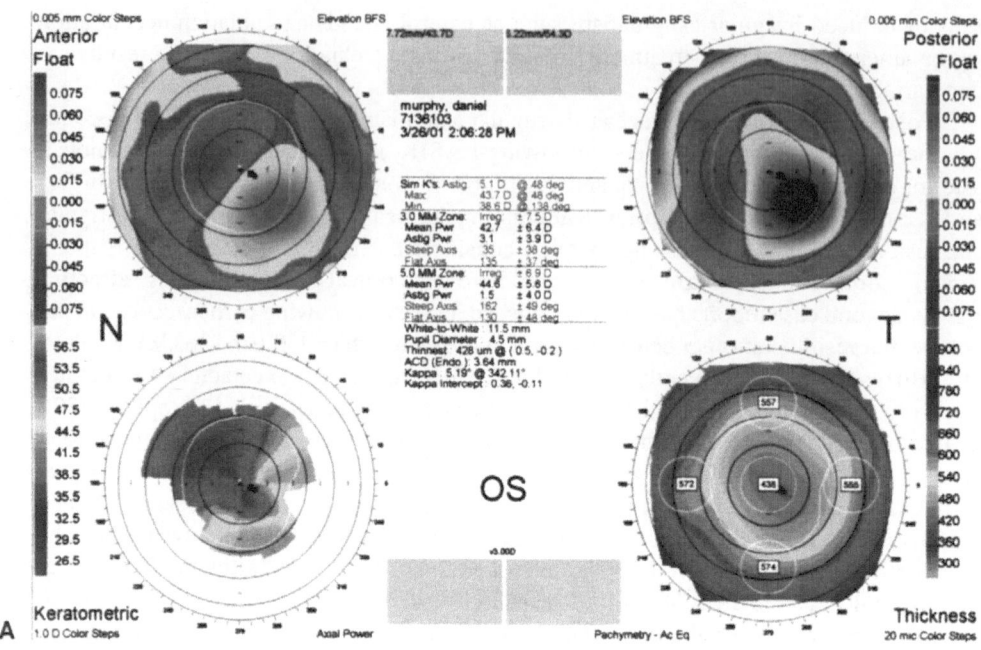

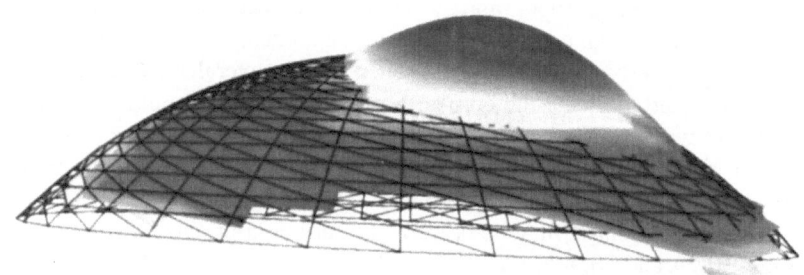

Figure 30.9 Forward bowing of the posterior corneal service. In this situation, additional laser treatment should be avoided.

specifically designed for these procedures, including the Pineda LASIK iron (American Surgical Instruments Corporation, Westmont, IL), can be utilized, or a murocel sponge may suffice.

Once the issue of flap striae is addressed, visual acuity and corneal topography are monitored for improvement. If improvement in flap appearance does not provide sufficient visual acuity improvement, and topographical evidence of irregular astigmatism persists, then the previous guidelines regarding irregular astigmatism apply.

If deferring further laser treatment is not possible and irregular astigmatism treatment is to be attempted, the most common method is to use a modulating agent to absorb selectively a portion of the laser beam energy. Once the corneal flap is retracted, a small amount of moderately viscous fluid is placed on the stromal bed. Examples of appropriate solutions include 0.1% dextran 70 (Tears Naturale II, Alcon Opthalmics, Fort Worth, TX) and car-

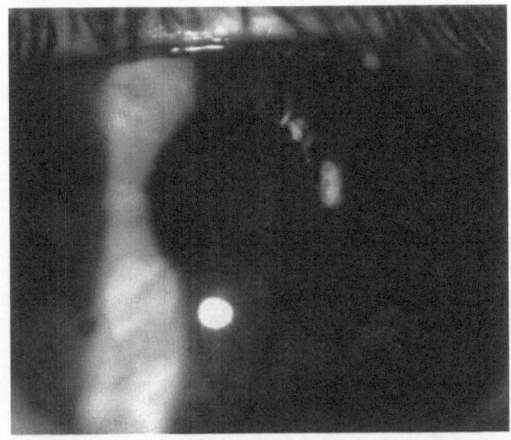

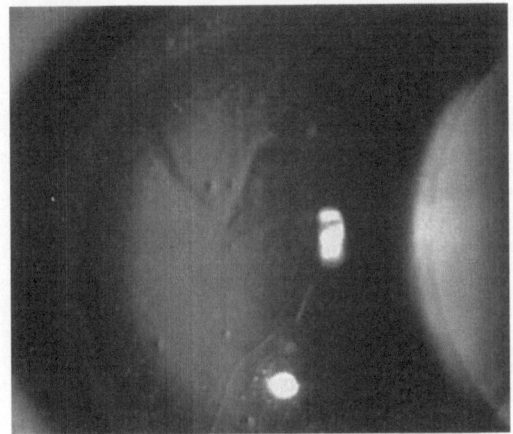

Figure 30.10 Prior to pupillary dilatation, the corneal striae are barely visible (top). After dilatation, retroillumination facilitates visualization of the striae (bottom).

boxymethylcellulose sodium (Celluvisc, Allergan Pharmaceuticals, Irvine, CA) (40). This solution should then be lightly dispersed over the stromal bed using a lint-free sponge (such as a merocel spear) to distribute the fluid evenly. The goal is to allow the modulating agent to pool in the low spots on the irregular stromal surface and transiently produce a smooth corneal surface. The laser treatment is then applied, and the high corneal points are ablated, while the lower points are protected by the pooled fluid, which selectively absorbs the laser energy. Following laser application, the high points will have been eliminated, while the lower points remain unaffected and a more regular stromal surface is created.

Again, corneal topography and manifest refraction should be monitored for stabilization. Once stabilization occurs, further laser application, if necessary, can be performed for a refractive effect. This would be the final step in the process of eliminating irregular astigmatism. While in theory this approach should successfully eliminate any irregular astigmatism, clinically it is not always successful. A conservative approach is necessary in these cases, and for some patients deferring further treatment may be the best option.

REFERENCES

1. SG Farah, DT Azar, C Gurdal, J Wong. Laser in situ keratomileusis: literature review of a developing technique. J Cataract Refract Surg 1998;24:989–1006.
2. SW Kang, ES Chung, WJ Kim. Clinical analysis of central islands after laser in situ keratomileusis. J Cataract Refract Surg 2000;26(4):536–542.
3. PS Hersh, KS Scher, R Irani. Corneal topography of photorefractive keratectomy versus laser in situ keratomileusis. Ophthalmology 1998;105:612–619.
4. S Levin, CA Carson, SK Garrett, HR Taylor. Prevalence of central islands after excimer laser refractive surgery. J Cataract Refract Surg 1995;21:21–26.
5. A El-Maghraby, T Salah, GO Waring III, S Klyce, O Ibrahim. Randomized bilateral comparison of excimer laser in situ keratomileusis and photrefractive keratectomy for 2.50 to 8.00 diopters of myopia. Ophthalmology 1999;106:447–457.
6. MC Knorz, B Wiesinger, A Liermann, V Seiberth, H Liesenhoff. Laser in situ keratomileusis for moderate and high myopia and myopic astigmatism. Ophthalmology 1998;105:932–940.
7. MC Knorz, A Liermann, V Seiberth, H Steiner, B Wiesinger. Laser in situ keratomileusis to correct myopia of −6.00 to −29.00 diopters. J Refract Surg 1996;12:575–584.
8. RR Krueger, NF Saedy, PJ McDonnell. Clinical analysis of steep central islands after excimer laser photorefractive keratectomy. Arch Ophthalmol 1996;114:377–381.
9. DTC Lin. Corneal topographic analysis after excimer photorefractive keratectomy. Ophthalmology 1994;101:1432–1439.
10. CNJ McGhee, IC Bryce. Natural history of central topographic islands following excimer laser photorefractive keratectomy. J Cataract Refract Surg 1996;22:1151–1158.
11. SE Wilson. LASIK: management of common complications. Cornea 1998;17:459–467.
12. L Probst. Response. In: T Kohnen, ed. Consultations section: refractive surgical problem. J Cataract Refract Surg 1998;24:1177–1178.
13. Y Tsai, JM Lin. Natural history of central islands after laser in situ keratomileusis. J Cataract Refract Surg 2000;26:853–858.
14. EE Manche, RK Maloney, RJ Smith. Treatment of topographic central islands following refractive surgery. J Cataract Refract Surg 1998;24:464–470.
15. LB Szczotka, M Aronsky. Contact lenses after LASIK. J Am Optom Assoc 1998;69:775–784.
16. I Schipper, U Businger, R Pfarrer. Fitting contact lenses after excimer laser photorefractive keratectomy for myopia. CLAO J 1995;21:281–284.
17. K Zadnik. Contact lens management of patients who have had unsuccessful refractive surgery. Current Opinion in Ophthalmology 1999;10:260–263.
18. MA Aronsky, T Aggarwal, WJ Reinhart. Application of videokeratographic data for fitting reverse geometry contact lenses in post–corneal surgery patients. Invest Ophthalmol Vis Sci 1998;39:1545.
19. T Bufidi, AG Konstas, IG Pallikaris. Contact lens fitting difficulties following refractive surgery for high myopia. CLAO J 2000;26:106–110.
20. CR Munnerlyn, SJ Koons, J Marshall. Photorefractive keratectomy: a technique for laser refractive surgery. J Cataract Refract Surg 1988;14:46–52.
21. K Buzzard, BR Fundingsland. Treatment of irregular astigmatism with a broad beam excimer laser. J Refract Surg 1997;13:624–636.
22. JL Alio, A Artola, FA Rodriguez-Mier. Selective zonal ablations with excimer laser for correction of irregular astigmatism induced by refractive surgery. Ophthalmology 2000;107: 662–673.
23. B Seitz, A Langenbucher, MM Kus, M Harrer. Experimental correction of irregular corneal astigmatism using topography based flying-spot-mode excimer laser photoablation. Am J Ophthalmol 1998;125:252–256.
24. B Wiesenger-Jendritza, MC Knorz, P Hugger, A Liermann. Laser in situ keratomileusis assisted by corneal topography. J Cataract Refract Surg 1998;24:166–174.

25. C Moser, J Kampmeier, P McDonnell, D Psaltis. Feasibility of intraoperative corneal topography monitoring during photorefractive keratectomy. J Refract Surg 2000;16:148–154.

26. MC Knorz, B Jendritza. Topographically-guided laser in situ keratomileusis to treat corneal irregularities. Ophthalmology 2000;107:1138–1143.

27. S Wilson. LASIK: management of common complications. Cornea 1998;17(5):459–467.

28. YY Tsai, JM Lin. Ablation centration after active eye-tracker-assisted photorefractive keratectomy and laser in situ keratectomy. J Cataract Refract Surg 2000;26:28–34.

29. JB Lee, JI Jung, YK Chu, JH Lee, EK Kim. Analysis of the factors affecting decentration in photorefractive keratectomy and laser in situ keratomileusis. Yonsei Med J 1999;40:221–225.

30. W Verdon, M Bullimore, RK Maloney. Visual performance after photorefractive keratectomy. Arch Ophthalmol 1996;114:1465–1472.

31. DT Azar, PC Yeh. Corneal topographic evaluation of decentration in photorefractive keratectomy: treatment displacement vs intraoperative drift. Am J Ophthalmol 1997;124:312–320.

32. N Alkar, U Genth, T Seiler. Diametral ablation—a technique to manage decentered photorefractive keratectomy for myopia. J Refract Surg 1999;15:436–440.

33. MD Rachid, SH Yoo, DT Azar. Phototherapeutic keratectomy for decentration and central islands after photorefractive keratectomy. Ophthalmol 2001;108:545–552.

34. JH Talamo, MD Wagoner, SY Lee. Management of ablation decentration following excimer photorefractive keratectomy. Arch Ophthalmol 1995;113:706–707.

35. NM Taylor, RH Eikelboom, PP van Sarloos, PG Reid. Determining the accuracy of an eye tracking system for laser refractive surgery. J Refract Surg 2000;16(5):S643–S646.

36. T Seiler, AW Quurke. Iatrogenic keractasia after LASIK in a case of forme fruste keratoconus. J Cataract Refract Surg 1998;24:1007–1009.

37. T Seiler, K Koufala, G Richter. Iatrogenic keratectasia after laser in situ keratomileusis. J Refract Surg 1998;14:312–317.

38. CFM Schmitt-Bernard, C Lesage, B Arnaud. Keratectasia induced by laser in situ keratomileusis in keratoconus. J Refract Surg 2000;16:368–370.

39. KA Buzard, A Tuengler, JL Febbraro. Treatment of mild to moderate keratoconus with laser in situ keratomileusis. J Cataract Refract Surg 1999;25(12):1600–1609.

40. EW Kornmehl, RF Steinert, CA Puliafito. A comparative study of masking fluids for excimer laser phototherapeutic keratectomy. Arch Ophthalmol 1991;109:860–863.

31

LASIK and TopoLink for Irregular Astigmatism

MICHAEL C. KNORZ

University of Heidelberg, Heidelberg, Germany, and Baylor College of Medicine, Houston, Texas, U.S.A.

Laser in situ keratomileusis has become the procedure of choice in the treatment of low and moderate myopia. In the early days, LASIK was also widely used to treat high myopia (1,2). Decentration of the ablation, central islands in broad-beam lasers, and other factors have contributed to induce irregular astigmatism in a certain number of eyes treated. Irregular astigmatism caused by surface asymmetries of the cornea may only be corrected with hard contact lenses. In many cases fitting of these lenses is very difficult, and many are not tolerated by the patients. The use of a customized ablation pattern like in TopoLink LASIK is aimed just in the same direction. Spot-scanning or flying-spot excimer lasers provide the technological platform to perform ablations of any shape (3). Corneal topography enables us to measure the shape of the individual cornea with great precision. Could we combine corneal topography and scanning lasers to create customized ablations? This question posed quite a challenge when we started to treat our first patients with so-called TopoLink LASIK a few years ago (4). Several systems, including the C-Scan (Technomed Co., Baesweiler, Germany) and the Orbscan II corneal tomography system (Bausch & Lomb Surgical, Claremont, CA) were used. We initially treated eyes that had previously undergone refractive surgery ("repair procedures") (5) and then also included so-called normal eyes, which underwent a routine LASIK procedure. In this chapter, I will describe the technique of TopoLink LASIK based on corneal topography and present some examples as well as the results of the repair procedures and of the normal eyes.

A. TECHNIQUE OF TOPOLINK

Surgical technique involves the use of the Hansatome microkeratome (Bausch & Lomb Surgical, St. Louis, MO) and the Technolas 217 excimer laser (Bausch & Lomb Surgical

Technolas, Munich, Germany) with an active eye tracker. The laser ablation was based on the preoperative corneal topographic map obtained with the Orbscan II corneal analysis system (Bausch & Lomb Surgical, Irvine, CA). Three different maps were taken, and the one featuring the fewest eye movements was used. The maximum eye movement considered acceptable during data acquisition was 200 μm. Patients who did not comply with this requirement owing to poor cooperation were excluded. Once the topography was taken, data were copied and the ablation profile was calculated using a special software called TopoLink (Version 2.9992TL; Bausch & Lomb Surgical Technolas, Munich, Germany). Input values were manifest refraction in minus cylinder format and corneal thickness as measured by the Orbscan II. The target K-value was determined by the software by subtracting the manifest sphere from the K-value in the steep corneal meridian. The target K-value and a preset shape factor of −0.25 defined the target asphere which we planned to achieve after LASIK. The TopoLink software basically compares the shape of the target asphere to the corneal shape actually measured. Simplified, the target shape is fitted from beneath to the actual cornea for a given planned optical zone size. The difference between the two shapes is then ablated. Any overlap between target and actual shape must thus be outside the planned optical zone, as tissue cannot be added but ablated only. The TopoLink software therefore represents a new and different approach that is not based on Munnerlyn's formula. It rather calculates a certain "lenticle" of corneal tissue to be removed, and the scanning laser used provides the means to remove this tissue even if its shape is asymmetrical or even irregular. The diameter of the planned optical zone was 6 to 7 mm. Only if the ablation required to achieve these optical zones left a residual corneal stromal bed of less than 250 μm, the diameter of the planned optical zone was decreased to maintain a residual stromal bed of at least 250 μm. Based on these data, TopoLink calculated a session file that basically contained information for the scanning laser on which ablation pattern to perform. The session file was transferred via disc and loaded into the Keracor 217 excimer laser just prior to treatment. We used the Keracor 217 excimer laser, manufactured by Bausch & Lomb Surgical Technolas, Munich, Germany. This laser uses a 2 mm beam, which is scanned across the cornea at a shot frequency of 50 Hz. It was modified by including an aperture that allows the use of both a 1 mm beam and a 2 mm beam.

B. EXAMPLES OF TOPOLINK

Patient 1. Irregular Astigmatism after PKP and RK

This patient had a penetrating corneal graft because of recurrent stromal herpetic keratitis in 1992. He was first referred in 1993. Manifest refraction was +0.25 sphere −6 cyl axis 135°. Corneal astigmatism was −8 D axis 135° and slightly asymmetric. Initially, astigmatic keratotomy was performed in 1994. After AK, manifest refraction was −2.5 sphere −4 cyl axis 165°. UCVA was 20/400 and BCVA was 20/60. Corneal topography showed marked irregularity and axis shift (Fig. 31.1, upper left, see color insert). We therefore decided to perform TopoLink LASIK. Average refractive power of the cornea overlying the entrance pupil was estimated to be 45 D. The spherical equivalent of manifest refraction was −4.5 D. We therefore selected a target K-value of 40.5 D. A 5.4 mm optical zone was used, and the ablation depth was 150 μ. Corneal thickness was 610 μ centrally, and both the internal and the external margins of the graft were well aligned with the host cornea. It is very important to check alignment prior to the lamellar cut. In poor alignment

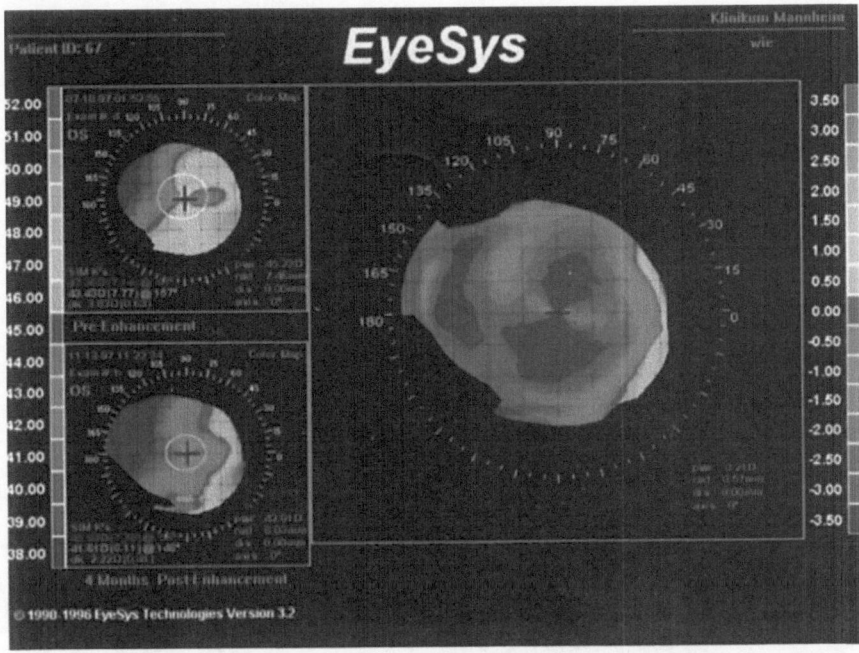

Figure 31.1 Topographic workplace used to design the ablation of patient 1. The preoperative topographic map (scale in diopters) is on the upper left, and the ablation profile suggested by the TopoLink LASIK software (scale in μm) on the upper right. On the lower left, the surgeon can add individual fudge factors, and the expected result is displayed on the lower right hand side.

or localized ectasia at the edge, corneal thickness might be reduced, and the keratome cut may cause further weakening of the cornea, inducing more ectasia, or even a penetration of the anterior chamber. In this patient, alignment was perfect, and the LASIK procedure performed in July 1997 was uneventful. A 160 μ flap was used. One day after TopoLink LASIK, UCVA had improved to 20/30, and BCVA was 20/25 (correction: +0.75 sphere). After 4 months, UCVA was 20/30 and BCVA 20/25, but manifest refraction had changed slightly to +1 sphere −2.0 cyl axis 10°. Corneal topography 4 months after TopoLink LASIK showed marked improvement of the irregularity (Fig. 31.1). Some residual WTR astigmatism was still present, but the irregular astigmatism that was present preoperatively had virtually disappeared, as shown by the differential map (Fig. 31.1, see color insert).

Patient 2. Irregular Astigmatism

This patient had irregular astigmatism due to a peripheral scar caused by a corneal ulcer in prolonged contact lens wear in his right eye. The preoperative topographic map (Fig. 31.2) shows marked asymmetry of the astigmatism. Refraction was −2.5 sphere −0.5 cylinder axis 5°. Uncorrected visual acuity was 20/200, and spectacle-corrected visual acuity was 20/25. We performed a TopoLink LASIK. One month after surgery, uncorrected visual acuity was 20/20 and refraction was plano. Corneal topography showed no irregularities (Fig. 31.3.

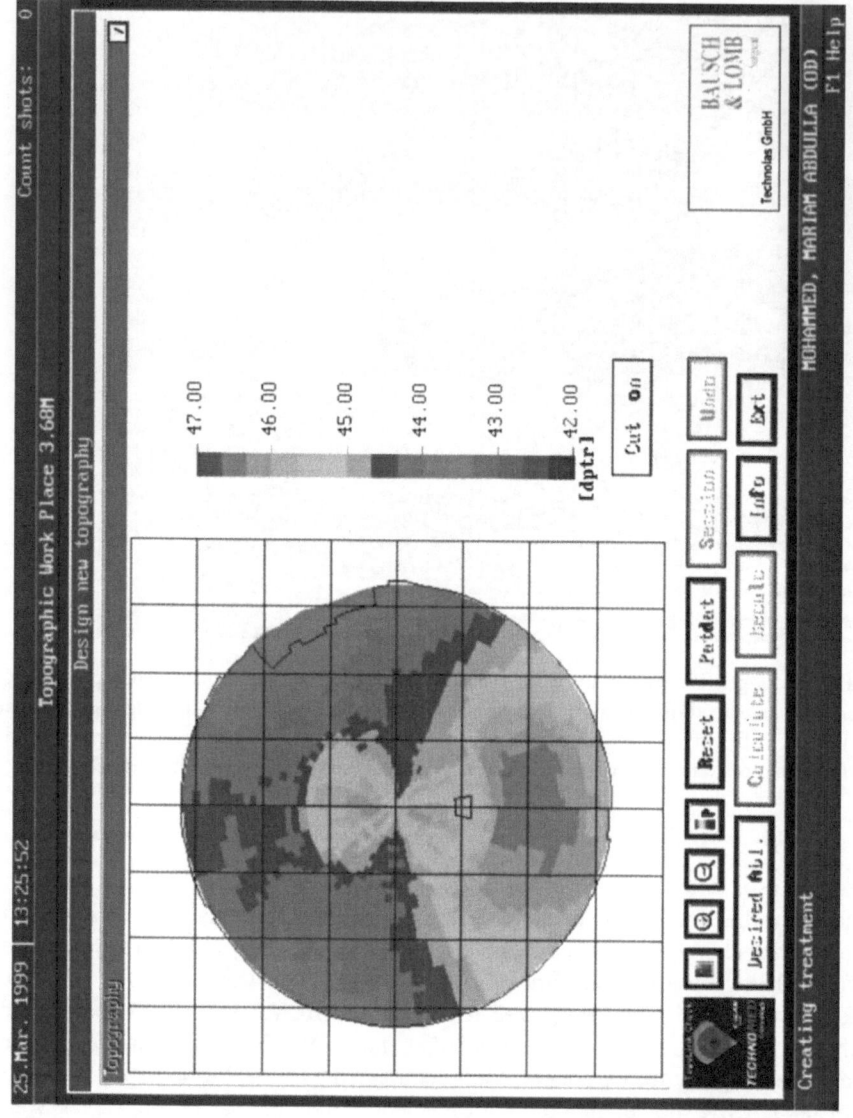

Figure 31.2 Pre- and postoperative topographic maps and differential map of patient 1 (penetrating injury with irregular astigmatism).

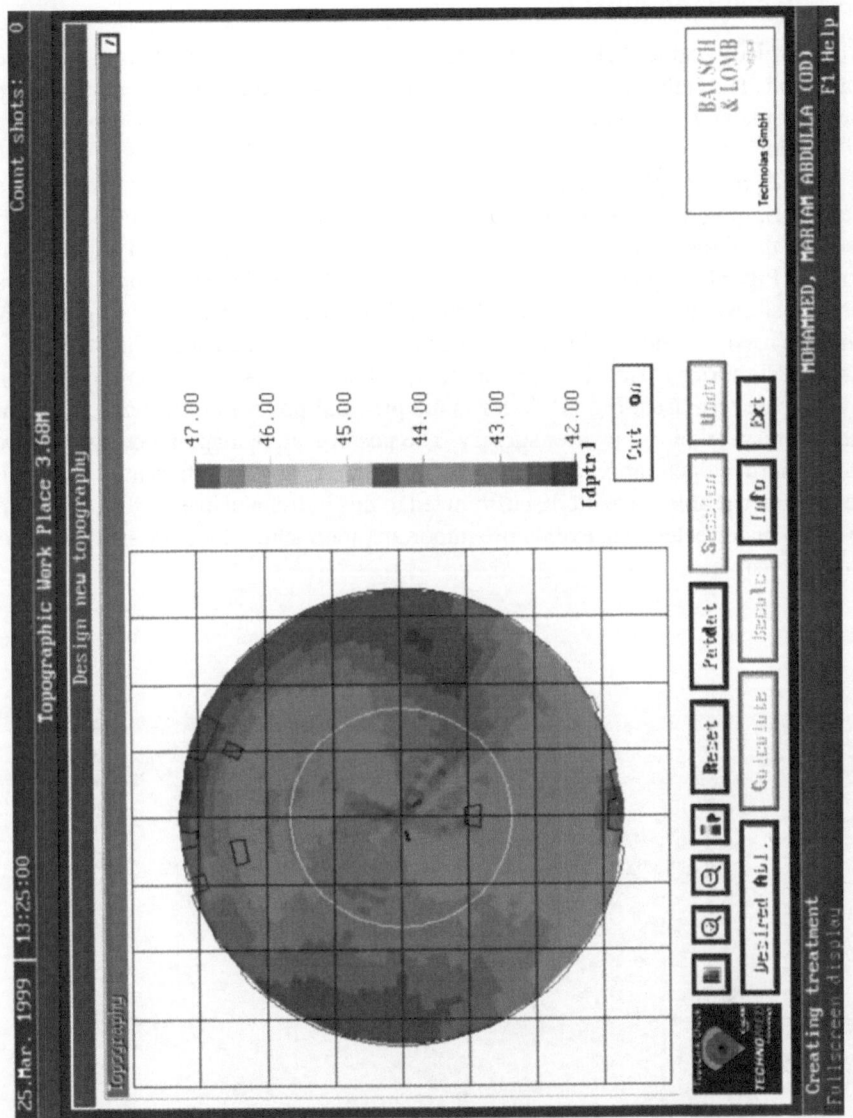

Figure 31.3 Pre- and postoperative topographic maps and differential map of patient 2 (irregular astigmatism after PKP and RK).

Patient 3.   Decentered Ablation

This 36 year old lady had LASIK in both eyes in 1998 and was referred because of a decentered ablation. The right eye was perfect, but she complained bitterly about permanent monocular diplopia and distorted halos in her left eye. A TopoLink LASIK was planned. The corneal topography taken prior to the TopoLink LASIK is shown in Fig. 31.4, lower left, and Fig. 31.5, lower right. A decentered myopic ablation is visible. The ablation is decentered about 1.5 mm downward and 1 mm temporally. We calculated a customized ablation based on the Orbscan II topographic map just described. The planned ablation pattern is shown in Fig. 31.4, upper right. The scale is in μm. The predicted outcome of corneal topography is shown in Fig. 31.4, lower right. The scale is in diopters again. The Hansatome was used to create a new flap with a thickness of 160 μm and a diameter of 8.5 mm (8.5 mm suction ring). The ablation was centered on the center of the entrance pupil, and the eye tracker was used. Fig. 31.5 shows the pre- and postoperative maps as well as the differential map, taken 1 day after surgery. The postoperative map, upper right, shows significantly improved centration and no residual astigmatism. The differential map, left, shows the asymmetric ablation pattern, customized to this individual eye. Visual acuity improved to 20/25 uncorrected, and even more important, monocular double vision and halos were no longer visible.

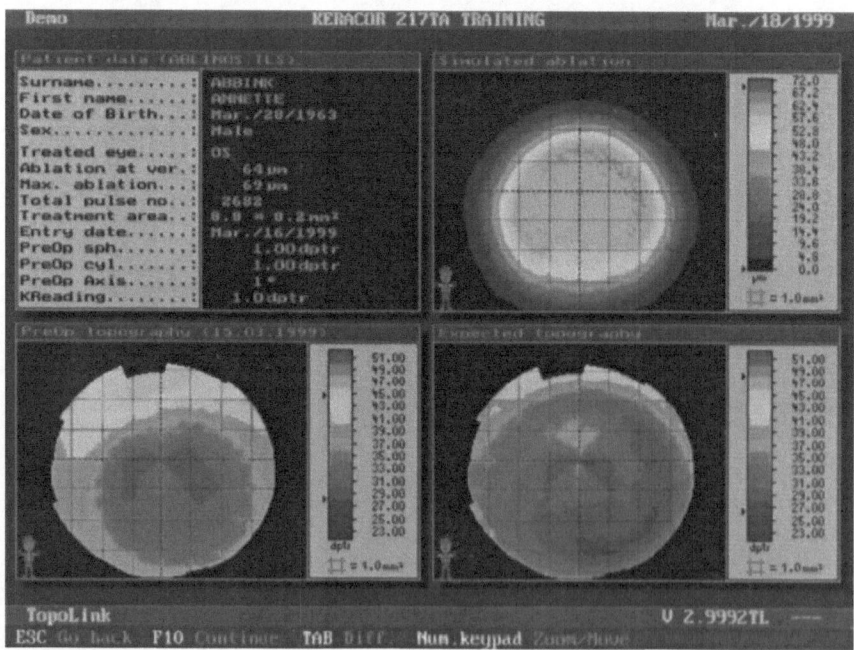

Figure 31.4   Treatment plan in TopoLink LASIK. This plan is shown on the screen of the Keracor 217 excimer laser when the treatment is loaded. It features patient data, upper left, preoperative topography, lower left, the simulated ablation pattern, upper right, and the expected postoperative topography, lower right.

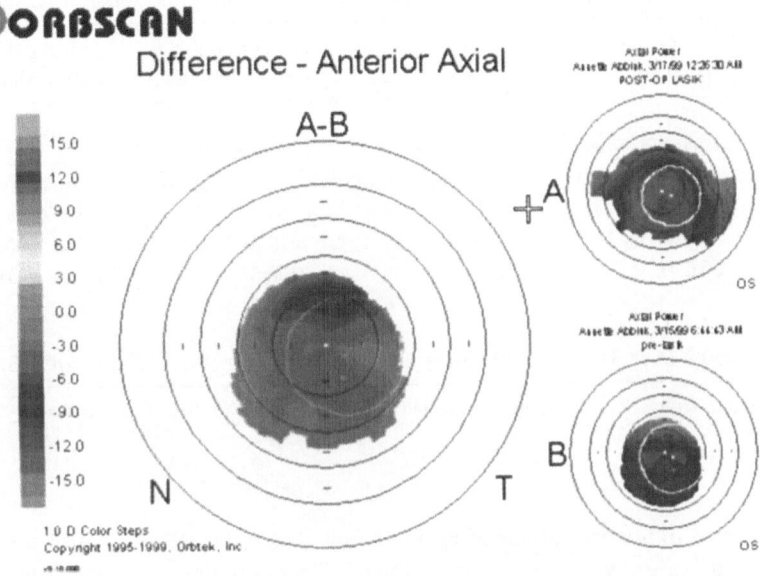

Figure 31.5 Orbscan II differential map after treatment. The preoperative map, lower right, shows a decentered ablation, the postoperative map, upper right, shows improved centration. The differential map is shown on the left.

C. RESULTS OF TOPOLINK IN REPAIR PROCEDURES

In our initial prospective study we evaluated 29 eyes of 27 patients treated between July 1996 and July 1997 (5). Inclusion criteria were irregular corneal astigmatism due to trauma or previous corneal surgery. We considered TopoLink LASIK as their last option prior to performing a corneal graft. Eyes were divided into four groups:

Group 1 (the postkeratoplasty group) consisted of six eyes (in five patients) with irregular corneal astigmatism after penetrating keratoplasty. All grafts were performed more than 2 years ago. Group 2 (the posttrauma group) consisted of six eyes (in six patients) with irregular corneal astigmatism after corneal trauma. The trauma dated back more than 2 years in all eyes. Group 3 (the decentered/small optical zones group) consisted of 11 eyes (in 10 patients) with irregular corneal astigmatism after PRK (one eye) or LASIK (10 eyes) due to decentered or small optical zones. All patients complained about halos and image distortion even during the day. Group 4 (the central islands group) consisted of six eyes (in six patients) with irregular astigmatism after PRK (two eyes) or LASIK (four eyes) due to central islands or keyhole patterns. All patients complained about blurred vision or image distortion even during the day.

The results of our initial study are shown in part in Table 1. In the postkeratoplasty group and in the posttrauma group, corrective cylinder was significantly reduced as compared to the preoperative value. The topographic success rate was defined as either the planned correction fully achieved or the attempted correction partially achieved (decrease of irregularity of more than 1 D on the differential map and/or increase of optical zone size by at least 1 mm). The success rate was highest in the decentered/small optical zones group, being 91%, followed by the posttrauma group with a success rate of 83%. The lowest suc-

Table 1 Refraction, Visual Acuity, and Corneal Topography 12 Months After TopoLink LASIK

	Group 1, postkeratoplasty	Group 2, posttrauma	Group 3, decentered/small	Group 4, central islands
No. of eyes	6	6	11	6
Cylinder preoperatively	5.83 ± 1.25 D (4.00 to 8.00 D)	2.21 ± 1.35 D (1.00 to 5.00 D)	0.73 ± 0.71 D (0 to 2.00 D)	1.42 ± 1.13 D (0 to 3.50 D)
Cylinder at 12 months	2.96 ± 1.23 D* (1.50 to 4.50 D)	0.50 ± 0.84 D** (0 to 2.5 D)	0.36 ± 1.05 D (0 to 3.5 D)	0.50 ± 0.84 D* (0 to 2.00 D)
Success rate (topo as planned or improved)	66% (n = 4)	83% (n = 5)	91% (n = 10)	50% (n = 3)
Reoperation rate	50% (n = 3)	50% (n = 3)	36% (n = 4)	50% (n = 3)

UCVA: uncorrected visual acuity; SCVA: spectacle-corrected visual acuity; *: $p = 0.01$; **: $p = 0.001$.

cess rate was observed in the central island group, being 50% only. Overall, 14 of the 29 eyes were reoperated (48%) owing to the regression of effect or undercorrection. The rate of reoperation was lowest in the decentered/small optical zones group, being 36% as compared to 50% in all other groups (Table 1).

These results demonstrate that TopoLink LASIK works. We were able to significantly reduce irregularities in these extremely irregular corneas. On the other hand, our results demonstrated that most eyes were undercorrected, and we had to adjust the algorithm to take care of the undercorrection. Finally, the problem of targeting the right spot on the cornea must be addressed. The results of group 4 (central islands) were poor, which suggests that we may not have hit the right target in these eyes featuring small and circumscribed irregularities. Ideally, the laser should be locked on a topographic map of the cornea prior to treatment, and that is what we are currently working on to improve the results in the rare cases.

D. RESULTS OF TOPOLINK IN NORMAL EYES

In a prospective, noncomparative case series, we operated on 203 eyes of 203 patients between January 1999 and July 1999. Results were presented at the American Academy of Ophthalmology Annual Meeting in Orlando 1999 and accepted for publication in *Ophthalmology*. Inclusion criteria were myopia of −1.00 to −12.00 D with or without astigmatism of up to −4.00 D. The patients were divided into two groups:

Group 1 (low myopia) consisted of 114 patients with myopia of −1.00 to −6.00 D (mean, −3.83 ± 1.67 D) and astigmatism of 0 to −4.00 D (mean, −1.32 ± 1.06 D).

Group 2 (high myopia) consisted of 89 patients with myopia of −6.10 to −12.00 D (mean, −7.83 ± 1.38 D) and astigmatism of 0 to −3.50 D (mean, −1.06 ± 0.92 D).

No reoperations were performed in these series and no complications occurred. Three months after surgery, 51 patients of the low myopia group and 40 patients of the high myopia group were available for follow-up. In the low myopia group, 96.1%, and in the high myopia group, 75% were within ±0.50 D of emmetropia. Uncorrected visual acuity was 20/20 or better in 82.4% of the low myopia group and in 62.5% of the high myopia group, 20/25 or better in 98.0% of the low myopia group and in 70.0% of the high myopia group, and 20/40 or better in 100% of the low myopia group and in 95.0% of the high myopia group. In low myopia, spectacle-corrected acuity at the higher levels improved as compared to preoperative values, and 13.7% ($n = 7$) had a spectacle-corrected visual acuity of 20/12.5 or better, and 47.1% ($n = 24$) saw 20/15 or better after TopoLink LASIK as compared to the preoperative values of 5.9% ($n = 3$) and 37.3% ($n = 19$), respectively. Differences were statistically significant ($p < 0.01$). However, comparing mean values (log scale) of spectacle-corrected visual acuity, differences were not significant ($p = 0.2$).

The larger percentage of patients seeing 20/12.5 or 20/15 three months postoperatively than preoperatively in the low myopia group may indicate an improvement of spectacle-corrected visual acuity owing to the customized LASIK. In the high myopia group, no improvement was observed, whereas a one-line improvement should be expected owing to higher magnification (3). The lack of improvement in the high myopia group is most likely because corneal refractive surgery in high myopia causes a significant decrease in optical quality of the eye, and consecutively in quality of vision, because of the relationship of optical zone size, reversed asphericity, and pupil size (4,5). We were able to demonstrate that the new approach, customizing ablation based on corneal topography, works clinically at least as well as a standard ablation in normal eyes. This is a significant finding, as our approach is based on a totally different calculation of the ablation. Instead of ablations based on Munnerlyn's formula we defined a target asphere and ablated the differences between this target and the actual cornea.

E. SUMMARY

We have presented the technique of TopoLink in the treatment of irregular astigmatism, either occurring naturally or caused by trauma or surgical procedures. The presented data demonstrate that TopoLink showed some promise. Comparative studies also indicated that TopoLink LASIK improved best corrected visual acuity in a certain number of normal eyes, as shown above. On the other hand, we observed significant undercorrection and regression that are unexplained to date. TopoLink needs further refinement before it can be incorporated in routine clinical use. It remains to be seen if ablations based on wave front technology yield similar or even better results.

REFERENCES

1. MC Knorz, A Liermann, V Seiberth, H Steiner, B Wiesinger. Laser in situ keratomileusis to correct myopia of −6.00 to −29.00 diopters. J Refract Surg 1996;12:575–584.
2. MC Knorz, B Wiesinger, A Liermann, V Seiberth, H Liesenhoff. LASIK for moderate and high myopia and myopic astigmatism. Ophthalmology 1998;105:932–940.
3. MC Knorz. Broad-beam versus scanning-beam lasers for refractive surgery. Ophthalmic Practice 1997;15:142–145.
4. B Wiesinger-Jendritza, MC Knorz, P Hugger, A Liermann. Laser in situ keratomileusis assisted by corneal topography. J Cataract Refract Surg 1998;24:166–174.
5. MC Knorz, B Jendritza. Topographically-guided LASIK to treat corneal irregularities. Ophthalmology 2000;107:1138–1143.z

32

Management of Flap Complications in LASIK

MANOLETTE R. ROQUE and SAMIR A. MELKI

Massachusetts Eye and Ear Infirmary and Harvard Medical School, Boston, Massachusetts, U.S.A.

DIMITRI T. AZAR and EMILY YEUNG

Massachusetts Eye and Ear Infirmary, Schepens Eye Research Institute, and Harvard Medical School, Boston, Massachusetts, U.S.A.

A decade after the initial LASIK-related journal report publication (1), more than 370 published LASIK articles (to August 2000) have appeared in peer-reviewed publications. Of particular interest are LASIK flap complications. In this chapter we summarize the information obtained through an Advanced PubMed (National Library of Medicine) search for all articles reporting on LASIK flap complications as well as their management. The literature was searched using Advanced PubMed (under key words "LASIK" or "laser assisted in situ keratomileusis") and using citations from the articles obtained (2–38). All abstracts presenting a flap complication were incorporated in the review. We have also included information gathered from selected presentations at scientific meetings, from personal communications with other surgeons, and from our own personal experience.

Although effective methods have emerged to deal with LASIK flap complications, others are still subject to investigation. A comprehensive awareness of the potential flap complications of LASIK and the numerous strategies to handle them are fundamental for surgeons performing the procedure. This will aid not only in improving surgical outcomes and in offering patients comprehensive informed consent but also in future refinements of our current surgical techniques.

A. CORNEAL PERFORATION (FULL THICKNESS ANTERIOR CHAMBER ENTRY)

Anterior chamber penetration may occur during lamellar dissection (36–38) or through laser ablation (39,40). Globe perforation may range from a simple corneal perforation to perforation with damage to the iris and crystalline lens with or without vitreous loss. This potentially catastrophic complication is primarily related to flawed microkeratome assembly. The plate may be absent or erroneously inserted into the microkeratome. Some keratome models require the placement of a thickness footplate to achieve a certain flap thickness. If left out, a full thickness corneal incision with serious damage to anterior and/or posterior segment structures could develop. Alternatively, corneal perforation may result from excessively thin corneas, for instance following old corneal wounds, ulcers, previous refractive surgery, or in keratoconus. In one published report, a thin preexisting keratoconic cornea was suspected as the etiology for the full thickness laser ablation.

1. Intraoperative Management

Immediate closure of a corneal wound with 10-0 nylon sutures should be performed. Further management depends on the severity of the damage caused to the globe (Table 1). An ocular protective shield should be placed and the patient be asked to try to relax and minimize straining and coughing. The patient should be transferred to the major operating room and given general anesthesia after ensuring adequate closure of the corneal entry site. Administration of local periocular anesthesia increases the risk of ocular damage during surgical repair of an open globe. Repair may involve corneal repair, iris repair, lensectomy with or without intraocular lens implantation, and anterior and/or posterior vitrectomy.

2. Postoperative Rehabilitation

A contact lens may be necessary. Aphakic contact lenses with or without an artificial pupil may be required. There may be a need for a secondary intraocular lens implantation (posterior chamber, iris sutured, or transscleral sutured). In some instances a rotational or penetrating keratoplasty may be required for visual rehabilitation.

3. Prevention

Meticulous adherence to the instructions of keratome assembly cannot be emphasized enough to prevent this catastrophic event. For microkeratomes requiring assembly, a double check system, involving the technician and the surgeon, should be implemented in order to avoid any untoward incidents. Habitual checking will prove beneficial in the long run. Acquiring a modern microkeratome with an integrated plate will decrease the risk. Stringent screening of patients for possible corneal thinning (keratoconus, old corneal wound, old corneal ulcer scar) is important to minimize the risk of perforation.

B. FREE CAP (ABSENT HINGE)

A free cap results from unintended complete dissection of the corneal flap (Fig. 32.1). The cumulative mean incidence from early studies is reported to be about 4.9%. More recent studies report an incidence between 0.01% and 1%. Intraoperative factors leading to a free cap include (1) loss of adequate suction secondary to machine malfunction, kink or obstruction in the tubing, or handpiece malposition, (2) absence, malposition, or maladjust-

Table 1 Management of Corneal Perforation

Types	Acute intervention	Follow-up	Long term management	Outcomes of surgery
Simple corneal perforation	Stop suction ASAP and remove microkeratome carefully Reform the anterior chamber with viscoelastics and suture with 10–0 nylon	Monitor wound healing and suture tightness	Corneal scare management if perforation occurs in visual axis	Depends on the degree of astigmatism
Perforation with damage to the iris and lens without vitreous loss	Stop suction ASAP and remove microkeratome carefully Protect the eye with a plastic shield and transfer the patient to an operating room Reform the anterior chamber with viscoelastics Lens surgery as needed Repair the iris and cornea	Manage like a globe perforation IOL implantation if deemed safe		Astigmatism Corneal scarring Photophobia if significant amount of iris is damaged Loss of BCVA
Perforation with posterior segment damage including vitreous loss	Stop suction ASAP and remove microkeratome carefully Protect the eye with a plastic shield Transfer the patient to an operating room and administer general anesthesia A vitreoretinal surgeon should be available if posterior segment damage renders such needful Anterior vitrectomy followed by reformation of anterior chamber by viscoelastics Repair the iris and cornea	Aphakic contact lens Vitreoretinal follow-up	Secondary scleral-fixated IOL	Prolonged rehabilitation Loss of BCVA

Prevention
1. Good preop assessment to identify irregular corneal thickness, keratoconus, and previous refractive surgery.
2. Proper assembly of the microkeratome making sure that the depth plate and the stopper are inserted correctly.
3. Use of modern microkeratome with integrated plate.

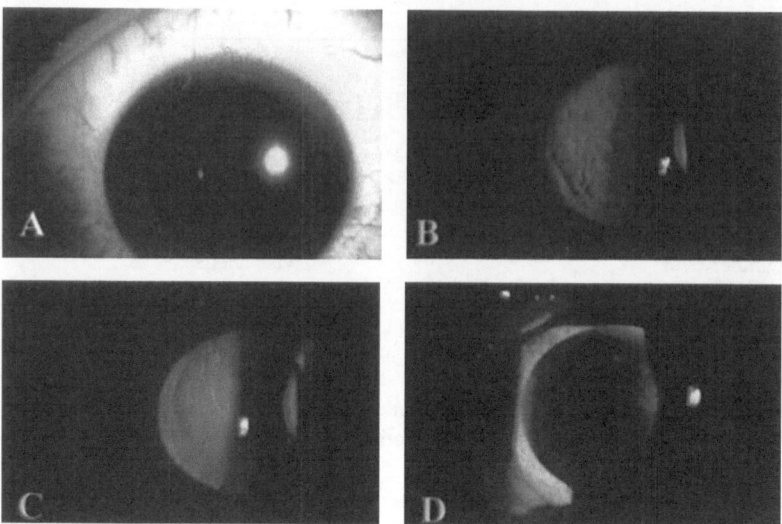

Figure 32.1   31/M 3 years S/P LASIK OD with residual myopia and astigmatism. VscOD was 20/70 SP 1° LASIK. A deeper (180 μm) LASIK flap was fashioned with a Hansatome, and laser ablation was made to correct for −1.4 D sphere. The patient's VscOD was 20/20 2 days later. (A) Anterior view with no apparent anatomic problems, OD. (B, C) On retroillumination, the corneal flap is noted to be small with interface debris and fibers near the hinge, OD. (D) On slit beam, there is note of a stromal scar, OD.

ment of the thickness footplate or the "stop" mechanism during assembly of certain microkeratomes, (3) flat corneas (<41 D) (41), and (4) inadequate corneal exposure. In certain instances, the microkeratome can jam, preventing microkeratome head reversal to free the flap. This might prompt the surgeon to release the suction and lift an incarcerated flap within the microkeratome head, resulting in a free cap. Postoperatively, external trauma can theoretically lead to a free cap (Table 2).

1.   Intraoperative Management

Preplaced fiducial corneal marks with gentian violet used for proper orientation and careful attention during retrieval of the cap from the microkeratome head allow for favorable management of a free cap (42). The anatomy of the free corneal tissue should be respected, and it should be handled gently. While transferring the cap into an antidesiccation chamber using a perforated spatula (such as a Barraquer fenestrated spatula), it is important to ensure that the epithelial side of the free cap is placed facing down. If the small size of the cap does not permit laser ablation to the underlying stroma, the ablation should be deferred to allow adequate healing time. If the diameter of the exposed stroma is equal to or larger than the intended laser ablation zone, then laser treatment may proceed as planned. The cap is then retrieved from the antidesiccation chamber and repositioned using the preplaced paracentral marks preserving the original. The width of the gutter should be uniform; a Merocel sponge sweep can be used for this purpose. It is important that the cap be replaced, epithelial side up, on the stromal bed. It has been suggested that the free cap be floated on a bed of BSS and allowed to adhere spontaneously to the stroma, assisted by careful placement of a microsponge at different gutter positions. The bed of BSS will slowly disappear

Table 2 Management of Free Caps

Types	Acute intervention	Follow-up	Outcomes
Small cap (Cap size < optical zone)	Abort the laser ablation Reposition the cap	May recut in 3 months' time if refraction is stable	Usually good
Large cap (Cap size ≥ optical zone)	Respect anatomy of tissue and handle the cap gently, transfer to antidesiccation chamber with perforated spatula on a drop of BSS with epithelial surface down (No BSS on stromal side) Proceed with laser Transfer the cap from the chamber with the perforated spatula Reposition the cap with blunt atraumatic instrument such as the Merocel sponge using the paracentral marks as well as the width of the gutter as guides Suturing is not usually needed Wait for at least 6 minutes Bandage contact lens is optional as some believe that a poorly fitted contact lens may predispose to cap displacement Keep the patient in the office for at least 1 hour to monitor the cap before discharge	Watch out for dislocation Stress importance of eye shield and the avoidance of mechanical disruption	Usually good
Loss of cap	Measure the stromal bed with pachymetry Place a bandage contact lens	Monitor refraction	Possible hyperopic shift depending on diameter/ thickness of the cap

Prevention
1. Eyeshield while sleeping during first two weeks.
2. Avoidance of trauma and eye rubbing.

by capillary action towards the dry sponge, assuring an even, wrinkle-free adherence of the free cap to the corneal stroma. Care must be exhibited in aligning the preplaced fiducial marks. Cap and stromal adhesion should be ensured by allowing adequate time of contact. Five to 8 minutes should be sufficient for this purpose. Performing the striae test to check for adherence may be valuable: a dry Merocel sponge is used to exert light pressure on the outer section of the gutter of resection. Good adhesion will manifest as formation of striae that radiate from the point of pressure toward the center of the cornea across the gutter. Sutures are seldom necessary but may be placed in an antitorque fashion. A bandage contact lens may be placed in order to protect the cap, especially if the epithelium has been damaged. Some authors prefer to avoid the use of bandage contact lenses, if the epithelium is intact, because the lens may dislocate the cap (43).

2. Postoperative Rehabilitation

Regular follow-up for cap displacement should be performed, as the cap may be lost secondary to vigorous blinking or with fall of the contact lens. The latter is removed a few days postoperatively or when reepithelialization occurs. Wearing eye shields at night and special protective polycarbonate eyewear for sports activities are helpful. If needed, a recut may be performed at least 3 months later. The new cut should start more peripheral and go deeper than the original one. The surgical outcome is usually good.

3. Prevention

Asymmetry in the placement of the fiducial marks will allow for proper alignment at the end of the surgical procedure. If the marks do not traverse the angle of resection, they are not helpful. The microkeratome should be checked prior to surgery. The suction ring should also be inspected and tested. The same measures described later to prevent thin and small flaps also will help avoid free cap complications. Meticulous care should be made in the proper assembly of the microkeratome.

C. CAP LOSS

Cap loss may occur intraoperatively or during the early postoperative period. Factors that may lead to the loss of the corneal cap include incomplete adherence of the cap to the stroma, eye rubbing, loosening and removal of the pressure patch, excessive blinking, and trauma. In addition to patients with a free cap, cap loss may also occur following trauma in patients with normal corneal flaps.

1. Surgical Management

If the cap cannot be retrieved, attempts at fashioning a lamellar flap from a donor eye should not be attempted as a primary procedure. The corneal epithelium is allowed to grow centrally in a manner similar to that after other "superficial" keratectomy procedures such as PRK with possibly a more profound central applanation effect. A bandage contact lens is placed and the surface is evaluated over a period of 3 to 4 days or until the cornea is fully reepithelialized. Any excimer laser treatment should be aborted and retreatment deferred until refractive stability is achieved. However, some authors advocate immediate suturing of a lamellar homograft to the stromal bed (43,44) whenever possible. A slightly smaller cap is produced to serve as a lamellar homograft to the recipient stromal bed. Prophylactic topical antibiotics and steroids should be given. Secondary enhancement procedures may be performed later (44,45).

2. Prevention

Although most LASIK surgeons do not wait more than 5 minutes for the flap to adhere at the end of an uncomplicated LASIK procedure, adherence of the free cap to the underlying stroma may require air-drying for a period of at least 8 minutes. Application of a bandage contact lens or a pressure patch may also be needed. In addition to wearing a protective shield, the patient should avoid forceful blinking to reduce the chance of cap loss.

D. INCOMPLETE FLAP

Incomplete flaps occur when the microkeratome blade comes to a halt before reaching the intended location of the hinge. Visual aberrations are more likely to occur when the new hinge results in scarring in proximity to the visual axis (Fig. 32.2). The incidence of this complication reported in large series ranges between 0.3% and 1.2%. Eyelashes, eyelids, eyelid specula, surgical drapes, and conjunctival folds may cause mechanical obstruction of the microkeratome head. Debris along the track such as loose epithelium, eyelid makeup, and precipitated salt from the irrigating solution have been recognized as possible impediments to smooth gear progression. Microkeratome jamming due to either electrical failure or mechanical obstacles on the microkeratome edge or footpedal may be the most common etiology of incomplete flaps. Incomplete flaps also occur when the gear advancement mechanism jams or is inadequate (46). Loss of adequate suction in some microkeratomes may lead to automatic abortion of the dissection or to a premature arrest of the microkeratome head advancement.

1. Intraoperative Management

In cases where the microkeratome head is jammed, the suction should be released followed by careful removal of the suction–microkeratome complex from the eye. If the exposed

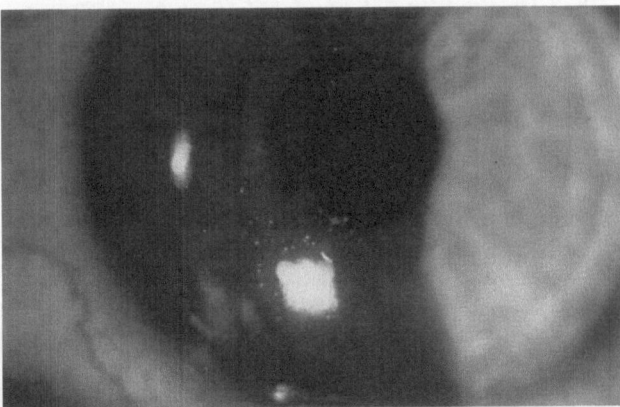

Figure 32.2 Stromal scarring in an incomplete flap after an aborted LASIK. (Reproduced from Ref. 1, with permission.)

Table 3   Management of Incomplete Flap

Types	Acute intervention	Follow-up	Outcomes
Incomplete flap (with enough stromal bed for laser)	Proceed to laser if hinge is beyond optical zone Protect the flap from laser exposure by a metallic plate or a surgical sponge	Routine	Most cases do well Visual distortion from induced astigmatism occurs rarely
Incomplete flap (with hinge near the optical zone)	Withhold laser and reposition the flap Reverse the jammed microkeratome instead of pushing through with forward cutting Avoid completing the work by manual dissection	Recut in 3 months with a larger ring and a deeper blade if the corneal thickness permits	Most cases do well Visual distortion from induced astigmatism occurs rarely

Prevention

1. Double check to ensure no mechanical obstruction such as lashes, lids, lid drape, conjunctiva along the microkeratome track to cause jamming.
2. Perform a dry run on the keratome prior to each cut.

stromal bed is not large enough to allow adequate laser ablation, the flap should be repositioned and the laser procedure postponed (Table 3). Irrigation of the flap–stromal interface is performed in a manner similar to that of uncomplicated LASIK. The flap is then flattened carefully and dried. Resuming forward cutting after stoppage may result in an irregular stromal bed and irregular astigmatism.

If the created hinge is beyond the visual axis, some surgeons may consider manually extending the dissection with a blade. Caution is advised when attempting such a maneuver because of the risk of uneven bed creation and flap buttonhole formation. When the laser ablation is performed, the flap should be protected from laser exposure. Placement of a metallic plate or a surgical sponge over the flap may prevent inadvertent laser ablation on the hinge and flap.

2. Postoperative Rehabilitation

Fashioning a LASIK flap may be performed 3 to 6 months later, assuming an uneventful postoperative course. It is advisable to attempt a deeper and more peripheral cut during the retreatment. Factors to consider in setting the depth for the second pass include corneal thickness and amount of tissue ablation contemplated.

3. Prevention

Prior to every case, the surgeon or a technician working on behalf of the surgeon should test the forward and reverse excursion of the suction ring–microkeratome complex. This will decrease the probability that a gear jam may take place during actual use. Microkeratome jamming can be minimized by meticulous cleaning of its components and by inspection of its electrical connections. The manufacturer's recommendations for cleaning procedures and solutions may differ over time as more is learned about a particular machine. A clear cutting path for the microkeratome can be achieved through adequate draping (to prevent lashes from getting into the cutting field), adjustable eye specula (to provide the widest interpalpebral opening tolerated by the patient) and by gently lifting the globe after vacuum activation (to provide better exposure and unhindered gear progression). This should be followed by the IOP measurement step to rule out inadvertent loss of suction pressure when lifting the globe.

Deep-set eyes may represent a challenge, as some keratome heads may not fit and may be stopped by the eyelid speculum. The risks and discomfort associated with more invasive techniques such as retrobulbar saline injections and lateral canthotomies may not be justified, given the elective nature of the procedure.

E. BUTTONHOLES

A buttonhole occurs when the microkeratome blade exits through the epithelium during mid-incision and then reenters to complete the flap (Fig. 32.3) (47). The incidence is reported to range between 0.2% and 2.6% of cases (48,49). This was the most common complication resulting in loss of BCVA among 1062 eyes studied by Stulting et al. (4). Buttonholed flaps can provide a channel for epithelial cells to infiltrate the flap–stroma interface (Fig. 32.4). There is also an increased risk of subepithelial scar formation in flaps with buttonholes. A flap buttonhole is more likely to occur when performing LASIK on eyes with previous incisional keratotomy (41). Thompson described a flap hydrodissection technique to minimize incision separation in this situation (49).

Inadequate coupling of the blade to the cornea may lead to buttonholes. Steep corneas (>46.7 D) have been compared to tennis balls that would buckle centrally upon applanating pressure. This results in a central dimple missed by the blade so that a buttonhole is formed. Another theory is that higher keratometric values offer increased resistance to cutting when applanated, so that there is an upward movement of the blade. The latter is

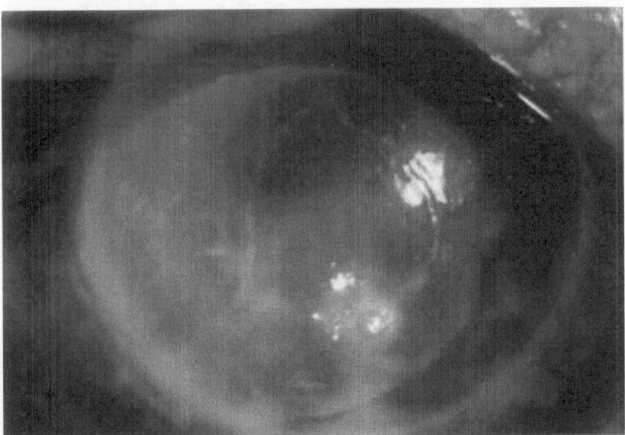

Figure 32.3 Buttonhole secondary to a lamellar dissection in a corneal graft with 49.0 D keratometry reading in the steep meridian. (Reproduced from Ref 1, with permission.)

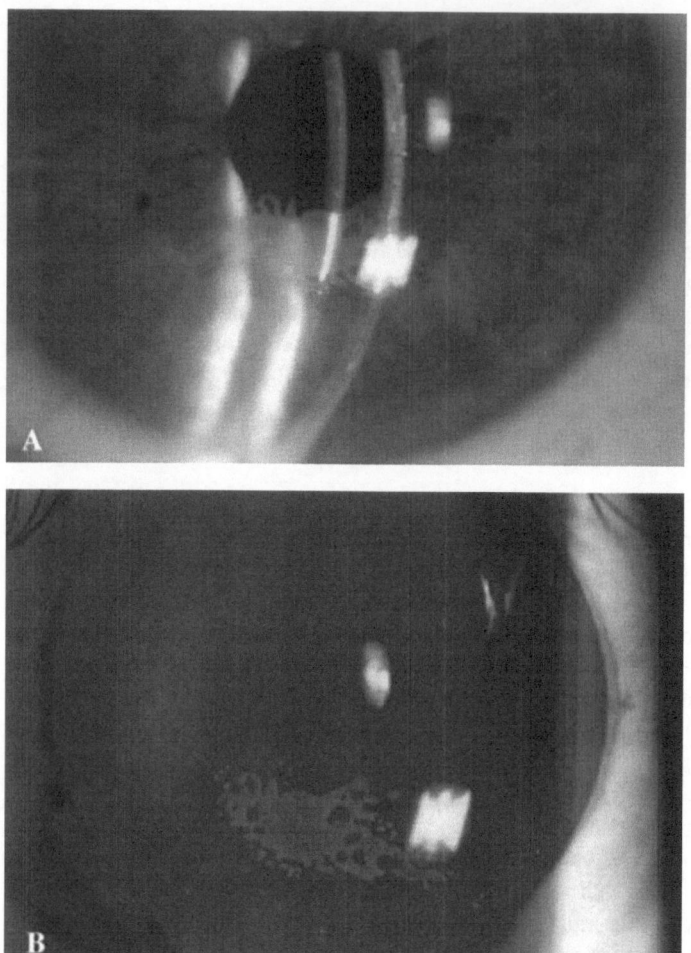

Figure 32.4   Epithelial ingrowth. (A) Slit lamp appearance. (B) Retroillumination. This condition requires flap lifting and epithelial scraping.

probably more applicable to keratomes with lower blade oscillation rates. Blunted blades, poor oscillation, and microflaws of blades have also been described as mechanical micro-keratome problems that may lead to buttonholes (51–53).

Inadequate coupling of the blade to the cornea is often due to poor suction. Suction may be poor in cases with sunken globes, small diameter corneas leading to inadequate suction ring placement, conjunctival incarceration in the suction port, conjunctival scarring, or eyes with previous surgery (54,55). Nonangled or low-angled microkeratome blades are more prone to move superficially during flap dissection, resulting in buttonholed cuts. These blades have equal likelihood of moving upwards (towards the surface) or downwards (towards the stromal side) when greater resistance is encountered. On the other hand, inferiorly angled blades are more likely to be driven towards the stroma.

Another possible risk factor for flap buttonhole occurrence is previous ocular surgery as shown by Stulting et al. (4). However, this did not reach statistical significance

($P=0.09$). Tham et al. reported a higher incidence of buttonholes with large size flaps when using the Hansatome. It is theorized that the larger area required for flattening may result in central dimpling if the IOP is not adequate (56).

1. Intraoperative Management

The safest way to proceed when a buttonholed flap is encountered is to avoid lifting the flap or immediately reposition the flap and abort the procedure. Epithelial debris should be gently irrigated out with BSS.

While some surgeons advocate proceeding with scraping the epithelium and performing a PRK laser ablation within 2 weeks (78), this approach may not be feasible in higher myopes owing to the appearance of subepithelial haze (which may require Mitomycin C treatment or prophylaxis) (58–60). A bandage contact lens should be used to protect the buttonholed flap from migration.

2. Postoperative Management

Table 4 summarizes the steps in managing buttonholes. Most patients with buttonholes end up with no significant loss of vision after adequate healing has occurred, especially if uncomplicated by epithelial ingrowth. Epithelial ingrowth after a buttonhole begins centrally and is associated with central corneal melting. Buttonholes may also be compounded by epithelial ingrowth in the periphery (43). Management of epithelial ingrowth of this type can be very frustrating. Oftentimes the only viable option is discarding what remains of the flap. Reepithelialization is then allowed to occur, delaying further refractive treatment till stability is achieved.

3. Prevention

The incidence of perforated flaps may be reduced if the surgeon ensures adequate suction, inspects the blades routinely and regularly, adjusts the plate thickness according to corneal curvature (i.e., deeper microkeratome footplates in cases of steep corneas), and pays attention to the following guidelines:

1. Avoid cutting the flap if the intraocular pressure (IOP) is low due to low suction. A pressure of at least 80 mm Hg may be essential for safest flap creation. Measurement is probably most valuable with a pneumotonometer (61–63), as other means may provide imprecise readings at times (47). Care should be taken to avoid conjunctival clogging of the suction port, which could lead to discrepancy between the intraocular pressure and the suction pressure recorded on the microkeratome vacuum console. Newer microkeratomes have a safety mechanism to abort the procedure automatically or to activate additional suction, but they are also prone to similar problems if direct IOP measurements are not obtained to ensure adequate suction.

2. Set the microkeratome to a deeper cutting depth if keratometry readings exceed 46 D, assuming that the amount of intended myopic correction to be treated allows such modification.

3. Use larger suction rings in flat corneas to prevent small flaps.

4. Avoid microkeratomes with nonangled blades.

5. Inspect the microkeratome blade under the operating microscope before engaging it in the suction ring in order to rule out manufacturing or other preoperative damage to

the blade. Keep the microkeratome away from hard surfaces after assembly to avoid subsequent blade damage.

   6.   Inspect previous keratotomy incisions to ensure adequate healing and lack of epithelial plugs prior to proceeding with LASIK. This can prevent intraoperative separation of incisions.

F.   THIN, IRREGULAR, AND DECENTERED FLAPS

The incidence of thin flaps after LASIK has been reported to vary between 0.3% and 0.75% in the three major studies (64). Lamellar flap creation in LASIK should be deeper than Bowman's layer (65), sparing it from laser ablation. A flap is considered thin when the keratome cuts within or above the 10 μm thick Bowman's layers. Intraoperatively, this finding is seen as a shiny reflex on the stromal surface. The use of pachymetry (66,67) before and after lifting the flap may also be helpful in recognizing this occurrence. A measurement below 60 μm is suspicious, as the thickness of the corneal epithelium is approximately 50 μm (68). Thin flaps seem to result from an inadequate coupling of the blade to the cornea. Nonangled or low-angled microkeratome blades are more prone to move superficially during flap dissection, resulting in thin cuts. Flat corneas may result in a thin flap, as they could be below the adequate cutting plane in certain locations. Other implicated reasons for this complication include epithelial sloughing, poor suction, conjunctival chemosis, and small lid fissures.

   Irregular flaps are bileveled flaps, bisected flaps, or notched flaps. The incidence of irregular flaps is lower than that of thin flaps. Irregular flaps may result from an inadequate coupling of the blade to the cornea and from damaged microkeratome blades. Blade damage may happen either during manufacturing or at the time of usage.

   Decentered flaps may be otherwise perfect. They may be caused by surgeon error in centering the suction ring to allow room for the desired ablation. The palpebral fissure may be small with difficult placement of the suction ring. It may also be caused by spontaneous decentration of the ring following activation of the pump. The activation of negative pressure on the suction ring somehow causes sliding of the mechanical apparatus over the cornea if the applanation of the ring is not even throughout. Lastly it may be caused by lack of patient cooperation during surgery.

1.   Intraoperative Management

The safest way to proceed when a thin or irregular flap is encountered is to reposition the flap and abort the procedure (Table 4).

   It may be tempting to lift a thin flap and treat with the laser. If the thin flap has sufficient stromal tissue (i.e., sparing the Bowman's layer) and is of sufficient size, then laser ablation may be possible (43).

   In the case of decentered flaps, if the ablation area is adequate one can immediately proceed with the laser correction. In some instances, the optical zone has to be decreased, to adjust to the decentered stromal surface. If the decentration is severe, the flap may have to be repositioned and the laser procedure deferred.

2.   Postoperative Management

In cases of thin, irregular, or decentered flaps, a deeper flap may be recut (20–60 μm deeper) approximately 10 to 12 weeks later (after confirming a stable refraction) and the

Table 4 Management of Buttonholes and Thin and Decentered Flaps

Types	Morphology	Acute intervention	Follow-up	Long-term	Outcomes of surgery
Buttonholes		Withhold laser and reposition the flap	Long term—defer laser for at least 3 months until refraction stabilized; some authors advise a deeper cut, while some use the same size blade	Transepithelial (esp. in low myopes) Gas: permeable contact lens or soft contact lens as alternatives	Loss of BCVA Risk of epithelial ingrowth and scarring
Thin flap	Small	Withhold laser and reposition the flap	Recut in 3 months with a deeper blade if corneal thickness permits	No long-term sequelae	Good
	Large	Proceed with laser if cut is below Bowman's layer	Routine	No long-term sequelae	Good
Variable depth	Linear vertical marks	Proceed with laser Careful replacement of the flap according to corneal marks and gutter width	Routine	No long-term sequelae	Good
	Irregular configuration	Abort laser and replace flap carefully	Consider recutting in 3 months with a deeper blade only if refraction stable with no induced astigmatism		Good
Irregular margins/ decentered	Clear visual axis	Proceed with laser if stromal bed is adequate for laser Take special precaution in replacing the flap	Routine		Good
	Through visual axis	Abort the laser Replace the flap	Consider recutting in 3 months	Routine	Usually good

Prevention
1. Preop assessment to identify predisposing factors (e.g., steep cornea). Modify surgical technique accordingly.

LASIK procedure completed. Three months seems to be the well-accepted time for reoperations. A deeper properly placed flap during reoperation is essential, especially in hyperopic procedures requiring large ablation zones.

Kapadia and Wilson advocate using a no-touch transepithelial PRK within 2 weeks of the initial irregular cut to prevent irregular astigmatism formation from the uneven ablation profile resulting from any late scar formation (47,68). This technique seems reasonable especially in low myopes. During the reoperation, one can perform transepithelial PRK to eliminate the scar. This is best performed in cases with a very superficial cut and within the first few weeks after the initial procedure.

3. Prevention

The incidence of thin or irregular flaps may be reduced if the surgeon ensures adequate suction, inspects the blades routinely and regularly, adjusts the plate thickness according to corneal curvature (i.e., deeper microkeratome footplates in cases of steep corneas), and pays attention to the guidelines presented for the prevention of buttonhole formation.

Prevention of decentration entails monitoring the preplaced corneal marks. The marks have to be placed properly, of course. Centration of the optical axis should be ascertained by observing the position and movement of a nondilated pupil. The surgeon should also be continuously conscious of the astigmatic axis. The keratometry values will guide the preoperative choice for the flap size. Once the suction ring is placed on the globe and all these factors have been taken into consideration, it is important that the ring be equally in contact to the globe at all points. Equal pressure placed on the suction ring while it is resting on the globe, prior to suction activation, will ensure a good equal hold of the suction ring device on the globe. If there is even a slight drift during this procedure, the surgeon should release the suction and repeat proper alignment once more. This should be done until proper alignment is attained.

G. FLAP WRINKLES (STRIAE AND FOLDS)

Authors have used the terms wrinkles, striae, and folds interchangeably so often that we sometimes think that they are referring to different entities. Now the confusion has even been more complicated with descriptions of peripheral or central "creases." Other qualifiers like macro and micro, and fixed and nonfixed, have made these reports even more colorful. Carpel et al. attempted to solve this terminology dispute by proposing a classification of "striae" types (69). We consider that striae are finer than folds and that folds are, in fact, wrinkles.

Flap folds can induce irregular astigmatism with optical aberrations and loss of BCVA (Fig. 32.5), especially if they involve the visual axis (71). "Macrofolds" are easily seen by slit lamp exam and represent full thickness flap tenting in a linear fashion (Fig. 32.6). On the other hand, "microfolds" within the flap itself may represent wrinkles in Bowman's layer or in the epithelial basement membrane (72). They are easily visualized as negative staining lines with sodium fluorescein (73). Carpel et al. described five types of folds and striae in LASIK flaps (69). While confocal microscopy reveals microfolds at the Bowman's layer in 97% of cases (74), the incidence of folds requiring intervention ranges between 0.2% and 1.5%. It is not clear why some folds may adversely affect vision while others with similar appearance may be asymptomatic.

Flap folds result from uneven alignment of the flap edge and the peripheral epithelial ring. This can occur with an unequally hydrated stromal bed prior to flap repositioning.

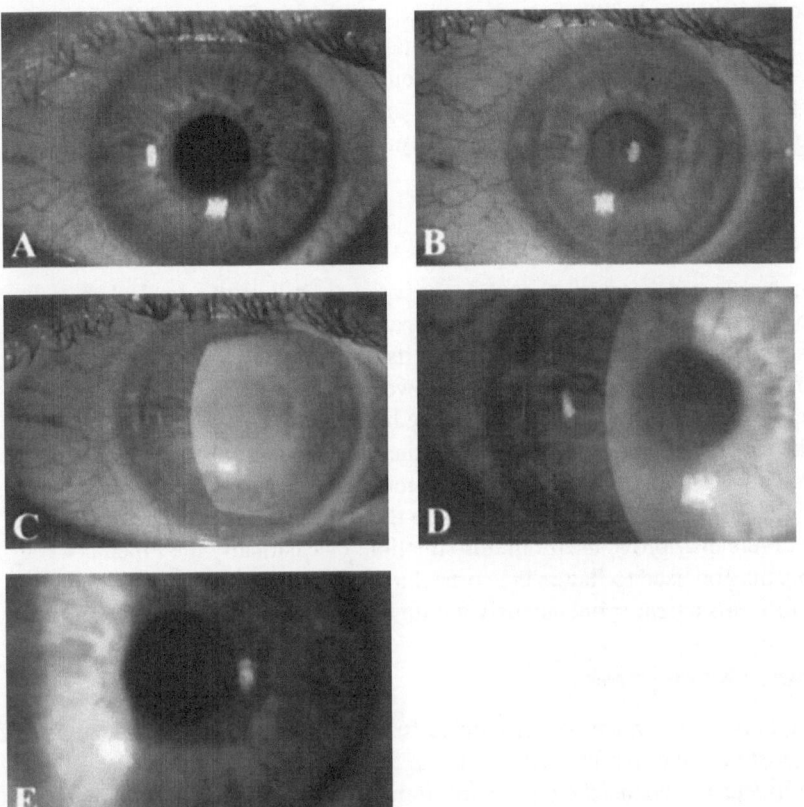

Figure 32.5 47/M 1 day S/P LASIK, OS flap wrinkles noted radiating from hinge. The nasal gutter margin was widened. VscOS was 20/60. A bandage contact lens was placed after scraping the epithelium at the area of the gutter. VscOS was 20/30 five days later. (A) Anterior view with no apparent corneal problems. There is, however, evident conjunctival injection. (B, C) Superior punctate keratopathy is seen on the anterior corneal flap surface. (D) Fluorescein staining reveals the LASIK flap margins, SPK, as well as the fine epithelial striae originating from the hinge. (E) A larger magnification of Fig. 2D. (F) An even larger view of 2D.

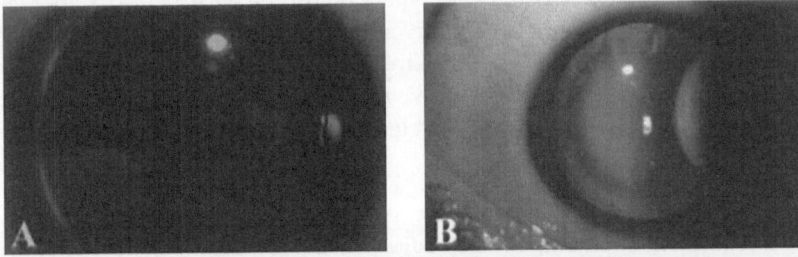

Figure 32.6 41/F S/P LASIK, OD 4 months prior. Her VscOD is 20/40-2 → NI. There is a note of nonvisually significant wrinkles on the flap. An enhancement ablative procedure was planned to improve the visual acuity. One day postenhancement her VscOD improved to 20/15-2. (A) Anterior view shows wrinkles on the flap. (B) On retroillumination, the wrinkles are more visible. The flap gutter is highly visible as well.

Thinner and larger flaps tend to shift more readily, causing surface wrinkling. Uneven sponge smoothing can result in radial (with centrifugal movement) folds or circumferential (with centripetal movement) folds. A higher incidence of flap folds is usually found in higher myopes and is sometimes unavoidable. This is owing to reduced central convexity and stromal support, which result in flap redundancy that may be quite difficult to flatten. This is referred to as the "tenting effect" (75).

1. Intraoperative Management

Flap striae, wrinkles, or folds may be seen while the patient is still on the surgical chair, immediately postop, or on early follow-up. The intraoperative management of flap wrinkles, striae, and folds is gentle replacement of the flap to its original neutral position. Gentle refloating of the flap may be attempted. This is followed by systematic sweeps of a moistened Merocel sponge to smoothen the flap from the hinge out. A single parallel direction technique may be used in attempting to smooth out the flap, or a central-to-periphery radial technique may be undertaken. Fluid in the flap–stroma interface should be eliminated. Air drying time should be at least 4 minutes to increase the likelihood of good adhesion. Mechanical hot air dryers may prove useful in this situation. Occasionally the Pineda or Caro LASIK flap irons may be used to flatten the corneal irregularities. Usually epithelial wrinkling, striae, or folds disappear spontaneously within a few days (Table 5).

2. Postoperative Management

The management of flap folds ranges from simple lifting and refloating of the flap to placement of sutures to stretch the flap in position (Table 5). It is likely that the earlier a flap is attended to, the higher the chances of quick resolution (75). Fixed folds probably occur when epithelial hyperplasia has time to form in the crevices formed by the folds. Flattening should aim towards an even distribution of forces applied to the flap (72,75–77). This can be performed with methylcellulose sponges or their equivalent. Instruments such as the Pineda or Caro LASIK Flap Iron can also be used to flatten isolated flaps at the slit lamp or under the operating microscope by gently pressing on them. Recalcitrant folds may respond well to placement of running antitorque sutures at the flap edge (78). However, this may result in significant astigmatism. Another strategy is to make superficial epithelial incisions or frank epithelial debridement over the wrinkled area. This may relieve contractures that occur secondary to epithelial hyperplasia in longer standing folds. Probst et al. described a technique using the red reflex as a way to better detect mild irregularities (75). Other reported strategies include hydrating the flap with hypotonic saline (60–80%) or deionized water (79,80), which may facilitate flattening. In extreme cases, removal of the corneal cap may be the most successful course of action (78). We have noted few instances where mere flap ironing will result in refractive error shift of at least one diopter.

3. Prevention

Preplaced surgical landmarks straddling the flap edge permit accurate repositioning of the flap in the immediate operative and postoperative period. The delicate balance of hydration and dehydration status of the corneal flap may play a role in the creation of striae and folds. The cornea should be adequately moist prior to the microkeratome cut. Once the flap is fashioned, it should not be allowed to dry. Buratto suggests that operating room humidity levels should even be checked and factored in (43). The flap lifting to flap repositioning

Table 5 Management of Flap Folds, Wrinkles, and Striae

Types	Acute intervention	Follow-up	Long-term management	Outcomes
Wrinkles/striae	Gentle repositioning of the flap on a damp stromal bed (no excessive hydration)	Vision not affected Decrease BCVA	Observe Lift and refloat	Good
Peripheral folds	Observe	No epithelial ingrowth	Observe	
		Epithelial ingrowth	Lift flap and scrape epithelial cells and debris	Good
Central folds	Refloat/iron	Resolved Recurrence	Observe Lift flap and refloat Consider debridement of overlying epithelium Suturing and removal of sutures early to avoid astigmatisms and infection	Decrease BCVA

Prevention
1. Reposition the flap using the preplaced fiducial marks and the gutter as guides.
2. Avoid eye squeezing or blinking in the early post-operative period with good pain control.

time should be minimized as much as possible. During ablation the epithelial side of the flap should be placed on a moistened Chayet sponge. Prior to replacing the flap, the stromal bed should be sufficiently moist. Once repositioned, the interface should be irrigated adequately.

Placing a wet microsponge on the stromal aspect of the flap during long ablations might minimize the dehydration effect. However, this may introduce fibrils and debris in the interface. We currently favor spreading one or two drops of fluid on the stromal aspect of the reflected flap after lifting.

Examination at the slit lamp 20 minutes after the procedure is useful to ensure adequate flap positioning. Care should be taken to ensure even distribution of the gap ("gutter") between the flap edge and the peripheral epithelial ring. This gap is noted after the procedure and usually disappears by the first postoperative day. This gap is probably due to flap dehydration and subsequent retraction. Contraction of intercellular adhesion complexes secondary to mechanical trauma might also contribute to the retraction of the flap. There has been no histological confirmation of these theories.

The presence of diffuse lamellar keratitis after LASIK may rarely lead to corneal scarring (Fig. 32.7) that can be confused with flap folds and wrinkles. Additional factors

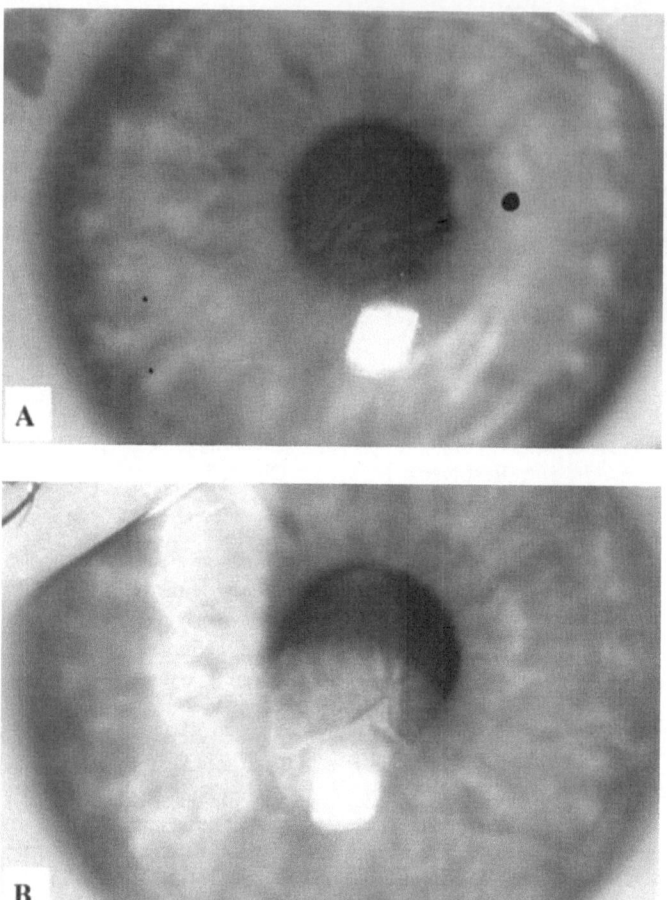

Figure 32.7 Diffuse lamellar keratitis (A) may require flap irrigation. (B) Progression to stromal scarring and flap wrinkles.

that may be associated with large wrinkles include surgery for epithelial ingrowth (Fig. 32.4) and DLK with or without loss of BCVA. Treatment of these conditions should include avoidance of postoperative striae and folds and may require the use of flap sutures to avoid secondary folds and striae.

H.   DISPLACED/DISLODGED/INCORRECT REPLACEMENT OF FLAP

A dislodged flap is an emergency. It should be repositioned as soon as possible to prevent fixed folds and epithelial ingrowth. This displacement can occur as late as many months after the procedure (81). The incidence of perioperative flap dislocation has been reported to vary between 1.1% and 2.0% in recent LASIK papers. The relatively high rate of dislodged flaps after LASIK in earlier publications has prompted many investigators to refine their techniques of flap repositioning with resultant positive impact on lowering the incidence of this complication (82–85).

Mechanical displacement by lid action is the main culprit in the early period. This may follow eyelid rubbing or squeezing. Larger diameter and thinner flaps are more prone to be displaced, especially if the hinge is small. The flap remains vulnerable to traumatic displacement several months after surgery (Fig. 32.8 and 32.9) (86). Two reports described dislocation of a LASIK flap during vitrectomy surgery (87,88). LASIK corneal flaps can be lifted for retreatment (89–94) as late as 12 months (95,96) after the primary procedure. This is in agreement with histological studies showing minimal healing at the stromal interface after LASIK (97–100).

Occasionally, the beginning or the high-volume surgeon may neglect to follow the salient guidelines in properly repositioning the corneal flap and ends up doing so improperly.

1. Intraoperative Management

Once flap dislocation is identified, it should be immediately addressed (Table 6). Gentle irrigation of the flap–stromal bed interface should be done with BSS. Afterwards the flap

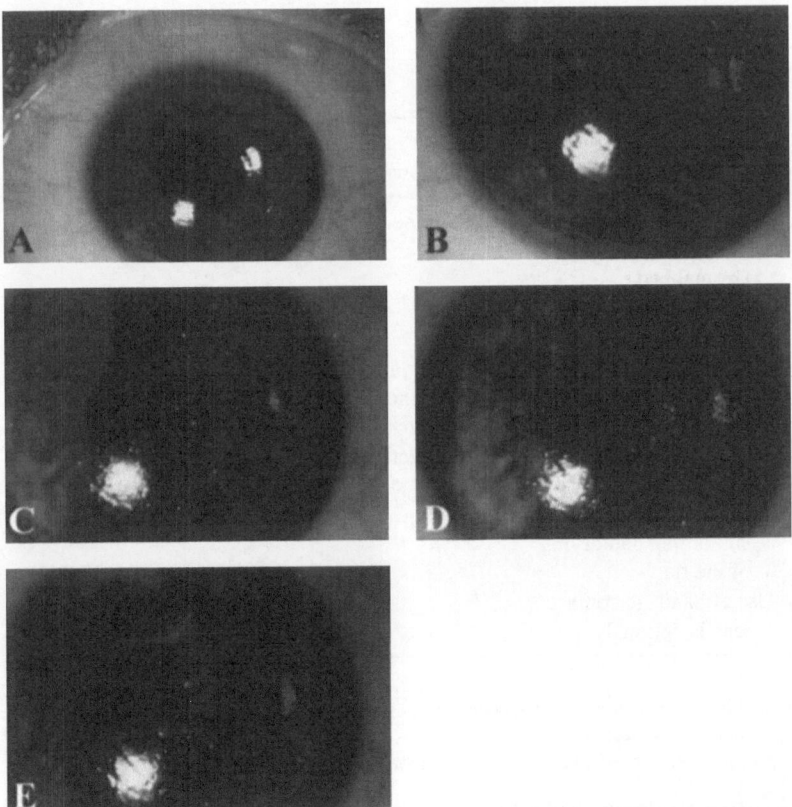

Figure 32.8   One day S/P LASIK, OS, this 46/F rubbed her postop eyes prior to sleeping. She failed to place her fox shield on. She presented the next day with a wrinkled flap nasally, nonmovable and epithelial patches on the surface. Reoperation was performed (exploration, unfolding of the flap fold, epithelial scraping of the flap surface, flap stretching, irrigation, and repositioning). (A) The gutter is widened and there are flap folds nasally. (B) Higher magnification of A. (C) Epithelial debris noted. (D) Diffuse side illumination showing epithelial defects and debris. (E) D with blue light filter. [Color in original]

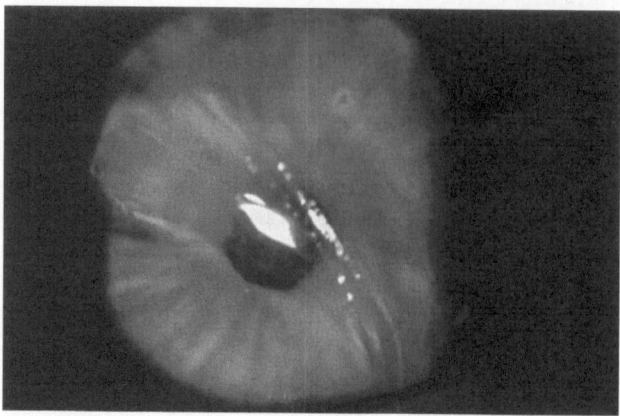

Figure 32.9   Dislocation of a corneal flap 3 weeks after LASIK secondary to trauma by finger to the eye. (Courtesy of Nada S. Jabbur, M.D.)

Table 6   Management of Displaced Flap

Timing	Acute intervention	Follow-up	Long-term management	Outcomes
Intraoperative	Reposition the flap after gentle irrigation of the stromal bed Use of bandage contact lens is optional	Routine	Routine	Good
Postoperative	Careful inspection and scraping of the stromal bed of epithelial cells or debris before repositioning of flap Allow additional time for smoothing and drying of the flap Use of bandage contact lens is optional	Observe for epithelial ingrowth, infection and striae	Keep eyes well lubricated Eye shield for first two weeks	Good

Prevention
1. Good communication with the patient to avoid sudden eye movement and blinking during the procedure as well as when the speculum is removed.
2. Superior hinged flap with the newer microkeratome can improve the flap stability by blinking, which circumvents upper edge displacement.
3. Patient education to avoid trauma and the use of eye shield at night for the first 2 weeks.

may be repositioned gently following the steps described in the management of striae, folds, and wrinkles. A bandage contact lens may be placed in order to prevent further friction on the flap.

2. Postoperative Management

The flap should first be reflected and the interface (stromal bed and stromal aspect of the flap) carefully examined for epithelial cells or other debris. They should be aggressively scraped prior to repositioning the flap (Fig. 32.10). A contact lens can be applied to provide added protection from further displacement (101). Techniques described above to flatten any associated folds should be used. Additional time in smoothing and drying the flap should be exercised. This is important to prevent epithelial cell migration from the healing periphery towards the flap interface under the tented folds.

The flap should be well lubricated for a couple of weeks. This will decrease the probability of friction causing further mischief. An eye shield may be suggested for an extended period of time.

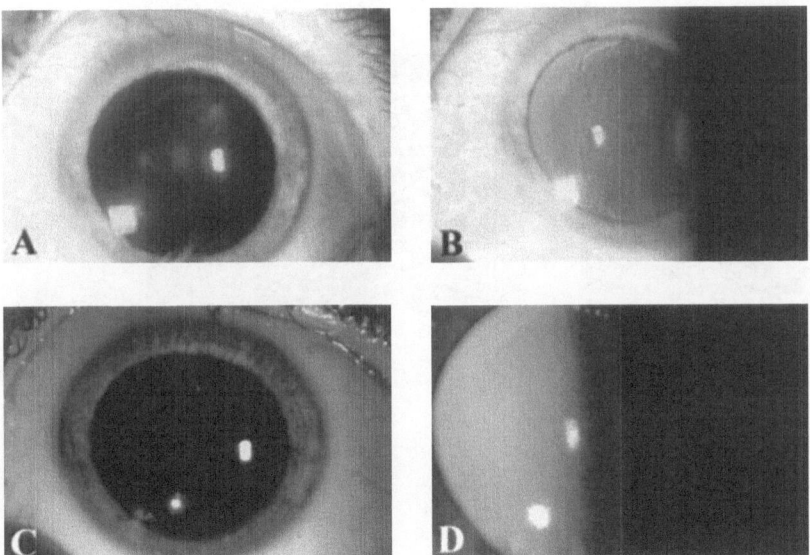

Figure 32.10 43/F S/P 1° LASIK, OS, 2 months prior to referral. One day postop, flap slippage was noted. The 1° surgeon refloated the flap with a note of residual wrinkles postop. VscOS was 20/30-2 despite this. Upon referral we noted that there was an epithelial ingrowth from 4 to 8 hours. There were residual wrinkles radiating from the 4 mm ACS hinge. We lifted the flap, scraped the epithelial ingrowth, flattened the flap with the Pineda iron, and irrigated the interface. VscOS was maintained at 20/30 after debridement and ironing. (A) Epithelial ingrowth noted at margins from 4 to 8 hours (preop). (B) On retroillumination, flap wrinkles and epithelial ingrowth are clearly seen. (C) Improvement noted on flap edge. There is no evidence of epithelial ingrowth 8 days after debridement and ironing. (D) On retroillumination, a clearer view shows the lack of epithelial ingrowth with residual wrinkles.

3. Prevention

Prevention of dislodged flaps rests mainly on using protective measures such as the superiorly hinged flaps, which were designed to circumvent upper flap edge displacement through blinking (102). It is not clear yet whether they have achieved their intended purpose. It helps to ask the patient not to blink while the drape and the speculum are removed. A technique for removing the eyelid speculum that may be useful is to rotate the speculum vertically while it is being removed. The LASIK flap would then be undisturbed. Other preventive steps include applying a contact lens after the procedure, lid taping, and encouraging eyelid closure in the first few hours following surgery. We advise our patients not to apply eyedrops soon after surgery to avoid any early mechanical disturbances. Wearing a protective shield when sleeping in the few weeks after the procedure can also minimize traumatic displacement through unintentional rubbing or mechanical pressure on the eyelids. Patients involved in contact sports and similar activities should be thoroughly counseled about the added risk of late flap displacement with LASIK. PRK might be a better alternative, if judged feasible, in these situations.

I. EPITHELIAL DEFECTS AND TEARS

On postoperative day #1, dilute sodium fluorescein is applied to detect epithelial defects that might have occurred during or after the procedure (Figs. 32.11, 32.12, and 32.13).

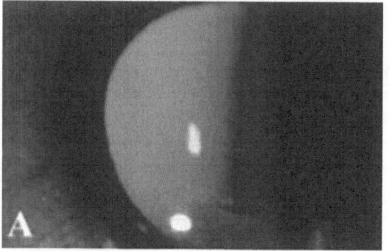
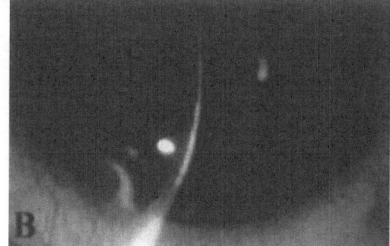
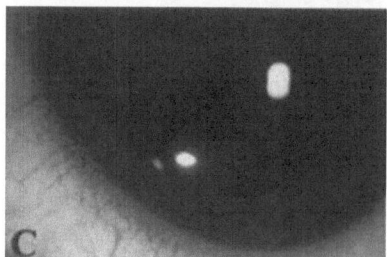

Figure 32.11   37/M S/P LASIK, OS 2 months prior to presentation. There was postlaser infection of the flap with swelling, redness, and pain and a decrease in vision OS. This was treated with steroids. The patient came in for an opinion and possible retreatment. Upon examination we noted an epithelial ingrowth at the edge of the LASIK flap. Surgical repair was discussed and agreed upon. The flap was lifted and the epithelial cells were scraped in order to avoid flap melting and progressive decrease in vision. After several follow-ups, there were no epithelial cells noted. (A) On retroillumination, the epithelial ingrowth is noted away from the hinge. There are wrinkles seen along the visual axis. (B) Slit beam photography across the epithelial ingrowth. (C) Follow-up image showing resolution of ingrowth. [Color in original.]

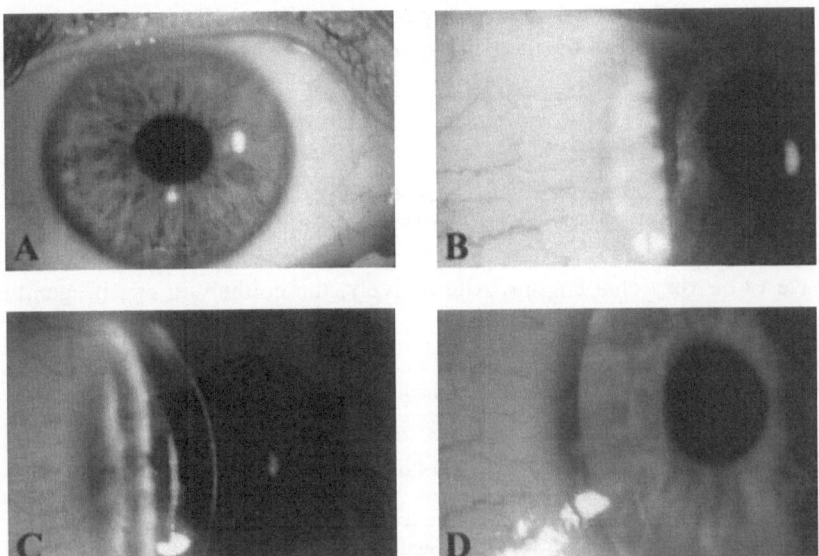

Figure 32.12 /F S/P LASIK. (A) Anterior view shows slight peripheral haze opposite the flap hinge. (B) On closer view, epithelial ingrowth is noted. (C) Slit beam shows the depth of involvement. (D) Three weeks after debridement, a peripheral flap melt is noted.

Many patients will demonstrate mild staining at the edge of the flap. Larger defects are more worrisome, especially those with a connection to the flap edge (Fig. 32.13 see color insert). The incidence of epithelial defects with LASIK was reported to be around 5% (103). As mentioned above, the proliferating epithelial cells may migrate under the flap edge (Figs. 32.11 and 32.12). Associated inflammation can also lead to melting of the surrounding flap tissue. Furthermore, we have observed an increased risk of diffuse lamellar keratitis in patients with epithelial defects (Fig. 32.7).

Patients with a history of recurrent erosions (104–107) and/or anterior basement membrane dystrophy (ABMD) (108,109) are at higher risk of developing epithelial abra-

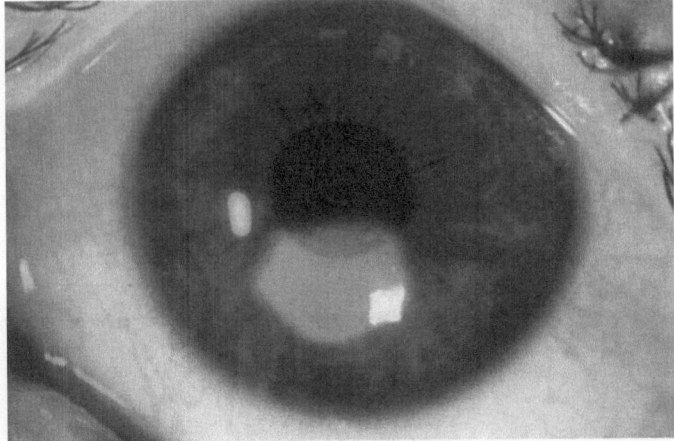

Figure 32.13 Epithelial abrasion noted after the microkeratome pass.

sions, especially with LASIK, and would probably be better PRK candidates. In fact, surface excimer laser ablation is one of the modalities used to treat patients with recurrent erosion syndrome (111–115).

1. Intraoperative Management

If an epithelial defect is noted intraoperatively, a higher index of suspicion for epithelial ingrowth should be maintained (Figs. 32.12 and 32.13). An attempt at repositioning the loose epithelium should be performed (Table 7). Carefully piecing the loose edges together may sometimes prove to be very challenging. Alternatively, the epithelium can be gently

Table 7   Management of Epithelial Tears/Defects/Edema

Types	Acute intervention	Follow-up	Long-term management	Outcomes
Epithelial tear	Reposition the epithelium if possible	Observe for epithelial ingrowth and infection Aggressive topical steroids for DLK prophylaxis	Lubrication	Good
Epithelial defect	Replace all adherent and loose epithelium and place a bandage contact lens	Lubrication Prophylaxis for infection with antibiotics Treatment of pain with BCL, topical NSAID Aggressive topical steroids for DLK prophylaxis	Remove BCL after adequate lubrication	Good
Stromal edema	Gentle pressure on the flap with a microsponge or blunt spatula	Aggressive topical steroids for DLK prophylaxis	Slight haze if persistent stromal edema	Good
Stretched flap	Gentle replacement of epithelium and eliminate redundant epithelium is rarely required Bandage contact lens if necessary	Lubrication	Routine	Good
Shrinked/contracted flap	Distend the flap with care Lift and rehydrate the flap Suturing as needed	Lubrication	Routine	Good

Prevention
1. Consider PRK in patients with anterior membrane dystrophy and symptoms consistent with recurrent corneal erosion syndrome.
2. Avoid excessive use of topical anesthetic as it may loosen the epithelium; use a glycerin-based preparation such as Proparacaine.
3. Place minimal fiducial marks and avoid the central 3.0 mm of cornea.

debrided and a contact lens applied (116–118). These measures help in pain control as well as improving flap adherence and preventing epithelial cell infiltration.

2. Postoperative Management

Topical nonsteroidal anti-inflammatory drugs (NSAIDS) may also be useful to ease the associated discomfort (119–125). A bandage contact lens may be placed in order to prevent the lids from abrading the cornea and enlarging the epithelial defect. Caution should be exercised when the contact lens is removed because of the risk of flap dislocation upon its removal.

3. Prevention

Candidates for LASIK surgery should be questioned for prior history or symptoms of recurrent erosion syndrome. Slit lamp examination should include careful inspection of the epithelial surface for signs of ABMD. Even when the corneal surface appears clear, negative or asymmetric fluorescein staining should alert the observer to an abnormality in corneal surface integrity. Some investigators recommend touching the corneal epithelium at the slit lamp with a microsponge applicator in patients with suspected loose epithelium. If movable epithelium is noted, PRK may be a more appropriate procedure. Anecdotal reports of delaying preoperative topical anesthesia on the cornea until just prior to the placement of the microkeratome may help protect the integrity of the corneal epithelium.

J. EDEMATOUS FLAPS

An edematous flap is sometimes associated with poor adhesion to the underlying stromal bed. Flap decentration or displacement may occur. This has been named the floating flap phenomenon (43). The main etiology is prolonged manipulation and fluid irrigation.

4. Intraoperative Management

Attempting to stroke the flap gently with a moist microsponge or a blunt spatula to displace the excess fluid may help. The use of the Pineda LASIK flap iron or the Johnstone Applanator may be useful in flattening edematous flats. Buratto recommends using a Thornton ring to stabilize the eye while fluid is being induced away from the intercellular spaces.

5. Postoperative Management

Persistent LASIK flap edema in the postoperative period should alert the surgeon to the possibility of an underlying epithelial ingrowth possibly requiring surgical intervention.

6. Prevention

Minimal manipulation and irrigation are the two key elements that would prevent the occurrence of corneal flap edema. Meticulous expression of interface fluid should be performed whenever copious irrigation is used intraoperatively.

K. SHRUNKEN FLAPS

Occasionally, after an otherwise uneventful LASIK surgical procedure a groove or gutter along the incision line is seen. We believe that this phenomenon of corneal flap shrinkage is a common yet underreported complication of LASIK surgery.

It is theorized that there are corneal tension lines that exert forces on the cornea that influence its configuration. This is clearly displayed by the gap that is sometimes seen after replacement of the corneal flap. A noticeable groove may be visualized despite the best efforts in replacing the corneal flap to its original location. More commonly, corneal shrinkage may be due to the corneal flap becoming edematous and subsequently thickening with resultant shrinkage in its diameter and circumference. Ironically, flap dehydration will also cause flap shrinkage. Delays during surgery will cause excessive dryness of the flap, which will cause it to shrink.

Corneal flap stretching, on the other hand, is mostly brought about by prolonged manipulation by an overeager surgeon. Excessive smoothing and flap positioning may contribute to the production of an aberrantly enlarged flap. Actually, epithelial defects may also be caused by these same faulty practices. Having an enlarged flap may actually produce a redundant epithelium. Difficulty in replacing the epithelium may be encountered. There may also be the production of some striae that may affect vision, especially if it is found centrally.

1. Intraoperative Management

It is rarely necessary for any intervention to be done in order to address the phenomenon of flap shrinkage (Table 7). Simple steps may be done in order to attempt to remedy the situation. The flap may be gently stretched and distended. This may be done by refloating the flap and rehydrating it once more. Additional smoothing and positioning exercises may be instituted in the hope that the rehydration will contribute to flap size normalization. Strategies used in the management of wrinkled flaps may be used in addressing this peculiar complication (Table 5). Suturing of the shrunken flap is rarely necessary but is an option. A bandage contact lens may be necessary in some cases in order to lessen the opportunity of ocular debris incisipating in between the corneal interface. Adequate topical antibiotic coverage is recommended. See Table 7 for a summary of steps to undertake.

Intraoperative management of a stretched flap entails gentle repositioning of the flap, approximating as natural a position as possible. In cases of stretched flaps, redundant epithelium is almost always present. Gentle repositioning of epithelium should be carried out. Redundant epithelium may be subjected to amputation in some cases, although it is rarely necessary. A bandage contact lens may be placed if necessary. Caution should be taken in removing this contact lens because of the risk of displacing the epithelium or the flap.

2. Postoperative Management

Shrunken and contracted flaps should be continuously exposed to generous amounts of lubrication. The possibility of epithelial ingrowth or debris in the interface is higher in these cases. The surgeon should be vigilant in the follow-up of these patients. One should be ready to approach it as any other epithelial ingrowth case.

Stretched flaps should also be given generous amounts of lubrication. There is rarely any problem with these cases in the long-term follow-up.

3. Prevention

Flap shrinkage is a peculiar phenomenon. It is impossible to determine where the ocular tension lines may be found. However, in cases of previous ocular trauma and/or surgery with notable scarring, such areas may be identified. Delays in surgery should be avoided. The time between flap reflection and stromal ablation should be kept to a minimum. The time between ablation and flap repositioning should be reduced as well. Nominal manipulation of the corneal flap and minimal irrigation may decrease the chances of corneal flap shrinkage. Speed is of the essence. Remember that both overhydration and dehydration may contribute to flap shrinkage. Keeping these things in check will decrease the likelihood of encountering any problem.

It is interesting to note that the steps in preventing flap shrinkage also are valid in preventing flap stretching. We believe that following the suggestions outlined above should decrease if not eliminate the occurrence of both flap shrinkage and stretching.

L. CONCLUSIONS

LASIK refractive surgery is a relatively new technique with a very high success rate, in which higher standards of safety are necessary because relatively healthy eyes are placed at risk every time the procedure is performed. These risks can be minimized by learning from mistakes, by analyzing outcomes, and by entering new territory thoughtfully and ethically.

Investigators have helped advance our knowledge of unexpected results and have prompted in-depth procedural review of this relatively recent surgical procedure by reporting their complications and sharing their experiences with the rest of the refractive community. This has allowed for continuous refinements in LASIK flap surgical technique and provided the basis for new and improved future vision correction strategies.

REFERENCES

1. S Melke, DT Azar. LASIK complications. Surv Ophthalmol 2001.
2. HV Gimbel, EE Penno, JA van Westenbrugge, M Ferensowicz, MT Furlong. Incidence and management of intraoperative and early postoperative complications in 1000 consecutive laser in situ keratomileusis cases. Ophthalmology 1998;105:1839–1847, discussion 1847–1848.
3. RT Lin, RK Maloney. Flap complications associated with lamellar refractive surgery [see comments]. Am J Ophthalmol 1999;127:129–136.
4. RD Stulting, JD Carr, KP Thompson, GO Waring, WM Wiley, JG Walker. Complications of laser in situ keratomileusis for the correction of myopia. Ophthalmology 1999;106:13–20.
5. L Buratto, M Ferrari. Indications, techniques, results, limits, and complications of laser in situ keratomileusis. Curr Opin Ophthalmol 1997;8:59–66.
6. SG Farah, DT Azar, C Gurdal, J Wong. Laser in situ keratomileusis: literature review of a developing technique. J Cataract Refract Surg 1998;24:989–1006.
7. IG Pallikaris, ME Papatzanaki, EZ Stathi, O Frenschock, A Georgiadis. Laser in situ keratomileusis. Lasers Surg Med 1990;10:463–468.
8. IG Pallikaris, DS Siganos. Excimer laser in situ keratomileusis and photorefractive keratectomy for correction of high myopia. J Refract Corneal Surg 1994;10:498–510.
9. SG Slade, SA Updegraff. Advances in lamellar refractive surgery. Int Ophthalmol Clin 1994;34:147–162.
10. SH Yoo, DT Azar. Laser in situ keratomileusis for the treatment of myopia. Int Ophthalmol Clin 1999;39:37–44.
11. JD Gottsch, EV Rencs, JL Cambier, D Hall, DT Azar, WJ Stark. Excimer laser calibration system. J Refract Surg 1996;12:401–411.
12. L Missotten, R Boving, G Francois, C Coutteel. Experimental excimer laser keratomileusis. Bull Soc Belge Ophthalmol 1986;220:103–120.
13. SL Trokel, R Srinivasan, B Braren. Excimer laser surgery of the cornea. Am J Ophthalmol 1983;96:710–715.
14. IG Pallikaris, ME Papatzanaki, DS Siganos, MK Tsilimbaris. A corneal flap technique for laser in situ keratomileusis. Human studies. Arch Ophthalmol 1991;109:1699–1702.

15. J Barraquer. Queratoplastia refractiva. Estudio Inform Oftal Inst Barraquer 1949;10:2–21.
16. JI Barraquer. [Autokeratoplasty with levelins for the correction of myopia (keratomileusis). Technique and results.] Ann Ocul (Paris) 1965;198:401–25.
17. JI Barraquer. The history and evolution of keratomileusis. Int Ophthalmol Clin 1996;36:1–7.
18. D Ainslie. The surgical correction of refractive errors by keratomileusis and keratophakia. Ann Ophthalmol 1976;8:349–367.
19. JI Barraquer. Keratomileusis. Int Surg 1967;48:103–117.
20. FA Jakobiec, P Koch, T Iwamoto, W Harrison, F Troutman. Keratophakia and keratomileusis: comparison of pathologic features in penetrating keratoplasty specimens. Ophthalmology 1981;88:1251–1259.
21. LF Rich. A technique for preparing corneal lamellar donor tissue using simplified keratomileusis. Ophthalmic Surg 1980;11:606–608.
22. JH Krumeich. [Keratomileusis. A new surgical technique in eye surgery. Information for the general practitioner.] ZFA (Stuttgart) 1981;57:1321–1326.
23. JH Krumeich. Indications, techniques, and complications of myopic keratomileusis. Int Ophthalmol Clin 1983;23:75–92.
24. Automated lamellar keratoplasty. American Academy of Ophthalmology [see comments]. Ophthalmology 1996;103:852–861.
25. S Esquenazi. Comparison of laser in situ keratomileusis and automated lamellar keratoplasty for the treatment of myopia. J Refract Surg 1997;13:637–643.
26. K Hanna, JC Chastang, Y Pouliquen, G Renard, L Asfar, GO Waring. A rotating slit delivery system for excimer laser refractive keratoplasty. Am J Ophthalmol 1987;103:474.
27. J Marshall, SL Trokel, S Rothery, RR Krueger. Long-term healing of the central cornea after photorefractive keratectomy using an excimer laser. Ophthalmology 1988;95:1411–1421.
28. MB McDonald, JM Frantz, SD Klyce, RW Beuerman, R Varnell, CR Munnerlyn, TN Clapham, B Salmeron, HE Kaufman. Central photorefractive keratectomy for myopia. The blind eye study. Arch Ophthalmol 1990;108:799–808.
29. CR Munnerlyn, SJ Koons, J Marshall. Photorefractive keratectomy: a technique for laser refractive surgery. J Cataract Refract Surg 1988;14:46–52.
30. SL Trokel, R Srinivasan, B Braren. Excimer laser surgery of the cornea. Am J Ophthalmol 1983;96:710–715.
31. EJ Velasco-Martinelli, FA Tarcha. Superior hinge laser in situ keratomileusis. J Refract Surg 1999;15:S209–S211.
32. J Blanckaert, G Sallet. Lasik learning curve: clinical study of 300 myopic eyes. Bull Soc Belge Ophtalmol 1998;268:7–12.
33. M Moretti. U.S. laser vision correction market explodes. Eye World 1999;12.
34. DV Leaming. Practice styles and preferences of ASCRS members—1998 survey. J Cataract Refract Surg 1999;25:851–859.
35. GO Waring III. A cautionary tale of innovation in refractive surgery. Arch Ophthalmol 1999;117:1069–1073.
36. EA Ansari, AJ Morrell, K Sahni. Corneal perforation and decompensation after automated lamellar keratoplasty for hyperopia [see comments]. J Cataract Refract Surg 1997;23:134–136.
37. JF Arevalo, E Ramirez, E Suarez, J Morales-Stopello, R Cortez, G Ramirez, G Antzoulatos, J Tugues, J Rodriguez, D Furenmayor-Rivera. Incidence of vitreoretinal pathologic conditions within 24 months after laser in situ keratomileusis [in process citation]. Ophthalmology 2000;107:258–262.
38. HV Gimbel, S Basti, GB Kaye, M Ferensowicz. Experience during the learning curve of laser in situ keratomileusis [see comments]. J Cataract Refract Surg 1996;22:542–550.
39. Y Hori, H Wantanabe, N Maeda, Y Inoue, Y Shimomura, Y Tano. Medical treatment of operative corneal perforation caused by laser in situ keratomileusis. Arch Ophthalmol 1999;117:1422–1423.

40. CK Joo, TG Kim. Corneal perforation during laser in situ keratomileusis. J Cataract Refract Surg 1999;25:1165–1167.

41. L Buratto, SF Brint. LASIK Principles and Techniques. SLACK 113–139, 371–379.

42. EK Kim, CM Choe, SJ Kang, HB Kim. Management of detached lenticule after in situ keratomileusis. J Refract Surg 1996;12:175–179.

43. L Buratto, S Brint, eds. LASIK Surgical Techniques and Complications.

44. I Pallikaris, D Siganos. LASIK complications and management. Cornea, 2d ed. Chap. 9, pp 227–243.

45. SA Melki, CE Proano, DT Azar. Optical disturbances and their management after myopic laser in situ keratomileusis. Int Ophthalmol Clin 2000;40:45–56.

46. V Filatov, JS Vidaurri-Leal, JH Talamo. Selected complications of radial keratotomy, photorefractive keratectomy, and laser in situ keratomileusis. Int Ophthalmol Clin 1997;37: 123–148.

47. SE Wilson. LASIK: management of common complications. Laser in situ keratomileusis. Cornea 1998;17:459–467.

48. GO Waring III, JD Carr, RD Stulting, KP Thompson, W Wiley. Prospective randomized comparison of simultaneous and sequential bilateral laser in situ keratomileusis for the correction of myopia. Ophthalmology 1999;106:732–738.

49. V Thompson. Flap management during LASIK after radial keratotomy [letter]. J Refract Surg 1997;13:128.

50. DSC Lam, ACK Cheng, ATS Leung. LASIK complications (letters). Ophthalmology 1999; 106:1455–1456.

51. AT Leung, SK Rao, AC Cheng, EW Yu, DS Fan, DS Lam. Pathogenesis and management of laser in situ keratomileusis flap buttonhole. J Cataract Refract Surg 2000;26:359–362.

52. EA Penno, G Kaye, J van Westenbrugge. LASIK complications (authors' reply). J Cataract Refract Surg 1999;106:1456–1457.

53. JM Davidorf, R Zaldivar, S Oscherow. Results and complications of laser in situ keratomileusis by experienced surgeons. J Refract Surg 1998;14:114–122.

54. R Zaldivar, JM Davidorf, S Oscherow. Laser in situ keratomileusis for myopia from −5.50 to −11.50 diopters with astigmatism. J Refract Surg 1998;14:19–25.

55. VMB Tham, RK Maloney. Microkeratome complications of laser in situ keratomileusis. Am J Ophthalmol 2000;107:920–924.

56. J Marshall, SL Trokel, S Rothery, RR Krueger. Long-term healing of the central cornea after photorefractive keratectomy using an excimer laser. Ophthalmology 1988;95:1411–1421.

57. GS Polunin, VV Kourenkov, IA Makarov, EG Polunina. The corneal barrier function in myopic eyes after laser in situ keratomileusis and after photorefractive keratectomy in eyes with haze formation [in process citation]. J Refract Surg 1999;15:S221–S224.

58. FW Price Jr, MW Belin, LT Nordan, PJ McDonnell, M Pop. Epithelial haze, punctate keratopathy, and induced hyperopia after photorefractive keratectomy for myopia. J Refract Surg 1999;15:384–387.

59. M Goggin, P Kenna, F Lavery. Haze following photorefractive and photoastigmatic refractive keratectomy with the Nidek EC5000 and the Summit ExciMed UV200. J Cataract Refract Surg 1997;23:50–53.

60. P Cernea, F Constantin, A Stefanescu, I Filipescu. [Determination of ocular pressure with the pneumotonometer.] Rev Chir Oncol Radiol O R L Oftalmol Stomatol Ser Oftalmol 1980;24: 37–41.

61. J Guildford, DM O'Day. Applanation pneumotonometry in screening for glaucoma. South Med J 1985;78:1081–1083.

62. MJ Hodkin, MA Pavilack, DC Musch. Pneumotonometry using sterile single-use tonometer covers. Ophthalmology 1992;99:688–695.

63. RT Lin, RK Maloney. Flap complications associated with lamellar refractive surgery [see comments]. Am J Ophthalmol 1999;127:129–136.

64. DS Lam, AT Leung, JT Wu, AC Cheng, DS Fan, SK Rao, JH Talamo, C Barraquer. Management of severe flap wrinkling or dislodgment after laser in situ keratomileusis. J Cataract Refract Surg 1999;25:1441–1447.

65. JJ Salz, SP Azen, J Berstein, P Caroline, RA Villasenor, DJ Schanzlin. Evaluation and comparison of sources of variability in the measurement of corneal thickness with ultrasonic and optical pachymeters. Ophthalmic Surg 1983;14:750–754.

66. RA Villasenor, VR Santos, KC Cox, DF Harris, M Lynn, GO Waring. Comparison of ultrasonic corneal thickness measurements before and during surgery in the Prospective Evaluation of Radial Keratotomy (PERK) study. Ophthalmology 1986;93:327–330.

67. T Nishida. Basic science: cornea, sclera, and ocular adnexa anatomy, biochemistry, physiology, and biomechanics (cornea). In: M Krachmer, Holland. Cornea: Fundamentals of Cornea and External Disease, St. Louis: Mosby Year Book, 1997, pp 3–28.

68. MS Kapadia, SE Wilson. Transepithelial photorefractive keratectomy for treatment of thin flaps or caps after complicated laser in situ keratomileusis. Am J Ophthalmol 1998;126: 827–829.

69. EF Carpel, KH Carlson, S Shannon. Folds and striae in laser in situ keratomileusis flaps. J Refract Surg 1999;15:687–690.

70. TL Steinemann, NC Denton, MF Brown. Corneal lenticular wrinkling after automated lamellar keratoplasty. Am J Ophthalmol 1998;126:588–590.

71. JS Pannu. Wrinkled corneal flaps after LASIK [letter; comment]. J Refract Surg 1997; 13:341.

72. YS Rabinowitz, K Rasheed. Fluorescein test for the detection of striae in the corneal flap after laser in situ keratomileusis. Am J Ophthalmol 1999;127:717–718.

73. M Vesaluoma, J Perez-Santonja, WM Petroll, T Linna, J Alio, T Tervo. Corneal stromal changes induced by myopic LASIK. Invest Ophthalmol Vis Sci 2000;41:369–376.

74. LE Probst, J Machat. Removal of flap striae following laser in situ keratomileusis. J Cataract Refract Surg 1998;24:153–155.

75. JS Pannu. Incidence and treatment of wrinkled corneal flap following LASIK [letter; comment]. J Cataract Refract Surg 1997;23:695–696.

76. JS Pannu, S Mutyala. Corneal flap adhesion following LASIK [letter] [in process citation]. J Cataract Refract Surg 1999;25:606.

77. T Ling. Osmotically induced central and peripheral corneal swelling in the cat. Am J Optom Physiol Opt 1987;64:674–677.

78. G Munoz, JL Alio, JJ Perez-Santonja, WH Attia. Successful treatment of severe wrinkled corneal flap after laser in situ keratomileusis with deionized water. Am J Ophthalmol 2000;129:91–92.

79. NA Chaudhry, WE Smiddy. Displacement of corneal cap during vitrectomy in a post-LASIK eye. Retina 1998;18:554–555.

80. M Montes, AS Chayet, A Castellanos, N Robledo. Use of bandage contact lenses after laser in situ keratomileusis. J Refract Surg 1999;13:S430–S431.

81. JS Pannu, S Mutyala. Corneal flap adhesion following LASIK [letter] [in process citation]. J Cataract Refract Surg 1999;25:606.

82. EP Perez, B Viramontes, P Schor, D Miller. Factors affecting corneal strip stroma-to-stroma adhesion. J Refract Surg 1998;14:460–462.

83. SE Wilson. LASIK: management of common complications. Laser in situ keratomileusis. Cornea 1998;17:459–467.

84. AT Leung, SK Rao, DS Lam. Traumatic partial unfolding of laser in situ keratomileusis flap with severe epithelial ingrowth. J Cataract Refract Surg 2000;26:135–139.

85. NA Chaudhry, WE Smiddy. Displacement of corneal cap during vitrectomy in a post-LASIK eye. Retina 1998;18:554–555.

86. EP Shakin, DM Fastenberg, IJ Udell, JL Shakin, PL Schwartz, BM Golub, G Neck. Late dislocation of a corneal cap after automated lamellar keratoplasty and epithelial debridement for retinal surgery [letter]. Arch Ophthalmol 1996;114:1420.

87. B Yang, J Chen, Z Wang. Enhancement ablation for the treatment of undercorrection after excimer laser in situ keratomileusis for correcting myopia. Chin Med J (Engl) 1998;111: 358–360.

88. AS Chayet, KK Assil, M Montes, M Espinosa-Lagana, A Castellanos, G Tsioulias. Regression and its mechanisms after laser in situ keratomileusis in moderate and high myopia. Ophthalmology 1998;105:1194–1199.

89. DS Durrie, AA Aziz. Lift-flap retreatment after laser in situ keratomileusis. J Refract Surg 1999;15:150–153.

90. E Martines, ME John. The Martines enhancement technique for correcting residual myopia following laser assisted in situ keratomileusis. Ophthalmic Surg Lasers 1996;27:S512–S516.

91. JJ Perez-Santonja, MJ Ayala, HF Sakla, JM Ruiz-Moreno, JL Alio. Retreatment after laser in situ keratomileusis. Ophthalmology 1999;106:21–28.

92. JL Febbraro, KA Buzard, MH Friedlander. Reoperations after myopic laser in situ keratomileusis. J Cataract Refract Surg 2000;26:41–48.

93. A Ozdamar, C Aras, H Bahcecioglu, B Sener. Secondary laser in situ keratomileusis 1 year after primary LASIK for high myopia. J Cataract Refract Surg 1999;25:383–388.

94. D Zadok, G Maskaleris, V Garcia, S Shah, M Montes, A Chayet. Outcomes of retreatment after laser in situ keratomileusis. Ophthalmology 1999;106:2391–2394.

95. T Kato, K Nakayasu, Y Hosoda, Y Watanabe, A Kanai. Corneal wound healing following laser in situ keratomileusis (LASIK): a histopathological study in rabbits. Br J Ophthalmol 1999;83:1302–1305.

96. CK Park, JH Kim. Comparison of wound healing after photorefractive keratectomy and laser in situ keratomileusis in rabbits. J Cataract Refract Surg 1999;25:842–850.

97. JJ Perez-Santonja, TU Linna, KM Tervo, HF Sakla, JL Alio y Sanz, TM Tervo. Corneal wound healing after laser in situ keratomileusis in rabbits. J Refract Surg 1998;14:602–609.

98. J Wachtlin, K Langenbeck, S Schrunder, EP Zhang, F Hoffmann. Immunohistology of corneal wound healing after photorefractive keratectomy and laser in situ keratomileusis. J Refract Surg 1999;15:451–458.

99. EJ Velasco-Martinelli, FA Tarcha. Superior hinge laser in situ keratomileusis [in process citation]. J Refract Surg 1999;15:S209–S211.

100. JM Davidorf, R Zaldivar, S Oscherow. Results and complications of laser in situ keratomileusis by experienced surgeons. J Refract Surg 1998;14:114–122.

101. MA Flynn, DB Esterly. Bilateral recurrent erosion of cornea. Am J Ophthalmol 1966; 62:964–966.

102. P Heyworth, N Morlet, S Rayner, P Hykin, J Dart. Natural history of recurrent erosion syndrome—a 4 year review of 117 patients [see comments]. Br J Ophthalmol 1998;82:26–28.

103. RF Lowe. Recurrent erosion of the cornea. Br J Ophthalmol 1970;54:805–809.

104. DE Puk, LE Probst, EJ Holland. Recurrent erosion after photorefractive keratectomy. Cornea 1996;15:541–542.

105. E Balestrazzi, V De Molfetta, L Spadea, P Vinciguerra, G Palmieri, G Santeusanio, L Spagnoli. Histological, immunohistochemical, and ultrastructural findings in human corneas after photorefractive keratectomy. J Refract Surg 1995;11:181–187.

106. JA Fogle, KR Kenyon, WJ Stark, WR Green. Defective epithelial adhesion in anterior corneal dystrophies. Am J Ophthalmol 1975;79:925–940.

107. DT Azar, RF Steinert. Phototherapeutic keratectomy, management of scars, dystrophies, and PRK complications. In: PTK in the Management of PRK Complications. Baltimore: Williams & Wilkins, 1997, pp 175–188.

108. W Forster, S Grewe, U Atzler, C Lunecke, H Busse. Phototherapeutic keratectomy in corneal diseases. Refract Corneal Surg 1993;9:S85–S90.

109. VP Kozobolis, DS Siganos, GS Meladakis, IG Pallikaris. Excimer laser phototherapeutic keratectomy for corneal opacities and recurrent erosion. J Refract Surg 1996;12:S288–S290.

110. CP Lohmann, H Sachs, J Marshall, VP Gabel. Excimer laser phototherapeutic keratectomy for recurrent erosions: a clinical study. Ophthalmic Surg Lasers 1996;27:768–772.
111. DP O'Brart, MG Muir, J Marshall. Phototherapeutic keratectomy for recurrent corneal erosions. Eye 1994;8:378–383.
112. MJ Orndahl, PP Fagerholm. Phototherapeutic keratectomy for map-dot-fingerprint corneal dystrophy. Cornea 1998;17:595–599.
113. ML McDermott, JW Chandler. Therapeutic uses of contact lenses. Surv Ophthalmol 1989;33: 381–394.
114. JJ Salz, AL Reader III, LJ Schwartz, K Van Le. Treatment of corneal abrasions with soft contact lenses and topical diclofenac. J Refract Corneal Surg 1994;10:640–646.
115. SA Arshinoff, MD Mills, S Haber. Pharmacotherapy of photorefractive keratectomy. J Cataract Refract Surg 1996;22:1037–1044.
116. PM Cherry. The treatment of pain following excimer laser photorefractive keratectomy: additive effect of local anesthetic drops, topical diclofenac, and bandage soft contact. Ophthalmic Surg Lasers 1996;27:S477–S480.
117. W Forster, I Ratkay, R Krueger, H Busse. Topical diclofenac sodium after excimer laser phototherapeutic keratectomy. J Refract Surg 1997;13:311–313.
118. AF Phillips, S Hayashi, B Seitz, WR Wee, PJ McDonnell. Effect of diclofenac, ketorolac, and fluorometholone on arachidonic acid metabolites following excimer laser corneal surgery. Arch Ophthalmol 1996;114:1495–1498.
119. S Tomas-Barberan, P Fagerholm. Influence of topical treatment on epithelial wound healing and pain in the early postoperative period following photorefractive keratectomy. Acta Ophthalmol Scand 1999;77:135–138.
120. MK Tutton, PM Cherry, PS Raj, MG Fsadni. Efficacy and safety of topical diclofenac in reducing ocular pain after excimer photorefractive keratectomy. J Cataract Refract Surg 1996; 22:536–541.

33

Management of Interlamellar Epithelium

NAN WANG and DOUGLAS D. KOCH

Cullen Eye Institute, Baylor College of Medicine, Houston, Texas, U.S.A.

Interlamellar epithelium is a common postoperative complication of LASIK. Although treatment is generally successful, recurrences are common, and progressive forms can be sight threatening. Keys to management are prevention, early recognition, and, when indicated, early surgical treatment.

A. INCIDENCE

There is wide variation in the reported incidence of interlamellar epithelium. Farah et al. (2) reviewed all literature published between 1990 and 1997 related to LASIK and found a 4.3% cumulative incidence of interlamellar epithelium (range: 0% to 20%). Subsequent reports have noted incidences ranging from 0% (Febbraro et al. [3]) to 31% (Perez-Santonja et al. [22]). However, the incidence is generally reported to be less than 10%, i.e., 1% by Gimbel et al. (5), 4% by Knorz et al. (13), 2.2% by Lin and Maloney (15), 7.1% by Forseto et al. (4), 3.4% by Lindstrom et al. (16), 9.1% by Stulting et al. (24), 3.3% by Lindstrom et al. (17). Indeed, three recent studies reported an incidence of less than 1%: 0.7% by Kawesch and Kezirian (11), 0.92% by Wang and Maloney (26), and 0.34% by Walker and Wilson (25). It should be noted that some of the differences among these reports might be attributable to the use of different criteria to define interlamellar epithelium.

B. CLASSIFICATION

Clinically, there are two patterns interlamellar epithelium:

1. The first consists of an isolated epithelial nest within the lamellar interface with-
    out any connection to epithelium at flap edge (Fig. 33.1). This can occur cen-
    trally or peripherally and can be single or multifocal.
2. The second is an advancing wave of epithelial cells growing in from the flap
    edge (epithelial ingrowth under lamellar bed), usually remote from the flap hinge
    (Fig. 33.2). In this form, the epithelium within the lamellar bed is connected to
    the surface epithelium (Wright et al. [29], Wang and Maloney [26]).

Therefore, we believe that interlamellar epithelium is a better term to describe both
patterns, while epithelial ingrowth is more specific for the latter form.

C. PATHOGENESIS

1. Isolated Epithelial Nest

Isolated epithelial nests are presumably caused by intraoperative implantation of epithelial
cells. Since these cells are not connected to the surface epithelium, they have limited
growth potential, and this process is therefore almost always self-limited. However, they
may release enzymes and cytokines, causing inflammation or apoptosis (Helena et al. [8],
Wilson et al. [28], Wilson [27]). The cells may gradually get absorbed or undergo fibrous
metaplasia.

Potential mechanisms for introducing epithelium into the interface include (1) Dragging of surface epithelial cells by the microkeratome blade (Helena et al. [9]), possibly
more likely if the blade quality is poor; (2) an irregular cut such as a buttonhole flap, where
the same blade exits and then reenters the stroma before completing the flap (Helena et al.

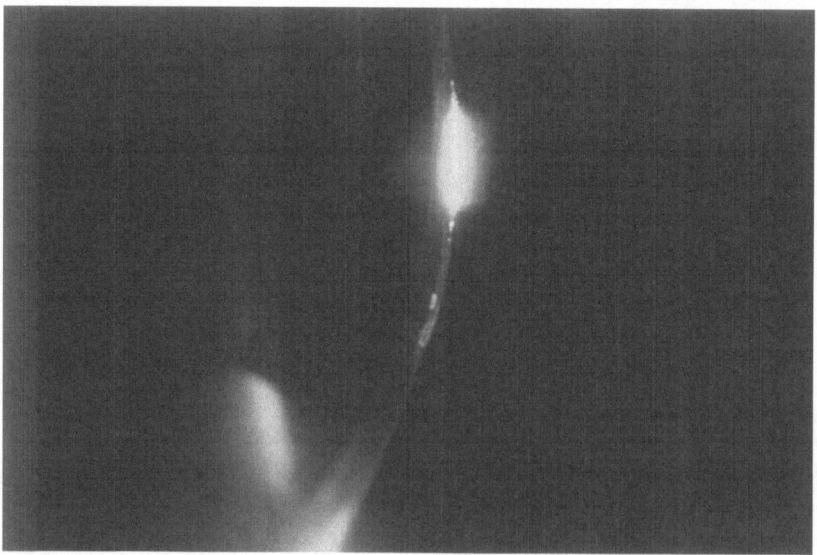

Figure 33.1   Epithelial nest following LASIK surgery.

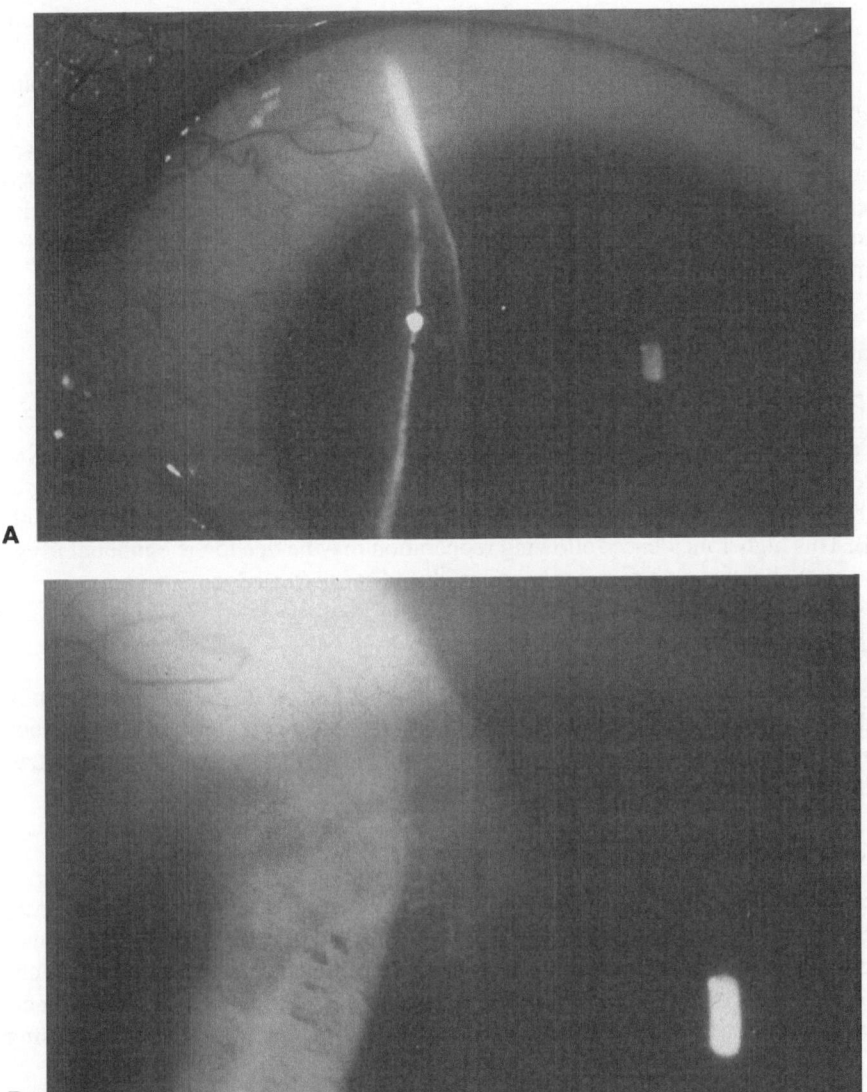

Figure 33.2   Epithelial ingrowth in a rim pattern (A). Higher magnification (B).

[9]); (3) temporary infolding of the flap with release of epithelial cells into the interface; and (4) backflow of irrigation, which allows epithelium to float into the interface. In each of these instances, inadequate irrigation would permit the introduced epithelial cells to remain in the interface.

2.   Epithelial ingrowth

With epithelial growth beneath the flap edge, the interface cells are connected to limbal stem cells and therefore have unlimited growth potential. The epithelial-stromal interactions are similar to those observed in isolated epithelial nests but to a larger scale. Cytokine-mediated inflammation and apoptosis could further hinder flap adherence, causing more epithelial ingrowth.

The two basic mechanisms of epithelial ingrowth are poor flap adherence and trapping of epithelial tags beneath the flap edge. Causes of poor flap adherence include (1) A malpositioned flap with striae, folds, dislocation, contraction or asymmetric gutter; (2) postoperative epithelial defect, which causes flap edema and therefore poor adherence; (3) high correction causing large disparity between the cap and the bed; and (4) interface debris and inflammation. Epithelial tags that are caught under the flap may act as tracks for epithelium to grow, in addition to causing poor flap adherence.

D. PREDISPOSING FACTORS

1. Reoperation

The incidence of interlamellar epithelium appears to be higher after enhancement. Reported rates following primary and enhancement procedures are 1.3% vs. 3.2% (Stulting et al. [24]), 8.5% vs. 31% (Perez-Santonja et al. [22]), and 0.92% vs. 1.7% (Wang and Maloney [26]). This higher incidence following reoperation may be due to the epithelial irregularity and epithelial tags that commonly are produced at the flap edge.

2. Epithelial Defects

Postoperative epithelial defects are associated with higher risk of interlamellar epithelium. Wang and Maloney (26) reported that, out of 43 eyes with postoperative epithelial defects, 14 (33%) subsequently developed epithelial ingrowth. The presumed mechanism is flap edema with reduced flap adherence.

3. Prior Incisional Refractive Surgery

LASIK after prior incision refractive surgery (RK, AK) may predispose to a higher incidence of interlamellar epithelium (Marotta [19]) (Fig. 33.3). Forseto et al. (4) reported that one of fourteen (7.1%) post-RK corneas developed epithelial ingrowth. At least two mechanisms are possible: (1) interface growth of preexisting epithelial cysts plugging the incision and (2) separation of incisions allowing a path for epithelial ingrowth or promoting poor flap adherence.

4. Hyperopic LASIK

The incidence of interlamellar epithelium may be higher following hyperopic LASIK (Marotta [19]). Lindstrom et al. (16,17) reported a rate of 3.3% to 3.4% after hyperopic LASIK. Although this again is in line with the overall incidence after myopic LASIK, it is higher than has been reported in recent studies (Kawesche and Kezirian [11], Wang and Maloney [26], Walker and Wilson [25]).

5. Buttonhole in Flap

A buttonhole in the flap may predispose to interlamellar epithelium (Marotta, 2000), presumably through poor flap adherence. However, there are no peer-reviewed studies documenting this, perhaps due to the relatively infrequent occurrence of this complication.

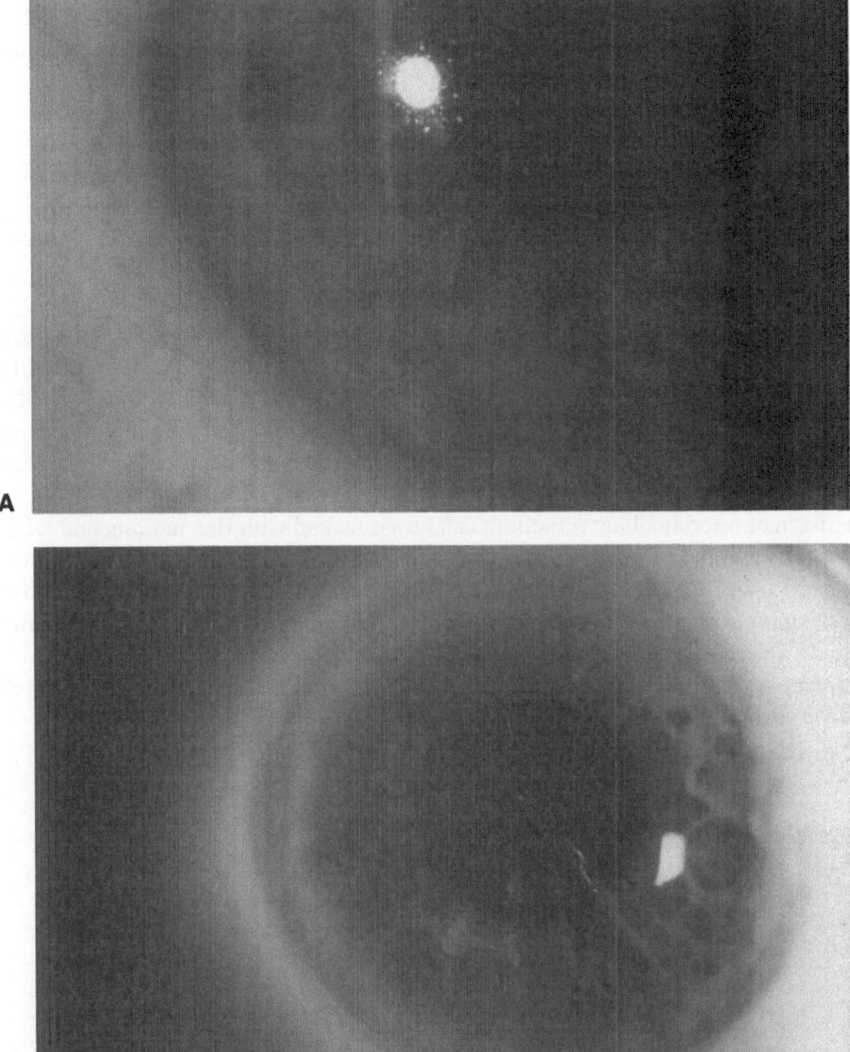

Figure 33.3 Epithelial ingrowth at junction of RK/AK incisions. High magnification of an RK incision shows the epithelial ingrowth (A). Scleral scatter can facilitate identification of the ingrowing area (B).

E. CLINICAL FEATURES

1. Appearance

On slit lamp examination, interlamellar epithelium may appear as loss of lamellar transparency with whitish gray patches or opalescent cysts. There may be overlying epithelial irregularity. With isolated epithelial nests, the entire perimeter of the interface epithelium can usually be discerned. For epithelial ingrowth, the most prominent sign may be only a faint arcuate line extending under the flap edge (Fig. 33.4); in some instances, particularly when the ingrowth is progressive, instillation of fluoroscein may reveal staining at the flap edge where the peripheral epithelium is continuous with interface epithelium. In more advanced cases, flap melting and scarring can be observed.

2. Progression

Isolated epithelial nests within lamellar interface can be seen as early as the day following surgery but are more often noted at 1 week postoperatively. This form usually does not enlarge significantly over time.

Epithelial ingrowth under the lamellar bed has been noted as early as 2 days postoperatively (Lin and Maloney [15]) but generally is first identified at 1 to 3 weeks. This form usually exhibits an early phase of growth, which can be either fast (Fig. 33.5) or slow. In some patients, over the next 4 to 8 weeks, the rate of growth slows and then stops, with the leading edge usually within 1 to 1.5 mm of the flap edge. In other eyes, the growth is more rapid and progressive, extending 2 mm or more beneath the flap edge, producing flap lysis and scarring.

Either form of interlamellar epithelium can be associated with flap melting and DLK (Lyle and Jin [18]), which in itself can result in inflammatory flap melting or stromal keratolysis (Figs. 33.6 and 33.7). Flap melting usually is restricted to the periphery (Castillo et al. [1], Perez-Santonja et al. [22], Perez-Santonja et al. [23]), since patients are sufficiently symptomatic to seek medical attention before central melting occurs. It is obviously imperative to treat progressive melting to prevent flap destruction in the papillary axis, which would produce severe visual loss.

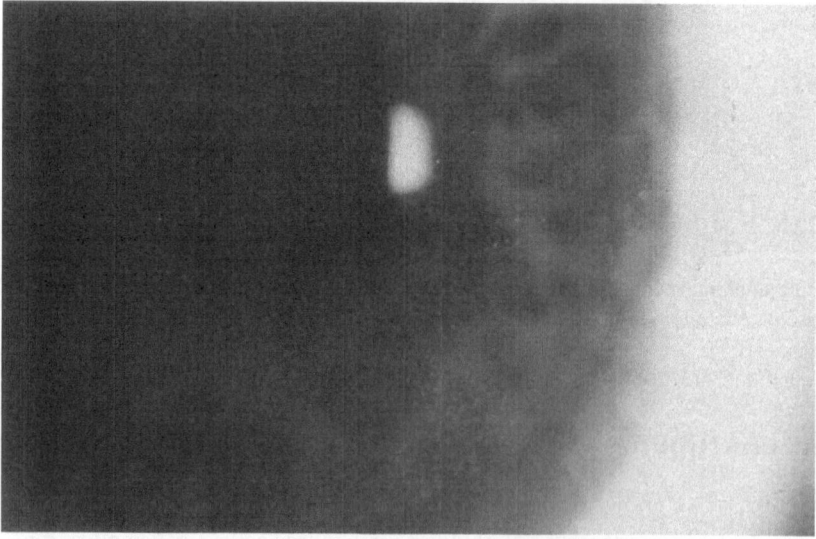

Figure 33.4 Patient presented complaining of decreased vision 4 weeks following enhancement. Note central margin of the interlamellar epithelium extending into the pupil. His uncorrected visual acuity (UCVA) was 20/80.

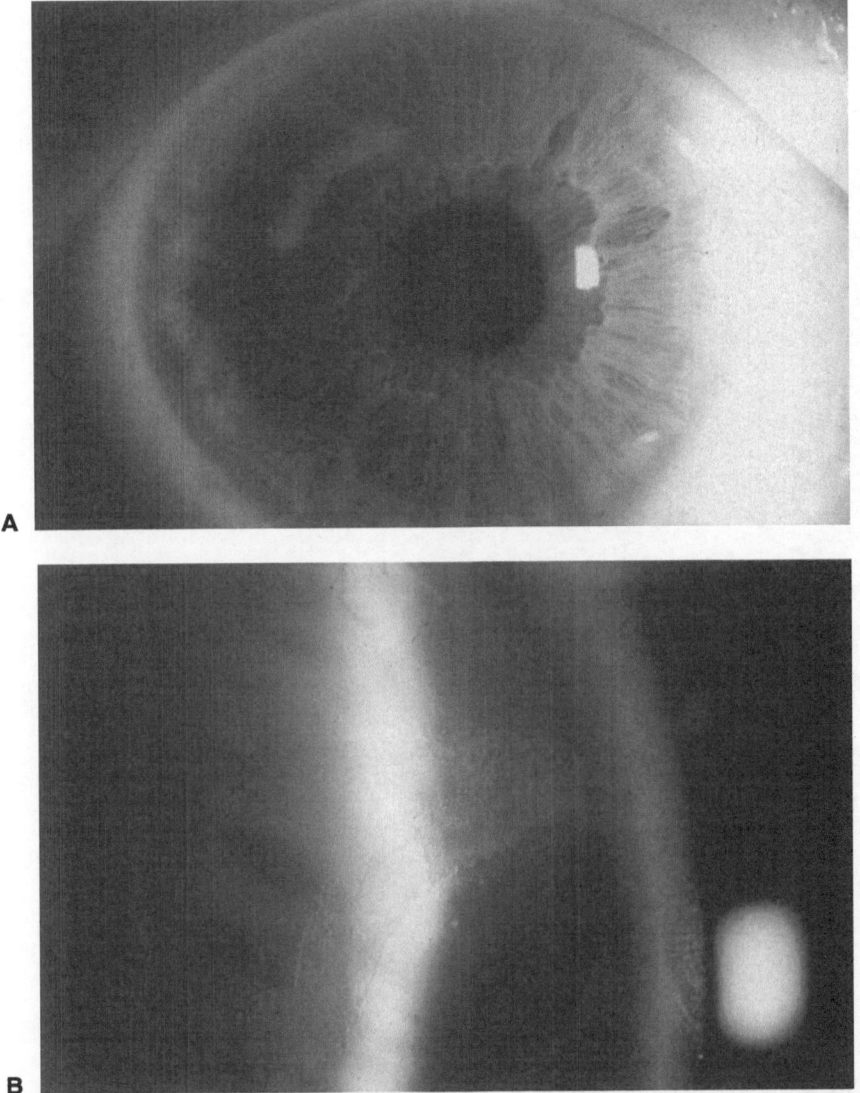

Figure 33.5 Aggressive epithelial ingrowth on day 11 after primary LASIK. (A) The superior edge of the flap is clearly involved with epithelial ingrowth. (B) Higher magnification shows the epithelial ingrowth within the pupillary area.

3. Symptoms

Interlamellar epithelium can be asymptomatic or can produce a wide range of symptoms, including foreign body sensation, photophobia, redness due to surface irregularity, and loss of vision due to irregular astigmatism (Fig. 33.8) produced by epithelial irregularity or central extension of flap melting (Fig. 33.9).

There have been reports of interlamellar fluid accumulation associated with interlamellar epithelium and elevated intraocular pressure (IOP) (Lyle and Jin [18], Najman-

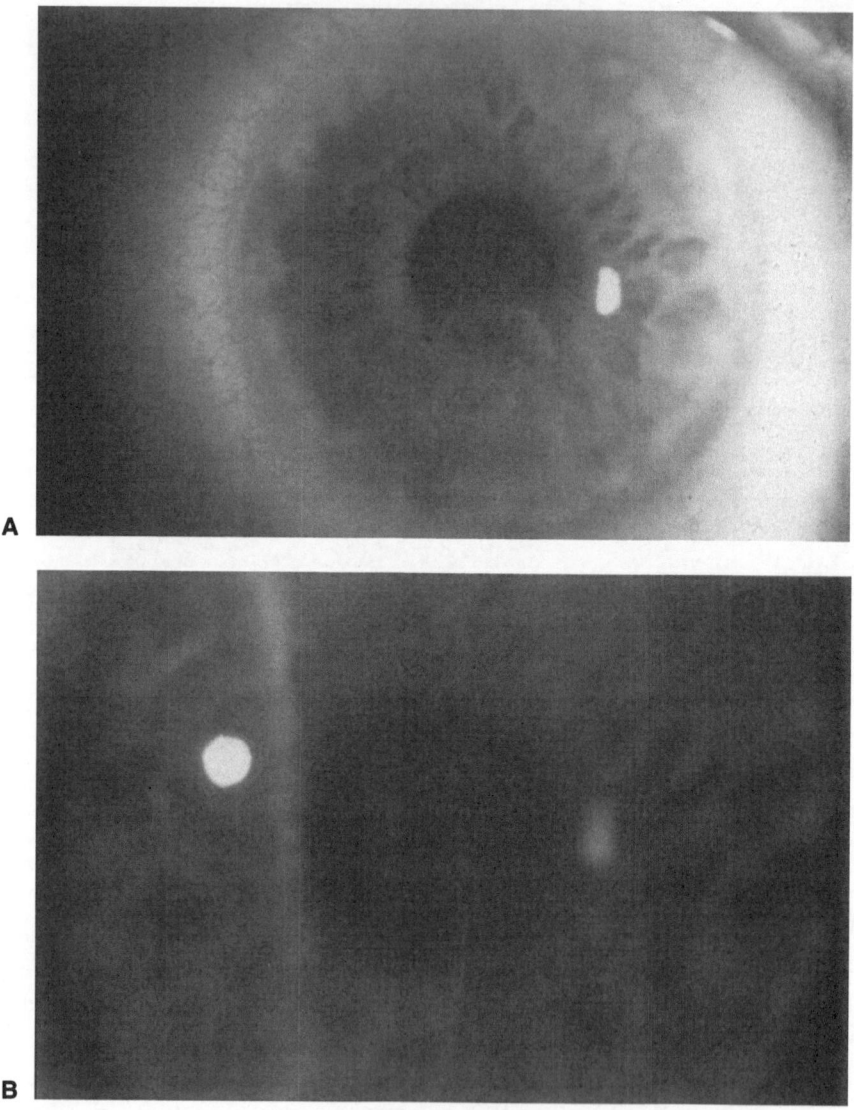

Figure 33.6   Active flap melt with epithelial ingrowth (A). Note irregular thinning of slit beam inferiorly (B).

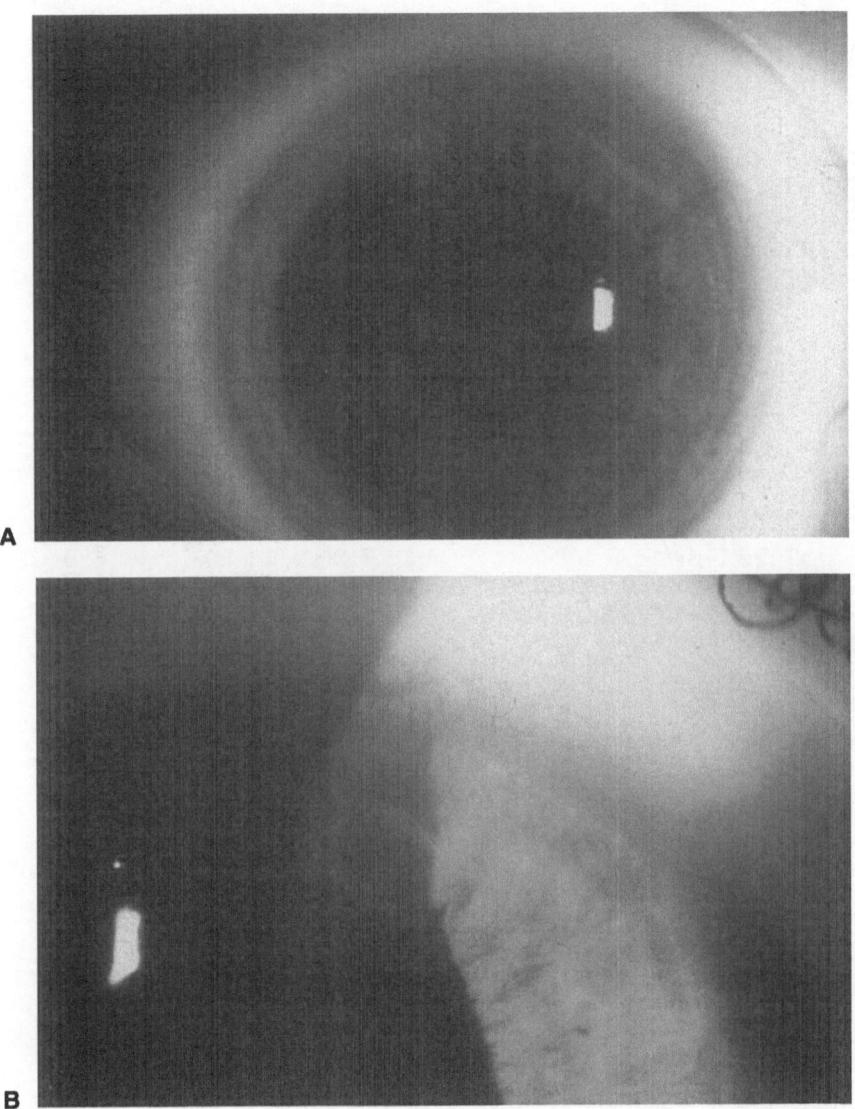

Figure 33.7   Scalloped flap edge is typical of resolved flap melt (A). Higher magnification of the same area showing the scalloped flap edge (B).

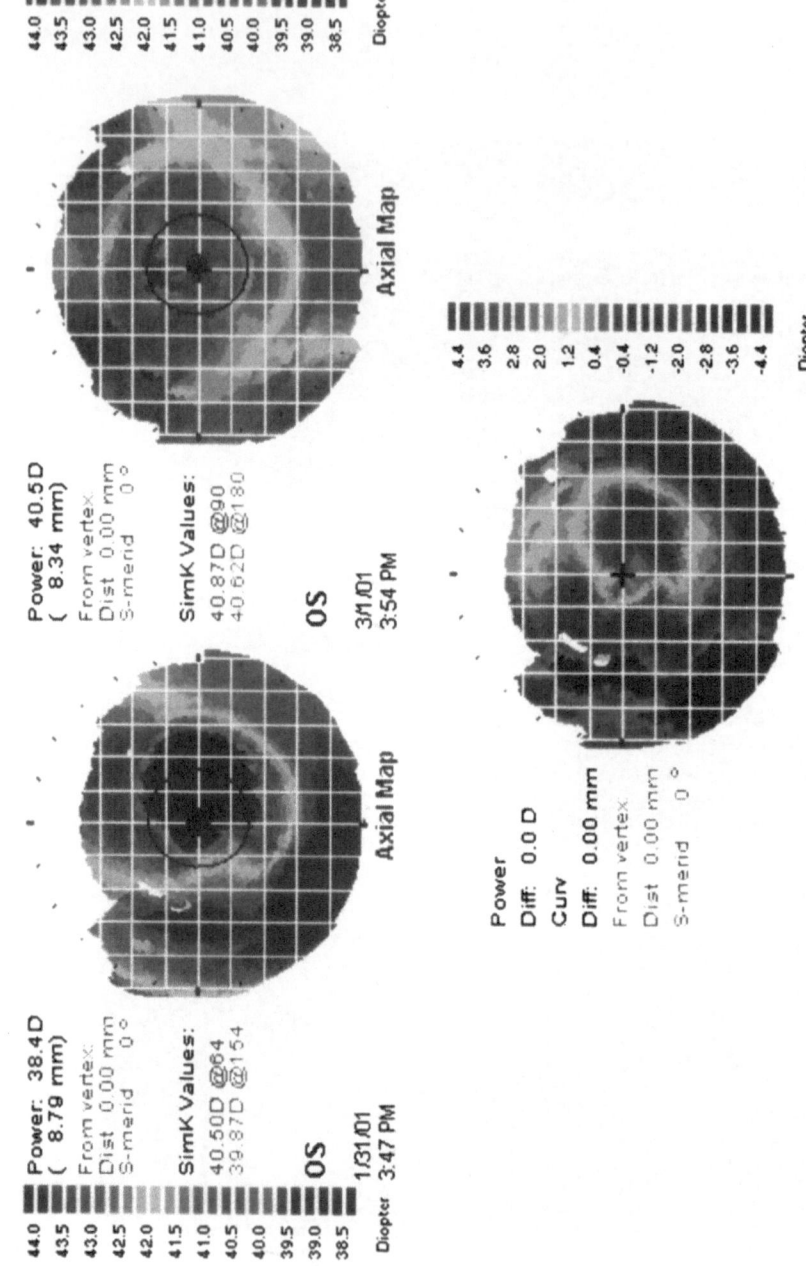

Figure 33.8 Axial topography of patient shown in Fig. 4 on presentation (upper left) and following removal of interlamellar epithelium (upper right). The difference map (bottom) shows that the irregularities were surgically corrected (1 month post op). Patient achieved UCVA of 20/16 1 month after treatment.

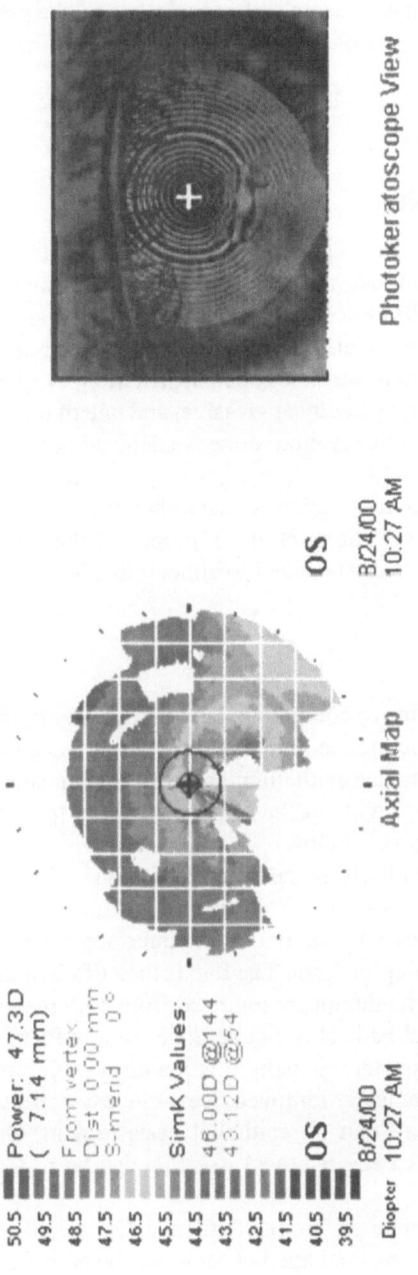

Figure 33.9 Irregular astigmatism due to central extension of flap melt. Axial map (left) and photokeratoscopic view (right) of patient shown in Fig. 33.6 on presentation.

Vainer et al. [21]). In addition to causing shifting refractions, the presence of this fluid produces falsely low IOP and can also cause falsely low IOP readings which can delay treatment of glaucoma.

F. TREATMENT

1. Indications and Timing

The three primary indications for treatment of interlamellar epithelium are (1) central progression of ≥ 2 mm, (2) visual loss, and (3) flap melting/interlamellar fluid. The appropriate time to intervene surgically is at the earliest point at which any of these complications occurs or is imminent. Surgery is also usually indicated when patients have symptoms of moderate-to-severe foreign body sensation, ocular irritation, or glare and photophobia; in these instances the ingrowth is typically aggressive, and one of the above three problems is presumably soon to develop. Observation alone is adequate for asymptomatic interlamellar epithelium.

Reports from several sources indicated that only a fraction of eyes with interlamellar epithelium requires treatment. Stulting et al. (24) reported that, of 9.1% of eyes with epithelial ingrowth, only 1.7% of eyes needed treatment; this is a 19% rate of surgical intervention.

2. Techniques

The goal of treatment is to remove completely the interlamellar epithelium and any factors that might predispose to its recurrence. In the authors' experience in surgically treating approximately 10 eyes, interlamellar epithelium has always been successfully cured (Fig. 8) by simple mechanical removal without the use of additional measures such as alcohol or phototherapeutic keratectomy (see below).

The technique begins with lifting the flap. This is done in the operating room by gently dragging a microhook (e.g., Sinskey) from the inferior limbus in a central direction in the area of the ingrowth. The hook will easily find the interface due to the poor flap adhesion produced by the interlamellar epithelium. The flap is then lifted in the standard fashion.

The epithelium is then meticulously removed from both the undersurface of the flap and the surface of the stromal bed. This can be done using a PRK spatula and dry Merocel sponges. In most instances, the epithelium is readily visible, making it easy to determine when it has been mechanically removed. Nevertheless, repeated scraping of the two surfaces is advisable to insure that no epithelial nests remain. Once it has been determined that all epithelium has been removed, the flap can be refloated and positioned in the standard fashion.

Careful attention should be paid to the flap edge. On the stromal surface, the epithelium should be removed until the cut edge is visible for the entire extent of the flap. When replacing the flap, redundant epithelium on either the flap or the cornea should be preserved if possible and carefully repositioned to span the gutter. This will essentially eliminate the risk of epithelial ingrowth in these regions. In these patients, it may be advisable to use a contact lens to promote flap adherence and facilitate more rapid epithelial healing.

The most common complication of surgical treatment of interlamellar epithelium is recurrence with rates reported as high as 23% (Wang and Maloney [26]). Results of retreatment may not be as favorable, presumably because recurrent epithelial ingrowth results in stromal damage that may hinder flap adherence. In refractory cases in which there are one or more occurrences, more extreme measures may be employed. These include suturing the flap to assure good flap adherence, application of 50% ethanol to ensure that all interlamellar epithelium has been killed, and phototherapeutic keratectomy (which would consist of a few pulses on both surfaces), again with the purpose of rendering all remaining epithelial cells nonviable.

In eyes with central epithelial ingrowth due to a buttonhole in the flap, lifting the flap is usually not indicated. An option in these eyes is transepithelial photorefractive keratectomy, if the residual myopia is sufficiently high to allow complete ablation of the flap and epithelial ingrowth (Kapadia and Wilson [10]).

G. PREVENTION

Prevention and early surgical intervention are the keys to preventing visual loss from interlamellar epithelium. The risk of epithelial ingrowth can be minimized by avoiding microkeratome complications, thoroughly (but not excessively) irrigating the interface, meticulously managing the flap edge and epithelial tags, carefully realigning the flap, ensuring that the flap is adherent before removing the lid speculum, and using a bandage contact lens when there are large epithelial defects or other factors that might impede good flap adherence. With appropriate management, loss of vision is fortunately an extremely uncommon outcome of interlamellar epithelium.

REFERENCES

1. A Casillo, D Diaz-Valle, AR Gutierrez, N Toledano, F Romero. Peripheral melt of flap after laser in situ keratomileusis. J Refract Surg 1998;14:61–63.
2. SG Farah, DT Azar, C Gurdal, J Wong. Laser in situ keratomileusis: literature review of a developing technique. J Cataract Refract Surg 1998;24:989–1006.
3. JL Febbraro, KA Buzard, MH Fridlander. Reoperations after myopic laser in situ keratomileusis. J Cataract Refract Surg 2000;26:41–48.
4. AS Forseto, RA Nose, CM Francesconi, W Nose. Laser in situ keratomileusis for undercorrection after radial keratotomy. J Refract Surg 1999;15:424–428.
5. HV Gimbel, EE Anderson-Penno, JA van Westenbrugge, M Ferensowicz, MT Furlong. Incidence and management of intraoperative and early postoperative complications in 1000 consecutive laser in situ keratomileusis cases. Ophthalmology 1998;105:1839–1848.
6. JL Guell, A Muller. Laser in situ keratomileusis (LASIK) for myopia from −7 to −18 diopters. J Refract Surg 1996;12:222–228.
7. WW Haw, EE Manche. Treatment of progressive or recurrent epithelial ingrowth with ethanol following laser in situ keratomileusis. J Refract Surg 2001;17:63–68.
8. MC Helena, F Baerveldt, WJ Kim, SE Wilson. Keratocyte apoptosis after corneal surgery. Invest Ophthalmol Vis Sci 1998;39:276–283.
9. MC Helena, D Meisler, SE Wilson. Epithelial growth within the lamellar interface after laser in situ keratomileusis. Cornea 1997;16:300–305.
10. MS Kapadia, SE Wilson. Transepithelial photorefractive keratectomy for treatment of thin flaps or caps after complicated laser in situ keratomileusis. Am J Ophthalmol 1998;126:827–829.
11. GM Kawesch, GM Kezirian. Laser in situ keratomileusis for high myopia with the VISX star laser. Ophthalmology 2000;107:653–661.
12. MC Knorz, A Liermann, V Seiberth, H Steiner, B Wiesinger. Laser in situ keratomileusis to correct myopia of −6.00 to −29.00 diopters. J Refract Surg 1996;12:575–584.
13. MC Knorz, B Wiesinger, A Liermann, V Seiberth, H Liesenhoff. Laser in situ keratomileusis for moderate and high myopia and myopic astigmatism. Ophthalmology 1998;105:932–940.

14. I Kremer, M Blumenthal. Myopic keratomileusis in situ combined with VISX 20/20 photore-fractive keratectomy. J Cataract Refract Surg 1995;21:508–511.

15. RT Lin, RK Maloney. Flap complications associated with lamellar refractive surgery. Am J Ophthalmol 1999;127:129–136.

16. RL Linstrom, DR Hardten, DM Houtman, B Witte, N Preschel, YR Chu, TW Samuelson, EJ Linebarger. Six-month results of hyperopia and astigmatic LASIK in eyes with primary and secondary hyperopia. Trans Am Ophthalmol Soc 1999;97:241–255.

17. RL Linstrom, EJ Linebarger, DR Hardten, DM Houtman, TW Samuelson. Early results of hy-peropia and astigmatic laser in situ keratomileusis in eyes with secondary hyperopia. Ophthal-mology 2000;107:1858–1863.

18. WA Lyle, GJ Jin. Interface fluid associated with diffuse lamellar keratitis and epithelial in-growth after laser in site keratomileusis. J Cataract Refract Surg 1999;25:1009–1012.

19. H Marotta. Treatment of epithelial ingrowth. In L Buratto, S Brint, eds. LASIK Surgical Tech-niques and Complications. Thorofare, NJ: Slack, 2000, pp 547–553.

20. A Marinho, MC Pinto, R Pinto, F Vaz, MC Neves. LASIK for high myopia: one year experi-ence. Ophthalmic Surg Lasers 1996;27(suppl):S517–S520.

21. J Najman-Vainer, RJ Smith, RK Maloney. Interface fluid after LASIK: misleading tonometry can lead to end-stage glaucoma. J Cataract Refract Surg 2000;26:471–472.

22. JJ Perez-Santonja, MJ Ayala, HF Sakla, JM Ruiz-Moreno, JL Alio. Retreatment after laser in situ keratomileusis. Ophthalmology 1999;106:21–28.

23. JJ Perez-Santonja, J Bellot, P Claramonte, MM Ismail, Alio JL. Laser in situ keratomileusis to correct high myopia. J Cataract Refract Surg 1997;23:372–385.

24. RD Stulting, JD Carr, KP Thompson, GO Waring III, WM Wiley, JG Walker. Complications of laser in situ keratomileusis for the correction of myopia. Ophthalmology 1999;106:13–20.

25. MB Walker, SE Wilson. Incidence and prevention of epithelial growth within the interface af-ter laser in situ keratomileusis. Cornea 2000;19:170–173.

26. MY Wang, RK Maloney. Epithelial ingrowth after laser in situ keratomileusis. Am J Ophthal-mol 2000;126:746–751.

27. SE Wilson. Keratocyte apoptosis in refractive surgery. CLAO J 1998;24:181–185.

28. SE Wilson, Y He, J Weng, Q Li, AW McDowall, M Vital, EL Chwang. Epithelial injury in-duces keratocyte apoptosis: hypothesized role for the interleukin-1 system in the modulation of corneal tissue organization and wound healing. Exp Eye Res 1996;62:325–333.

29. JD Wright, Jr, CC Neubaur, G Stevens, Jr. Epithelial ingrowth in a corneal graft treated by laser in situ keratomileusis: light and electron microscopy. J Cataract Refract Surg 2000;26:49–55.

34

Management of Infections, Inflammation, and Lamellar Keratitis After LASIK

BILAL F. KHAN

*Massachusetts Eye and Ear Infirmary and Harvard Medical School,
Boston, Massachusetts, U.S.A.*

MARGARET CHANG

*Columbia University College of Physicians and Surgeons,
New York, New York, U.S.A.*

SANDEEP JAIN, KATHRYN COLBY, and DIMITRI T. AZAR

*Massachusetts Eye and Ear Infirmary, Schepens Eye Research Institute,
and Harvard Medical School, Boston, Massachusetts, U.S.A.*

Over 1,000,000 laser in situ keratomileusis (LASIK) procedures were performed in the United States in the year 2000. Although our understanding of the inflammatory and infectious complications has improved, several questions remain about the etiology and management of these uncommon conditions.

A. DIFFUSE LAMELLAR KERATITIS (DLK) AFTER LASIK

Smith and Maloney first described the inflammatory condition called diffuse lamellar keratitis (DLK), a distinct syndrome of unknown cause characterized by noninfectious infiltrates in the lamellar interface (1). This syndrome has also been called the sands of the

Table 1 Alternate Names for
Diffuse Lamellar Keratitis (DLK)

Diffuse intralamellar keratitis
Delayed keratitis after LASIK
Sands of Sahara syndrome
Shifting sands
Sterile interface keratitis
Post-LASIK interface keratitis
Nonspecific diffuse lamellar keratitis
Lamellar keratitis

Sahara syndrome because of the characteristic wavy appearance at slit lamp examination; (2) several additional names have also been suggested (Table 1).

1. Frequency

Linebarger et al. (3) reported a post-LASIK frequency of mild DLK ranging from 2 to 4%; severe vision-threatening DLK was less frequent (0.02%). Holland et al. (4) reported a cluster of 52 DLK cases in a series of 983 LASIK cases, a frequency of 5.3%, and Johnson et al. (5) have reported a frequency of 1.3% in 2711 eyes.

2. Etiology

DLK can occur in an isolated case or in a cluster of cases (8), with a single factor or multiple factors. Several possible etiological factors (1,2,6–13) have been suggested (Table 2), and the etiology may be multifactorial.

Azar noted that sporadic cases of DLK are associated with the presence of an epithelial defect (Diffuse Lamellar Keratitis session, 2000, American Society of Cataract and Refractive Surgeons meeting, Boston, MA). Johnson et al. (5) reported that although epithelial defects occurred in only 3% of LASIK cases, they are associated with 38.9% of DLK

Table 2 Possible Etiologies of Diffuse
Lamellar Keratitis (DLK) after LASIK

---

 1. Oil, wax, metallic fragments, silicates
 2. Bacterial endotoxins
 3. Bacterial exotoxins
 4. Laser/contaminant interaction
 5. Meibomian gland secretion
 6. Transected corneal epithelial cells
 7. Overlying epithelial defects
 8. Red blood cells
 9. Tear film debris
10. Nonsteroidal anti-inflammatory drops
11. Surgical drape debris
12. Povidone-iodine
13. Lubricant or rust from microkeratome
14. Laser energy

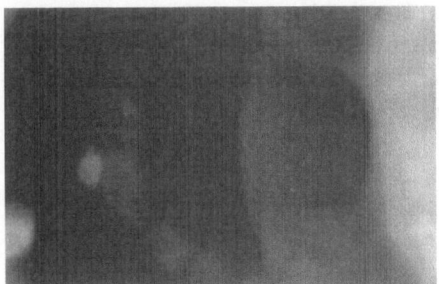

Figure 34.1 Diffuse lamellar keratitis (DLK) slit lamp photograph.

cases. This suggests that an epithelial defect following LASIK increases the risk of developing DLK.

Clusters of DLK may be related to endotoxins released from Gram-negative biofilms in sterilizer reservoirs. The sterilization process kills the bacteria, but their cell wall components (lipopolysaccharide subunits and possibly peptidoglycans) may initiate DLK. Holland et al. (4) reported an outbreak of DLK affecting 52 patients. The gram-negative bacterium, *Burkholderia pickettii,* was isolated from the sterilizer reservoir. Epidemiological investigation showed that biofilm control in the sterilizer reservoirs was associated with a significant reduction in the development of DLK.

3. Symptoms and Signs

In early to mild DLK the patient may be completely asymptomatic with no change in vision, and only a careful, detailed slit lamp examination will reveal the fine, rippled, white granular infiltrate (Fig. 34.1). It does not extend posteriorly into the stroma or anteriorly into the corneal flap. With increasing DLK severity, the patient may suffer pain, irritation, photophobia, and decreased vision. The symptoms of DLK may mimic microbial keratitis. However, as will be discussed later in this chapter, in microbial keratitis the conjunctiva could be inflamed with concomitant ciliary flush, and the infiltrate extends posteriorly in the corneal stroma or anteriorly into the corneal flap. Hypopyon could also be present. Meibomian gland secretions may mimic DLK, but the Meibomian secretions have a glistening, oily appearance, unlike the flat, white, granular appearance of DLK.

4. Classification

Azar and Johnson have developed a DLK classification system based on the extent and pattern of migration of inflammatory cells (Table 3). Type I DLK typically begins at the periphery and at the flap margin and may progress only mildly. Visual acuity is usually

Table 3 Classification of Diffuse Lamellar
Keratitis (DLK)

Type IA	Center-sparing, sporadic
Type IB	Center-sparing, cluster
Type IIA	Center-involved, sporadic
Type IIB	Center-involved, cluster

unaffected, and patients rarely have any complaints. They tend to respond well to high-dose steroids, with little risk of long-term sequelae. Type II DLK may initially begin at the flap margin but can advance across most of the stromal interface. Central involvement may be seen as early as day 1 or may take up to 5 days. Patients complain of decreased visual acuity, decreased contrast sensitivity, glare, and photophobia. Type II DLK may worsen even with hourly topical steroids and should be monitored closely. Rarely, inflammatory cells form clusters and may cause stromal degradation, flap melting, and irregular astigmatism.

5. Stages and Treatment

Several grading methods have been suggested in an attempt to characterize the severity of inflammation and appropriate management strategies (1,4,13). Linebarger et al. (3) divide DLK into four stages, each with specific management strategy (Table 4).

Table 4 Stages and Treatment of Diffuse Lamellar Keratitis (DLK) After LASIK (Linebarger Classification)

Stage	Time	Frequency	Clinical presentation and outcome	Treatment
1	Day 1	1 in 25–50 cases	Fine white granular cells in periphery No decrease in BCVA Self-limiting	Prednisone acetate 1% every h Topical fluoroquinolone TID Follow up 24–48 h
2	Day 2 or 3, occasionally day 1	1 in 200 cases	Fine white granular cells migrate from periphery to center Some cells still in periphery Involves central visual axis Shifting sands No decrease in BCVA	Prednisone acetate 1% every h Topical fluoroquinolone TID Follow-up 24–48 h IOP check to avoid DLK-masquerade syndrome
3	Day 2 or 3	1 in 500 cases	Increased density of clumped inflammatory cells in center Involves central visual axis Subjective haze felt by the patient 1 or 2 lines BCVA decrease Threshold DLK	Prednisone acetate 1% every h Topical fluoroquinolone TID Lift flap, irrigate bed and flap with BSS Wipe gently with moistened sponge Follow up in 24–48 h IOP check to avoid DLK-masquerade syndrome
4	Follow stage 3	1 in 5000 cases	Increased collagenase activity Fluid collection, bullae formation Stromal melting Corneal scarring BCVA decreased Irregular astigmatism Hyperopic shift	Prednisone acetate 1% every h Topical fluoroquinolone TID Lift flap, irrigate bed and flap with BSS Wipe gently with moistened sponge Follow-up in 24–48 h AVOID at Stage 3

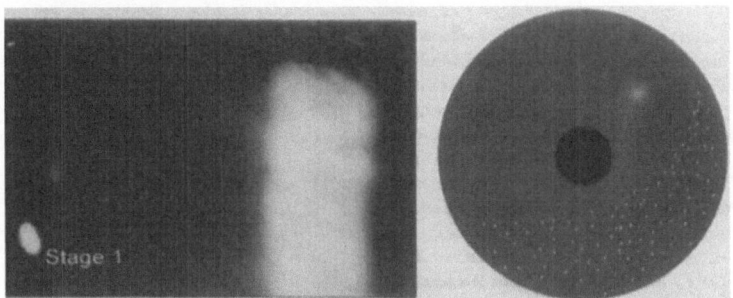

Figure 34.2   Stage 1 (Linebarger classification). Peripheral pattern of stage 1 DLK.

Stage 1: Presents on day 1 and occurs in 2 to 4% of cases of LASIK. There are fine, white, granular cells in the periphery of the flap interface with no involvement of the visual axis (Fig. 34.2). Stage 1 usually has a self-limiting course, resolving in 7 to 10 days. However, careful follow-up is needed, as it can progress to a higher stage. Prednisone acetate 1% administered topically every hour along with topical broad-spectrum fluoroquinolone antibiotic three times a day are used (see Figure 17.5).

Stage 2: Usually presents on day 2 or 3 and occurs in 0.5% cases. The inflammatory cells involve the visual axis (Fig. 34.3), although there is no decrease of visual acuity. Some cells may also be present at the periphery of the flap interface. This migration of cells has a shifting sands appearance. Treatment is similar to stage 1, but extremely careful follow-up is needed as progression to vision-threatening stage 3 may occur.

Stage 3: Usually presents on day 2 or 3 and occurs in 0.2% cases. Aggregation of the cells becomes more dense, white, and clumped in the central visual axis. The flap periphery is relatively clear (Fig. 34.4). Patients will often report a subjective haze and may experience a decrease of one or two Snellen lines of vision. If left untreated, this stage, also called threshold DLK, may cause permanent scarring. Treatment is more aggressive. The corneal flap is lifted. The stromal bed and the under surface of the flap are irrigated with balanced salt solution (BSS). Irrigation reduces the load of the inflammatory cells and the collagenolytic action of the PMNs. Prednisone acetate 1% is administered topically every hour along with broad-spectrum fluoroquinolone antibiotic three times a day. Prolonged use of steroids may raise IOP and cause DLK-masquerade syndrome (62).

Stage 4: Follows untreated stage 3 and has the most debilitating effect on visual outcome. It occurs in approximately 0.02% of cases. The aggregation of inflammatory cells in

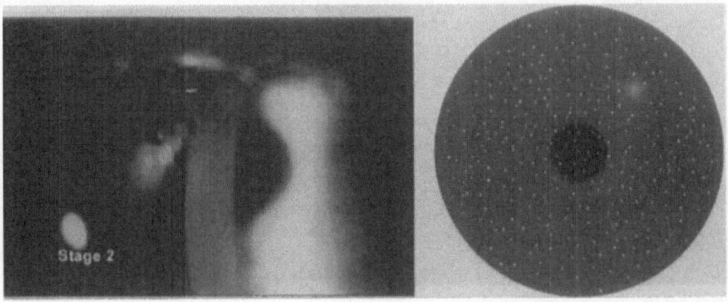

Figure 34.3   Stage 2 (Linebarger classification). Central involvement of stage 2 DLK.

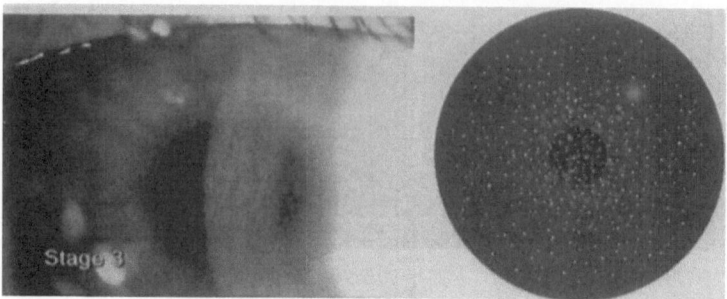

Figure 34.4   Stage 3 (Linebarger classification). Aggregation of more dense white and clumped cells in the visual axis of stage 3 DLK.

the central visual axis becomes denser. The release of collagens causes fluid collection in the central lamellae with resultant overlying bullae formation. This results in stromal melting and permanent scarring. The patient develops decreased visual acuity, irregular astigmatism, and hyperopia (Fig. 34.5). Treatment includes lifting the corneal flap for irrigation as in stage 3. Prednisone acetate 1% administered topically every hour along with broad-spectrum fluoroquinolone antibiotic three times a day are used. IOP needs to be monitored to prevent DLK-masquerade Syndrome (62).

B.   INFECTIONS FOLLOWING LASIK

Although LASIK is a relatively safe procedure (14,15), infection can be a rare but sight-threatening complication. Case reports of infection after LASIK have appeared periodically. Although they are limited in scope, a few descriptive reviews published as parts of articles reporting new cases (16–20) recognize the importance of effective management of this potentially serious complication after LASIK. Since the frequency of infections after LASIK is low (21–23), here we note all published case reports of such infection, to provide a better perspective. Similar integrative reviews have been published for infections after radial keratotomy (24,25).

We identified 36 original manuscripts describing infections after LASIK surgery. There were 25 case reports (21,26–51), nine original articles (16–20,22,52–54), and two letters to the editor (55,56). A search of ARVO and ASCRS abstracts yielded three unpublished case reports describing six cases of infection after LASIK (57–59).

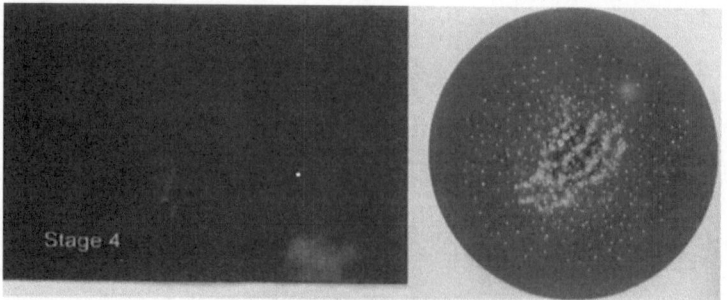

Figure 34.5   Stage 4 (Linebarger classification). Waves of increased density and permanent scarring associated with stage 4 DLK.

1. Frequency

A total of 39 infections involving 35 patients were described in the 26 articles analyzed. Four patients had bilateral infection, and 30 had unilateral infection. Thirty of the 39 (76.9%) infections occurred after primary LASIK; six (15.4%), after reoperations.

The frequency of post-LASIK infection varied among different case series (Table 5). Pirzada and Kalaawry (22) reported an infection frequency of 1.2% (1 of 83), Dada et al. (21) a frequency of 0.2% (1 of 500), Stulting et al. (54) a frequency of 0.19% (2 of 1062), Pérez-Santonja et al. (43) a frequency of 0.12% (1 of 801), and Lin and Maloney (53) a frequency of 0.1% (1 of 1019). In unpublished case series, Seedor et al. (58) documented one case of microbial keratitis out of 6312 eyes (0.02%) and Miller et al. (59) reported three cases of infection after LASIK in 1958 eyes (0.15%). However, several large LASIK case series have reported no infectious complications (23,60,61) (Figure 34.6).

2. Presenting Signs and Symptoms

Twenty-two (62.9%) of the 35 eyes presented with pain, 13 (37.1%) had photophobia, 12 (34.3%) had redness, 11 (31.4%) had decreased or blurry vision, 8 (22.9%) presented with foreign-body sensation, and 5 (14.3%) complained of discharge.

Corneal infiltrate was present in 35 of 39 (89.7%) eyes. Anterior chamber reactions were documented in 18 (46.2%) eyes. Twenty (51.3%) new-onset epithelial defects were found on initial presentation. Flap separation was noted in eight (20.5%) eyes, and two had epithelial ingrowth on presentation. One case of endophthalmitis was reported. In two cases, the lamellar flap melted due to the infection and was missing at the time of evaluation.

Gram-positive infections were more likely to present with pain and discharge and were significantly more associated with an epithelial defect than were infections with other microorganisms. Decreased vision, photophobia, and foreign-body sensation were nonspecific symptoms of infection that were not associated with any particular microorganism.

3. Microbiological Profile

Cultures were obtained in all but 1 case (Table 6). Gram-positive infections were found in 17 (43.6%) of the 39 eyes; included were *Staphylococcus aureus* (10), *Streptococcus pneu-*

Table 5 Frequency of Infection after LASIK

Source	Frequency of infection (cases/total)
Miller et al. (59)	0.15% (3/1958)
Pirzada et al. (22)	1.20% (1/83)
Dada et al. (21)	0.20% (1/500)
Stulting et al. (54)	0.19% (2/1062)
Pérez-Santonja et al. (43)	0.12% (1/801)
Lin and Maloney (53)	0.10% (1/1019)
Seedor et al. (58)	0.02% (1/6312)
Gimbel et al. (60)	(0/2142)
Kawesch and Kezirian (23)	(0/290)
Price et al. (61)	0 (0/1747)

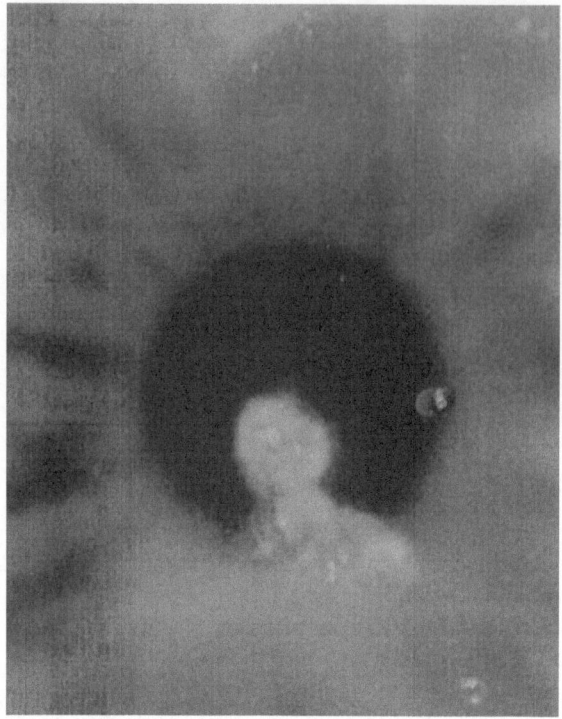

Figure 34.6   Bacterial keratitis after LASIK.

Table 6   Microbiological Profile of Post-LASIK Infections

Organism	No. of eyes	
Gram-positive bacteria	17	
Staphylococcus aureus		10
Streptococcus pneumoniae		2
Streptococcus viridans		2
Staphylococcus epidermidis		2
Nocardia		1
Fungus	4	
Aspergillus		2
Scedosporium		1
Curvularia		1
Mycobacterium	8	
M. chelonae		7
M. fortuitum		1
Coinfections	2	
S. epidermidis and *Fusarium solani*		1
Staphylococcus and *M. chelonae*		1

In one case, culture was not obtained; seven cultures were sterile.

moniae (2), *Streptococcus viridans* (2), *Staphylococcus epidermidis* (2), and *Nocardia* (1). Fungal infections, such as *Aspergillus* (2), *Scedosporium* (1), and *Curvularia* (1), were found in four (10.3%) eyes. Eight (20.5%) mycobacterial infections due to *M. chelonae* (7) and *M. fortuitum* (1) were found. There was one combined *S. epidermidis* and *Fusarium solani* infection and one combined *Staphylococcus* and *M. chelonae* infection. Seven (17.9%) cultures were sterile.

4. Risk Factors and Potential Associations of Infection

Two patients were HIV-positive; both had bilateral infections after LASIK. No other systemic associations were found. One patient had a history of glaucoma and another had a history of blepharitis. Three eyes had undergone previous radial keratotomy (RK), and one had previous RK and photorefractive keratectomy (PRK). Aseptic technique (sterile drapes, providone-iodine, sterile hand controls) was not used in one case of bilateral keratitis in an HIV-positive patient (34). Epithelial defects during the LASIK procedure occurred in three of the 38 eyes. Interface debris was noted perioperatively in three of the 38 eyes, and bandage contact lens was placed in three eyes. Postoperatively, there was a history of eye rubbing prior to the onset of infection in one case, and one case of an epithelial abrasion was caused by a fingernail.

Of the 25 unilateral cases of infection occurring after primary LASIK, seven (28.0%) occurred after sequential or unilateral LASIK and 12 (48.0%) after bilateral simultaneous treatment. All four cases of bilateral infection occurred after bilateral simultaneous LASIK, two of which involved no changing of the blade between eyes. Of these 20 eyes undergoing bilateral simultaneous LASIK, the microkeratome blade was changed between eyes in one case and not changed in 11 cases. Five of the 11 infection cases in which the blade was not changed occurred in the second eye treated and five in the first eye treated.

5. Treatment

Three of the four *Streptococcus* infections were treated with a cephalosporin–tobramycin combination; one was treated with ofloxacin, vancomycin, and ceftazidime. Four of the 12 *Staphylococcus* infections were treated with fluoroquinolones, three were treated with a cephalosporin combined with gentamicin or tobramycin, two were treated with ofloxacin and imipenem, two were treated with vancomycin and gentamicin or tobramycin, and one was treated with a cephalosporin–tobramycin–ciprofloxacin combination. The single case of *Nocardia* infection was treated with sulfacetamide and trimethoprim. Three of the seven *Mycobacterium* infections for which treatment was available were treated with amikacin and clarithromycin, two with amikacin and fortified cefazolin, one with clarithromycin and sulfacetamide, and one with tobramycin and erythromycin. Two of the four fungal infections were treated with natamycin and amphotericin B, one with natamycin and ketoconazole, one with a natamycin–cephalosporin–tobramycin combination, and one with a ketoconazole–fluoroquinolone–cephalosporin combination. Systemic antibiotics were used in 10 (29.4%) of the 34 eyes.

A flap lift for irrigation, scraping, and/or culture, with repositioning of the flap, was performed in 22 of the 39 (56.4%) eyes. Ten flaps were not lifted, and six flaps were removed. Of these latter six eyes, two flaps melted and sloughed secondary to infection, two were accidentally removed during corneal scraping or flap lift, and two were removed therapeutically. Information about flap lift was unavailable in one case.

Gram-positive infections were seen in 10 of the 13 early flap lift and repositioning cases (Table 7). Mycobacterium was implicated in four of the six late flap lift cases, and two cases involved fungus. The mean final Snellen visual acuity was 20/42 in the early flap lift group and 20/200 in the late flap lift group. Of the six cases that had late flap lifts, the decision to lift was spurred in three cases because there was sudden progression of infection after no improvement, two were lifted because no improvement occurred with medical therapy, and one was lifted after deterioration following initial improvement.

6. Outcomes and Sequelae

Final visual acuity was available for 35 of the 39 eyes. Clinically nonsignificant reductions in visual acuity occurred in 15 (38.5%) eyes, eight had moderate reductions, and 12 suffered severe reductions. Of the 15 infections resulting in nonsignificant reductions in acuity, 10 were caused by gram-positive bacteria, one each by fungus and mycobacterium, and three were culture-negative.

Of the eight eyes with moderate visual acuity reduction, five of the infections were due to Gram-positives, one to mycobacterium, and two were culture-negative. Gram-positives caused two infections in the severe acuity reduction group, three were due to fungus, three were mycobacterial, two were combined Gram-positive and mycobacterium or fungal infections, one eye was culture-negative, and one eye was not cultured.

Of the 19 Gram-positive infections, including the two coinfections with mycobacterium and fungus, the mean final Snellen VA was 20/59. The mean visual acuity of eyes after fungal infections was 20/2173 (worse than count fingers at 2 feet), and after mycobacterial infections 20/165. Severe reductions in vision are more likely to occur with fungal and mycobacterial infections than gram-positive infections (Table 8).

Nine total keratoplasties, including one lamellar keratoplasty and eight penetrating keratoplasties, were performed. Six were performed for therapeutic reasons and three for optical reasons (scarring and irregular astigmatism). Three of 39 cases developed epithelial ingrowth after resolution of infection. Information about scarring and irregular astigmatism was available for 30 eyes, after excluding those with therapeutic penetrating keratoplasty. Twenty-three of the 30 (76.7%) eyes were left with residual scars and eight with irregular astigmatism.

Table 7 Microbiological Profile and Outcomes After Early and Late Flap Lifting

Category of flap lift	No. of eyes	Microbiological profile	No. of keratoplasties	Mean final Snellen VA
Early (<3 days) Mean: 0.2 ± 0.6 Range: 0–2	13	10/13 Gram-positive (76.9%) 1/13 Mycobacterium (7.7%) 1/13 Negative culture (7.7%) 1/13 Not cultured (7.7%)	3/13 (23.1%)	20/42
Late (>7 days) Mean: 25.3 ± 6.7 Range: 14–32	6	4/6 Mycobacterium (66.7%) 1/6 Fungus (16.7%) 1/6 Negative culture (16.7%)	3/6 (50.0%)	20/200
Not lifted	10	4/10 Gram-positive (40.0%) 4/10 Negative culture (40.0%) 2/10 Fungus (20.0%)	1/10 (10.0%)	20/55

Table 8 Visual Outcomes of Infections by Specific Microorganisms

	Gram-positive	Fungus	Mycobacterium	Negative culture
No. of eyes	19	5	9	7
Mean final Snellen VA	20/59	20/2173	20/165	20/38

Total number of organisms is more than the total number of eyes, because more than one organism was isolated in two cases.

7. Summary of Infections After LASIK

Although infection after LASIK is a rare complications, serious consequences such as moderate or severe reductions in visual acuity are not uncommon after infection. About half of the infections were found to involve Gram-positive bacteria, with mycobacteria, fungus, and sterile cultures making up the remainder of cases. However, severe visual acuity reductions were significantly more associated with fungal and mycobacterial than with Gram-positive bacterial infections. Moderate or severe reductions in visual acuity occurred in a majority of cases, and keratoplasty was performed in almost a quarter of the eyes for either therapeutic or optical reasons. Both early identification of the infectious agent and early scraping and irrigation of the stromal bed by flap lifting and replacement were associated with better visual outcome. Based on this analysis, it seems likely that in cases of suspected infection, if no response or worsening is observed despite 7 days of broad-spectrum antibiotics, the possibility of a mycobacterial or fungal infection should be entertained. The importance of this lies in the severe visual acuity reductions that occur following infection with these organisms. Since early flap-lift and identification of the organism are significantly associated with a better outcome, our analysis supports early intervention in cases of suspected infection following LASIK.

It is generally accepted that aseptic technique, including sterile drapes, gloves, and povidone-iodine usage, may help prevent infection. One of the bilateral cases occurred in an HIV-positive patient when aseptic technique was not used. It is still unclear whether lack of microkeratome blade change between eyes in simultaneous bilateral LASIK is a risk factor for infection.

Perhaps the most important observation in this study is that 10 (28.6%) of the 35 corneal infiltrates were not accompanied by an epithelial defect. This is contrary to the dogma that an epithelial defect is necessary for the diagnosis of an infectious infiltrate. Epithelial defects usually serve as portals for organisms to establish infections in the stroma. However, in LASIK patients, creating the lamellar flap may introduce organisms into the stroma, and an infection may occur without an epithelial defect. Infection should be suspected if infiltrates are seen in LASIK patients, and antibiotic therapy should be commenced before an epithelial defect occurs.

Based on our analysis, we recommend lifting and repositioning the flap early after symptom onset for culture, scraping, and irrigation of the stromal bed, especially when the infiltrate involves the interface. However, infiltrates confined to the flap or those associated with full-thickness ulcers may not benefit greatly from early flap-lift, though scrapings for culture should still be taken. Cultures for fungus and mycobacteria should not be neglected. Additionally, Gram stains, Giemsa stains, and KOH preparations at the time of scraping may provide valuable insight into the proper antibiotic therapy before culture results become available.

C. CONCLUSIONS

As the popularity of refractive surgery increases, refractive surgeons will face newer challenges in the management of LASIK complications. Although DLK and infections are rare after LASIK, their prevention, early diagnosis, and effective management are the keys to a satisfactory outcome. Intraocular pressure should be monitored to prevent DLK-masquerade syndromes (62).

REFERENCES

1. RJ Smith, RK Maloney. Diffuse lamellar keratitis: a new syndrome in lamellar refractive surgery. Ophthalmology 1998;105:1721–1726.
2. R Maddox, A Hatsis. Shifting sands of the Sahara: interface inflammation following LASIK. In: HV Gimbel, EE Anderson Penno, eds. LASIK Complications: Prevention and Management. Thorofare, NJ: Slack, 1999, pp 30–36.
3. EJ Linebarger, DR Hardten, RL Lindstrom. Diffuse lamellar keratitis: diagnosis and management. J Cataract Refract Surg 2000;26:1072–1077.
4. SP Holland, RG Mathias, DW Morck, J Chiu, SG Slade. Diffuse lamellar keratitis related to endotoxins released from sterilizer reservoir biofilms. Ophthalmology 2000;107:1227–1234.
5. JD Johnson, MH Dagher, R Pineda, S Yoo, DT Azar. Diffuse lameller keratitis: incidence, associations, outcomes and a novel classification system. J Cataract Refract Surg 2001, In press.
6. SC Kaufman, DY Maitchouk, AGY Chiou, RW Beuerman. Interface inflammation after laser in situ keratomileusis: sands of the Sahara syndrome. J Cataract Refract Surg 1998;24: 1589–1593.
7. SC Kaufman. Post-LASIK interface keratitis, sands of the Sahara syndrome, and microkeratome blades (letter). J Cataract Refract Surg 1999;25:603–604.
8. KO Karp, PS Hersh, RJ Epstein. Delayed keratitis after laser in situ keratomileusis. J Cataract Refract Surg 2000;26:925–928.
9. PD Moyer, R Khanna, TG Berbos, AF Drew, D Schneider, AH Wander, AH Kaufman. Interface keratitis after LASIK may be caused by microkeratome lubricant deposits. Invest Ophthalmol Vis Sci 1998;39(suppl):S750.
10. DC Macaluso, LF Rich, SM MacRae. Sterile interface keratitis after laser in situ keratomileusis: three episodes in one patient with concomitant contact dermatitis of the eyelids. J Refract Surg 1999;15:679–682.
11. SM MacRae, DC Macaluso, LF Rich. Sterile interface keratitis associated with micropannus hemorrhage after laser in situ keratomileusis. J Cataract Refract Surg 1999;25:1679–1681.
12. A Lachance, M Tremblay. The sands of the Sahara. Can J Ophthalmol 1998;33:387–388.
13. DS Lam, AT Leung, JT Wu, DS Fan, AC Cheng, Z Wang. Culture-negative ulcerative keratitis after laser in situ keratomileusis. J Cataract Refract Surg 1999;25:1004–1008.
14. SG Farah, DT Azar, C Gurdal, J Wong. Laser in situ keratomileusis: literature review of a developing technique. J Cataract Refract Surg 1998;24:989–1006.
15. RY Choi, SE Wilson. Hyperopic laser in situ keratomileusis: primary and secondary treatments are safe and effective. Cornea 2001;20:388–393.
16. JL Alió, JJ Pérez-Santonja, T Tervo, KF Tabbara, M Vesaluoma, RJ Smith, B Maddox, RK Maloney. Postoperative inflammation, microbial complications, and wound healing following laser in situ keratomileusis. J Refract Surg 2000;16:523–538.
17. R Ambrosio Jr, SE Wilson. Complications of laser in situ keratomileusis: etiology, prevention, and treatment. J Refract Surg 2001;17:350–379.
18. P Garg, AK Bansal, S Sharma, GK Vemuganti. Bilateral infectious keratitis after laser in situ keratomileusis: a case report and review of the literature. Ophthalmology 2001;108:121–125.
19. PA Quiros, RS Chuck, RE Smith, JA Irvine, JP McDonnell, LC Chao, PJ McDonnell. Infectious ulcerative keratitis after laser in situ keratomileusis. Arch Ophthalmol 1999;117: 1423–1427.

20. SE Wilson. LASIK: management of common complications. Cornea 1998;17:459–467.
21. T Dada, N Sharma, VK Dada, RB Vajpayee. Pneumococcal keratitis after laser in situ keratomileusis. J Cataract Refract Surg 2000;26:460–461.
22. WA Pirzada, H Kalaawry. Laser in situ keratomileusis for myopia of −1 to −3.50 diopters. J Refract Surg 1997;13:S425–S426.
23. GM Kawesch, GM Kezirian. Laser in situ keratomileusis for high myopia with the VISX star laser. Ophthalmology 2000;107:653–661.
24. S Jain, DT Azar. Ocular infections after refractive keratotomy. J Refract Surg 1996;12: 148–155.
25. S Jain, I Arora, DT Azar. Success of monovision in presbyopes: review of the literature and potential applications to refractive surgery. Surv Ophthalmol 1996;40:491–499.
26. Early Treatment Diabetic Retinopathy Study Research Group. Early treatment diabetic retinopathy study design and baseline patient characteristics: ETDRS report number 7. Ophthalmology 1991;98:741–756.
27. JT Holladay. Proper method for calculating average visual acuity. J Refract Surg 1997;13: 388–391.
28. M Al-Reefy. Bacterial keratitis following laser in situ keratomileusis for hyperopia. J Refract Surg 1999;15:216–217.
29. C Aras, A Özdamar, H Bahçecioglu, B Sener. Corneal interface abscess after excimer laser in situ keratomileusis. J Refract Surg 1998;14:156–157.
30. MS Chung, MH Goldstein, WT Driebe Jr, B Schwartz. Fungal keratitis after laser in situ keratomileusis: a case report. Cornea 2000;19:236–237.
31. MS Chung, MH Goldstein, WT Driebe Jr, BH Schwartz. Mycobacterium chelonae keratitis after laser in situ keratomileusis successfully treated with medical therapy and flap removal. Am J Ophthalmol 2000;129:382–384.
32. H Gelender, HL Carter, B Bowman, WE Beebe, GR Walters. Mycobacterium keratitis after laser in situ keratomileusis. J Refract Surg 2000;16:191–195.
33. V Gupta, T Dada, RB Vajpayee, N Sharma, VK Dada. Polymicrobial keratitis after laser in situ keratomileusis. J Refract Surg 2001;17:147–148.
34. JA Hovanesian, EG Faktorovich, JD Hoffbauer, SS Shah, RK Maloney. Bilateral bacterial keratitis after laser in situ keratomileusis in a patient with human immunodeficiency virus infection. Arch Ophthalmol 1999;117:968–970.
35. KO Karp, PS Hersh, RJ Epstein. Delayed keratitis after laser in situ keratomileusis. J Cataract Refract Surg 2000;26:925–928.
36. HM Kim, JS Song, HS Han, HR Jung. Streptococcal keratitis after myopic laser in situ keratomileusis. Korean J Ophthalmol 1998;12:108–111.
37. EK Kim, DH Lee, K Lee, SJ Lim, IS Yoon, YG Lee. Nocardia keratitis after traumatic detachment of a laser in situ keratomileusis flap. J Refract Surg 2000;16:467–469.
38. GA Kouyoumdjian, SL Forstot, VD Durairaj, RE Damiano. Infectious keratitis after laser refractive surgery. Ophthalmology 2001;108:1266–1268.
39. IC Kuo, TP Margolis, V Cevallos, DG Hwang. Aspergillus fumigatus keratitis after laser in situ keratomileusis. Cornea 2001;20:342–344.
40. DSC Lam, ATS Leung, JT Wu, DSP Fan, ACK Cheng, Z Wang. Culture-negative ulcerative keratitis after laser in situ keratomileusis. J Cataract Refract Surg 1999;25:1004–1008.
41. MG Mulhern, PI Condon, M O'Keefe. Endophthalmitis after astigmatic myopic laser in situ keratomileusis. J Cataract Refract Surg 1997;23:948–950.
42. B Parolini, G Marcon, GA Panozzo. Central necrotic lamellar inflammation after laser in situ keratomileusis. J Refract Surg 2001;17:110–112.
43. JJ Pérez-Santonja, HF Sakla, JL Abad, A Zorraquino, J Esteban, JL Alió. Nocardial keratitis after laser in situ keratomileusis. J Refract Surg 1997;13:314–317.
44. RW Read, RSH Chuck, NA Rao, RE Smith. Traumatic Acremonium atrogriseum keratitis following laser-assisted in situ keratomileusis. Arch Ophthalmol 2000;118:418–421.

45. V Reviglio, ML Rodriguez, GS Picotti, M Paradello, JD Luna, CP Juárez. Mycobacterium chelonae keratitis following laser in situ keratomileusis. J Refract Surg 1998;14:357–360.
46. JC Rudd, M Moshirfar. Methicillin-resistant Staphylococcus aureus keratitis after laser in situ keratomileusis. J Cataract Refract Surg 2001;27:471–473.
47. MS Sridhar, P Garg, AK Bansal, U Gopinathan. Aspergillus flavus keratitis after laser in situ keratomileusis. Am J Ophthalmol 2000;129:802–804.
48. MS Sridhar, P Garg, AK Bansal, S Sharma. Fungal keratitis after laser in situ keratomileusis. J Cataract Refract Surg 2000;26:613–615.
49. H Watanabe, S Sato, N Maeda, Y Inoue, Y Shimomura, Y Tano. Bilateral corneal infection as a complication of laser in situ keratomileusis. Arch Ophthalmol 1997;115:1593–1594.
50. SK Webber, MA Lawless, GL Sutton, CM Rogers. Staphylococcal infection under a LASIK flap. Cornea 1999;18:361–365.
51. S Levartovsky, G Rosenwasser, D Goodman. Bacterial keratitis following laser in situ keratomileusis. Ophthalmology 2001;108:321–325.
52. SW Chang, FM Ashraf, DT Azar. Wound healing patterns following perforation sustained during laser in situ keratomileusis. J Formos Med Assoc 2000;99:635–641.
53. RT Lin, RK Maloney. Flap complications associated with lamellar refractive surgery. Am J Ophthalmol 1999;127:129–136.
54. RD Stulting, JD Carr, KP Thompson, GO Waring III, WM Wiley, JG Walker. Complications of laser in situ keratomileusis for the correction of myopia. Ophthalmology 1999;106:13–20.
55. N Sharma, T Dada, VK Dada, RB Vajpayee. Acute haemorrhagic keratoconjunctivitis following laser in situ keratomileusis. Clin Experiment Ophthalmol 2000;28:431–433.
56. A Tripathi. Fungal keratitis after LASIK. J Cataract Refract Surg 2000;26:1433.
57. SJ Kang, EK Kim, KY Seo, SE Jung, JB Lee, JW Park, XH Wan. Two cases of mycobacterial keratitis at the interface after LASIK. ARVO Abstract No. 2675, 2001.
58. JA Seedor, DE Shapiro, DC Ritterband, AJ Ross, MS Kresloff, RS Koplin. LASIK complication rates. ARVO Abstract No. 2668, 2001.
59. D Miller, J Newton, E Alfonso. Surveillance and infection control standards for refractive surgery centers? ARVO Abstract No. 1679, 2000.
60. HV Gimbel, JA van Westenbrugge, EE Anderson Penno, M Ferensowicz, GA Feinerman, R Chen. Simultaneous bilateral laser in situ keratomileusis: safety and efficacy. Ophthalmology 1999;106:1461–1468.
61. FW Price, L Willes, M Price, A Lyng, J Ries. A prospective, randomized comparison of the use versus non-use of topical corticosteroids after laser in situ keratomileusis. Ophthalmology 2001;108:1236–1244.
62. S Hannush. DLK-masquerade syndrome after LASIK. American Society of Cataract and Refractive Surgery meeting, Philadelphia, 2002.

35

The Future of LASIK

NAN WANG and DOUGLAS D. KOCH

Cullen Eye Institute, Baylor College of Medicine, Houston, Texas, U.S.A.

To address the issue of future advances, one must first ask a more fundamental question: Is there a future for LASIK? Is there a future for lamellar refractive surgery? If we reflect on lamellar refractive surgery and other options, such as intraocular implants, photorefractive keratectomy, thermal keratoplasty, and intracorneal ring segments, the advantages of LASIK and related procedures seem obvious. We can group these into three categories:

1.   Safety: Considering the incredible quantity of LASIK procedures being performed worldwide, the number of eyes losing significant amounts of vision is remarkably small. These numbers are likely to diminish as technology further improves.

2.   Quality of vision: As demonstrated in Chaps. 18 and 19, LASIK outcomes are generally excellent, and LASIK offers the opportunity to perform wave front–guided ablations that may improve best spectacle corrected visual acuity beyond that achievable with glasses or contact lenses. There are some arguments suggesting that PRK may be a better approach for this, but reduction in aberrations should certainly be achievable with LASIK.

3.   Patient acceptance: LASIK offers the advantage of minimal discomfort, rapid recovery of vision, and options for later retreatments. Again, the large number of LASIK procedures being performed is testimonial to patient acceptance of this procedure.

So what issues remain to be addressed? We believe that they fall into three categories and that advances in each of these will further improve the outcomes that can be obtained with LASIK and related procedures. These areas are patient safety, improvement in quality of vision, and options for lifelong adjustment of refractive error and aberrations.

1.   Safety: The sight-threatening complications of LASIK include microbial keratitis, keratectasia, and rare posterior segment complications such as ischemic optic neuropathy and subretinal hemorrhages. More common but less devastating complications include induction of irregular astigmatism, decentered ablation, dry eyes, and refractive inaccuracy.

491

Microbial keratitis occurs because of intraoperative introduction of organisms into the lamellar interface. Introduction of laser devices to make lamellar flaps will reduce the amount of instrumentation that is required and should minimize this risk. If technology permits the development of intrastromal keratomileusis, then tissue can be ablated without the creation of a lamellar flap, which should completely eliminate the risk of microbial keratitis.

Keratectasia occurs in patients who are predisposed to this due to abnormal topography or excessively thin corneas, or in patients in whom inadequate posterior corneal tissue is preserved. Further work is required to understand which types of patients are predisposed to developing keratectasia, but this clearly is an achievable goal. Laser microkeratomes again offer exciting possibilities, in that flap thickness can presumably be determined with great precision, which should eliminate the risk of ablating too deeply into the corneal stroma.

Retinal and optic nerve complications such as submacular hemorrhages and ischemic optic neuropathy are presumably related to the increase in intraocular pressure that is produced by the vacuum required by the mechanical microkeratome. Once again, laser microkeratomes hold the promise of eliminating these risks.

Refractive issues such as irregular astigmatism, decentered ablations, and under- and overcorrections will be addressed in the next section, but again these problems seem solvable.

Dry eye after LASIK is due primarily to corneal denervation caused by the cutting of corneal nerves. Altered corneal contour may contribute to this problem as well. It is still somewhat unclear if there is long-term reduction in tear production in all patients who undergo LASIK. Elimination of this problem will require development of nerve-sparing techniques for making the flap, which is again a potential advantage of intrastromal ablation. Another option would be the development of growth factors to stimulate corneal nerve regeneration.

2.   Quality of vision: This is certainly the area of greatest ongoing interest in LASIK and in refractive surgery overall. Several areas need to be addressed, but they fall into two large categories: accurate measurement and delivery of laser energy, and accurate prediction of postoperative wound healing.

The steps required to improve quality of vision and eliminate optical complications have been described in part in Chap. 9. Several key steps are required.

First, accurate measurement of wave front aberrations must be performed. However, we also believe that accurate measurement of the corneal contribution to wave front aberrations will be essential. If the causes of wave front aberrations are intraocular, then correction of these will require the induction of aberrations on the corneal surface. Depending upon the magnitude of these aberrations, the cornea may or may not be amenable to maintaining these corrections.

Registration of the measurement to the treatment will be essential. This will require linkage of the wave front measurement to the laser delivery and will include issues such as torque and rotation of the eye. We must remember that tracking systems that are driven by the pupil can be deceived in part by parallax. Ultimately, real-time measurement of ongoing treatment is desirable, but this is unlikely with current technology owing to the difficulty of obtaining intraoperative measurements. Factors such as corneal hydration and temporary flap irregularity are major barriers to achieving this goal.

Finally, we need to understand better the role of the LASIK flap and wound healing in altering postoperative aberrations. Will we develop new flap-making techniques that either eliminate new aberrations or are predictable in generating known changes? What will be the role of PRK and its associated wound-healing response?

3. Lifelong refractive adjustments: The ultimate procedure will provide a lifetime (or close to it) of excellent vision. The refractive error of most people varies from their teens throughout the remainder of their lives. There is a trend toward myopia between the ages of 20 and 40, and a shift toward hyperopia between ages 40 and 60. In addition, the aberrations of the eye change owing to both corneal and lenticular factors. Patients who obtain "super vision" will naturally wish to maintain this quality of vision throughout their lifetimes. Therefore a truly adjustable procedure is required.

For lifelong adjustments, LASIK as currently practiced has the major disadvantage of being a subtractive procedure. As a result, many patients might eventually run out of tissue that could be safely ablated. A better option would therefore be an additive, e.g., lamellar surgery with implantation of an intracorneal lens. This lens could be replaced or modified in situ as needed to maintain quality of vision. Periodic replacement of the lenses would introduce the risks of reopening a lamellar flap and predisposing the patient to the vagaries of corneal wound healing. Therefore the ideal solution would be a material that could be modified in situ, presumably using some form of laser technology to adjust or modify the optical characteristics of the synthetic lens. Recent advances in intracorneal lenses offer at least the possibility of the exchangeable implant, and early work with a new type of silicone intraocular lens suggests that at least one modification of a lens might be obtainable using external laser irradiation.

Conclusion: LASIK is currently state-of-the-art for the correction of a wide range of refractive errors. New advances offer the promise of improved safety, enhanced postoperative quality of vision, and the opportunity for lifelong adjustment of refractive errors and ocular aberrations. The Holy Grail of lamellar refractive surgery lies in the attainment of these goals.

Index

Ablation, depth, 183
Ablation efficiency, 42
Ablative decomposition, approaches, 43
ABMD, 453–454
Absent hinge, 432–436
Accommodation, 103–104
ACS, 27
ACS microkeratomes, 61, 68
Acutane, 92
Adaptive optics, 143–144
Adjustable refractive surgery (ARS), 329–331
Age, nomograms, 195–196
AK, 11–12
    retreatment, 307
ALK (*see* Automated lamellar keratoplasty
        (ALK))
Alphagan, decentration, 412
Altered index of refraction, 14–15
Ametropia
    spectacle-correction, 102
    types, 3–4
Amikacin, 485
Amiodarone, 92
Amphotericin B, 485
Analysis of Radial Keratotomy, 9
Anesthesia, 176
Angle lambda, 203–206
Anisometropia, 105–106
Anterior basement membrane dystrophy
        (ABMD), 453–454
Anterior chamber reaction, 373
Apex, 112

Apex/OmniMed, 43
Aphakia, H-Lasik, 291
Applanation tonometry, 96–97
Argon fluoride excimer laser, 2, 41, 46
    ablation, 57
    electromagnetic spectrum, 40
ARS, 329–331
Artificial tears, 256
Artisan lens implantation, 330
Astigmatic keratotomy (AK), 11–12
    retreatment, 307
Astigmatism, 3–5
    corneal topographic pattern, 123
    LASIK, 98, 376–377
        after PKP, 320
    maps for patient with, 124
    myopia, 267
    refractive evaluation, 104
Automated lamellar keratoplasty (ALK), 5,
        27, 28, 164–165
    excimer, 33
    hyperopic, 5
    keratomileusis, 22–27
Automatic corneal shaper (ACS), 27
Autorefractors, 74–75
Axial decentration, measurement, 210–211
Axial maps
    curvature, 113–116
    myopic patterns, 120–122
Axial topography, 210, 213
Azar-Lu MEEI keratoconus scoring system,
        155

Bacterial keratitis, 484
Baley-Lovie distance visual acuity chart, 72
Bandage contact lenses, 256–257
Barraquer, Jose, 1, 21, 57
Barraquer-Krumeich-Swinger (BKS)
  refractive system, 25–26
  technique, 25
Barraquer tonometer, 180
Barraquer wire speculum, 85
BAT, 108
BCVA (*see* Best corrected visual acuity
    (BCVA) loss)
Beam, homogeneity, 194
Bell's phenomenon, 218
Best corrected visual acuity (BCVA) loss, 3
  extremely high myopia, 271
  low and moderate hyperopia, 272
  low myopia, 268
  moderate and high myopia,
    267–268
Betadine, 177
Bilateral simultaneous LASIK
  advantages, 244–245
  comparative studies, 246–247
  disadvantages, 245–246
  informed consent, 247–251
  patient counseling, 247–251
  surgical considerations, 251
Bioptics, 329–334
  contraindications, 332
  indications, 332
  possible combinations, 331–332
  preoperative examination, 332
  results, 333
BKS
  refractive system, 25–26
  technique, 25
Blade selection, 193–194
Blepharitis, 248
Brau, Charles, 28
Brightness Acuity Test (BAT), 108
Broad beam ablation, 43
Broad beam excimer laser, ablation, 52
BSS cannula, interface irrigation, 185
Buratto, Lucio, 32
Burkholderia pickettii, 479
Buttonhole, 439–442
  intraoperative management, 441
  management, 443
  postoperative management, 441
  prevention, 441–442

Buttonhole flap
  interlamellar epithelium, 466
  microkeratome, 232
Buzard Barraqueratome, 67

Cap, loss, 436–437
Carriazo-Barraquer, 62
Ceftazidime, 485
Centering, corneal light reflex,
    205–207
Central axial keratometry maps,
    156–157
Central islands, 389, 403–410
  maps, 134
  nonsurgical management, 404–406
  photoablation, 236–237
  prevention, 409–410
  surgical intervention, 406–409
Centration, 199–222
  accurate, importance, 208–209
  current techniques, 202–203
  entrance pupil, 202, 207–208
  future directions, 217
  improper, 199–200
  initial techniques, 200–202
  prevailing method, 207–208
  recommended technique, 209–211
  techniques, controversy, 205–207
Cephalosporin-tobramycin, 485
Chayet ring, 84, 85
  application, 182
Chiron-Technolas Keracor 116, 43
Choroidal complications, 361
Choroidal neovascularization, 399–400
Clarithromycin, 485
Clinical outcomes, decentration, 212
Coherence, definition, 40
Coherent-Schwind Keratom, 43
Colvard pupillometer, 80
Computerized videokeratography (CVK),
    95, 108
  monitoring postoperative outcomes,
    130–132
  refractive surgery, 125–130
  reoperation, 135
  selecting optimal surgical procedure, 130
  topographically driven corneal ablation,
    130
Connective tissue disease, 153
Consent, LASIK, 98
Consultation, LASIK, 93

Contact lens, 102
  induced corneal warpage, 126
  topographic stabilization, 125–127
Contact LTK, 13
Contrast sensitivity, 108–109, 379–380,
    387–388
  reduced, 279
Cornea
  biomechanical properties,
      163–168
  poor access, 356–357
  preplaced marks, 178, 179
  shape, 3
  tensile strength, 171
  topography, 112
  wavefront system, 147
Corneal asphericity, 123–125
Corneal biomechanics
  after LASIK, 165–166
Corneal bleed, microkeratome, 234
Corneal ectasia, 378, 389–390
Corneal epithelial defect, 357–358
  microkeratome, 233–234
Corneal haze, 373
Corneal light reflex, 111
  centering, 205–207
Corneal light scattering, 391–392
Corneal pachymetry, 118
Corneal penetration, inadvertent, 192
Corneal perforation
  intraoperative management, 432
  management, 433
  microkeratomes flap complications, 356
  postoperative rehabilitation, 432
  prevention, 432
Corneal radius of curvature, 171
Corneal relaxing incisions, postkeratoplasty
    astigmatism, 321
Corneal scarring, 129, 131
Corneal subtractive procedures, 5–8
Corneal surface remodeling, 9–14
Corneal topography, 75, 111–125, 210
  LASIK, 94
  predicting patient complaints, 216–217
  principles, 111–119
  terminology, 111–112
Corneal uniformity index (CUI), 116
Corneal warpage, contact lens induced, 126
Cross cylinder aberroscope, 141
Cryolathe keratomileusis, 1
CUI, 116

Curvature maps
  axial radius, 113–116
  instantaneous radius, 114–115
CVK (see Computerized videokeratography
    (CVK))
Cycloplegic refraction, 103

Debris interface, 238
Decentered ablation, 236
  elevation map, 132
  TopoLink, 426
Decentered cut, microkeratome, 235
Decentered flaps, 442–444
  management, 443
Decentration, 389, 410–414
  clinical outcomes, 212
  defined, 210–211
  nonsurgical management, 412
  photoablation, 235–236
  prevention, 414
  surgical intervention, 412–413
Diabetes, 103
Difference maps, 115
Diffuse lamellar keratitis (DLK), 250–251,
    257, 370–371, 448, 477–482
  alternate names, 478
  classification, 479–480
  etiology, 478–479
  frequency, 478
  optical aberrations following,
      390–393
  slit lamp photograph, 479
  stages and treatment, 480–482
  symptoms and signs, 479
Dim oblique illumination, 183–184
Direct illumination, 186
Directional displacement, 221
Discharge, 188
Dislodged flap, 369
  management, 448–452
Displaced flap, management, 448–452
Disposable microkeratomes, 64
  design, 64
  examples, 65
  safety, 64
  technical features, 65
Distance charts, 72
Distant design, 112
DLK (see Diffuse lamellar keratitis (DLK))
Down's syndrome, 153–158
Drift, 211

Drift effect, visual acuity outcomes, 212–214
Drift index measuring, 211–212
Dry eye, 248
   LASIK, 96
   surface light scattering, 393

E-ALK, 33
Early Treatment Diabetic Retinopathy Study
      (ETDRS) chart, 73
EBMD, 357
Eccentric pupil, 223
Ectatic corneal disorders, detection, 127–128
Edematous flaps, 455–457
   intraoperative management, 455
   postoperative management, 455
   prevention, 455
Effective refractive power (EffRP), 116
EffRP, 116
Electromagnetic spectrum, argon fluoride
      (ArF) excimer laser, 40
Elevation-based systems, 117
Elevation-based topographical unit, 78
Elevation map, 115
   decentered ablation, 132
Emmetropia, 1, 2
Endothelial cell loss, 377
Energy, definition, 39
Entrance pupil
   centration, 202, 207–208
Epi (see Epikeratophakia)
Epikeratophakia, 8–9, 24–26
Epikeratoplasty (see Epikeratophakia)
Epithelial basement membrane dystrophy
      (EBMD), 357
Epithelial defects
   interlamellar epithelium, 466
   management, 452–455
Epithelial ingrowth, 249–250, 374–375, 440,
      465–466
   optical aberrations following, 390–393
Epithelial tears, management, 452–455
Equipment, preoperative familiarity, 180
Erythromycin, 485
ETDRS chart, 73
Ewing, James, 28
ExciMed, 43
Excimer ALK (E-ALK), 33
Excimer laser, 46
   ablation, 51–53
   beam degradation, 51
   calibration, 51–53
   calibration techniques, 52–53

[Excimer laser]
   development, 28–29
   disadvantages, 49
   examples, 149
   gas impurities, 51–52
   indications, 92
   intrastromal keratomileusis, 32
   ocular electrophysiology, 398
   optics degradation, 51
   postkeratoplasty astigmatism, 321
   strong beams, 49
Excimer 193 nm UV laser, 1–2
Excited dimer (excimer) 193 nm UV laser,
      1–2
Extremely high myopia, 270–271
   BCVA loss, 271
   postoperative UCVA, 271
   preoperative refraction, 270–271
   refractive outcome, 271
   visual outcome, 271
Eye
   length, 3
   simplified schematic, 200
Eyelash scrubbing, 176–177
Eyelid drape, 83–84
EyeSys Corneal Analysis System,
      116
Eye tracking systems
   early development, 219–220
   first FDA approved, 220
   laser, 53

Fechtner conjunctival ring forceps, 86
Femtosecond, definition, 40
Flap
   apposition, 187
   dislocation during surgery, 239
   displaced/dislodged/incorrect placement,
      448–452
   edema, 239
   irreversible damage, 240
   lifting, 183
   refloating, 185
   repositioning, 185
   shrinkage, 239
   thickness, 191–192
Flap buttonhole, microkeratomes, flap
      complications, 353–354
Flap centration, 221
Flap complications
   management, 360–361
   microkeratome, 351–356

Flap decentration, 222–223
  indication, 224
Flap forceps, 87
Flap melt, 375
Flap-related complications, optical aberrations
        following, 390–393
Flap wrinkles, management, 444–448
Flap wrinkling, 359, 369–371
Fluence, definition, 39
Flying spot ablation, 45
F-MKM, 22
Folds, 444–448
Fornices, drying, 182
Fornix, proparacaine, 178
Free cap, 432–436
  intraoperative management, 434–436
  microkeratome, 231–232
  microkeratomes flap complications, 354
  postoperative rehabilitation, 436
  prevention, 436
Free keratomileusis, 23
Freeze keratomileusis, for myopia and
        hyperopia, 23
Freeze-myopic keratomileusis (F-MKM), 22
Full thickness anterior chamber entry, 432
Fyodorov, Svyatoslav, 9

Gas lasers, 46
Glare, 250, 278, 387–388
Glare testing, 108–109
Glaucoma, LASIK, 96–97
Globe
  microkeratome
    inadequate exposure, 233
    perforation, 232
    poor coupling to, 233
  surgeon assisted fixation, 218
Gutter
  murocel, 186

Haag Streit slit lamp, 81
Halos, 250, 278, 379, 387–388
Hansatome, 68
Hansatome microkeratome, 229
  hyperopic astigmatism, 290
Hartmann-Shack sensor, 141–142
Head holding, 184
HEPA (high efficiency particulate air) filter,
        194
Herpes simplex keratitis, 92
Herpes zoster ophthalmicus, 92
Hexagonal keratotomy, 12

High ametropia, 34
High efficiency particulate air filter, 194
Highest rate of steepening (HRS), 129
High myopia, 266–268 (see also Extremely
        high myopia)
  astigmatism, 267
  BCVA loss, 267–268
  follow-up, 266
  LASIK, 103
    ICRS with, 342–345
  postoperative refraction, 266
  postoperative UCVA, 267
  preoperative refraction, 266
  refractive outcome and predictability,
        266–267
  visual outcome, 267
High-order aberrations, 141
Hinge location, 59
H-Lasik
  aphakia, 291
  complications, 292–293
Homogeneity, definition, 39–40
HRS, 129
Humphrey Atlas, 116
Humphrey ultrasonic pachometer model 8050,
        81–82
Hunkeler hook, 300
Hydrops, keratoconus, 154
Hyperope, LASIK, 97
Hyperopia, 92, 286–289 (see also Low
        hyperopia; Moderate Hyperopia)
  corneal topographic pattern, 123
  residual, RK, 314
  secondary focal point, 3
  spherical, ablation profiles, 287
Hyperopic ALK, 5
Hyperopic astigmatism, 289–290
Hyperopic LASIK, 198
  interlamellar epithelium, 466

Iatrogenic keratectasia, 93
  after LASIK, 167–170
Iatrogenic keratoconus, 5, 378
ICRS (see Intracorneal ring segments (ICRS)
Inadvertent corneal penetration, 192
Incipient cataract, LASIK, 96
Incisional keratotomies retreatments, 304
Incisional refractive surgery, 164
Incisional surgery, 9–12
Incomplete flap, 437–439
  intraoperative management, 437–438
  management, 438

[Incomplete flap]
   microkeratome, 230
   postoperative rehabilitation, 438
   prevention, 438–439
   stromal scarring, 437
Increased intraocular pressure, steroids, 250
Induced aberrations, 388
Induced keratoconus, 378
Infectious keratitis, 248–249, 371–373
Inferior-superior value, 128
Informed consent, bilateral simultaneous
     LASIK, 247–251
Infrared pupillometry, 79–80
In situ keratomileusis, 5
Instantaneous maps
   curvature, 114–115
   myopic patterns, 120–122
INTACS, retreatments, 305
Intensity, definition, 39
Intentional flap displacement, 223
Interface
   debris, 238, 360–361
   irrigation, 185
   reirrigation, 186
Interferometric system, 119
Interlamellar epithelium
   appearance, 467–468
   classification, 464
   clinical features, 467–475
   incidence, 463
   management, 463–475
   pathogenesis, 464–466
   predisposing factors, 466
   prevention, 475
   prior incisional refractive surgery, 466
   progression, 468
   symptoms, 469–474
   treatment, 474–475
Intracorneal ring segment (ICRS), 8–9
Intracorneal ring segments (ICRS),
     335–336
   after LASIK, 345, 346–347
   implantation, 329
   vs. LASIK, 337–342
   LASIK with high myopia, 342–345
   myopia complications, 339
Intraocular lens (IOLs), 14–16
   phakic implantation, 329
   retreatment, 306–307
     implantation, 305
Intraocular pressure (IOP), check, 180
Intraoperative adjunctive instrumentation, 84

Intraoperative complications, 229–240,
     351–362
Intraoperative flap complications,
     management, 361–362
Intraoperative pachymetry, 161
Intraoperative tonometry, 87–88
Intrastromal corneal ring segment, 8–9
Intrastromal corneal segments (INTACS)
   retreatments, 305
IOLs (*see* Intraocular lens (IOLs))
IOP, check, 180
Iowa Pupillometer, 79–80
Iron, 88
Irradiance, 42
   definition, 39
Irregular astigmatism, 5, 389, 414–419
   TopoLink, 421–426
     after PKP and RK, 421–422
Irregular flaps, 193, 442–444
Irrigating cannulae, 86, 87
Isolated epithelial nest, 464–465

KCI, 128
KeraMetrics Corneal Laser Analysis System
     1000, 119
Keratectasia, 492
Keratoconus, 153–158
   classification, 158
   complications, avoidance, 161
   detection, 127–128
   diagnosis, 154
   with hydrops, 154
   LASIK, 95–98
   LASIK/PRK, 160
   Orbscan findings, 158–160
   spot patterns, 142
   systemic diseases, 153
   topographic map, 127
Keratoconus index (KCI), 128
Keratoconus predictability index (KPI), 128
Keratoconus scoring system, Azar-Lu MEEI,
     155
Keratoconus severity index (KSI), 128
Keratoglobus, 129
Keratometer, manual *vs.* automated, 76
Keratometry, 75
Keratomileusis to ALK, 22–27
Keratopathy, central toxic example, 133
Keratophakia, 8, 24
Keratoscopy, 75
Ketoconazole, 485
KISA % index, 129

KPI, 128
KSI, 128

LADAR, 220
LADARVision system, clinical results, 54
Lamellar corneal surgery, 164–165
Lamellar procedures, 5
LASEK, 6–8
Laser
    centration, 182–183
    eye tracking systems, 53
    frequency, 40–41
    history, 40
    homogeneity, 41
    intensity, 42
    irradiance, 42
    LASIK, 39–53
    physics, 39–40
    properties, 40–41
    readiness, 178–179
    settings, guidelines, 194–198
Laser ablation, 301–302
Laser astigmatic treatment, outcomes, 273
Laser drift, comparison, 215
Laser epithelial keratomileusis (LASEK), 6–8
Laser heads, types, 45–47
Laser in-situ keratomileusis (LASIK)
    adjunctive instrumentation, 71–81
    after ICRS, 346–347
    astigmatism, 376–377
    bandage contact lenses, 256–257
    contraindications, 92
    corneal biomechanics after, 165–166
    corneal ectasia after, 389–390
    definition, 1–2
    development, 30–32
    ectasia following, 160
    epidemiology, 2–3
    eye tracking, 53
    flap complications, management, 431–457
    future trends, 34, 491–493
    history, 21–32
    iatrogenic keratectasia after, 167–170
    vs. ICRS, 337–342
    ICRS after, 345
    ICRS with high myopia, 342–345
    indications, 92
    infections following, 482–487
        associations, 485
        frequency, 483
        microbiological profile, 483–485
        outcomes, 486

[Laser in-situ keratomileusis (LASIK)]
    risk factors, 485
        signs and symptoms, 483
        treatment, 485–486
    instrumentation, 83–84
    intraocular pressure monitoring after, 380
    keratoconus, 160
    lasers, 39–53
    long term follow-up, 260–261
    optical aberrations after, 387–393
    optical quality, 145–146
    overcorrection, 365–369
    posterior corneal changes after, 166–167
    posterior segment complications, 397–401
    postoperative complications, 365–380
        early, 365–375
        late, 376–380
    postoperative management protocols,
        255–263
    postoperative medications, 256
    preoperative considerations, 102–104
    vs. PRK, 33
    procedures, centration, 199–222
    regression, 376
    routine postoperative visits, 257–260
    safe corneal bed thickness after, 170
    stage I, 175–178
        preparation, 175–178
    stage II, 180–183
    stage III, 183–186
    techniques, 175–184
    topographical irregularities following,
        403–419
    undercorrection, 365–369
    vision quality after, 277–280
    wound healing, 31
Laser microkeratome, 66
Laser nomograms
    adjustments, 194–197
    updating, 196
Laser room environment, 194
Laser thermokeratoplasty (LTK), 13, 388
    retreatment, 304–306, 308
LASIK (see Laser in-situ keratomileusis
        (LASIK))
Leber's congenital amaurosis, 153
Lens power, 3
Liebermann Adjustable wire speculum, 85
Lifelong refractive adjustments, 493
Lift flap retreatments, 299–300
Lighthouse Distance Visual Acuity Chart, 73
Limbal bleeding, 358–359

Line of sight, 112, 203
Loktal Medical Clear Corneal Molder, 66–67
Low and moderate hyperopia, 271–272
    BCVA loss, 272
    postoperative refraction, 272
    postoperative UCVA, 272
    preoperative refraction, 272
    refractive outcome and predictability, 272
    visual outcome, 272
Low myope, LASIK, 97
Low myopia, 268–269
    BCVA loss, 268
    LASIK vs. ICRS, 337–342
    postoperative UCVA, 268, 270
    preoperative refraction, 268
    visual outcome, 268, 270
LTK, 13, 304–308, 388

Machat adjustable speculum, 85
Machat LASIK retreatment spatula, 87
Macular hemorrhage, 399–400
Maps
    central axial keratometry, 156–157
    central islands, 134
    corneal scarring, 131
    curvature, 113–116
    difference, 115
    elevation, 115, 132
    myopic patterns, 120–122
    pachymetry, 156–157
    patient with astigmatism, 124
    refractive, 115
    topographic
        keratoconus, 127
        pellucid marginal degeneration, 130
        pre-LASIK, 168–169
Markers, 85
Marking pens, 85
Mechanical immobilization vs. patient
        fixation, 218–219
Medjet Hydrokeratome, 64
Medjet Hydrorefractive Keratectomy
        hydrokeratome, 64
MEEI keratoconus system, 158
Meridian, 112
Merocel rings, 85
Merocel sponges, 85, 86
Microbial keratitis, 492
Microkeratome, 57–69
    advance/reverse, 181
    buttonhole flap, 232
    complications, 58, 229–235

[Microkeratome]
    components, 58
    corneal bleed, 234
    corneal epithelial defect, 233–234
    flap complications, 351–356
        corneal access, 356–357
        corneal perforation, 356
        flap buttonhole, 353–354
        free cap, 354
        incomplete, short or irregular flaps,
            355–356
        ocular anatomy, 352
        surgeon experience, 352–353
    free cap, 231–232
    gear-driven, 61
    globe, poor coupling to, 233
    globe perforation, 232
    inadequate globe exposure, 233
    incomplete cut, 230–231
    incomplete flap, 230
    inspection, 176, 181
    intraocular penetration, 232
    irregular cut, 230–231
    lubrication, 181
    perforated lenticule, 232
    pizza slicing, 234
    readiness, 178–179
    settings, 189–191
    testing, 176
    types, 58
    wound dehiscence, 234
MKM, 22
Moderate hyperopia, 271–272
    BCVA loss, 272
    postoperative refraction, 272
    postoperative UCVA, 272
    preoperative refraction, 272
    refractive outcome and predictability, 272
    visual outcome, 272
Moderate myopia, 266–268
    astigmatism, 267
    BCVA loss, 267–268
    follow-up, 266
    postoperative refraction, 266
    postoperative UCVA, 267
    preoperative refraction, 266
    refractive outcome and predictability,
        266–267
    visual outcome, 267
Moire interference system, 119–120
Monovision, 105–106
Monovision refractive surgery, 106–108

Moria Carriazo-Barraquer microkeratome, 229
Moria LSK-1 microkeratomes, 61
Murocel, gutter drying, 186
Mutagenicity, 213 nm wavelength, 50
Mycobacterium, 485
Myopia (*see also* High myopia; Low myopia;
    Moderate myopia)
   complications, 292–293
   corneal topographic pattern, 119–123
   residual, RK, 314
   secondary focal point, 3
Myopic automated lamellar keratoplasty, 6
Myopic keratomileusis (MKM), 22
Myopic LASIK, 197
Myopic patterns, 120–122

Nanosecond, definition, 40
Natamycin, 485
Nd:glass (femtosecond) laser, 50–51
Nd:YLF laser, 49
Near charts, 73–74
Near design, 112
Near vision, optical requirements, 106
New keratectomy, 300–301
Night glare, 378–379
Night vision
   LASIK effect on, 280
   problems, 378–379
Nocardia, 485
Nondisposable microkeratomes
   horizontal, 58–59
      design, 61
      examples, 60
      gears *vs.* sliding, 59
      oscillation, 62
      safety, 61–62
   vertical, 62–64
      design, 62–64
      examples, 63
      safety, 64
Nonfragmenting sponges and rings, 85
Nonsteroidal anti-inflammatory agents
    (NSAIDs), 256
Nontoothed forceps, 86
NSAIDs, 256

Obscan Topography System, 82
Ocular motility, 103
Oculocardiac reflex, 238–240, 360
Ofloxacin, 485
Ophthalmic Technologies Inc./Loktal Medical
    Clear Corneal Molder, 66–67

Optical aberrations, 278–279
   wavefront technology, 279
Optical axis, centration, 200–202
Optical zone, 203
Orbscan keratoconus, 158–160
Orbscan corneal topographer, 167, 415
Orbtek ORBSCAN, 117–120
Orthokeratology, 13–14

Pachymetry, 81, 158–159, 176, 183
   corneal, 118
   intraoperative, 161
   maps, 156–157
   ultrasonic, 81, 82
Pain, 238
Pallikaris, Ioannis, 30
Pararadial sweeping, 186, 187
PAR Corneal Topography System, 119
Patient counseling, bilateral simultaneous
    LASIK, 247–251
Patient fixation
   vs. mechanical immobilization, 218–219
   refractive surgery, 217
Patients
   complaints
      corneal topography, 216–217
   reassurance, 180–181
Patient satisfaction, 277–278
   studies of, 278
Patient selection, LASIK, 98
Patient self-fixation, 218
PCA, 116
Pellucid marginal degeneration, 129
   topographic map, 130
Penetrating keratoplasty (PK)
   LASIK after, 319–327
      astigmatism, 320
      complications, 326
      studies, 324–326
   photorefractive keratectomy after, 323–324
   retreatment, 306
Perforated lenticule, microkeratome, 232
PERK, 9, 164
Peyman, Gholam, 31
Phakic IOLs, 14–16
   implantation, 329
Photoablation
   central islands, 236–237
   complications, 235–237
   decentration, 235–236
   inadequate suction, 236
Photoablative rate, 42

Photorefractive keratectomy (PRK), 6–9, 45
  ectasia following, 160
  eye tracking, 53
  keratoconus, 160
  vs. LASIK, 33
  LASIK after
    complications, 316
    residual refractive errors management,
      314–316
  retreatment, 308
  retreatments, 304
Phototherapeutic keratectomy (PTK), 45
Picosecond, definition, 40
Pilocarpine, decentration, 412
Pineda LASIK Iron, 86, 88
Pizza slicing, microkeratome, 234
PK (*see* Penetrating keratoplasty (PK))
Placido-based topography, 77
Placido disk system, 112–117
  data acquisition, 112–113
  data processing and map display,
    113–116
  indices, 116–117
PMMA, 8
PNAC, 74
Pneumatonometer, 83, 88
Polymethyl methacrylate (PMMA), 8
Posterior corneal changes after LASIK,
  166–167
Posterior corneal ectasia, 415
Postkeratoplasty astigmatism
  corneal relaxing incisions, 321
  excimer laser, 321
  incisional surgical procedures, 320–321
  management, 320–324
  refractive aids, 320
  RK, 320–321
Postoperative medications, 256
Postoperative UCVA
  extremely high myopia, 271
  low and moderate hyperopia, 272
  low myopia, 268, 270
  myopia, 267
Power, definition, 39
Power map corneal scarring, 131
Practical near acuity chart (PNAC), 74
Predicted corneal acuity (PCA), 116
Pre-LASIK topography, 168–169
Preoperative screening, computerized
    videokeratography, 125–128
Presbyopia, 5
  LASIK, 97

Presbyopic LASIK, 293
Primary LASIK
  retreatment after, 299–306
  visual outcomes, 265–273
Prior refractive surgery
  LASIK after, 291–292
PRK (*see* Photorefractive keratectomy (PRK))
Proparacaine, fornix, 178
Prospective Evaluation of Radial Keratotomy
    (PERK), 9, 164
PTK, 45
Punctal occlusion, 256
Pupil
  centration, 184
  size, 103
Pupillary axis, 203–206
Pupillometry, 79–80
Purkinje-Sanson image, 205

Rabinowitz-McDonnell indices, 127
Radial keratotomy (RK), 9–11
  LASIK after
    complications, 316
    residual refractive errors management,
      314–317
  marker, 84
  postkeratoplasty astigmatism, 320–321
  retreatment, 307
Radial sweeping, 186, 187
Rasterphotogrammetry, 77, 119
Refraction, LASIK, 93–94
Refractive errors, 101–104
  epidemiology, 5–15
  etiology, 5–15
  treatment, 1–15
  types, 3–4
Refractive evaluation, 104–106
Refractive maps, 115
  myopic patterns, 120–122
Refractive surgery
  computerized videokeratography,
    125–130
  patient fixation, 217
Refractive surprises, 388
Refractors, automated, 74–75
Regular astigmatism, 5
Reoperation, interlamellar epithelium, 466
Residual bed, calculation, 183
Residual hyperopia, RK, 314
Residual myopia, RK, 314
Residual posterior stromal thickness (RPST),
  191

Retina
  detachment, 380, 398–399
  tears, 398–399
Retinal complications, 361
Retinal nerve fiber, layer thickness, 400
Retinoscopy, 104–105
Retreatments, 297–309
  after primary LASIK, 299–306
  complications, 303
  incisional keratotomies, 304
  indications, 297–299
  INTACS, 305
  intraocular lens implantation, 305
  laser ablation, 301–302
  laser thermokeratoplasty, 304–305
  new keratectomy, 300–301
  PRK, 304
  results, 302–303
  secondary LASIK after other procedures,
    306–308
Reveyes, decentration, 412
Rigid gas permeable contact lens,
    decentration, 412
Ring image, corneal scarring, 131
Rings, 85
  suction, 175–180, 189–191
RK (see Radial keratotomy (RK))
Rosenbaum card, 79
Routine postoperative visits, 257–260
RPST, 191
Ruiz, Luis, 27
Ruiz automated microkeratome, 27

Safety, future, 491–492
SAI, 116
Sato, Tsutomu, 9
Scanning slit ablation, 43–45
Scanning slit beam system, 78
Scanning slit imaging system, 117–120
SCMD microkeratomes, 61
Scrapers, 88
Searles, Stuart, 28
Secondary keratectomy, 301
Setser, Donald, 28
Shrunken flaps, 455–457
  intraoperative management, 456
  postoperative management, 456
  prevention, 456–457
Simulated Keratometry (Sim K), 116–117
Skin, scrubbing, 176–177
Skin laceration, 360
Slade speculum, 85

Slap, stretching, 239
Sliding flap, 369
Slit bean scanning technology, advantages,
    118–119
Snellen chart, 72
Snellen near chart, 73–74
Software
  data analysis, 196
  outcomes, 196
Solid-state lasers, 49
Spasm of accommodation, 106
Spatulas, 87
Spectacle-correction, ametropias, 102
Speculum, 83–84, 178
  removal, 187
Spherical hyperopia, ablation profiles, 287
Sponges, 85, 86
Spot patterns, 142
SRI, 116
Standardized visual acuity charts, 71–72
Sterile drapes, 177
Steroids, increased intraocular pressure, 250
Streptococcus, 485
Striae, management, 444–448
Styles-Crawford effect, 103
Subhyaloid hemorrhage, 400
Subjective ray tracing, 141
Suction ring, 175–178
  application, 179–180
  size, 189–191
Summit Apex Plus, 43, 286
Summit Excimer Laser, 33
Superficial epithelial abrasions, 370
Surface asymmetry index (SAI), 116
Surface laser ablation, 6–8
Surface light scattering, dry eyes, 393
Surface regularity index (SRI), 116
Swinger's technique, 57

Taco fold, 183
Tangential displacement, measuring, 211
Tangential topography, 210, 216
Tear film, 112
Temperature, laser room, 194
Tensile strength, normal cornea, 171
Thermal surgery, 13
Thin flaps, 442–444
  management, 443
Tight lens syndrome, 256–257
TMS-2 videokeratoscope, 154
Tobramycin, 485
Tomey unit, 116

Topcon Hartmann-Shack sensor, 142
Topcon wavefront analyzer, 149
Topographical unit, elevation-based, 78
Topographic map
   keratoconus, 127
   pellucid marginal degeneration, 130
   pre-LASIK, 168–169
TopoLink
   irregular astigmatism, 421–426
   results, 427–430
Treatment displacement, 211
Trokel, Stephen, 29
Tscherning aberroscope, 141
213 nm wavelength, mutagenicity, 50

Ultrasonic pachymetry, 81, 82
Uncorrected daytime vision, LASIK effect on,
   279
Uncorrected visual acuity (UCVA)
   extremely high myopia, 271
   low and moderate hyperopia, 272
   low myopia, 268, 270
   myopia, 267
Unilateral LASIK, scheduling second eye
   after, 257
Unintentional flap displacement, 224
United States Air Force (USAF) School of
   Aerospace Medicine, 29

Vacuum, setting, 193
Vancomycin, 485
Vasovagal reflex, 238–240, 360
Vertex, 112
Very high myope, LASIK, 97
Videokeratoscopes, 76
Video Vision Analyzer (VIVA) pupillometer,
   80
VISC laser, calibration, 52

Visijet hydrokeratome, 64
Vision, quality of, future, 492
Visual acuity, 71
   LASIK, 93–94
Visual acuity outcomes, drift effect, 212–214
Visual axis, centration, 200–202
VISX Star S2, 43, 286–287
   hyperopic astigmatism, 290
VISX WaveScan, 148
Vitreous loss, 399

Water jet microkeratomes, 64–66
Wavefront
   analysis, 140–141
   defined, 139–140
   refractive errors, 141
   sensors, examples, 146
Wavefront analyzer, Topcon, 149
Wavefront-guided ablation, LASIK, 145–147
Wavefront sensing, principles, 139–143
Wavefront system, cornea, 147
Wavefront technology, LASIK, 139–148
213 nm wavelength, mutagenicity, 50
Wavelength-modulated Nd:YAG, 49
Wavelight Allegretto excimer laser, 147–148
Wide area (broad beam) ablation, 43
Wire speculum, 84, 85
Wound dehiscence, 358
   microkeratome, 234
Wound healing
   LASIK, 31
Wrinkled flap, 237
Wrinkles, complications, 237

Young's modulus, 163

Zernike polynomials, 143
   graphical representation, 144